Department for Economic and Social Information and Policy Analysis
Population Division

Family Planning, Health and Family Well-Being

Proceedings of the United Nations Expert Group Meeting
on Family Planning, Health and Family Well-Being
Bangalore, India, 26-30 October 1992

Convened as part of the substantive preparations
for the International Conference on
Population and Development, 1994

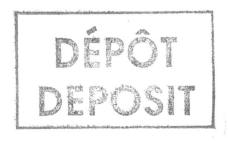

 United Nations   New York, 1996

NOTE

The designations employed and the presentation of the material in this publication do not imply the expression of any opinion whatsoever on the part of the Secretariat of the United Nations concerning the legal status of any country, territory, city or area or of its authorities, or concerning the delimitation of its frontiers or boundaries.

The designations "developed" and "developing" economies are intended for statistical convenience and do not necessarily express a judgement about the stage reached by a particular country or area in the development process.

The term "country" as used in the text of this publication also refers, as appropriate, to territories or areas.

The views expressed in signed papers are those of individual authors and do not imply the expression of any opinion on the part of the United Nations Secretariat.

Papers have been edited and consolidated in accordance with United Nations practice and requirements.

ST/ESA/SER.R/131

UNITED NATIONS PUBLICATION

Sales No. E.96.XIII.12

ISBN 92-1-151308-1

PREFACE

The Economic and Social Council, in its resolution 1991/93, decided to convene the International Conference on Population and Development in 1994, with population, sustained economic growth and sustainable development as the overall theme. Through its resolution 1992/37, the Council accepted the offer of the Government of Egypt to host the Conference and decided to hold it at Cairo from 5 to 13 September 1994.

At the request of the Council, the Secretary-General appointed the Executive Director of the United Nations Population Fund (UNFPA) to serve as the Secretary-General of the Conference and the Director of the Population Division of the Department of Economic and Social Development* as Deputy Secretary-General.

Also, in its resolution 1991/93, the Council authorized the Secretary-General of the Conference to convene, as part of the preparation for the 1994 International Conference on Population and Development, six expert group meetings corresponding to the six groups of issues that it had identified as those requiring the greatest attention during the forthcoming decade. One of those six expert group meetings was on family planning, health and family well-being; it was convened at Bangalore, India, from 26 to 30 October 1992. The Meeting was organized by the Population Division, in consultation with UNFPA.

Contained in this volume are the report and recommendations of the Meeting and the papers submitted to the Meeting. These materials not only made a valuable contribution to the 1994 Conference itself but will serve as useful tools for future research on family planning programmes, health and family well-being, as well as contribute to the work of the United Nations in those areas.

It is acknowledged with appreciation that the Government of India, which hosted the Meeting, contributed significantly to both the substantive and the organizational aspects of the Meeting. Thanks are also due to the experts and other participants who prepared invited papers and contributed to the discussions.

---

*Now the Department for Economic and Social Information and Policy Analysis.

CONTENTS

TABLES

ANNEX TABLES

FIGURES

Explanatory notes

Symbols of United Nations documents are composed of capital letters combined with figures.

The following symbols have been used in the tables throughout this report:

Two dots (..) indicate that data are not available or are not separately reported.
An em dash (—) indicates that the amount is nil or negligible.
A hyphen (-) indicates that the item is not applicable.
A minus sign (–) before a number indicates a decrease.
A point (.) is used to indicate decimals.
A slash (/) indicates a crop year or financial year, e.g., 1995/96.
Use of hyphen (-) between dates representing years (e.g., 1995-1996), signifies the full period involved, including the beginning and end years.

Details and percentages in tables do not necessarily add to totals because of rounding.

Reference to "dollars" ($) indicates United States dollars, unless otherwise stated.

The term "billion" signifies a thousand million.

The following abbreviations have been used in this publication:

AIDS	acquired immunodeficiency syndrome
AVSC	Association for Voluntary Surgical Contraception
BKKBN	National Family Planning Coordinating Board (in Indonesia)
BRAC	Bangladesh Rural Advancement Committee
CBD	community-based distribution
CBS	community-based services
CEDPA	Center for Development and Population Activities
CELADE	Centro Latinoamericano de Demografía
CIS	Commonwealth of Independent States
CONRAD	Contraceptive Research and Development Program
CPO	Center for Population Options
CPR	Center for Population Research
CPS	Contraceptive Prevalence Survey
CSM	contraceptive social marketing
CYP	couple-years protection
DAWN	Development Alternatives with Women for a New Era
DHS	Demographic and Health Surveys
DMPA	depot-medroxy progesterone acetate
ECA	Economic Commission for Africa
ECE	Economic Commission for Europe
ECLAC	Economic Commission for Latin America and the Caribbean
ESCAP	Economic and Social Commission for Asia and the Pacific
ESCWA	Economic and Social Commission for Western Asia
FDA	Food and Drug Administration (United States of America)
FHI	Family Health International
FPA	family planning association
FSH	follicle stimulating hormone
GNP	gross national product
GnRH	gonadotrophin hormone-releasing hormone
hCG	human chorionic gonadotrophin
HIV	human immunodeficiency virus
ICAF	International Center for Adolescent Fertility

ICMR	Indian Council of Medical Research
IEC	information, education and communication
IIRI	International Institute for Rural Reconstruction
IMR	infant mortality rate
IMSS	Instituto Mexicano del Seguro Social
IND	Investigational New Drug (FDA application form)
IPPF	International Planned Parenthood Federation
IRD	Institute for Resource Development
ISTI	International Science and Technology Institute
IUD	intra-uterine device
IUSSP	International Union for the Scientific Study of Population
JFPA	Japanese Family Planning Association
JFPPA	Jordan Family Planning and Protection Association
JOICFP	Japanese Organization for International Cooperation in Family Planning
KAP	knowledge, attitude and practice [survey]
MCH	maternal and child health
MCH/FP	maternal and child health and family planning
MWRA	married women of reproductive age
NET-EN	norethisterone enanthate
NICHD	National Institute of Child Health and Development (United States of America)
NIH	National Institutes of Health (United States of America)
NIHFW	National Institute of Health and Family Welfare (India)
PAHO	Pan American Health Organization
PATH	Program for Appropriate Technology in Health
PIACT	Program for the Introduction and Adaptation of Contraceptive Technology
PID	pelvic inflammatory disease
SBC	school-based clinic
SDP	service delivery point
SIV	simian immunodeficiency virus
SLC	school-linked clinic
SMC	social marketing of contraceptives
STD	sexually transmitted disease
THP	traditional health practitioner
TFR	total fertility rate
UNESCO	United Nations Educational, Scientific and Cultural Organization
UNFPA	United Nations Population Fund
UNICEF	United Nations Children's Fund
USAID	United States Agency for International Development
WFS	World Fertility Survey
WHO	World Health Organization
WHO/HRP	World Health Organization/Special Programme of Research, Development and Research Training in Human Reproduction
ZNFPC	Zimbabwe National Family Planning Council

Part One

REPORT AND RECOMMENDATIONS OF THE EXPERT GROUP MEETING

INTRODUCTION

A. BACKGROUND

The Economic and Social Council, in its resolution 1991/93 of 26 July 1991, decided to convene an International Conference on Population and Development under the auspices of the United Nations and decided that the main theme of the Conference would be population, sustained economic growth and sustainable development. The Council authorized the Secretary-General of the Conference to convene six expert group meetings as part of the preparatory work.

Pursuant to that resolution, the Secretary-General of the Conference convened the Expert Group Meeting on Family Planning, Health and Family Well-being at Bangalore, India from 26 to 30 October 1992. The Meeting was organized by the Population Division of the Department of Economic and Social Development of the United Nations Secretariat in consultation with the United Nations Population Fund (UNFPA). The participants, representing different geographical regions, scientific disciplines and institutions, included 18 experts invited by the Secretary-General of the Conference in their personal capacity; representatives of the five regional commissions; representatives of United Nations offices and specialized agencies, including the Office at Vienna, the United Nations Children's Fund (UNICEF), the United Nations Educational, Scientific and Cultural Organization (UNESCO), the World Health Organization (WHO) and the World Bank. Also represented were the following non-governmental organizations: International Institute for Rural Reconstruction (IIRI); International Planned Parenthood Federation (IPPF); International Union for the Scientific Study of Population (IUSSP); Population Council; Center for Development and Population Activities (CEDPA); Population Institute; Program for Appropriate Technology in Health (PATH); Association for Voluntary Surgical Contraception (AVSC); Family Health International (FHI); Institute for Resource Development (IRD)/Macro Systems, Inc.; Japanese Organization for International Cooperation in Family Planning (JOICFP); Pathfinder International; Population Crisis Committee; and Rockefeller Foundation.

As a basis for discussion, 16 experts had prepared papers on the agenda items. The views expressed by the experts were their own and did not necessarily represent the policies of their Governments or organizations. The Population Division of the Department of Economic and Social Development prepared a background paper entitled "Key issues in family planning, health and family well-being in the 1990s and beyond". UNFPA contributed a paper on future contraceptive requirements and logistics management needs. Discussion notes were provided by the United Nations Office at Vienna, the regional commissions and a number of specialized agencies and non-governmental organizations.

B. OPENING STATEMENTS

Opening statements were given by the Honourable Smt. D. K. Thara Devi Siddartha, Union Minister of State for Health and Family Welfare of the Government of India; Dr. Nafis Sadik, Secretary-General of the International Conference on Population and Development; and Mr. Shunichi Inoue, Deputy Secretary-General of the Conference.

In her opening remarks, Dr. Sadik noted that India provided an ideal setting for the Meeting because India had been the first developing country in the world to have a national population programme and had continued its commitment to planned population growth and voluntary family planning since 1951. She also commended the efforts of the Government of India in placing family planning in the wider context of health and family welfare and agreed with the national strategy, which emphasized the development of human resources rather than controlling human numbers. Smt. Thara Devi Siddartha reaffirmed the position of the Government of India that, for the future well-being of the country, the highest priority had been accorded to the population stabilization efforts. In that regard, she took note that fertility behaviour could not be understood in isolation without reference to the sociocultural context, nor could family planning policies be successfully pursued without promoting conducive socio-economic conditions, such as female literacy, the general quality of life, reproductive health and family well-being. She further stated that there was a need to shift the emphasis from quantitative to qualitative assessment of the population, which would require a "holistic approach" to population control.

Women's total health must become the central concern of planning. When a woman was given the opportunity of choosing her time of conception, the size of her family and the time period between births, very large benefits were likely to accrue.

In her speech, Dr. Sadik emphasized the need to place family planning in a wider context of quality of life of women and children, health and family welfare. She also pointed out the need to enhance the status of women, which was crucial for achieving sustainable development. To realize that goal women must have equal access to education and equal participation in social, economic, cultural and political life. Those considerations implied the need for universal access to a broad range of safe, affordable and effective contraceptive alternatives to meet the vast unmet demand for family planning. Considering the growing problem of adolescent fertility, she stressed the necessity of preventing teenage pregnancy and removing the widespread ignorance among young people of the risks of unprotected sexual activity. She emphasized the need to involve men in family planning and to provide them with the necessary information, education and encouragement to take greater responsibility in contraceptive practice and responsible parenthood. She noted that family planning programmes could contribute substantially to the reduction of maternal mortality and improvement of the reproductive health of women. She hoped that strategies for the prevention of the acquired immunodeficiency syndrome (AIDS) could be found within the framework of family planning and the Safe Motherhood Initiative, with particular focus on the needs of women and adolescents. She stressed the importance of high quality of services for expanding the levels of acceptance and continuation of contraceptive practices. She stated

that special efforts were needed to bring high-quality family planning services to vulnerable and/or underserved sections of the population, including people in minority communities, rural areas and urban slums. In order to improve the quality of care, the clients must be given a wide choice of contraceptive methods and must be treated with dignity and respect by well-trained service providers. She stressed that more research, development and training were necessary to widen the range and improve the quality of available contraceptive methods. It was also necessary to ensure that contraceptive supplies should be available at the right time and place and in the right quantity. She underscored the necessity of directly involving local communities to ascertain the family planning needs of communities with widely different backgrounds and suggested that this "people-centred approach" might encourage clients to share the cost of services. She observed that the pool of international resources for development was not growing as rapidly as the demand for resources. It was therefore essential to increase coordination and collaboration between national family planning programmes, non-governmental organizations, the private sector and international organizations.

Mr. Inoue, while enumerating the notable progress made in family planning practice in the past decade, pointed out that the current level of fertility and the rate of population growth in many developing countries were still too high and incompatible with the goal of achieving sound social and economic development. He stressed the importance of women's choice of the number of children or family size and the matching of individual fertility goals to national goals. He suggested that family planning should be seen as a means to improve the health and well-being of the family.

I. REPORT OF THE EXPERT GROUP MEETING

In addition to a more general exchange of views concerning the key issues in family planning, health and family well-being in the 1990s and beyond, and the linkages between family planning, health and family well-being, the Expert Group devoted particular attention to the following areas: society and family planning; review of existing family planning programmes and lessons learned; issues related to implementation of family planning programmes (quality of services and human resource development, unreached population groups, adolescent fertility, diffusion innovative activities, community-based distribution systems (CBD) and social marketing of contraceptives (SMC), and future contraceptive requirements and logistics management needs); family planning and health (safe motherhood and child survival, the interdependence of services, family planning, sexually transmitted diseases (STDs) and AIDS); family planning and family well-being (family size, structure and child development, fertility decline and family support systems); people's involvement in family planning programmes (community participation in family planning, cost of contraceptive supplies and services and cost-sharing, contraceptive research and development and re-examination of the roles of Governments, non-governmental organizations and the private sector in family planning). Situations in both developed and developing countries were considered, although the latter group dominated the discussion.

In formulating recommendations, the Expert Group focused on identifying practical measures that could be taken to broaden the scope of family planning programmes in order to make them more effective and efficient, that would help meet the unmet reproductive health needs of women and that would also have desirable effects on the status of women and health and the well-being of the family. The Expert Group also reviewed the state of knowledge about the topics mentioned above and made recommendations regarding needs for research and data collection.

The contributions of family planning towards improving the quality of life of the population, particularly the health and well-being of the family, have been the focus of increasing international attention in a variety of contexts, including human rights and equity and the participation of women in the process of social and economic development. There was currently an array of international declarations and agreements concerning the roles of family planning in improving the status of women, health of mothers and children, and the environment. Those instruments included the World Population Plan of Action (1974) and the Recommendations for its further implementation of the Plan (1984), the Nairobi Forward-looking Strategies for the Advancement of Women (1985), the Safe Motherhood Initiative (1987) and the Amsterdam Declaration on a Better Life for Future Generations (1989). The Expert Group took note that international declarations and agreements provided necessary support and sound guidelines for charting the future course of action and urged that necessary action be taken in implementing them.

A. GENERAL ISSUE OF SOCIETY AND FAMILY PLANNING

The Expert Group Meeting considered the general issues of fertility transition, women's status and sociocultural milieu and how women's status had affected the practice of family planning. The status of women needed to be examined in relation to social organizations and cultural contexts which varied from society to society; hence, it remained an elusive concept, further complicated by varied definitions of status, such as prestige, power, autonomy and rights. It was suggested that identification of the factors underlying gender inequality might help in understanding fertility behaviour, because fertility goals were likely to depend upon the extent to which women relied upon their male kin and sons for status and security. It was recommended that the removal of gender inequalities would enhance the status of women, which, in turn, would have a positive impact on family planning. The Expert Group Meeting further considered the reverse side of the relation, namely, the effect of reduced fertility on women's status. The reduction of time spent in reproduction and child care allowed women to expand their participation in public sphere. It followed that family planning was a major avenue to improve women's status by providing greater control over reproductive decisions. It also provided control over fate and thus empowered women. Those independent effects of family planning at microstructural levels needed to be emphasized.

The Expert Group Meeting also considered issues related to fertility transition and socio-economic development, including status of women and associated policy questions on investments in social sectors. More specifically, the questions raised concerned which social sector investments were likely to strengthen the impact of family planning and reproductive health services and how the design of services could be better tailored to the socio-economic structure in which they all expected to be effective. The Meeting was of the view that social development might be contributing more to fertility decline than economic development. The Meeting emphasized, however, that there was no point in presenting socio-economic development and family planning programmes as competitive or alternative approaches. Changes in fertility behaviour that derived from increased acceptance of family planning and socio-economic development should be seen as a gradual process with synergistic effects. It would therefore be productive to identify the linkages between social change, family planning programme effort and reproductive behaviour. One such linkage was established through research on "proximate" determinants of fertility, where the effects of socio-economic factors on fertility were usually seen to be mediated through such proximate factors as use of contraception and rising age at marriage.

A second line of inquiry that had helped clarify the understanding of synergies between socio-economic forces and programmatic variables in accelerating fertility decline was the series of cross-national studies. Those studies showed that fertility declined most rapidly in countries with high scores with both sets of indicators. Those synergies were also found in country-level studies of fertility transitions that were currently occurring in many developing countries, particularly in Asia and Latin America. Those studies illustrated that even in ostensibly unfavourable conditions, fertility decline could be accelerated by programme efforts which were sensitive to local conditions, responsive to community needs and designed to encourage social change. For instance, in Bangladesh, the recruitment of female outreach workers had contributed to changes in the status of women. In the light of recent empirical evidence, the Meeting made an important assertion that the progress of family planning programmes was not dependent upon levels of socio-economic development, because programmes were more than the mere supply of contraceptives; they had evolved to respond to particular needs of a particular society. Thus, two decades of programme experience had shown that the linkages

between programme effort and socio-economic setting involved a variety of synergies that needed to be better understood and strengthened in order to guide social sector investments in health and family planning, female education and other factors that would improve the status of women.

B. REVIEW OF EXISTING FAMILY PLANNING PROGRAMMES: LESSONS LEARNED

A comprehensive overview of the family planning situations in various regions of the developing world was presented at the Expert Group Meeting. This overview highlighted the process of socio-economic changes affecting different parts of the world in terms of gross national product (GNP) per capita, literacy, primary- and secondary-school enrolment, percentage of men in the non-agricultural labour force, life expectancy, total fertility rate and infant mortality rate. Particular attention was paid to the current situation in the least developed countries. In most regions, there had been socio-economic progress, notably in Eastern and South-eastern Asia, with simultaneous progress in the development of family planning programme efforts. It was quite apparent that, in general, programme improvements had not matched the progress in socio-economic development. Nevertheless, there was a positive relation between the improvement in socio-economic conditions and programme strength. There were also exceptions to those relations, where there had not been much socio-economic improvement but programmes had become stronger and where fertility decline was in progress (for example, Bangladesh and Botswana). On the other hand, notable changes had taken place in socio-economic conditions among the Arab States; yet fertility decline had not been observed owing, in part, to the absence of organized family planning programmes, except in Algeria, Egypt, Morocco and Tunisia. In a third set of countries (sub-Saharan Africa), neither had socio-economic conditions changed to any appreciable extent nor had programme efforts gained much strength. In most of those regions, fertility levels still remained high and contraceptive practice very low. The primary impetus to adoption of policies to reduce fertility in Latin America and the Caribbean had come from the medical profession, who were greatly concerned about large number of septic abortions. Governments were slow to react; hence, the private sector and non-governmental organizations had played a very important role in supporting the cause of family planning and also in the provision of services. Latin America, in general, with better socio-economic conditions compared with developing countries in other regions, showed a relatively high contraceptive prevalence throughout most of the region.

The general conclusions drawn from the above broad assessment were that family planning programmes could have an independent effect on fertility rates and their effectiveness was greatly enhanced when socio-economic development occurred simultaneously. Organized family planning programmes and socio-economic development together produced synergistic effects on fertility. In the overview, several important programme characteristics were identified as crucial for the success of family planning programmes. A selected few of them drew the attention of the Meeting more than the others. Those characteristics were: political commitment and strong leadership; adoption of a client's perspective; contraceptive availability/accessibility; quality of services; wide choice of methods; modes of delivery of services; and information, education and communication (IEC) campaigns. It was said that political commitment was fundamental to the success of the programmes but its importance diminished as socio-economic conditions improved. In high socio-economic settings, favourable to low fertility, political commitment was necessary only to remove barriers to family planning programmes. It was also pointed out that political commitment in the developed countries was necessary to ensure sufficient international financial aid. Concern was expressed at the Meeting that current design and ethos of many family planning programmes emphasized quantitative aspects of achievement at the cost of quality of care, clients' needs and preferences; therefore, women's reproductive health needs were neglected. To further raise contraceptive prevalence, it would be necessary to increase the participation of women in the decision-making process for programme design and implementation. Furthermore, women should be given the choice of meeting their reproductive goals. It was noted that as abortion played important roles in maternal mortality and fertility decline, the question of abortion could not be put aside.

C. ISSUES RELATED TO IMPLEMENTATION OF FAMILY PLANNING PROGRAMMES

The Expert Group Meeting again stressed the need to improve the quality of services in all stages of programme development. The success of family plan-

ning programmes had usually been evaluated on the basis of their quantitative impact on fertility. In these circumstances, there had been overwhelming concern for quantitative achievements—number of clients; births averted; and so on. The issue of quality of services had become all the more important since it had been recognized that improvement in the quality of services would result in increased contraceptive use and a subsequent reduction in fertility. The Meeting therefore emphasized that a shift to quality services had emerged as an important area of programme development during the 1990s. It was often claimed that calls for greater quality of services could not be met due to lack of resources, but the Meeting observed that the critical bottleneck with respect to quality was not resources but lack of commitment on the part of the top management. A significant part of that lack of commitment could be traced to the difficulties in defining the quality of services and the absence of readily measurable indicators of quality. The Expert Group then considered various elements of quality of service: choice of contraceptive methods; information given to clients; technical competence; client/provider relations; mechanisms to encourage continuity; and appropriate constellation of services. These six elements were regarded as fundamental but their relative importance and precise form should be adjusted according to specific country situation. A first, important step in the right direction would be to shift the focus from demographic targets to individual needs. With regard to measures for improvement of quality of services, the Expert Group also emphasized the necessity of human resource development with provision for continuous supervision and a management style that emphasized enhancement of skills rather than punitive measures. Quality of care and human resource development were generally linked.

The Expert Group noted that although levels of contraceptive use had increased substantially throughout the developing countries during the past decade, there remained many sectors of the population, such as minorities, remote rural areas or adolescents, that had not been reached by programmes because of resource constraints and other reasons. More importantly, men represented the "forgotten 50 per cent of family planning clientele". The critical constraint in reaching men was the providers, not men themselves. Men had not received the attention they deserved. Empirical evidence suggested that men had played a major role both as facilitators and as inhibitors for female contraceptive use. The role of men in family planning was becoming increasingly important in the context of raising contraceptive prevalence and further reduction of the level of fertility. Men, when approached, were often willing to support family planning practice, either by practising themselves or by helping their wives practise. Therefore, men should be approached with more assertive motivational campaigns that stressed the sharing of contraceptive responsibility, choices of contraceptive methods and parenthood responsibilities. That new direction implied more research on male methods of contraception and male attitudes.

A growing concern was expressed in the Meeting about the necessity of reaching the minority populations with family planning services. The Meeting recognized that the strategies that had succeeded in increasing contraceptive use in the majority population might not have much effect on those special groups. Family planning providers needed to understand better the barriers to family planning acceptance in those communities before undertaking vigorous promotional activities. Community and religious leaders and husbands might be helpful in overcoming the barriers to contraceptive use in those communities.

Another important category that had not been reached sufficiently constituted the people in remote areas: a neglect that had given rise to pronounced regional differences in contraceptive use. The Expert Group stated that every effort should be made to reach those areas in order to remove regional disparities. The Group also recognized the special unmet need of young couples, within or outside marriage, to have access to family planning services. Despite Governments' declared intentions, access to appropriate services by that particular group remained problematic. Furthermore, the need for family planning counselling services (for postponement or spacing of births) for that group could not be overemphasized.

The Expert Group expressed concern about the level of adolescent pregnancies. Precocious child-bearing continued to be a major impediment to improvements in the status of women. The social cost of adolescent fertility was high: it hindered possibilities for educational attainment and self-fulfilment, and led to greater health risk. It was observed that the percentage of women under age 20 that gave birth was quite high in many developing countries. The actual number of teenage pregnancies was unknown because of lack of statistics on abortion and miscarriages, but it was

undoubtedly very high. There was ample evidence showing that much of that early child-bearing—whether within or outside marriage—was unwanted. High rates of unsafe abortion among adolescent women also attested to the issue of unwanted pregnancies. Adolescents were, in many countries, increasingly at high risk of contracting and transmitting STDs, including the human immunodeficiency virus (HIV) and AIDS; and they were often poorly informed about how to protect themselves. It was observed that many adolescents were sexually active and family planning programmes should be sensitive to their needs because they were the future users. The Group therefore emphasized the importance of involving youth in identifying their special needs and urged Governments to make provision for sex education, family life education and HIV/AIDS education, and to ensure easy access to reproductive health services, including family planning services. In that regard, nongovernmental organizations might play important partnership roles with Governments in developing innovative programmes for that segment of the population. The Group encouraged further research for better understanding of those adolescent concerns. In considering adolescent issues, the Group also focused on the related issue of abortion.

With regard to the issue of diffusion of innovative behaviour and IEC activities, the Expert Group noted that there was a substantial amount of unmet need for family planning; many women wanted no more children and were exposed to the risk of pregnancy but were not practising family planning. The intervention most suited to transforming those high levels of need into effective demand was IEC activities. The Meeting also took note that two important aspects of IEC activities—research on development of IEC material, and management and evaluation of the dissemination process—were often neglected. There was much concern that IEC materials were designed on the basis of feelings rather than on research. It was also noted that IEC activities needed to be better managed, taking into consideration the existing IEC infrastructure, the relevance of different IEC strategies and the mixing of messages in appropriate media formats. Another important aspect that drew the attention of the Expert Group was IEC activities directed to providers, policy makers and informal leaders. For the purpose of institutionalizing family planning in society, IEC programmes must identify the motivational needs of health-care providers, policy makers and informal leaders and must meet those needs; their support was essential for effective implementation of programmes.

The Expert Group noted that community-based distribution of contraceptives had played an important role in making contraceptives available to people living in areas not covered by commercial networks or institutional services. In a related area, social marketing of contraceptives to low-income groups in developing countries had been met with mixed results. The impact of SMC in terms of increased contraceptive prevalence or fertility decline was still very uncertain but it undoubtedly constituted a way to complement other supply channels. Both of those modes of delivery of supplies, CBD and SMC, had great potential which needed to be properly evaluated to determine their cost effectiveness, the scope of their contribution and the extent to which subsidies were necessary. The question of combining those two approaches to reduce cost needed to be examined.

The future contraceptive requirements and logistic management needs of family planning programmes were considered at the Meeting. In order to achieve the United Nations medium-variant population projection by the year 2000, contraceptive prevalence in developing countries must rise from 51 per cent in 1990 to 59 in 2000. Thus, an estimated 567 million couples must be using some form of contraceptive at the end of the century. According to that projection, the following contraceptives would be needed in developing countries by the decade 1991-2000: 151 million surgical procedures for female and male sterilization; 8.76 billion cycles of oral pills; 663 million doses of injectables; 310 million intra-uterine devices (IUDs) and 44 billion condoms.

If the contraceptives required for the period 1991-2000 were purchased in the market, they would cost about $5 billion. From an annual cost of $399 million in 1990, the cost for contraceptives would rise to $627 million by the year 2000. It should be noted that the total did not include the much larger cost of delivery of services. The total cost would vary according to the method mix; for example, wider use of the Norplant implant would increase costs considerably. It was projected that between 1990 and 2000, Governments' share of the cost would be reduced from 60 to 52 per cent; the private sector share would remain the same at 17 per cent and the share of international donors would rise from 22 to 31 per cent from 22. Large though those sums were, the costs of contraceptive supplies constituted only about one fifteenth, or 7 per cent, of the total required by the year 2000 for supporting population activities, which was set at $9 billion by the Amsterdam Declaration on a Better Life for Future Generations, adopted by the International Forum on Population in the Twenty-first Century.

Contraceptives were currently being manufactured locally in at least 23 developing countries and local production was under consideration in four or more countries. It was encouraging to note that in four large countries (Brazil, China, India and Indonesia), at least three methods (pills, condoms and IUDs) were produced locally with capacity approaching or exceeding their respective estimated commodity requirements. External assistance agencies had been active in supporting the local production of contraceptives.

D. FAMILY PLANNING AND HEALTH

The Expert Group observed that the issue of safe motherhood should not be discussed in the context of health only because motherhood was an important social function and not a disease. Rather it should be considered in the wider context of the role and status of women. Women that wanted to avoid unwanted pregnancies should be provided with family planning services, including access to safe abortion in order to protect their health and well-being. As family planning contributed substantially to child survival and reduction of maternal mortality, the relevance of family planning in any strategy for safe motherhood and child survival was undeniable. Another essential component of a safe motherhood strategy was good maternal care, which was not complete without preconception care and postpartum care, in which birth planning was a basic component. In that connection, it was observed that progress towards safe motherhood should be measured in terms of lifetime risk of maternal death and not in terms of the commonly used maternal mortality rate, which measured only obstetric risk. Equally important was the question of child survival, which was considered a desirable social goal in itself. Research evidence showed that family planning contributed substantially towards child survival. Women seeking preventive and promotive care for their children should have easy assess to family planning care. The Expert Group was of the opinion that reproductive health care should be provided as integrated package of services that were mutually strengthening, cost-effective and convenient to users. An important point to note in that respect was that users should be the ones to determine the type of integration most suited for their needs.

The Expert Group focused on the linkages between family planning, STDs and AIDS. Family planning was practised by sexually active men and women of child-bearing age. Those groups were at risk of coming into contact with STD as well as heterosexually transmitted HIV infection. The practice of family planning should play a crucial role in the prevention of vertical transmission of HIV from mother to child, through prevention of pregnancy among HIV-infected women. Another important linkage between family planning and STDs/AIDS was that some of the contraceptive methods did have a protective effect against those infections. These important linkages implied the need to widen the scope of family planning programmes to encompass reproductive health care, including STD and AIDS control. Efforts to control those diseases could be enhanced by utilization of the widespread network of family planning clinics, especially in the rural areas of developing countries. The facilities offered unparalleled opportunity to reach women of child-bearing age when the risk of exposure to STD and AIDS was greatest. Integration of those services would permit optimal use of the limited resources available in developing countries for the control of those infections as well as for family planning.

The obvious disadvantage of integration was that services might not reach men directly, and that area required reorientation of the family planning approach, which had hitherto relied mainly upon contact with women, to permit more interaction with men. For the purpose of integration, there was need to initiate training activities for the personnel involved in family planning and STD/AIDS control services, directed to making them realize the interrelation between the services they offered and thereby promoting closer working relations. The Meeting, however, cautioned about possible dangers of hasty integration. It could be an error to integrate STD-control programmes into existing family planning structures without making sure that the current facilities could provide quality services, that adequate staff were present and that they had the necessary training and orientation. It was also considered necessary to encourage research in sexual behaviour in different cultural settings to provide information that could be used in intervention programmes. Lastly, future research in contraceptive technology development should focus on methods that might have additional benefit in the prevention of STD/AIDS and especially on those methods which were women-controlled.

E. FAMILY PLANNING AND FAMILY WELL-BEING

Under the theme of family planning and family well-being, the Expert Group considered two important issues: changes in family size and structure; and fertility decline and family welfare systems. The Meeting recognized the importance of the family as a fundamental unit of society. The characteristics of the basic family types found in the East and the West were discussed and compared. The families in the East were characterized by a "feedback model" of intergenerational relations in which the older generation at first fostered the younger generation but was then cared for by the younger generation. The Western model was described as a "continued linear model", in which there was usually no feedback from younger to older generation. Consequently, the typical family pattern of Western society was the so-called "nuclear family", consisting of husband, wife and unmarried children. In many Eastern societies, married children did not necessarily leave their parental home to form nuclear families and thus three-generation families were common in the East. The family size was therefore relatively larger than that of the West.

As elsewhere in Eastern Asia, the traditional Chinese family had undergone substantial transformations during the past half-century. Both family size and family structure had been affected by the process of modernization and by the profound structural changes experienced by the Chinese society. The average family size had been 5.3 until the 1950s; it had declined to 4.43 by the 1982 census and it had decreased further to 3.97 by the 1990 census. The decline in family size during the 1950s and 1960s was mainly associated with social structural changes, such as land reform. By contrast, family size reduction in the 1970s and 1980s could primarily be attributed to fertility decline, although other factors, such as improved housing supply and census underenumeration, had also played a role. A process parallel to the decline in family size had been the trend towards family nuclearization. However, although the proportion of extended families had been decreasing substantially over the past five decades, the three-generation family still constituted about 20 per cent of Chinese families, and it was not certain that it would experience further reduction in the near future. Although there was no officially stated policy that promoted three-generation families, that family form had been viewed as beneficial for old-age care. However, the rapid fertility reduction would undoubtedly affect family structure in the coming years. When the children born under the current low-fertility programme reached the age of family formation, some elderly parents would not be able to live with married children, if they had only one married daughter, assuming that current cultural practices persisted. It was also noted that the policy with respect to number of children a couple could have led to large difference in fertility levels and family sizes between rural and urban areas, and between minorities and the Han majority. The Chinese case-study served as an illustration of how government policies along with changing socio-economic conditions affected the size and structure of the family. The attention of the Meeting was drawn to some undesirable consequences of the rapid fertility reduction experienced in the Chinese society: one child was sometimes raised as a "little emperor", with yet unknown consequences for child's development; and a strict one-child policy might lead to sex-selective abortion practices. The impact of rapid decline in fertility on child development was not yet fully known.

Lower fertility levels resulting in smaller families were thought to benefit both parents and their children directly. That view assumed that decisions about family size and family welfare were made simultaneously at the beginning of child-bearing. In recent years, that conventional wisdom had been increasingly challenged. The Meeting therefore examined the linkages between reduced family size and family welfare systems, including economic well-being of the family, welfare of the children, wife's employment opportunities and parental old-age security. Whether the number of children was positively or negatively correlated with the economic well-being of the family would vary with the life-cycle stage of both the parents and the children, as well as the existing social settings. A study in a village in Bangladesh found that male children became net producers at age 12 and could compensate for their cumulative consumption by age 15. Similar results were found in Northern Ghana. Other studies had shown that in a peasant society, at the aggregate level, the net worth of children was negative. A large family gained economic benefits from its size only in certain stages of the family life cycle. These studies, however, did not show the cumulative effect of actual family size on the economic well-being of the family. In a recent study in Thailand, where rapid socio-economic development had been taking place, an assessment of the impact of a reduced number of children on family economic well-being had been carried out by comparing couples whose reproductive years corresponded with the period of decline of

fertility in Thailand but who had small and large families. The study had found reduced family size to have positive effects on a couple's ability to accumulate wealth, participate in new forms of consumption and thus have more material possessions and better quality houses. In terms of welfare of the children, empirical evidence, from both developed and developing countries, showed a negative link between the educational attainment of the children and the size of the family. That relation had also been found to be true in Thailand. It was important to remember that, in the process of development, Thailand was experiencing rising costs of living and costs of rearing children. Thai parents also had high aspirations for their children in terms of educational attainment. It could be said, therefore, that economic benefits were not the only guiding factors on family size decisions. The nature of the linkages between fertility and women's employment varied according to a number of factors. Role incompatibility between reproduction and production was found to be stronger in urban areas as compared with rural areas. A recent study on parental care in Thailand had shown that fertility decline did not significantly reduce the proportion of the elderly that would co-reside with an adult child. It was generally felt that there was a serious scarcity of research to explore the linkages between fertility decline and family welfare systems, and that was an important area for future research.

F. FUTURE DIRECTIONS: PEOPLE'S INVOLVEMENT IN FAMILY PLANNING

During the 1960s, most of the public sector family planning programmes were centrally organized with a vertical delivery system and quantitative demographic targets rather than welfare goals. The past 15 years had seen an appreciable shift away from target-oriented vertical programmes. In their place, a growing concern had arisen that family planning services should be tailored to meet the needs and preferences of their clients. The concept of "user's perspective" had gradually come into prominence with the attendant emphasis on community participation. In the early 1980s, community participation had received strong endorsement as a cornerstone of family planning programmes. At this Meeting, such issues as community participation, individual needs and preferences, quality of care rather than quantity and welfare aspect of programmes became the recurrent themes of discussion. All of those themes had direct or indirect bearing on community participation. The essential ingredient of the community participation concept was empowerment: the notion that communities should have a degree of control over the nature of development goals and implementation of activities. The participation of the community in planning, decision-making and programme implementation was its underlying and fundamental feature. The application of the concept in family planning had led to various forms of participation. Contributory participation, where communities assisted pre-set programmes by means of labour (volunteers), cash or provision of other resources, such as land, was relatively common. The second most common form found was organizational participation where formal or informal structures existed to facilitate contributions by the community. The limited empirical evidence suggested that genuine community participation in family planning in terms of "empowerment" was still extremely limited. The following reasons for that situation were discussed: family planning was perceived to be a need of a small fraction of the community; inflexibility of centralized programmes did not allow for local variations; family planning might lack a ready appeal to community élites, typically older men whose wives had passed beyond the reproductive age span; and family planning as an innovation might create antagonism based on religious beliefs, moral issues etc. Participatory programmes were often found in the private sector and they had met with relatively greater success, because non-governmental organizations tended to be more adaptable and accommodating to community wishes than were government departments. It was interesting to observe that, in the non-governmental organization programmes, integration was a common characteristic of community participation projects that involved family planning. It seemed reasonable to conclude that an integrated package of services with a decentralized programme development mechanism and the use of local institutions would ensure greater participation of community in family planning and related activities and would make family planning services more responsive to people's needs. However, the Group was of the opinion that there was also need to make a serious objective evaluations of those activities, particularly in terms of cost/benefit analysis.

With regard to cost of contraceptive supplies and services and cost-sharing, the evidence presented at the Meeting pointed to some important conclusions. First, the reproductive age cohort was increasing rapidly even as overall population growth declined. Simultaneously, donor resources were not expected to increase as rapidly as the increase of women/couples of reproductive age. Secondly, more work needed to be done to measure accurately the extent of unmet need for contraceptives in developing countries, because available data were inadequate and measures were yet to be perfected. As a result, projections of unmet needs must be viewed as orders of magnitude. Thirdly, cost data were also troublesome because of the assumptions underlying them and the inaccuracy built into equating costs and expenditures. Determination of financial needs in the future, therefore, was complicated by the data limitations just mentioned. However, under the assumption that resources would be constrained in future, efforts should be made to assess alternative financing arrangements and to improve resource allocation and efficiency of service delivery. Available evidence suggested that among countries that charged for family planning, fees were a small proportion of per capita GNP. Moreover, studies showed that upward adjustments to modest fees had little effect on utilization, which indicated possible scope for establishing or raising fees for family planning. In addition, third-party payers (e.g., insurance companies) for health care represented another potential financier to share costs with Governments and users. The Meeting had seen that cost and unmet need data deserved more consideration and more careful interpretation to guide decision-making processes to promote efficiency and appropriate targeting for subsidies. To promote cost-sharing, Governments must have better information on price sensitivity of consumers. By removing impediments to private investment in family planning, Governments should encourage private sectors to expand their share of service delivery. Innovations in modes of delivery of family planning services were essential.

In the agenda item on contraceptive research and development, the Group reviewed the most important existing contraceptive methods with respect to safety and efficiency and emphasized their effects on women's reproductive health. The Meeting took note that women in their different life-cycle stages had different needs for different types of contraceptive methods. The current research agenda on contraceptive methods included the relation between hormonal methods and neoplasia, barriers methods for protection against STD/HIV, breast-feeding and contraceptive methods, and the use of modern IUDs with high efficiency and few side-effects. Through the collaboration between national and international agencies and non-governmental organizations, promising research was continuing on antifertility vaccines, methods for the regulation of male fertility and antiprogestins for early pregnancy termination. Research needs had been identified which would be critical in the future. In the light of that review and discussion, a few conclusions were reached at the Meeting. First, there had been a general decline in expenditures on research in fundamental reproductive physiology, new contraceptive methods and safety evaluation. Secondly, there had been large reduction in the involvement of pharmaceutical companies in contraceptive research for various reasons: belief that the market was already "mature"; the long time required to develop a new method; and the even longer period before there was any return on investment and the regulatory problems imposed by drug administrations and the legal liabilities. To encourage future research in new contraceptive methods, those barriers needed to be removed. Thirdly, non-governmental organizations had an important role to play in contraceptive research by creating a global partnership of scientists that would work together in the development of new methods, thus filling the gap left by the Governments and the commercial sector. Fourthly, there should be an emphasis in research on new methods for men.

In re-examining the role of Governments, non-governmental organizations and the private sector in family planning, the Meeting observed that despite recent progress in family planning, there were still many challenges, including a growing demand for services. Governments must at least sustain, or increase, support for family planning and try to remove legal and other barriers to expanding services. They should aim to be flexible, recognize the needs of adolescents and replicate successful models of service delivery. The existing role of non-governmental organizations in innovative service delivery should be extended to offer appropriate reproductive and sexual health services to those most in need, to improve quality of care and community involvement, to demonstrate cost effectiveness and address women's concern. Non-governmental organizations still had a advocacy role, particularly to reduce unsafe abortion and to increase services for young people. The private sector must cooperate with Governments and non-governmental organizations, price contraceptives for retail distribution on the basis of price sensitivity of consumers and participate in community-based distribution and social marketing.

II. RECOMMENDATIONS OF THE MEETING

A. PREAMBLE

The World Population Plan of Action, adopted by consensus at the World Population Conference at Bucharest in 1974, affirms that all couples and individuals have the basic right to decide freely and responsibly the number and spacing of their children and to have the information, education and means to do so. This right should be assured in all countries, irrespective of their demographic objectives.

The use of safe and appropriate fertility regulation methods has immediate benefits for the health, well-being and autonomy of women. Family planning also promotes the health and welfare of children, adolescents and men, and the well-being of the family as a unit. Lastly, family planning contributes to achieving other societal goals, such as advancement of women, improvements in overall health status, stabilization of population growth, preservation of the environment, sustainable economic and social development and overall quality of life. Indeed, as stated in the UNICEF report, *State of the World's Children, 1992*, the responsible planning of births is one of the most effective and least expensive ways of improving the quality of life on earth, both currently and in the future, and one of the greatest mistakes of the times is the failure to realize this potential.

Empirical evidence reaffirms strong linkages between socio-economic development and fertility trends. Family planning programmes tend to be most successful where social and economic conditions encourage the adoption of small family norms. Recent experience, however, has demonstrated that even in poor socio-economic conditions, considerable desire to regulate family size exists and fertility has fallen in countries with well-organized programmes. Persons in all settings should not be denied access to the information and means to regulate their fertility and improve the quality of life.

In the past two decades, a reproductive revolution has occurred. Countries have made dramatic progress in expanding the availability of family planning services, increasing use of contraception and accelerating the pace of fertility decline beyond what would have occurred in the absence of services. Based on data for women of reproductive age, 53 per cent of couples are currently estimated to be using contraception; however, between regions there are enormous disparities in levels of contraceptive use. The availability of family planning services has itself contributed to a dramatic downward adjustment of desired family size in many countries. In less developed regions, where fertility has been highest, total fertility rates have declined from approximately 6.1 in the 1950s to about 3.7 currently.

Despite this progress, major challenges remain. As a consequence of earlier high fertility in developing countries, more and more men and women are entering their reproductive years, and the need for family planning services in these countries will therefore continue to increase rapidly. During the 1990s, just to maintain current levels of contraceptive use, approximately 100 million more couples will need family planning services. If fertility declines according to the medium variant of the United Nations population projections, then a further 75 million couples will need access to family planning information and services by the year 2000.

In addition, large disparities remain both within and among countries in the practice of family planning. Sociocultural, economic and other institutional constraints often prevent couples and individuals from making informed decisions concerning child-bearing. Millions of men and women of reproductive age in both more developed and less developed regions still do not have access to safe and effective methods of fertility regulation, as well as information on how to use them. In many countries, high abortion rates reflect these conditions.

The adoption of family planning has contributed to safe motherhood and child survival. However, the death and suffering of women in fulfilling their child-bearing responsibilities continues to be a major scandal. Each year more than 500,000 women die due to causes related to pregnancy and childbirth. There has been very little progress towards the goal of reducing maternal mortality by one half by the year 2000. Avoiding unwanted pregnancies and proper planning of births lowers maternal mortality. However, safe motherhood will only be achieved through concerted national and international efforts to make quality maternal health services, including safe abortion, readily accessible to all women. This should be a high priority for the next decade.

The quality of family planning services is also uneven. A major challenge in the coming decade will be to expand currently available contraceptive choices for persons in many countries and to improve the interpersonal skills and technical competence of family planning providers. There is also an urgent need to develop new and improved contraceptive methods.

The revolution in contraceptive technology has stalled because of inadequate allocation of resources and the retrenchment of the pharmaceutical industry. Concerted efforts are needed to launch a second revolution in contraceptive technology to provide a new generation of contraceptives for the twenty-first century.

One of the most serious problems of the coming decade is the spread of the AIDS pandemic, which jeopardizes the well-being of humankind. Family planning programmes have an important role to play in the prevention of HIV.

The Expert Group Meeting on Family Planning, Health and Family Well-being, having reviewed the progress made in achieving the goals and objectives of the World Population Plan of Action, adopted the following recommendations, which are intended to reaffirm as well as extend or update previous recommendations adopted by Governments in various international forums. They seek to identify actions that Governments can take to support couples and individuals in making informed and voluntary choices about the timing, number and spacing of children, through family planning programmes and other social policies. Because these issues are of global concern, the recommendations are also addressed to intergovernmental and non-governmental organizations as well as to the donor community.

B. RECOMMENDATIONS

Recommendation 1. Governments are invited to note the growing evidence that all individuals and couples, regardless of their socio-economic status, value the opportunity to space and limit their families, and that family planning can be promoted successfully where levels of socio-economic development are low, provided that the design of services takes into account the sociocultural setting. Family planning programmes should be regarded as a cost-effective component of a broader development strategy, one that has significant independent effects on family well-being and individual and social welfare, particularly of women.

Recommendation 2. Governments should strive to develop social and political institutions and norms that are oriented to providing women opportunities, through formal and informal education, for personal development and greater autonomy both within the family and in the society as a whole. Governments should support the involvement of women at all levels of the public policy process and especially in the design, management, implementation and evaluation of social welfare, health and family planning programmes.

Recommendation 3. Recognizing the fundamental role of the family in reproduction and in the socialization of future generations, Governments are urged to support the family through public policies and programmes, taking into consideration changes in family forms, size and structure. Governments should promote family life education for responsible parenthood for both men and women, high-quality child-care arrangements to enable people to combine their dual roles as parents and workers, and adequate support for the children of single parents.

Recommendation 4. To save the lives of mothers, children and adolescents and to improve their general health, Governments and the international community are urged to increase their investment in family planning, reproductive and maternal and child health services. Governments are also urged to monitor progress in safer motherhood and child survival and to take the necessary actions to enhance the interventions effectiveness.

Recommendation 5. Governments and donors are urged to increase their support to the social sectors, foremost health and education, to a level where basic human rights in these areas can be satisfied.

Recommendation 6. Governments and intergovernmental and non-governmental organizations are urged to recognize that abortion is a major public-health concern and one of the most neglected problems affecting women's lives. Women everywhere should have access to sensitive counselling and safe abortion services.

Recommendation 7. Given the high prevalence of STDs and the AIDS pandemic which threatens the well-being of men, women and children, family planning programmes need to widen their scope to include reproductive health care including STD/HIV education and prevention.

Recommendation 8. Political leaders at all levels should play a strong, sustained and highly visible role in promoting and legitimizing voluntary adoption of family planning, and in ensuring a legal and regulatory climate that is favourable for the expansion of family planning services of high quality. National and local leaders should translate their commitment to family planning into the allocation of substantially increased budgetary, human and administrative resources required to meet the increasing demand for services.

Recommendation 9. Family planning programmes at both national and local levels should seek to increase awareness of the importance of family planning and commitment to the expansion of good quality family planning services on the part of key influence groups, including the media, women's and voluntary organizations, local and religious leaders and the private business community. The involvement of non-governmental groups in these advocacy efforts, wherever feasible, may greatly facilitate the process of consensus and coalition-building in support of family planning efforts.

Recommendation 10. Family planning programmes should aim to help individuals to achieve their reproductive goals, and should be based on voluntary, free and informed choice.

Recommendation 11. Governments should establish family planning goals on the basis of the unmet demand and need for information and services. Demographic goals, although legitimately the subject of government policies and programmes to achieve sustainable development, should not be imposed on family planning providers in the form of targets or quotas for recruitment of clients. Family planning services should be framed in the context of the needs of individuals, especially women. Over the long term, meeting unmet need appears to be the best strategy for achieving national demographic goals.

Recommendation 12. At a national level, the major institutions involved in family planning should periodically undertake a systematic examination of the strengths and weaknesses of family planning efforts, including the competence of national and regional managers. This process should include an assessment of how major programme elements are contributing in a cost-effective manner to overall goals and result in the development and implementation of coordinated strategies for programme improvement.

Recommendation 13. Family planning programme managers should consult with and encourage the partici-

pation of local community groups in the design, financing and delivery of family planning services wherever feasible. Promising strategies for increasing community participation include the following: increased involvement of social organizations such as men's, women's and youth groups; cooperatives and religious organizations and use of local volunteers; greater decentralization of decision-making to local administrative structures that are better placed to respond to community needs; and increased pluralism of institutions in the delivery of services.

Recommendation 14. Governments and non-governmental organizations are urged to improve the quality of family planning services by incorporating the user's perspective and respect for the dignity and privacy of the client. Programmes should provide: the broadest possible range of contraceptive methods; thorough and accurate information to enable clients to make informed choices; systematic follow-up; easy availability of and accessibility to services; and technically competent service providers who receive proper training and supervision, with additional emphasis on communication and counselling skills. Unnecessary medical and regulatory barriers restricting access to services should be removed. Strategies should be carefully designed and tailored according to local conditions, and the cost of services and contraceptives should be subsidized for people that cannot afford the full cost.

Recommendation 15. Governments, donors and non-governmental organizations are encouraged to increase the provision of family planning services through multiple channels to unserved and underserved populations, such as adolescent, minority, migrant and refugee groups. Effective outreach approaches include promotional activities, community-based strategies and local health and commercial networks.

Recommendation 16. Governments are urged to recognize the special needs of the young and adolescent population and to strengthen programmes to minimize the incidence of high-risk and unwanted pregnancies and STD/HIV infection. Special efforts need to be made to reach this target population with information, education and motivational campaigns through formal and informal channels, including the involvement of young people themselves. In view of the fact that adolescents tend to avoid or underutilize maternal and child health/family planning and STD services, often with disastrous consequences, it is important that service providers be trained to be more receptive to adolescents and that legislation not inhibit the use of services by adolescents. Programmes should provide confidential services to adolescent men and women without regard to marital status or age. Young people should be involved in the planning, implementation and evaluation of programmes designed to serve them in order for services to be sensitive to their needs.

Recommendation 17. Governments, donors and non-governmental organizations are called upon to provide resources for social marketing of contraception in order to create demand for family planning services, especially in underserved areas and among traditional communities and population groups where demand is low or non-existent. Emphasis should be placed on using consumer-oriented approaches, such as careful targeting and segmentation of unserved populations, proper design of education and communication strategies based on research and an appropriate mix of media and interpersonal communications.

Recommendation 18. Governments, donors and non-governmental organizations should encourage greater involvement in and responsibility for family planning on the part of men, through research on male attitudes and motivation, messages specifically tailored for men, strategies to encourage responsible fatherhood, sharing of responsibilities between men and women, research on male methods of contraception and innovative clinical services adapted to the needs of men.

Recommendation 19. Governments and non-governmental organizations are encouraged to support information, education and communication activities in order to increase awareness of the benefits of family planning for both individuals and the larger community, through comprehensive education efforts utilizing a wide variety of communications channels. Such programmes have played a crucial role in bringing about the transformation of traditional attitudes and social behaviour necessary for the adoption of modern contraception. Public education programmes should develop a clear communications strategy based on empirical research on social values and reproductive behaviour.

Recommendation 20. Governments and education administrators are called upon to expand and strengthen population and family life education at all levels of formal education as well as literacy programmes. Such programmes should be designed to help children and youth in making informed decisions regarding their

sexual behaviour, responsible parenthood and family planning. Special emphasis should be placed on training teachers and developing relevant communication methodologies.

Recommendation 21. Governments and international organizations are urged to increase their support to non-governmental organizations working in family planning, particularly in two ways: first, by facilitating the development of public/non-governmental organization partnerships directed to expanding access to family planning services; and secondly, by supporting these organizations to address in innovative ways such important issues as reproductive health of adolescents, women's empowerment, community participation, broader reproductive health services, quality of care and outreach to marginalized groups. Once shown to be effective and acceptable, new approaches can then be integrated into wider national family planning programmes.

Recommendation 22. Non-governmental organizations are encouraged to coordinate their activities at national and international levels and to continue to emphasize their areas of comparative advantage, including voicing to policy makers the real concerns and needs of women and local communities with regard to sexual and reproductive health.

Recommendation 23. Governments should identify and remove legal and regulatory barriers impeding private sector involvement in family planning, including regulations that constrain contraceptive options; tax and importation policies; advertising and promotion restrictions; patent and trade mark laws; pricing policies; and restrictions on fees charged by non-profit organizations.

Recommendation 24. Governments and non-governmental organizations should support public/private partnerships directed to expanding access to family planning services. Such arrangements include financing private services through insurance or other third-party mechanisms and facilitating commercial enterprises to provide family planning as part of the health benefit plans provided to employees. Public sector programmes should seek to complement the existing family planning activities of the private non-profit and commercial sectors, including private health-care providers.

Recommendation 25. Governments, non-governmental organizations and donors are urged to improve forecasting of contraceptive requirements based not only on current use but on plans for future programme directions and priorities. Increased efforts must be directed to coordinating planning for contraceptive needs and putting systems in place which minimize the need for emergency responses, as well as helping countries reduce their reliance upon donors.

Recommendation 26. In meeting future contraceptive requirements, the partnership between the public and commercial sectors should be strengthened. The role of the commercial sector should be expanded in producing, procuring and delivery of contraceptives.

Recommendation 27. National Governments, international and non-governmental organizations are called upon to provide additional resources for family planning in order to satisfy the rapidly increasing demand for services. With a view to reaching the United Nations medium-variant population projections, the cost of contraceptive commodities alone has been estimated at $627 million in the year 2000. The associated logistics, management and service delivery costs are likely to increase this figure as much as 10-fold.

Recommendation 28. In order to better address the quantity of resources required, further work is needed to estimate all the component costs of family planning programmes. At the same time, more attention must be paid to cost effectiveness, efficiency, cost recovery, cost subsidization, community-resource mobilization; local production of contraceptives, where appropriate, and other mechanisms to ensure the optimum use of existing resources, thereby lowering costs, targeting subsidies and promoting financial solvency.

Recommendation 29. Governments of developed and developing countries and intergovernmental organizations are thus urged to increase significantly their proportions of development assistance for family planning to meet resource requirements. In so doing, it should be noted that costs of programmes and sources of financing will vary by such factors as social and economic setting, programme maturity, programme coverage and delivery modes, including the extent of involvement of the private and non-governmental sectors.

Recommendation 30. Governments and donors are urged to increase support for research on improving existing contraceptive technology as well as developing new technology that will be affordable in developing countries, focusing on methods that may have additional benefits in the prevention of STD/AIDS, male methods to increase men's involvement in family planning and methods appropriate for breast-feeding women. Efforts should be made to remove constraints hindering progress in this field, including inappropriate litigation practices and unjustified regulatory requirements, and to enhance the involvement of private industry in this effort.

Recommendation 31. Governments and donors are encouraged to support social science research on human sexuality and sexual behaviour in different cultural settings to provide information useful in intervention programmes to prevent unwanted pregnancies and STD/HIV infections.

Recommendation 32. In order to improve the efficiency of limited resources available for family planning programmes, Governments and donors are urged to support field studies at the subnational level in different cultural settings to ascertain the relative cost effectiveness of various approaches.

Recommendation 33. Governments, non-governmental organizations and donors are urged to support ongoing applied research efforts in family planning. Special emphasis should be given to evolving definitions, standards and indicators of quality of services appropriate to a country/programme setting; and to including quality of service in the description, monitoring and evaluation of family planning programmes.

Recommendation 34. In view of the importance attached to the role of family planing programmes in enabling persons to achieve their reproductive goals, Governments and donors should support research efforts to develop indicators of programme performance to capture this crucial dimension.

Recommendation 35. Governments are urged to attach higher priority to the utilization of available data and information for programme planning and implementation, to the collection of timely and reliable data and information especially on cost; and to the strengthening of human resources in various countries in order to facilitate data collection, analysis and utilization for programme planning and implementation.

ANNEXES

ANNEX I

Agenda

1. Opening of the Meeting.

2. Election of officers.

3. Adoption of the agenda and organization of work.

4. Key issues in family planning, health and family well-being in the 1990s and beyond.

5. Society and family planning:

   (*a*) Sociocultural milieu, women's status and family planning;

   (*b*) Socio-economic development, importance of social sectors and fertility behaviour.

6. Review of existing family planning programmes: lessons learned: experiences in Asia, Latin America and the Caribbean, Africa, the Arab States and the least developed countries.

7. Issues related to implementation of family planning programmes:

   (*a*) Quality of services and human resource development;

   (*b*) Family planning services and unreached population groups;

   (*c*) Adolescent fertility;

   (*d*) Diffusion of innovative behaviour and information, education and communication activities;

   (*e*) Community-based delivery systems and social marketing of contraceptives;

   (*f*) Future contraceptive requirements and logistics management needs.

8. Family planning and health:

   (*a*) Safe motherhood and child survival: the importance of family planning and the interdependence of services;

   (*b*) Family planning, sexually transmitted diseases and AIDS.

9. Family planning and family well-being:

   (*a*) Family size, structure and child development;

   (*b*) Fertility decline and family support systems.

10. Future directions: people's involvement in family planning programmes:

    (*a*) Community participation in family planning;

    (*b*) Cost of contraceptive supplies and services and cost-sharing;

    (*c*) Contraceptive research and development;

    (*d*) Re-examination of the role of Governments, non-governmental organizations and the private sector in family planning.

11. Adoption of the recommendations.

12. Closing of the Meeting.

ANNEX II

List of participants

John Cleland, London School of Hygiene and Tropical Medicine, London, United Kingdom

Mahmoud F. Fathalla, Special Programme of Research, Development and Research Training in Human Reproduction, World Health Organization, Geneva, Switzerland

J. P. Gupta, Director, National Institute of Health and Family Welfare, Munirka, New Delhi, India

Kerstin Hagenfeldt, Department of Obstetrics and Gynaecology, Karolinska Hospital, Stockholm, Sweden

Napaporn Havanon, Graduate School, Srinakharinwirot University, Sukhumvit, Bangkok, Thailand

Tirbani P. Jagdeo, Chief Executive Officer, Caribbean Family Planning Affiliation Limited, St. John's, Antigua

Maureen A. Lewis, The World Bank, Washington, D.C., United States of America

Alfonso López Juárez, Director-General, Fundación Mexicanapara la Planificación Familiar, A.C., Tlapan, Mexico

Japhet Mati, The Rockefeller Foundation, Nairobi, Kenya

Elizabeth Maguire, Deputy Director, Office of Population, United States Agency for International Development, Washington, D.C., United States of America

W. Parker Mauldin, Consultant to Population Sciences, The Rockefeller Foundation, New York, New York, United States of America

Thomas W. Merrick, Senior Population Adviser, Population and Human Resources Department, The World Bank, Washington, D.C., United States of America

Marvellous Mhloyi, Department of Sociology, University of Harare, Harare, Zimbabwe

Asha A. Mohamud, Director, International Center on Adolescent Fertility, Center for Population Options, Washington, D.C., United States of America

Anna Runeborg, Population Coordinator, Health Division, Swedish International Development Agency, Stockholm, Sweden

Pramilla Senanayake, International Planned Parenthood Federation, London, United Kingdom

Peter Sumbung, Deputy Chairman, National Family Planning Coordinating Board, Jakarta, Indonesia

Jiang Zhenghua, Deputy Minister, State Family Planning Commission, Beijing, China

SECRETARIAT OF THE INTERNATIONAL CONFERENCE ON POPULATION AND DEVELOPMENT

Nafis Sadik, Executive Director, United Nations Population Fund (UNFPA); and Secretary-General of the Conference

Shunichi Inoue, Director, Population Division of the Department of Economic and Social Development of the United Nations Secretariat; and Deputy Secretary-General of the Conference

Jyoti Shankar Singh, Chief, Technical and Evaluation Division, United Nations Population Fund; and Executive Coordinator of the Conference

German A. Bravo-Casas, Coordinator, World Population Conference Implementation, Population Division of the Department of Economic and Social Development of the United Nations Secretariat; and Deputy Executive Coordinator of the Conference

Petri Tiukkanen, Junior Professional Officer, United Nations Population Fund

UNITED NATIONS

Department of Economic and Social Development
Population Division
Aminur R. Khan, Technical Secretary of the Meeting; and Chief, Fertility and Family Planning Studies Section
Maurice Szykman, Population Affairs Officer, Fertility and Family Planning Studies Section
Teresa Castro Martin, Associate Population Affairs Officer, Fertility and Family Planning Studies Section

United Nations Office at Vienna
Jacques du Guerny, Senior Social Affairs Officer, Division for the Advancement of Women
George Puthuppally, Social Affairs Officer, Centre for Social Development and Humanitarian Affairs

Economic Commission for Africa (ECA)
  Z. W. Kazeze, Population Division

Economic Commission for Europe (ECE)
  Erik Klijzing, Population Expert, Population Activities Unit, General Economic Analysis Division

Economic Commission for Latin America and the Caribbean (ECLAC)
  José Miguel Guzmán

Economic and Social Commission for Asia and the Pacific (ESCAP)
  Iqbal Alam, Population Division

Economic and Social Commission for Western Asia (ESCWA)
  Ahmed Abdel Ghany Al-Ayyat, First Population Affairs Officer

United Nations Population Fund (UNFPA)
  Mohammed Nizamuddin, Deputy to the Director and Chief, Population Data, Policy and Research Branch, Technical and Evaluation Division
  Nicholas Dodd, Chief, Maternal and Child Health/Family Planning Branch, Technical and Evaluation Division

SPECIALIZED AGENCIES

United Nations Educational, Scientific and Cultural Organization (UNESCO)
  R. C. Sharma, Regional Population Adviser for Asia

World Health Organization (WHO)
  Leila Mehra, Chief, Family Planning and Population
  H. Friedman, Chief, Adolescent Health

The World Bank
  Thomas W. Merrick, Senior Population Adviser, Population and Human Resources Department

NON-GOVERNMENTAL ORGANIZATIONS IN CONSULTATIVE STATUS WITH THE ECONOMIC AND SOCIAL COUNCIL

Category I
International Planned Parenthood Federation (IPPF)
  Fred Sai, President

Category II
International Union for the Scientific Study of Population (IUSSP)
  John Cleland, Center for Population Studies, London School of Hygiene and Tropical Medicine

The Population Council
  Anrudh K. Jain, Senior Associate; and Deputy Director, Program Division

Program for Appropriate Technology in Health
  Sabita Tejuja, Secretary, Board of Directors

Roster
  Association for Voluntary Surgical Contraception
  Hugo Hoogenboom, President

The Center for Development and Population Activities
  Mary Luke, Director of Programs

International Institute of Rural Reconstruction
  Goturi Narayana Reddy

The Population Institute
  Werner Fornos, President

Other non-governmental organizations
  Family Health International
  William P. Schellstede, Executive Vice-President

Institute for Resource Development/Demographic and Health Surveys
  Martin T. Vaessen, Director

Japanese Organization for International Cooperation in Family Planning, Inc.
  Yasuo Kon, Deputy Executive Director
  Sumie Yamaguchi Ishii, Programme Officer

Pathfinder International
  Daniel E. Pellegrom, President

Population Crisis Committee
  Shanti R. Conly, Director, Population Policy Analysis

The Rockefeller Foundation
  Steven Sinding, Director, Population Sciences

OBSERVERS

Government of India
  Sumita Kandpal, Principal Secretary (Health), Government of Uttar Pradesh
  S. S. Kapur, Director (Policy), Department of Family Welfare Ministry of Health and Family Welfare

International Institute for Population Sciences
  K. B. Pathak, Director

Indian Council of Medical Research
  Badri N. Saxena, Senior Deputy Director General

Parivar Seva Sanstha
  Sudha Tewari, Managing Director

ANNEX III

List of documents

Document No.	Agenda item	Title and author
ESD/P/ICPD.1994/EG.IV/1	-	Provisional agenda
ESD/P/ICPD.1994/EG.IV/2	-	Annotated provisional agenda
ESD/P/ICPD.1994/EG.IV/3	4	Key issues in family planning, health and family well-being in the 1990s and beyond United Nations Secretariat
ESD/P/ICPD.1994/EG.IV/4	5(*a*)	Sociocultural milieu, women's status and family planning Marvellous Mhloyi
ESD/P/ICPD.1994/EG.IV/5	5(*b*)	Social development, program effort and fertility transitions Thomas W. Merrick
ESD/P/ICPD.1994/EG.IV/6	6	Review of existing family planning programmes: lesson learned W. Parker Mauldin and Steven W. Sinding
ESD/P/ICPD.1994/EG.IV/7	7(*a*)	Quality of services and human resource development J. P. Gupta and Helen H. Simon
ESD/P/ICPD.1994/EG.IV/8	7(*b*)	Family planning services and unreached population Peter Sumbung
ESD/P/ICPD.1994/EG.IV/9	7(*c*)	Adolescent fertility and adolescent reproductive health Asha A. Mohamud
ESD/P/ICPD.1994/EG.IV/10	7(*d*)	Diffusion of innovative behaviour and information, education and communication (IEC) activities Tirbani P. Jagdeo
ESD/P/ICPD.1994/EG.IV/11	7(*e*)	Community-based delivery systems and social marketing of contraceptives Alfonso López Juárez
ESD/P/ICPD.1994/EG.IV/12	7(*f*)	Future contraceptive requirements and logistics management needs United Nations Population Fund
ESD/P/ICPD.1994/EG.IV/13	8(*a*)	Safe motherhood and child survival: the importance of family planning and the interdependence of services Mahmoud F. Fathalla
ESD/P/ICPD.1994/EG.IV/14	8(*b*)	Family planning, sexually transmitted diseases and AIDS Japhet Mati
ESD/P/ICPD.1994/EG.IV/15	9(*a*)	Changes in family size and structure in China Jiang Zhenghua
ESD/P/ICPD.1994/EG.IV/16	9(*b*)	Fertility decline and family support system Napaporn Havanon
ESD/P/ICPD.1994/EG.IV/17	10(*a*)	Community participation in family planning

ESD/P/ICPD.1994/EG.IV/17	10(*a*)	Community participation in family planning John Cleland
ESD/P/ICPD.1994/EG.IV/18	10(*b*)	Cost and cost-sharing in family planning programmes: review of the evidence and implications for the future Maureen A. Lewis
ESD/P/ICPD.1994/EG.IV/19	10(*c*)	Contraceptive research and development Kerstin Hagenfeldt
ESD/P/ICPD.1994/EG.IV/20	10(*d*)	Re-examination of the role of Governments, non-governmental organizations and the private sector in family planning Pramilla Senanayake
ESD/P/ICPD.1994/EG.IV/INF.1	-	Provisional organization of work
ESD/P/ICPD.1994/EG.IV/INF.2	-	Provisional list of participants
ESD/P/ICPD.1994/EG.IV/INF.3	-	Provisional list of documents
ESD/P/ICPD.1994/EG.IV/INF.4A	-	Information for participants travelling at United Nations expense
ESD/P/ICPD.1994/EG.IV/INF.4B	-	Information for participants travelling at their own expense
ESD/P/ICPD.1994/EG.IV/DN.1	5(*a*)	Gender perspective in family planning programmes United Nations Office at Vienna
ESD/P/ICPD.1994/EG.IV/DN.2	10(*c*)	Barriers to contraceptive development J. Joseph Speidel
ESD/P/ICPD.1994/EG.IV/DN.3	6	Making family planning work: a policy maker's check-list Population Crisis Committee
ESD/P/ICPD.1994/EG.IV/DN.4	6	Family planning policies and programmes in African countries Economic Commission for Africa
ESD/P/ICPD.1994/EG.IV/DN.5	6	Use of DHS data for family planning programme evaluation and health assessment Martin T. Vaessen
ESD/P/ICPD.1994/EG.IV/DN.6	7(*f*)	Future contraceptive requirements: the potential role of local production in meeting developing country needs Program for Appropriate Technology in Health
ESD/P/ICPD.1994/EG.IV/DN.7	7(*d*)	Diffusion of innovative behaviours and information, education and communication Scott Wittet and Elaine Murphy
ESD/P/ICPD.1994/EG.IV/DN.8	7(*a*)	Institution-building for quality services The Center for Development and Population Activities
ESD/P/ICPD.1994/EG.IV/DN.9	6	World Bank assistance in population The World Bank
ESD/P/ICPD.1994/EG.IV/DN.10	6	Family planning programmes in Latin America: present situation and new challenges Economic Commission for Latin America and the Caribbean

ESD/P/ICPD.1994/EG.IV/DN.11	10(*b*)	Economics of family planning Barbara Janowitz
ESD/P/ICPD.1994/EG.IV/DN.12	8(*a*)	Problems and prospects of integrating family planning with maternal and child health with special emphasis on adolescents World Health Organization
ESD/P/ICPD.1994/EG.IV/DN.13	6	Family planning and reproductive health in selected Member States of the Economic Commission for Europe Erik Klijzing
ESD/P/ICPD.1994/EG.IV/DN.14	5	Women: the essential constituency Daniel E. Pellegrom
ESD/P/ICPD.1994/EG.IV/DN.15	6	Family planning policies and programmes: lessons learned; the ESCWA region experience Economic and Social Commission for Western Asia
ESD/P/ICPD.1994/EG.IV/DN.16	6	Population policies and programmes in Asia and the Pacific Economic and Social Commission for Asia and the Pacific
ESD/P/ICPD.1994/EG.IV/DN.17	7(*d*)	Elements of family planning in population education programmes United Nations Educational, Scientific and Cultural Organization
ESD/P/ICPD.1994/EG.IV/DN.18	7 and 10	International family planning: charting a new course Werner Fornos
ESD/P/ICPD.1994/EG.IV/DN.19	7(*a*)	Potential constraints to and prospects of improving quality of care in family planning programs in developing countries Anrudh K. Jain
ESD/P/ICPD.1994/EG.IV/DN.20	9(*a*)	Family well-being: an International Year of the Family perspective United Nations Office at Vienna
ESD/P/ICPD.1994/EG.IV/DN.21	10(*d*)	Market-based services: strategic role in family planning services expansion Janet M. Smith and Vijay Rao
ESD/P/ICPD.1994/EG.IV/DN.22	7(*b*)	Extending family planning services to unreached population groups United States Agency for International Development
ESD/P/ICPD.1994/EG.IV/DN.23	7(*e*)	Community-based distribution and contraceptive social marketing United States Agency for International Development
ESD/P/ICPD.1994/EG.IV/DN.24	7(*e*)	Sustainable Community-based family planning programs Japanese Organization for International Cooperation in Family Planning, Inc.
ESD/P/ICPD.1994/EG.IV/DN.25	7(*b*)	Family planning for the underserved: an IPPF perspective International Planned Parenthood Federation
ESD/P/ICPD.1994/EG.IV/DN.26	7(*a*)	Medical quality assurance through development of local system Association for Voluntary Surgical Contraception

Part Two

GENERAL OVERVIEW

III. KEY ISSUES IN FAMILY PLANNING, HEALTH AND FAMILY WELL-BEING IN THE 1990s AND BEYOND

*United Nations Secretariat**

The evolution of human societies in the past several decades has, on the one hand, brought about considerable improvement in the level of living and the welfare of world populations; and has, on the other hand, created a considerable number of hardships and problems which Governments are painfully attempting to alleviate. Excessive population growth, in particular, has often been considered a major hindrance to rapid progress in economic development and hence to the betterment of people's lives. This view, in turn, raised great concern in countries where population growth was deemed too fast. Population policies to reduce fertility were formulated and family planning programmes were regarded as the best means of achieving those goals. Awareness of the population factors in development planning increased continuously among Governments. By 1974, when the World Population Conference was held at Bucharest, 55 countries considered their fertility level too high and 40 had formulated a policy to lower that level; by 1991, the number of countries that considered their fertility too high had increased to 80 and 70 were implementing policies to lower their fertility (United Nations, 1992).

Increasingly, however, family planning needs to be viewed in a larger societal context. Indeed, access to family planning is not solely a demographic and economic issue. It is also a question of individual and national health, of preservation of the environment and of the well-being of the family and the population at large. Likewise, it is also concerned with improving the status of women and the recognition of human rights, and through them, greater equity for all people.

As no policy can be implemented in a social and economic vacuum and pathways to solutions can gain from exchanging experiences, the United Nations convened, in the past two decades, two major population conferences which addressed the main population and development issues of the time. The first, the World Population Conference, held at Bucharest in 1974, adopted the World Population Plan of Action; the second, the International Conference on Population, held at Mexico City in 1984, reviewed the progress made during the preceding decade and adopted a series of recommendations for further implementation of the 1974 Plan of Action (United Nations, 1975 and 1984). In addition, the International Forum on Population in the Twenty-first Century, convened in 1989, produced the Amsterdam Declaration: A Better Life for Future Generations, which also recommends that key population issues be addressed to ensure a better life for future generations of humankind (UNFPA, 1989a). The more recent European Agenda for Action on World Population, adopted in February 1992 by parliamentarians of 20 European countries and the European Parliament, also recognizes the "fundamental right of access to family planning choices" and notes the "tragic gap between the legal assertion of the equality of women and the gender discrimination which continues to be almost universal" (UNFPA, 1992a).

These recommendations and positions set the stage for the International Conference on Population and Development, to be held in 1994. It is thus in the context of these previous efforts and concerns that this Conference plans to re-examine the past demographic issues, take stock of the existing experience and plan for future action, bearing in mind that new problems have emerged in the field of population and development and that new approaches will have to be adopted. The present background paper is intended to provide a framework within which the discussion papers presented at the various sessions of the Expert Group Meeting can be examined. It focuses on a number of specific issues and suggests discussion points, in addition to providing information on the evolution of past and current family planning programme activities. In particular, it gives priority to the empirical and operational aspects of family planning programme implementation and offers

---

*Population Division, Department of Economic and Social Development (now the Department for Economic and Social Information and Policy Analysis).

a frame of reference useful in examining implementation problems and issues in different sociocultural and economic contexts.

As underscored above, these issues need to be viewed in a new light. Some of these issues are not new, but others are recent and result from the continuous evolution of the context of family planning programmes. Still other issues arise from the need to improve the existing programmes to achieve better quality of services, reach larger segments of the population and increase the efficiency and effectiveness of activities. In all cases, however, new and better solutions need to be devised and implemented. For that purpose, greater involvement of a wider segment of the population in the design and implementation of programme activities and greater mobilization of resources are the key issues. Each of the discussion papers is geared to looking forward to the decade of the 1990s in the light of these new objectives and key issues.

The approach adopted in this background paper distinguishes, on the one hand, the societal conditions of family planning programme activities, and, on the other hand, the programme activities proper as represented by the scope and strength of the programme effort undertaken. Within this framework, a number of issues are addressed, of which the most critical are discussed in papers prepared by participants in this Expert Group Meeting, who offer empirical evidence and specific recommendations for future implementation. This background paper is divided into eight sections, which correspond to the substantive items of the provisional agenda.

In section A, fertility and contraceptive prevalence, estimates and projections are presented for the period 1975-1995. This overview provides the demographic background for the regions and countries of the world. The family planning programme aspects discussed relate only to the situation in the developing countries where fertility rates are considered too high by Governments and where family planning activities are usually carried out on an official and/or private basis. Section B, society and family planning, examines the societal aspects, particularly certain aspects of the political, economic and sociocultural context that are especially relevant to programme implementation. Special attention is devoted to the status of women. These aspects constitute the background against which the family planning programme activities are carried out

and which facilitates or hampers the success of the measures proposed.

Section C, family planning policies and programmes, briefly describes the current status of policies and programmes in the less developed regions and appraises the successes achieved. The focus of this chapter is on identifying the programme elements that could be replicated in further programme developments. Section D, family planning programme implementation, briefly examines various aspects of the management of a family planning programme, such as organization, administration and implementation. These aspects reflect the programme effort undertaken to lower fertility; their outcome is shaped by the societal context in which they are carried out. Section E, family planning and health, overviews briefly how family planning practice affects the health of mothers and children. Special attention is devoted to the problem of sexually transmitted diseases (STDs) including the acquired immunodeficiency syndrome (AIDS). Section F, in the same vein as section E, is devoted to an examination of the consequences of family planning programmes for the well-being of children and the family. Section G, people's involvement in family planning programmes, outlines family planning programme aspects wherein greater involvement of various sectors of the population might improve the outcome of family planning programme activities. Special attention is devoted to the role of the community, the Government and non-governmental organizations. Section H presents a brief conclusion concerning the issues reviewed.

A. FERTILITY AND CONTRACEPTIVE PREVALENCE

Total fertility rates (TFRs) for the periods 1980-1985 and 1985-1990, based on the most recent fertility data available, and the United Nations fertility assumptions for the period 1990-1995 are presented in table 1. The overall data show that TFRs have continued to decline in most major areas of the less developed regions, except in Eastern, Middle and Western Africa, where the declines between 1980-1985 and 1985-1990 were nil; and they are expected to remain negligible in Middle Africa during the period from 1985-1990 to 1990-1995. On the other hand, in Northern and Southern Africa, the fertility decline was substantial between 1980-1985 and 1985-1990, with fertility rates falling to about 5.0 births per woman, corresponding to a percentage reduction of almost 10 per cent in the former region

Major area and region	Total fertility rate			Percentage change		Required reduction in total fertility rate to achieve replacement level (per woman)[b]
	1980-1985	1985-1990	1990-1995[a]	1980-1985 1985-1990	1985-1990 1990-1995[a]	
World	3.64	3.43	3.26	-5.77	-4.96	1.16
More developed regions ...	1.93	1.92	1.92	0.52	0.52	-
Less developed regions ...	4.23	3.90	3.64	-7.80	-6.67	1.54
Africa	6.40	6.25	6.00	-2.34	-4.00	3.9
Eastern Africa	6.81	6.86	6.76	0.73	-1.46	4.66
Middle Africa	6.53	6.53	6.47	0.00	0.92	4.37
Northern Africa	5.66	5.10	4.66	-9.89	-8.63	2.56
Southern Africa	4.92	4.50	4.22	-8.54	-6.22	2.12
Western Africa	6.87	6.85	6.53	0.29	-4.67	4.43
Asia	3.77	3.45	3.21	-8.49	-6.96	1.11
Eastern Asia	2.44	2.30	2.15	5.74	-6.52	0.05
South-eastern Asia	4.20	3.73	3.38	-11.19	-9.38	1.28
Southern Asia	5.16	4.66	4.30	-9.69	-7.73	2.2
Western Asia	5.33	5.04	4.69	-5.44	-6.94	2.59
Europe	1.81	1.71	1.71	-5.52	0.00	-
Eastern Europe	2.18	2.10	2.01	-3.67	-4.29	-
Northern Europe	1.81	1.84	1.91	1.66	3.80	-
Southern Europe	1.82	1.54	1.48	-15.38	3.90	-
Western Europe	1.61	1.58	1.64	1.86	3.80	-
Latin America and the Caribbean	3.92	3.40	3.05	-13.27	-10.29	0.95
Caribbean	3.18	2.96	2.84	-6.92	-4.05	0.74
Central America	4.55	3.92	3.48	-13.85	-11.22	1.38
South America	3.78	3.27	2.91	-13.49	-11.01	0.81
Northern America	1.80	1.89	2.04	5.00	7.94	-
Oceania	2.62	2.52	2.51	-3.82	-0.40	0.41
USSR[c]	2.35	2.43	2.25	3.40	-7.41	0.15

Source: *World Population Prospects: The 1992 Revision* (United Nations publication, Sales No. E.93.XIII.7).

[a]Data for 1990-1995: medium-variant assumption rates are averages for five-year period.

[b]Replacement level is assumed to be TFR = 2.1, assuming mortality levels commensurate with those of the more developed regions.

[c]Former Union of Soviet Socialist Republics.

and almost 9 per cent in the latter. However, TFR for Africa as a whole still exceeded 6.0 births per woman, on average, during 1985-1990, compared with about 3.5 births in Asia and Latin America and the Caribbean.

From 1980-1985 to 1985-1990, declines in fertility rates were sharpest in Latin America (except in the Caribbean) with percentage declines exceeding 13 per cent. In Asia, only South-eastern Asia, with 11 per cent, experienced a decline close to this magnitude. Reductions are expected to be somewhat smaller during the following quinquennial period. By 1985-1990, Eastern Asia emerges with the lowest average TFR (2.3 births per woman) and Western Asia with the highest (5.0 births per woman). In Latin America and the Caribbean, the averages range from 3.0 in the Caribbean to 3.9 in Central America (table 1).

By 1985-1990, at the country level, three Asian countries or areas—Hong Kong, the Republic of Korea and Singapore, thus excluding Japan—had reached the status of low-fertility countries, with fertility rates below replacement level. Conversely, with an estimated 8.5 births per woman, Rwanda emerges as the country with the highest fertility during that period. Estimates of TFRs for individual countries or areas are presented in annex table A.1.

The population goal recommended in the Amsterdam Declaration calls for a reduction in the average number of children born per woman commensurate with the median-variant population projections of the United Nations (UNFPA, 1989a). Such a goal remains, however, quite far from achieving replacement level in the short term in most less developed regions. The last column of table 1 presents the reduction in TFRs to be realized in order to achieve the 2.1 replacement level.

As concerns contraceptive use, the data in table 2 show that estimates of contraceptive prevalence rates among women of reproductive age currently in a marital union in the less developed regions were highest in Asia and in Latin America and the Caribbean and lowest in sub-Saharan Africa. Within each of these, however, regional differences are substantial. In Eastern Asia (excluding Japan, where use rates are generally high),contraceptive prevalence rates exceed 70 per cent. In the other Asian countries, prevalence rates range, in general from 30 to 70 per cent, although they sometimes fall below 30 per cent in certain countries of Southern and Western Asia (annex table A.2).

In sub-Saharan Africa, prevalence levels usually remain below 20 per cent with some exceptions. Mauritius, with 75 per cent contraceptive use, is one exception; it has the highest contraceptive prevalence level in Africa. In Northern Africa, contraceptive prevalence rates exceed 30 per cent and even reach almost 50 per cent in Tunisia. On the other hand, prevalence levels of less than 10 per cent are not uncommon, notably in several countries of Eastern and Western Africa. In Latin America and the Caribbean, rates of contraceptives use vary within a narrower interval; in most countries, they fall between 30 and 60 per cent of women in a marital union. Rates vary with country and year of observations; most recent estimates show that in a number of countries, notably in Costa Rica and Colombia, contraceptive use rates exceed 60 per cent; and even reach 70 per cent, for example, in Cuba and Puerto Rico (annex table A.2).

It should be borne in mind that prevalence rates sometimes show imperfectly the birth regulation status in these countries. Indeed, non-clinical methods are not always properly recorded while, on the other hand, the overall prevalence levels shown include the less effective traditional methods. Hence, it is somewhat difficult to relate precise contraceptive prevalence and fertility levels, although these two factors are generally inversely related (Weinberger, 1991).

B. SOCIETY AND FAMILY PLANNING

Reproductive behaviour is influenced by two large groups of factors: the societal factors (discussed in the present chapter); and the programme factors (examined in the following chapters). The societal factors affects reproductive behaviour, and hence family planning programme success, in many ways (see, for example, Warwick, 1987). It is thus important, for policy purposes, to identify these factors to achieve a better understanding of the social process of procreation and, in particular, to identify those which can be more amenable to policy measures directed to facilitating contraceptive behaviour. Moreover, in the case of family planning programmes, aside from the social and economic factors, political factors also play an important role and need to be explicitly taken into consideration.

Three prerequisites of fertility decline have been identified: first, fertility must be within the conscious choice of individuals; secondly, reduced fertility must be advantageous to the individual or the family; and thirdly, effective techniques of fertility regulation must be available (Coale, 1973).

The first two conditions are inherent in the societal setting. The third condition underscores the fundamental role that family planning programmes can play in providing birth regulation methods to meey an already existing demand, and information and education to meet a latent or yet unaware demand for birth regulation. In addition, the programme can also provide efficient contraceptive methods when only less effective methods or no methods at all are available, to provide easier access to those methods if required and to make those methods affordable to population groups that cannot meet its cost.

Region	All methods (1)	Modern methods[b] (2)	Sterilization Female (3)	Sterilization Male (4)	Pill (5)	Inject-able (6)	Intra-uterine device (7)	Condom (8)	Vaginal barrier methods (9)	Rhythm (10)	With-drawal (11)	Other methods (12)
A. Percentage of couples with the wife of reproductive age												
World	53	44	16	4	7	1	11	5	1	4	4	1
More developed regions[c]	71	47	8	4	14	—	6	13	2	9	13	2
Less developed regions	48	44	18	5	5	1	12	3	0.3	2	1	1
China	72	71	28	8	3	0.2	30	2	0.3	0.5	—	0.3
Other countries	38	32	14	3	6	1	4	3	0.3	3	2	1
Africa	17	13	1	—	7	1	3	10.2	2	1	1	
Northern Africa	31	27	2	—	16	0.3	8	1	0.3	2	2	1
Sub-Saharan Africa	13	9	1	—	4	2	1	0.5	0.2	2	1	1
Asia and Oceania[d]	53	49	21	6	4	1	14	3	0.3	2	1	1
East Asia[c]	72	71	28	8	3	0.2	29	2	0.4	1	0.2	0.3
Other countries	40	34	16	5	4	1	4	4	0.3	2	2	2
Latin America and the Caribbean	57	47	20	1	16	1	6	2	1	5	3	1
B. Percentage of contraceptive users												
World	100	83	29	8	14	2	20	9	1	7	8	2
More developed regions[c]	100	66	11	6	20	—	8	18	3	13	19	2
Less developed regions	100	91	37	9	11	2	25	5	1	4	3	2
China	100	99	38	11	5	0.3	41	3	0.4	1	—	0.4
Other countries	100	84	36	8	16	4	12	8	1	7	5	4
Africa	100	79	9	—	40	8	18	4	1	9	5	6
Northern Africa	100	88	6	—	51	1	25	4	1	5	5	2
Sub-Saharan Africa	100	70	11	—	28	16	10	4	1	13	6	11
Asia and Oceania[d]	100	92	39	11	7	2	27	6	1	3	2	2
Eastern Asia[c]	100	98	39	11	5	0.3	40	3	1	1	0.2	0.4
Other countries	100	85	39	11	11	4	11	9	1	6	5	4
Latin America and the Caribbean	100	84	36	1	28	2	11	4	1	9	6	2

Source: Mary Beth Weinberger, "Recent trends in contraceptive behavior", in *Demographic and Health Surveys World Conference, August 5-7, 1991, Washington, D.C., Proceedings*, vol. I (Columbia, Maryland, IRD/Macro International, Inc., 1991).
NOTE: These estimates reflect assumptions about contraceptive use in countries with no data.
[a]Based on most recent available survey data; average date, 1987.
[b]Including methods in columns (3)-(9).
[c]Australia-New Zealand, Europe, Northern America and Japan.
[d]Excluding Japan.

The sociocultural and economic context

Motivation for small families

The first prerequisite formulated above refers to the sociopsychological approach to life as expressed by generally held values and implies, from the standpoint of fertility norms, a rational approach to reproductive decision-making. The second precondition is directly derived from the social and economic value attributed by parents and family to large numbers of children. Models attempting to account for the factors that create demand for children and give children their value (for example, Caldwell, 1982; and Bulatao and Lee, 1983), as well as for the conditions under which motivation for smaller families arises (for example, Easterlin, 1975), have been proposed and are invaluable for understanding, theoretically, both the desire for fewer children and the obstacles to resort to birth control to achieve that end.

Various cultural and religious beliefs and traditions are generally involved in shaping individual reproductive behaviour and family size norms, and norms are not all determined only by the perceived economic advantages of a large family. In fact, the rational approach to procreation is often rational only within the upper and lower limits of reproductive norms established by society (see, for example, Freedman, 1966; and Caldwell, 1980). Hence, the motivation for smaller families and that for use of birth regulation methods are not always closely linked, and family planning programmes need to adopt the view that gaps between the expressed desire not to have children and the lack of contraceptive use can be accounted for, at least in part, by both normative and rational behaviour. In many African countries, for instance, the persistence of high fertility is attributed mainly to factors of social organization (Lesthaeghe, 1989), and therein lies part of the limits of current family planning programmes.

In order to implement sound policies to reduce fertility, it is not only necessary to identify the general societal factors favourable to lower fertility but also important to understand the mechanism whereby such factors affect fertility, if only to facilitate the effectiveness of programme measures directed to increasing contraceptive use. The relations between the educational and work status of women and fertility are such factors, and their modes of action on fertility have not yet been satisfactorily accounted for on a cross-cultural basis.

Status of women

The status of women is an important factor related to fertility because it is generally held that the higher the woman's status, the lower her number of children ever born. This status is identified by various indicators, but most often by education and work (for example, United Nations, 1985). The importance of these two characteristics is derived from their effect on the timing and prevalence of marriage and on the fertility size norms.

As concerns the labour force factor, it is generally held that working women tend to have fewer children than non-working women. As stated, this hypothesis properly considers neither the direction of the relationship nor the sociocultural context in which it is supposed to apply.[1] Indeed, in many societies with traditional value systems, not only in sub-Saharan Africa but also in Asia and in other major areas, a large number of women participate in the labour force (United Nations, 1989b) while also having large families. Thus, in practice, the policy of involving women more in the process of development through their greater participation in the labour force emerges more as a policy to achieve equality of rights than one to achieve lower fertility.

Education, as women's other status indicator, appears as a necessary, although not always sufficient, condition to achieve lower fertility. Education is assumed to exert its effect on fertility not only as a result of delayed marriage but also at the normative level (Caldwell, 1980). In addition, education also affects fertility through occupation outside the household.

The magnitude of the impact of women's work on fertility varies. The lowest fertility rates are often observed among the most highly educated women and among those working in modern occupations (for example, United Nations, 1987). A certain duration of studies and a certain type of work are thus more likely to induce lower fertility and these two characteristics are obviously linked. Education and employment policies thus underlie the success of policy measured directed to improving the status of women. From this standpoint, their impact on fertility emerges as a prerequisite of improved health and family life.

Greater consideration to the status of women in family planning programme would undoubtedly improve performance of operations. In practice, it means greater

32

efforts devoted to meet women's individual needs and expectations within a specific cultural context: for instance, by ensuring the accessibility of contraceptive information and supplies to women without anyone's authorization; by providing family planning services at days and/or hours that meet women's availability; by ensuring availability of contraceptives acceptable to women; by providing proper privacy; by having female rather than male personnel available when appropriate; and by improving female counselling and follow-up. In addition, pertinent family planning activities could eventually be better designed, managed and implemented by qualified female personnel, notably to cope with obstacles of which men are not usually aware or are not in a position to remove easily.

Socio-economic development, importance of social sectors and fertility behaviour

The developing countries have experienced many socio-economic changes during the past decades. It is therefore important to identify the channels through which socio-economic forces other than population policies and family planning programmes affect fertility change. In particular, this statement implies not only that the impact on fertility of socio-economic factors must be properly distinguished from the impact of population policy factors. It will also be necessary, through continuous evaluation, to assess the relative contribution of individual socio-economic and policy determinants on any fertility decline. It is becoming increasingly apparent that social development contributes considerably to economic development and fertility change. Therefore, greater emphasis must be placed on the study of the role of social development factors in observed fertility declines. The Expert Group Meeting may wish to recommend that greater emphasis should be placed on social development.

The political context

Political support

Active political support to family planning programmes is imperative (Sadik, 1991). Such support can take many aspects. Clear priorities need to be set for demographic planning in order to facilitate programme implementation. Programme implementation should be carried out without political interference or administrative obstacles. Even more important,

official support needs to be expressed at all governmental levels through action and speeches by high-ranking officials, cultural role models, religious leaders, village chiefs etc. Only in this way can innovative family planning programme measures be perceived as legitimate and acceptable by the population at large.

Political support also encompasses enacting not only legislation repealing existing legal obstacles to the use of birth regulation methods but also legislation facilitating the availability of and accessibility to efficient modern contraceptive methods. Easy access to information and distribution of birth regulation methods, fiscal advantages, low-cost importation of contraceptive methods and ready licensing of local production of birth control devices are some of the important prerequisites of programme success. Likewise, regulations to help overcome cultural obstacles to access to contraception need to be enacted and enforced.

Human rights

The human rights aspect transcends demographic considerations. In this respect, the World Population Plan of Action affirms emphatically that the right to decide the number and spacing of children should be respected and ensured, regardless of any demographic goal. In the field of procreation, human rights encompass three main dimensions. First, there is the right of couples and individuals to achieve responsible parenthood and to have the number of children they want when they want them, which includes the right of medical assistance in case of subfecundity problems. This right also implies education and access to information, as well as availability of safe, acceptable and affordable birth regulation methods. Secondly, the human rights aspect also requires that couples and individuals be able to meet their reproductive goals without legal obstacles. Thirdly, the human rights aspect also needs to ensure that family planning programmes, especially their components dealing with motivation activities, as well as incentive and disincentive measures, shall be applied with equity and fairness towards both family planning personnel and family planning recipients and shall not create or increase disparities among different social groups. The rights of mothers and children to protection against illnesses or death related to child-bearing and protection against the threat of AIDS also bear on human rights (United Nations, 1990a).

C. FAMILY PLANNING POLICIES AND PROGRAMMES

The dissemination of population policies and programmes in the less developed regions reflects the keen awareness by Governments of the importance of the population factor in development planning (United Nations, 1990b). In countries where the population rate of growth is deemed too high, Governments have adopted such policies. As of 1990, in Africa, 48 out of 52 countries were providing direct or indirect support to the dissemination of modern methods of contraception; in Latin America and the Caribbean, 32 out of 33 countries were providing such support; and in Asia, 28 out of 38 countries (United Nations, 1991c).

Although many of the family planning programmes are integrated into the national health system, there is also a wide variety of delivery systems established through the cooperation with non-governmental organizations and private medical and commercial outlets. These family planning programmes have been carried out in a large array of cultural settings and economic and social conditions and from this wide spectrum of experiences lessons can to be learned.

Not all programmes realized all their objectives completely. In general, however, comparative studies in developing countries show that: (a) countries with family planning programmes experienced greater fertility reductions than countries without programmes; (b) among countries with fertility reductions, the greater the intensity of the programme effort, the larger the fertility decline; and (c) among these latter countries, the more advanced the level of development, the stronger the effect of the programme effort (Mauldin and Ross, 1991).

However, because time and human and financial resources are limited, it is important, in the next decade of programme implementation, to devote greater efforts to programme quality and coverage and to achieve greater and faster success. Consequently, new priorities may have to be set and revisions of current programmes undertaken in order to make them more effective in reducing fertility. Estimating programme impact on fertility remains thus a priority component of programme implementation.[2]

Such evaluations should be undertaken at the country level rather than at the cross-country level if country-specific implications need to be drawn for programme improvement. In addition, qualitative evaluation of programme activities under different conditions is needed to complement such quantitative evaluation. Indeed, the human factor, not easily quantifiable, often generates formidable obstacles to the success of well-planned, well-designed family planning programmes (see, for example, UNFPA, 1989b). Given the human and financial constraints noted above, priorities need to be set on the basis of clearly defined criteria.

D. FAMILY PLANNING PROGRAMME IMPLEMENTATION

Views, recommendations and suggestions about the effective management of family planning programmes (for example, In-Joung Whang, 1976; UNFPA, 1980; and UNESCO, 1982) and ways to improve performance are abundantly available in the specialized literature (for example, Lapham and Simmons, 1987; and Seidman and Horn, 1991). A large body of literature on techniques to evaluate the efficiency and the efficacy of family planning programmes is also available (for example, United Nations, 1979 and 1986; and United Nations, ESCAP, 1976).

For the decade of the 1990s, the issues to be addressed with regard to programme implementation concern: (a) a number of operational aspects which still hamper the empirical success of family planning programmes; and (b) the means of generating increased human and financial resources to meet increased programme needs (Sadik, 1991). Obstacles at various levels can be the focus of such concern, such as badly planned programme activities, well-planned activities that are not properly implemented or well-planned and well-implemented activities that could still benefit from improvement. From this management standpoint, two criteria guide any revision for improvement—increase in performance and lowering of costs. Discussion papers pertaining to the following six topics offer material, ideas and recommendations concerning these various operational issues.

Quality of service and human resource development

Although the 1990s will call for a considerable increase in the scope of family planning programmes, such a shift is not likely to be successful without a substantial shift from quantity to quality (for example, Bruce, 1990). Quality of service has been identified as a fundamental determinant of fertility decline in regions where family planning programmes are implemented (for example, Jain, 1989; Simmons and Phillips, 1990). Quality of service consists of a series of varied and interacting factors such as quality of training, skills, qualifications and especially attitude of personnel, availability of and accessibility to modern contraceptive methods, success of promotional activities and follow-up to prior services.

The performance of different programme components thus need to be closely monitored. A breakdown in quality of service is often disclosed by studies on trends in new contraceptive acceptance and on the duration of contraceptive use, the patterns of which can show shortcomings and directions of improvements (Jejeebhoy, 1989; United Nations, 1991b). Personnel training, field supervision and training evaluation are key approaches to improve the quality of personnel. Lastly, relationships between patients and service personnel are fundamental components of service quality. Occurrences of incorrect or inadequate information provided to clients by family planning service providers or workers, lack of courtesy and tact, class-oriented or group-oriented prejudices at contraceptive delivery systems, lack or inadequate information about possible side-effects and insufficient or lack of follow-up etc. (UNFPA, 1989a, 1989b, 1990a and 1990b) are causes of contraceptive use discontinuation, unfounded fears and lack of progress in contraceptive acceptance. Personnel shortcomings need to be identified immediately (through period evaluations), and incentives and disincentives for programme personnel should address quality of service rather than quantity, such as quota fulfilment.

Family planning services and unreached populations

As concerns delivery systems, availability of family planning services is a necessary but not a sufficient condition for good family planning programme performance. Indeed, availability of services needs to be combined not only with adequate staffing and management but, most of all, with easy accessibility. This question of accessibility has raised a number of problems because the physical presence of a delivery system post in a given area is not always perceived as such. Indeed, the perception of non-contracepting population groups concerning access to family planning services is sometimes incorrect; in various cases, knowledge of contraceptive outlets is simply associated with the need for contraceptive services (for example, Chamratrithirong and Kamnuansilpa, 1984; Laily and others, 1984).

Besides, the existence of contraceptive outlets is only part of contraceptive accessibility. Actual location, time needed to reach outlets, distance to outlets, availability of transportation, ease of travel, climatic obstacles and days and hours of availability of services all concur to facilitate or complicate access to contraceptive services.

The provision of family planning services to population groups not yet reached by family planning activities might considerably improve programme performance, provided that there is some demand for contraception. Studies on unmet needs of contraception find high percentages of married women that, at the time of the interview, did not want additional children but, nevertheless, did not use a contraceptive method (Westoff and Pebley, 1984; Johnson-Acsadi and Szykman, 1984).[3] Women of this group who claim lack of accessibility to contraceptive services could easily become contraceptive acceptors if adequate services are made available. Other population subgroups are not using contraception because delivery systems are not geared to serving them. This is the situation notably for adolescents, men, populations living in slums or in remote areas and low-income population.

Specific strategies to reach these subgroups need to be recommended, including the design of cultural innovations, for instance, to persuade adolescent couples—and their families—to delay the first birth, to obtain men's approval and support for women's birth regulation practices, to motivate men to utilize male contraceptive methods; and to approach unreached populations in remote, slum and overcrowded areas.

With acceptors properly informed about risks and side-effects, properly counselled and properly followed up by competent personnel, contraceptive acceptance and continuing use of effective contraceptive methods could be considerably increased. Likewise, services where potential demand exists (notably among postpartum women) could also be expanded. This approach appears to have worked notably with voluntary female sterilization in recent years (Church and Geller, 1990).

Adolescent fertility

The situation described above is particularly crucial as concerns adolescent population. With fertility rates at ages 15-19 years often fewer than 150, even 100, per 1,000, their fertility represents only a relatively small part of TFR (United Nations, 1991c). But for this subgroup, the contraception issue is not merely a demographic one (United Nations, 1989a). The social and health cost of adolescent fertility is of much greater concern. Indeed, maternal mortality and child mortality are generally much higher among adolescent mothers than among mothers in the higher age groups (WHO, 1989). Adolescent fertility may also constitute an obstacle to women's prolonged education and skill development. Furthermore, when adolescent fertility is illegitimate, as is the case in a number of countries, it creates tension and personal distress which lead to family crises, single-parent household and clandestine abortion with all its ill effects.

Diffusion of innovative behaviour and information, education and communication activities

In many cultural situations, the adoption of family planning may be considered a process of innovative behaviour. This action implies: first, a desire to limit and/or space the number of births; secondly, the conviction that it has become socially, culturally or religiously acceptable to interfere with the reproductive process; and thirdly, the acceptance of using artificial methods to regulate births. Because behaviour is exercised within the constraints of social norms, innovative behaviour always benefits from support in adopting new attitudes, which can sometimes be achieved by special motivational techniques (for example, Havelock and others, 1971).

Two of the main obstacles to adopting innovative reproductive behaviour are norms and lack of information. Dealing with the norms calls for more specific approaches. Motivation campaigns describing the family and health advantages of smaller families and information and educational activities concerning contraceptives (United Nations, ESCAP, n.d.) directed to individuals and couples are necessary but not sufficient. To be efficient, messages need to be coordinated at the individual, interpersonal, organizational and societal levels and need to persuade as much as to convince couples to approach procreation from a different point of view.[4] Once properly designed, messages need to be increasingly directed to specific populations and closely monitored.[5] An overall reassessment of the information, education and communication (IEC) approaches currently resorted to thus need to be recommended in light of past experiences and lessons learned.

Community-based delivery system and social marketing of contraceptives

The advantages and disadvantages of utilizing community-based delivery (CBD) systems and social marketing of contraceptives (SMC) depend notably upon the sociocultural environment, the programme infrastructure and the geographical conditions of any particular community. The major advantage of CBD system is, of course, the proximity of the delivery point to the contraceptive users. It is thus recommended in remote areas or when access is difficult. But it is also advantageous when there are cultural barriers and local support is needed to promote family planning and inspire confidence in the programme. Social marketing is more appropriate to service mass markets of contraceptive users at reasonable prices.[6]

The CBD system and SMC are thus two important and sometimes underused components of family planning programme delivery systems. It is believed that they can contribute considerably to future programme performance and help those programmes become more self-sufficient. Their implementation, however, encompasses a variety of difficulties which need to be better addressed in the coming years. One particularly fundamental issue of community-based activities is not only to initiate the involvement of the members of the community but to ensure their continuous motivation and continuity of operations. For these purposes, incentives (rather than disincentives), both individual and collective, can be used, but strict provisions need to be established and respected to prevent abuses. Likewise, even under optimum conditions of community cooperation, the provision of supplies, equipment and IEC support needs to be ensured by the official programme at all times (UNFPA, 1991a).

With regard to social marketing, the key issues are to identify the most relevant target populations and to obtain funding to support lower contraceptive prices, which, again, will depend upon the particular circumstances of the programme. Cooperation with private outlets and the feasibility of cost-sharing with institutions and contraceptive users that can afford it need to be examined along with cost-effective methods of managing this delivery system.

Future contraceptive requirements and logistics management needs

The future operational management of family planning programmes requires, first, estimates of the size of the populations to be served and the number and type of contraceptive methods that will be needed; and, secondly, an expansion of the organizational and management means of producing and delivering the contraceptives to the increasing number of users in an efficient way.

As concerns the estimates, a variety of methodologies have been proposed to assess the level of contraceptive prevalence needed to achieve a given fertility level at any given point in time (Nortman, 1978; Bongaarts, 1984; Mauldin, 1991). A recent estimation concluded that to achieve the United Nations medium-variant population projections of 6.2 billion people by the year 2000, the rate of contraceptive use among married women aged 15-49 should rise from 51 per cent in 1990 to 59 per cent in 2000. This estimate implies that in Africa, during that period, prevalence among women of reproductive age should increase from 9.1 to 17.7 per cent; and in Asia and the Pacific, from 57 to 65.4 per cent. It is thus estimated that by the end of the century, 567 million couples for whom adequate supplies need to be provided, should be using some method of contraception (UNFPA, 1991b).

Once contraceptive requirements are estimated, supplies will have to be produced and delivered to the population at the grass-roots level. Given the size of future requirements, new approaches to procurement will have to be adopted and new priorities set. Can production of modern contraceptives by local manufacturers be increased?[7] Can quantities of modern contraceptives purchased abroad and obtained from national and international donor organizations also be increased? As of 1990, it wss reported that only five countries (Brazil, China, India, Indonesia and Mexico) were either completely autonomous or about to be as concerns their requirements for condoms, intra-uterine devices (IUDs), oral contraceptives and injectables (PATH, 1991). Increasing quantities of contraceptives offered by donors imply increased funding of those donors.

The logistics of managing a family planning programme are even more challenging as a result of the various constraints that must be taken into consideration. Among these limitations, the particular geographical, sociocultural and economic conditions prevailing in any given country at any given time are of the essence. Services should provide a proper mix of socially acceptable contraceptive methods to the population and should ensure quality of contraceptives, proper storage, on-time delivery, affordable cost, meaningful distribution points etc.

If needed, mobile family planning clinics, mobile family planning teams and pick-up arrangements can be established to support or back up community-delivery systems and social marketing systems or to reach remote areas. In addition, sound management information system and decision-making processes need to be adopted (Keller, 1991).

Thus, ensuring the efficiency and effectiveness of programme logistics management is a multidimensional task which requires not only an accurate knowledge of current national and local conditions but a realistic assessment of the future. Because the future is generally associated with a wide range of unknowns and uncertainties, family planning logistics for the coming decade need to be flexible and adaptable, and to rely upon planning procedures that can be easily modified and readily revised or adjusted.

E. FAMILY PLANNING AND HEALTH

The health aspect of family planning is as fundamental as the demographic and social aspects. The practice of family planning, whether for limiting or spacing births, is important for good health of both children and mothers. Moreover, by using barrier methods, such as the condom, family planning is also efficient in preventing infection by STDs, notably AIDS (for example, Trussell and Pebley, 1984; United Nations, 1991a).

Health of children

Three aspects of family planning are related to child mortality: age of the mother; parity; and length of the birth interval. Births to adolescent mothers (those under age 20) are often associated with higher infant and child mortality than those occurring to older women (WHO, 1989). When the mother is under age 18, the excess risk of death of the first-born child is even higher (for example, Hobcraft, 1991). As concerns parity, mortality tends to be higher among first births (although there are exceptions), to be relatively low for second and third births and then to increase with increasing parity. Lastly, the length of the preceding birth interval increases the risk of death of the last child born (for example, Hobcraft, 1992); and it is suggested that close spacing of births may affect not only the health of the last child born but also that of the previous child, who may be prematurely weaned if the mother gets pregnant again too soon (UNFPA, 1992b).

Health of mothers

Studies have shown that in various circumstances, family planning, by reducing illegitimate pregnancy risks, also reduces abortion-related mortality. Although certain contraceptives have medical side-effects and in certain cases constitute serious health risks, studies also show that—depending upon prevailing medical and health conditions—maternal health risks associated with pregnancy are much higher than risks associated with contraceptive use (for example, Lettenmaier and others, 1988; WHO, 1989).

As a result of these findings, specific population subgroups can be targeted for family planning practice, notably the high-risk groups mentioned in section A. Among adolescent women, mortality could be reduced by delaying conceptions, especially when these conceptions are unwanted and may result in abortion-related deaths. Likewise, older and high-parity women, and women with short post-partum sterility, all at higher mortality risk, can also be subject to more intensive programme activities. In addition, women delivering children under unsafe conditions are also primary targets for birth regulation methods (for example, Isaacs and Fincancioglu, 1989; WHO, 1989).[8]

Sexually transmitted diseases

Family planning programmes could greatly contribute to the prevention of STDs, particularly the human immunodeficiency virus (HIV) causing AIDS. Greater emphasis needs to be put on the important role of the condom in preventing the spread of STDs and AIDS.[9] Couples at risk, especially those involved with more than one sexual partner, endanger not only their own health and that of their mates and newborn children but also family life and the stability of the community at large.

Family planning programmes attempting to address these problems might do so at two levels. At the institutional level, programmes need to be modified so that contraception is encouraged not only to space or limit the size of the family but also to escape the dangers of STDs and AIDS. This effort implies a greater emphasis on barrier contraceptives, such as the condom, as well as programmes to alert couples about the symptoms of the infections and to provide care or referrals for care in cases of need. It also implies greater awareness of those problems by the programme personnel, thus meaning extended personnel training to provide accurate information for counselling and offering the needed medical advice and services,[10] while ascertaining that these new activities do not negatively affect the family planning programme itself.

At the individual level, the programme could be concerned with the means of convincing people to change and/or adapt their contraceptive habits (Gordon and Klouda, 1989; Worth, 1989).

Interdependence of services

Achieving the combined aims of family planning and health policies calls, of course, for a genuinely efficient organization. Although family planning services are, to a large extent, integrated into the existing national public-health system in most countries, alternative means of contraceptive delivery should be established whenever appropriate.

The integration of family planning and health programmes has many advantages, notably use of the existing health infrastructure for contraceptive distribution and services and the financial support provided by the Government. On the one hand, integration has experienced a variety of limitations and pitfalls, which are addressed in the discussion papers.

After years of experience, the question as to the overall benefits and limitations of the integration approach is still debated. It is, however, the mode of integration of the various management components, not its principle, which is often questioned: decision-making; responsibilities; management; supervision; definition of objectives; etc. Current integrated programmes with unsatisfactory performance have to be redesigned; even satisfactory integration may require changes, as family planning programmes and socio-economic conditions evolve and as more is learned from past experience.[11]

Interdependence of family planning services need not be limited to health services. Linking family planning activities with rural development projects, agricultural projects, disease eradication programmes, cooperative programmes etc. has also been attempted so as to appeal to the specific interests of the target populations. Experience drawn from these various attempts are also briefly examined in the discussion paper.

F. FAMILY PLANNING AND FAMILY WELL-BEING

Family size, structure and child development

Family size and structure are undergoing radical changes in the developing countries due to forces of social change. These changes have many and varied implications for the welfare of the family, notably in terms of single-parent families and the risk for their children, reduced family size, better education and health of the children, making offspring a major components of the well-being of the family.

The Expert Group will review the changes in size and structure of the family, consider the implications of those changes and recommend measures to ensure family well-being, including good child development.

Fertility decline and family support system

The relation between fertility decline and family support systems is not very clear. On the one hand, with the reduction in family size, families tend to become more self-supporting. They are in a better position, financially and otherwise, to support themselves; and the possibilities of getting support from children is greatly enhanced as the life conditions of these children improve. On the other hand, when fertility declines, women tend to participate more in the labour force and their role in the family support system changes. The Group will examine the various aspects of the relation between fertility decline and the family support system.

G. PEOPLE'S INVOLVEMENT IN FAMILY PLANNING PROGRAMMES

An important means of improving programme efficiency and effectiveness is to increase the involvement of certain categories of people (e.g., women and persons in influential positions) and social institutions (women's organizations, labour unions, employers etc.) in the implementation of family planning programmes. Mobilization of these categories of manpower emerges as a major means of improving programme impact in the 1990s and beyond.

Community participation

Community participation may well be the most promising approach to people's involvement in family planning programmes. It is also the most complex to institute if a successful outcome is expected. In particular, community involvement, more than any other popular participation in a social programme, can only be successful if due consideration is given to the prevailing sociocultural conditions of that community. Community participation has been practised in many countries implementing family planning programmes, with varying levels of success. The question is how successful has this approach been so far and what are its advantages and disadvantages. Among the critical issues to be examined, one could mention the problem of identifying the stage of the family planning programme in which community programmes should be initiated and under what conditions, the importance of qualitative rather than quantitative aspects of community participation, the type of institutional links with public-health services and private family planning activities, and the flexibility and adaptability of community participation. Furthermore, means of motivating the community to sustain its effort in the long term need to be recommended.[12] Lastly, because some views suggest that this approach may be both difficult and costly (for example, Askew, 1989), alternative strategies must be recommended.[13]

A discussion paper presents the advantages and disadvantages and the successes and failures experienced with community participation in different programmes and under various conditions.

Cost of contraceptive supplies and services and cost-sharing

Funding of programmes will be one of the most critical issues of the 1990s. As populations grow and demand for family planning services increases, family planning programmes will have to expand their efforts and services. As reported above in section D, contraceptive requirements for the next decade are expected to be considerable. Consequently, the cost of contraceptive supplies, one of the largest component of programme cost, will also increase. The cost to meet the projected contraceptive needs was recently estimated at nearly $5 billion, not including service delivery costs (UNFPA, 1991b).

Programme costs can be met from three main sources: governmental budgets; national and international donors; and cost-sharing with contraceptive users.

39

With regards to governmental and non-governmental funding, previous experience and prevailing conditions will shape this aspect. But what is the feasibility of increasing cost-sharing by contraceptive users during the 1990s? Although family planning users are estimated currently to contribute no more than 10 per cent of total cost of family planning programmes, this contribution may have to double by the year 2000 (Lande and Geller, 1991). As cost to couples is already often considered a barrier to contraceptive practice, even among motivated couples, this alternative needs to be examined closely, particularly in terms of cost of contraception in relation to income.[14]

Alternatives must also be examined. For instance, to what extent should users that can afford it bear a greater share of the cost? How could the public and private sectors share the cost in order to make these services available to the needy free of charge? Many possibilities are open to make family planning more cost-effective (Lande and Geller, 1991).

The discussion papers presented to this Expert Group examine the funding potential of governmental and non-governmental organizations and the cost-sharing possibilities that could be recommended to obtain the needed financial resources for the future.

Contraceptive research and development

A considerable number of means have been and are being explored to render prevention of conception easier, cheaper and more use-effective. Research has progressed in two directions: improving the performance of current contraceptive methods; and developing new improved methods (WHO, 1990). Subcutaneous implants and injections of hormonal contraception have already facilitated adoption in a variety of situations. Likewise, low-dose oral contraceptives have also gained ground in the developing countries. But a variety of obstacles have hindered the offering of a number of new contraceptive technologies (e.g., hormonal male contraception and post-coital contraception) and have affected the dissemination and acceptance of methods already being distributed (Hatcher and others, 1989).[15] In a number of countries, side-effects of contraceptives have discouraged adoption of certain contraceptive methods, often as a result of inadequate information and follow-up.

As research continues in the next decade, the issues will pertain primarily to the question of national self-

reliance in reproductive health research, the strengthening of the research capabilities of countries and individual institutions and the greater coordination of research. The problem of the increasing demand for funding for research versus the diminishing availability of financial resources also needs to be addressed (WHO, 1990).

Role of governmental and non-governmental organizations and the private sector

In any discussion of population policies and programmes, special mention should be made of those responsible for their formulation, implementation and support. Prominent among this group are the major international donors (multilateral and bilateral). However, because the Expert Group Meeting on Population Policies and Programmes, held at Cairo, Egypt, in April 1992, gave particular attention to the topic of international population assistance, such discussion is not repeated in this paper.

Three social sectors share responsibilities for implementation of programmes: Governments; non-governmental (non-profit) organizations; and the private commercial sector.

During the 1990s, the magnitude of their participation needs to be reassessed in the light of the increasing effort required to meet the future demand for family planning services and the financial constraints to support this demand. In addition, the need to increase popular participation in the cost of family planning programmes overlaps these two aspects (Ross and Isaacs, 1988; UNFPA, 1990c). A discussion paper examines past experiences and the feasibility of shifting implementation and funding responsibilities between these three social sectors.

National Governments

Given their sovereignty, their access to financial resources and their ability to mobilize and organize institutions and manpower, national Governments are the key for successful implementation of family planning programmes during the 1990s.

Two major constraints, however, should be re-examined—the cost and cost effectiveness of governmental activities. Although self-reliance can be a long-term goal as concerns funding and national contraceptive production, considerable support still needs to be obtained in those areas from both national and international non-governmental organizations.

Integration of family planning activities into health and other type of activities has given rise to a variety of administrative, managerial and logistics problems which also call for a re-examination of the nature of such integration and coordination of current activities.

How could Governments, in the 1990s, increase their contribution to the cost of family planning services? Although the obvious means of government participation is an increment in family planning programme budgeting, countries can also resort to alternatives that do not involve increased disbursements of funds. Such measures as elimination of import duties, production taxes, sales taxes and licensing fees, for instance, could lower the cost of contraceptive supplies to users. Likewise, more efficient logistics management could lower the cost of delivery systems, storage and transportation. Lastly, Governments can play a major role in overcoming certain social obstacles which hinder access to birth regulation, notably with regard to discrimination against women, improved levels of education, greater participation of women in the labour force and greater accessibility of women to contraceptive services.

United Nations and non-governmental organizations

The international community and all major United Nations bodies, especially the United Nations Population Fund (UNFPA), the United Nations Children's Fund (UNICEF) and the World Health Organization (WHO), have been assisting Governments in carrying out their family planning programmes. But these efforts should be further strengthened and should call for increased population assistance.

To what extent can Governments depend upon international funding and assistance from non-governmental organizations during the 1990s? Can international and non-governmental donor organizations devote more efforts to assist national policies directed to reducing population growth? Many international organizations and agencies have called for greater assistance to national programmes. The United States Agency for International Development (USAID) has already announced a new population assistance strategy; several European donors are expected to increase significantly their population assistance; and contribu-

tions to UNFPA are expected to exceed the 1991 level (Population Crisis Committee, 1992).

Non-governmental organizations, such as the International Planned Parenthood Federation (IPPF) and the Population Council, and many others, have been pioneers in family planning activities, often preceding official policies. They still supplement family planning activities because of their efficient networks, special skills and adaptability to changing situations. These various advantages should be further utilized, and the activities of non-governmental organizations need to be further taken into consideration by the governmental strategies for implementation of their population policy.

In addition, other organizations could make their own contribution. Women's associations, youth organizations, employee and workers' unions also could eventually contribute in giving couples access to information and services on contraception. If necessary, guidance, training and other resources can be provided to willing non-governmental organizations.

Such expanded activities imply a decentralization of responsibilities and an increase in monetary resources. The mandates and functions of collaborating governmental and non-governmental organizations and international organizations, as well as their relationships, need to be clearly defined and coordinated to avoid costly overlapping activities.

The private sector

Established retail outlets for the promotion and delivery of contraceptive methods have been utilized in a number of programmes. More than in any other area, the experience gained from existing commercial outlets needs to be carefully assessed if the assistance of this sector is to be expanded during the 1990s. Indeed, marketing requirements, promotional efforts and the cost of contraceptives offered may not always be cost-effective. Private delivery systems for modern contraceptives are called for, especially in order to increase the use of non-clinical contraceptives, although demand has to be sufficient and sociocultural conditions favourable to make such an approach successful. Social marketing rather than complete privatization can make the private sector a viable alternative although management, provision and control over distribution need to be properly addressed. Here, too, lessons can be learned from the experience of such countries as Bangladesh, Colombia, India, Nepal and Pakistan.

Contraceptive promotion and delivery at the workplace, a system which has been successful in a variety of situations, is another possibility. Likewise, physicians and midwives have been used as contraceptive providers in various countries and can be instituted in more countries during the next decade if social conditions are favourable to these approaches. Here, too, government subsidies and incentive programmes for providers and recipients of contraceptive methods might be needed to achieve a more efficient diffusion of certain types of contraceptives (injectables or implants, for instance), provided such programmes are properly managed and supervised. Again, lessons need to be drawn from past experience, as shown in the discussion paper, in order to ascertain the most favourable and cost-effective conditions for such undertaking.

H. Conclusion

The framework presented in this overview addresses a number of general areas in which the Expert Group Meeting could offer recommendations to underscore and redirect efforts intended to improve the efficiency and effectiveness of family planning programmes. Despite the success of a number of family planning programmes and the decline in fertility rates observed in most countries of the less developed regions, the number of births in absolute term continues to increase. Hence, the main aspect to be borne in mind in making recommendations for expanding and revising family planning programmes is population size and the demands that a number of people impose on governmental responsibilities. Given the variety of national conditions within which programmes are carried out, those recommendations could merely point to directions, especially new directions, in which action is required. Priorities can only be set by the respective countries, taking into consideration their current and future societal conditions, demographic objectives, family planning needs and resources.

Some priorities are common to all programmes. One is that programmes should focus not merely on fertility reduction but more so on the well-being of the population and on individual and family life. Family planning activities thus need to encompass a broader perspective to include increasingly the status of women, health of mothers and children, condition of adolescent women, child development etc.

Another priority is that the national Government should increase its efforts to mobilize resources and personnel, facilitate funding and promote administrative cooperation.

Still another common priority is the individual's and the family's right of access to birth regulation services and the ethical aspects associated with the promotion of family planning practice. These rights need to be strongly reaffirmed if population measures are to find popular acceptance and if the health of individuals, the status of women, the well-being of the family and the welfare of the population are to be further improved through population policies.

That the management of family planning programme operations needs to be established on a solid administrative and logistic foundation is not a new issue. But achieving success in programme performance is hampered by cultural and technical obstacles. Because programme implementation is carried out in well-defined sociocultural and economic milieux, a reassessment of the societal conditions favourable to specific programme management styles is needed at the smallest geographical level to ensure optimum conditions of programme performance. Therefore, programme designs should not only be improved but should be made flexible and adaptable to different and changing conditions.

Ultimate and intermediate objectives need to be set goals realistically so as to avoid disappointments; appropriate training facilities should be provided so that qualified personnel are available to implement the programme measures; delivery systems (whether official or private) need to be suited for the local cultural and geographical conditions and should meet the particular needs of the contraceptive users. Areas of improvement should also include, more generally, quality of services, unmet contraceptive needs and outreach to specific population subgroups (such as adolescents, lower social strata, men and husbands, and populations of remote areas). Although new reliable management techniques to improve programme performance need to be adopted, it should also be borne in mind that better techniques are a necessary but not a sufficient condition to achieve better results; personnel motivation and qualifications are the key to good results. This aspect thus calls for expansion of personnel training activities. Furthermore, in the field of family planning programmes, which involve primarily women as contraceptive acceptors, it is important that more women be involved in the management and supervision of such activities.

In order to improve programme performance, it is evident that programme shortcomings and limitations first need to be identified. It is thus imperative that periodic evaluation be undertaken at all programme implementation levels (training, promotion, delivery, follow-up, discontinuation of contraceptive use) because without continuous feedback, immediate programme corrections and revisions cannot be undertaken, which can result in waste of financial and human resources. Lastly, the impact of the programme on fertility (which is the ultimate policy objectives) needs to be assessed to ascertain the contribution of the programmes to the fertility decline.

Estimates of needs for contraceptive services for the next decade suggest that programmes will have to widen the scope of their operations to satisfy the increasing potential of new acceptors. Hence, increased funding by Governments, international and national organizations will be required, and non-governmental organizations (national and international) could then be called upon to increase their contributions to governmental activities. Past experience suggests that the contribution of these institutional partners to the success of family planning programmes can be greatly increased through better cooperation and coordination.

Lastly, the diversity and complexity of carrying out family planning operations under different societal and programme conditions call for a more institutionalized means of centralizing information on past and current experiences in order to draw lessons for the future.

NOTES

[1] The common approach is that greater percentages of women that want to work away from home tend to limit the size of their family. On the other hand, research also supports the view that women that cannot have or do not want to have more children tend to enter the labour force in greater proportions. Still other conclusions consider that there are reciprocal effects of these two types of interrelations (for example, Krishnan, 1991). It is thus fundamental to know which causal relation is at work in a particular context if policy measures are to be successful.

[2] The first step needs to ascertain whether fertility declined at all during the evaluation period. The second step needs to distinguish the part of the decline, if any, which can be attributed to non-programme contraception and the part attributable to family planning programme contraception. The third step is to identify the specific programme elements that contributed to fertility decline and the specific socio-economic factors that facilitated the impact of these programme elements on the fertility decline (United Nations, 1979 and 1986). Data on new acceptors and continuing users used as proxies in programme evaluation are only approximate indicators of fertility impact and need to be utilized with great caution (United Nations, ESCAP, 1969; Chandrasekaran and Hermalin, 1975).

[3] The size of the unmet family planning needs may vary considerably according to the method of computation used to obtain quantitative estimates. Likewise, the legitimate reasons for not using a contraceptive method while not wanting more children can also vary greatly according to the base population used and specific situations (Szykman, 1982).

[4] It has previously been recommended that both women and men be approached in birth control campaigns. Beyond the couples, however, communication needs to be extended to an even wider population group, for the adoption of innovative behaviour is not only an individual matter but also requires both social legitimization and individual acceptability. Indeed, even when smaller family size is desired, modern contraceptive methods are not always acceptable if they can be used by women without male supervision, or if male methods are the less costly in a society where women traditionally are responsible for fertility control or if modern methods require introduction of foreign bodies (IUDs) or substances (injections, pills) into the human body and break taboos etc. The acceptance of innovative behaviour thus requires not only education but also reassurance, supervision and follow-up, which can be achieved only through proper organization. High contraceptive drop-out levels are often related to such pitfalls. While the sources of innovative behaviour are not always easy to trace (for example, Basu and Sundar, 1988), the efficacy of IEC activities cannot be increased if the motivational aspects of the adoption of new behaviour are not better known.

[5] New mass media and communication techniques can now be utilized to reach more people and for fast changes and modification of family planning messages (see, for example, Church, 1989).

[6] It was estimated in 1989 that pharmacies in developing countries served 15 million family planning customers, although it is estimated that more than 85 million couples could be served by this type of outlet (for example, Lande and Blackburn, 1989). One of the issues associated with social marketing, however, is its competition with regular commercial outlets. It is important that the smallest possible substitution effect takes place.

[7] The advantages and disadvantages of local production of contraceptives versus importation need to be rigorously assessed in each situation on the basis of priorities and cost. One basic prerequisite is that demand must remain constantly high so as to warrant investment in local production. Assessment models are actually needed to cope with such situations.

[8] It would not be advisable, for instance, to promote delaying births in societies where early marriage norms imply immediate conceptions. In these societies, adolescent births are legitimate and wanted births; hence, even when contraception is an acceptable practice, few couples will delay a first birth (Trussell and Reinis, 1989). Furthermore, subfecundity among adolescent women makes any target population very difficult to identify. In such circumstances, family planning programmes could encounter resistance and result in low success. On the other hand, if there are unwanted conceptions among unmarried adolescents, who are then likely to interrupt their pregnancy through illegal, unsafe abortions, mortality and morbidity risks are high and pregnancy prevention through family planning education could be highly successful.

[9] A simulation study suggests that under specified assumptions "an acceleration in the reduction in condom non-use of 1 percentage point [...] leads to a reduction of from 1.5 to 2.0 percentage points in zero prevalence after 20 years, as well as to a substantial reduction, in the thousands, in cumulative AIDS cases and deaths" (Bulatao, 1991, p. 95).

[10] Designing training curricula and manuals, developing specific skills and attitudes needed for HIV/AIDS prevention, training of counsellors and motivators for condom use, development of HIV/AIDS terms in local languages etc. are among the main tasks at hand.

[11] When family planning objectives are added to health objectives, one cannot expect the former health structure automatically to fit the new goals. (For instance, health objectives do not have to meet quantitative targets as family planning objectives demand for new acceptors.)

Likewise, the management of health is not identical to the management of family planning activities and, to a certain extent, policy-making and decision-making for family planning activities are to be the responsibility of family planning officials. Unlike health services, contraceptive services require more privacy, provided in a manner acceptable to the recipients. A salary policy to prevent rivalries, special training to achieve cooperation between medical and family planning personnel and equity in status and career prospects for all civil servants involved need also to be instituted if effective integration is expected.

[12]Incentive programmes in such circumstances need, however, to be instituted with caution. Ethical issues arise when cash payments exceed the purpose of compensation for the costs incurred, especially in cultures unfavourable to the methods offered or when the target populations are poor, or when exceeding social pressure is exerted by community leaders who are promised benefits for reaching specific

goals. Much can be learned from past experiences (see, for example, Cleland and Mauldin, 1991).

[13]The problem of obtaining midwives' cooperation has often been a critical issue. Since in many cultures births generally occur with a midwife's assistance, incentives to obtain help from this occupational group need to be continuously upheld.

[14]For instance, the cost of condoms is reported to be high in most developing countries (Liskin and others, 1990). Sterilization, which appears to be in the process of becoming an acceptable contraceptive means in an increasing number of societies, is an even more costlier procedure. If this is the case with most of the other modern contraceptive methods, the logical solution of increasing prices and fees could be self-defeating.

[15]Opposition was voiced to trials of subdermal implants in Bangladesh and Brazil (Population Crisis Committee, 1992).

ANNEX

TABLE A.1. United Nations estimates of total fertility rates, the world, major areas, regions, and countries or areas, and percentage change, 1980-1985—1990-1995[a]

Major area, region and country or area	Total fertility rate			Percentage change	
	1980-1985	1985-1990	1990-1995	1980-1985—1985-1990	1985-1990—1990-1995
World	3.64	3.43	3.26	-5.77	-4.96
More developed regions	1.93	1.92	1.91	-0.52	-0.52
Less developed regions	4.23	3.90	3.64	-7.80	-6.67
Africa	6.40	6.25	6.00	-2.34	-4.00
Eastern Africa	6.81	6.86	6.76	0.73	-1.46
Burundi	6.80	6.80	6.80	0.00	0.00
Comoros	7.05	7.05	7.05	0.00	0.00
Djibouti	6.60	6.60	6.60	0.00	0.00
Ethiopia	6.50	7.00	7.00	7.69	0.00
Kenya	7.50	6.80	6.28	-9.33	-7.65
Madagascar	6.60	6.60	6.60	0.00	0.00
Malawi	7.60	7.60	7.60	0.00	0.00
Mauritius	2.45	2.10	2.00	-14.29	-4.76
Mozambique	6.50	6.50	6.50	0.00	0.00
Réunion	2.90	2.54	2.32	-12.41	-8.66
Rwanda	8.49	8.49	8.49	0.00	0.00
Somalia	7.00	7.00	7.00	0.00	0.00
Uganda	7.00	7.30	7.30	4.29	0.00
United Republic of Tanzania	6.80	6.80	6.80	0.00	0.00
Zambia	7.00	6.75	6.33	-3.57	-6.22
Zimbabwe	6.19	5.79	5.33	-6.46	-7.94
Middle Africa	6.53	6.53	6.47	0.00	-0.92
Angola	7.00	7.20	7.20	2.86	0.00
Cameroon	6.34	6.10	5.70	-3.79	-6.56
Central African Republic	6.10	6.20	6.20	1.64	0.00
Chad	5.89	5.89	5.89	0.00	0.00
Congo	6.29	6.29	6.29	0.00	0.00
Equatorial Guinea	5.79	5.89	5.89	1.73	0.00
Gabon	4.51	4.99	5.34	10.64	7.01
Zaire	6.70	6.70	6.70	0.00	0.00
Northern Africa	5.66	5.10	4.66	-9.89	-8.63
Algeria	6.35	5.43	4.87	-14.49	-10.31
Egypt	5.06	4.53	4.12	-10.47	-9.05
Libyan Arab Jamahiriya	7.17	6.87	6.39	-4.18	-6.99
Morocco	5.43	4.82	4.37	-11.23	-9.34

Major area, region and country or area	Total fertility rates			Percentage change	
	1980-1985	1985-1990	1990-1995	1980-1985— 1985-1990	1985-1990— 1990-1995
Sudan	6.58	6.44	6.05	-2.13	-6.06
Tunisia	4.88	3.94	3.40	-19.26	-13.71
Southern Africa	4.92	4.50	4.22	-8.54	-6.22
Botswana	6.50	5.50	5.07	-15.38	-7.82
Lesotho	5.50	5.00	4.71	-9.09	-5.80
Namibia	6.00	6.00	6.00	0.00	0.00
South Africa	4.78	4.38	4.09	-8.37	-6.62
Swaziland	6.30	5.25	4.93	-16.67	-6.10
Western Africa	6.87	6.85	6.53	-0.29	-4.67
Benin	7.10	7.10	7.10	0.00	0.00
Burkina Faso	6.50	6.50	6.50	0.00	0.00
Cape Verde	6.29	4.83	4.26	-23.21	-11.80
Côte d'Ivoire	7.41	7.41	7.41	0.00	0.00
Gambia	6.50	6.50	6.06	0.00	-6.77
Ghana	6.50	6.39	5.96	-1.69	-6.73
Guinea	7.00	7.00	7.00	0.00	0.00
Guinea-Bissau	5.79	5.79	5.79	0.00	0.00
Liberia	6.80	6.80	6.80	0.00	0.00
Mali	7.10	7.10	7.10	0.00	0.00
Mauritania	6.50	6.50	6.50	0.00	0.00
Niger	7.10	7.10	7.10	0.00	0.00
Nigeria	6.90	6.90	6.42	0.00	-6.96
Senegal	6.70	6.50	6.06	-2.99	-6.77
Sierra Leone	6.50	6.50	6.50	0.00	0.00
Togo	6.58	6.58	6.58	0.00	0.00
Asia	3.77	3.45	3.21	-8.49	-6.96
Eastern Asia	2.44	2.30	2.15	-5.74	-6.52
China	2.52	2.38	2.20	-5.56	-7.56
Democratic Republic of Korea	2.77	2.50	2.37	-9.75	-5.20
Hong Kong	1.80	1.36	1.44	-24.44	5.88
Japan	1.76	1.68	1.65	-4.55	-1.79
Mongolia	5.25	5.00	4.64	-4.76	-7.20
Republic of Korea	2.40	1.73	1.75	-27.92	1.16
South-eastern Asia	4.20	3.73	3.38	-11.19	-9.38
Brunei Darussalam	3.80	3.40	3.07	-10.53	-9.71
Cambodia	4.80	4.60	4.50	-4.17	-2.17
East Timor	5.84	5.41	4.88	-7.36	-9.80
Indonesia	4.05	3.48	3.10	-14.07	-10.92
Lao People's Democratic Rep.	6.69	6.69	6.69	0.00	0.00
Malaysia	4.24	4.00	3.62	-5.66	-9.50
Myanmar	4.90	4.50	4.16	-8.16	-7.56
Philippines	4.74	4.30	3.93	-9.28	-8.60
Singapore	1.69	1.69	1.75	0.00	3.55
Thailand	2.96	2.57	2.21	-13.18	-14.01
Viet Nam	4.69	4.22	3.87	-10.02	-8.29
Southern Asia	5.16	4.66	4.30	-9.69	-7.73
Afghanistan	6.90	6.90	6.90	0.00	0.00
Bangladesh	6.15	5.10	4.72	-17.07	-7.45
Bhutan	5.89	5.89	5.89	0.00	0.00
India	4.73	4.20	3.85	-11.21	-8.33
Iran (Islamic Republic of)	6.50	6.50	5.95	0.00	-8.46

ANNEX TABLE A.1 (*continued*)

Major area, region and country or area	Total fertility rates			Percentage change	
	1980-1985	1985-1990	1990-1995	1980-1985—1985-1990	1985-1990—1990-1995
Maldives	6.75	6.50	6.17	-3.70	-5.08
Nepal	6.25	5.95	5.47	-4.80	-8.07
Pakistan	7.00	6.75	6.17	-3.57	-8.59
Sri Lanka	3.25	2.67	2.48	-17.85	-7.12
Western Asia	5.33	5.04	4.69	-5.44	-6.94
Bahrain	4.63	4.08	3.75	-11.88	-8.09
Cyprus	2.37	2.36	2.25	-0.42	-4.66
Iraq	6.35	6.15	5.70	-3.15	-7.32
Israel	3.13	3.05	2.85	-2.56	-6.56
Jordan	6.76	6.15	5.70	-9.02	-7.32
Kuwait	4.87	3.94	3.68	-19.10	-6.60
Lebanon	3.79	3.42	3.09	-9.76	-9.65
Oman	7.17	7.17	6.71	0.00	-6.42
Qatar	5.00	4.80	4.41	-4.00	-8.12
Saudi Arabia	7.28	6.80	6.37	-6.59	-6.32
Syrian Arab Republic	7.38	6.66	6.15	-9.76	-7.66
Turkey	4.10	3.79	3.45	-7.56	-8.97
United Arab Emirates	5.23	4.82	4.50	-7.84	-6.64
Yemen[b]	7.71	7.69	7.18	-0.26	-6.63
Europe	1.81	1.71	1.71	-5.52	0.00
Eastern Europe	2.18	2.10	2.01	-3.67	-4.29
Bulgaria	2.01	1.92	1.83	-4.48	-4.69
Czechoslovakia	2.09	2.00	1.97	-4.31	-1.50
Hungary	1.81	1.82	1.83	0.55	0.55
Poland	2.33	2.15	2.05	-7.73	-4.65
Romania	2.22	2.28	2.10	2.70	-7.89
Northern Europe	1.81	1.84	1.91	1.66	3.80
Denmark	1.43	1.54	1.70	7.69	10.39
Estonia	2.08	2.18	2.05	4.81	-5.96
Finland	1.69	1.66	1.80	-1.78	8.43
Iceland	2.25	2.12	2.20	-5.78	3.77
Ireland	2.87	2.28	2.10	-20.56	-7.89
Latvia	2.00	2.09	2.00	4.50	-4.31
Lithuania	2.03	2.09	2.00	2.96	-4.31
Norway	1.69	1.80	2.00	6.51	11.11
Sweden	1.65	1.91	2.07	15.76	8.38
United Kingdom	1.80	1.81	1.88	0.56	3.87
Southern Europe	1.82	1.54	1.48	-15.38	-3.90
Albania	3.40	3.08	2.70	-9.41	-12.34
Greece	1.96	1.53	1.47	-21.94	-3.92
Italy	1.55	1.33	1.31	-14.19	-1.50
Malta	1.96	2.02	2.07	3.06	2.48
Portugal	1.99	1.60	1.48	-19.60	-7.50
Spain	1.86	1.46	1.38	-21.51	-5.48
Yugoslavia	2.08	1.96	1.90	-5.77	-3.06
Western Europe	1.61	1.58	1.64	-1.86	3.80
Austria	1.62	1.45	1.50	-10.49	3.45
Belgium	1.59	1.56	1.65	-1.89	5.77
France	1.87	1.82	1.82	-2.67	0.00
Germany[c]	1.46	1.44	1.50	-1.37	4.17
Luxembourg	1.45	1.47	1.60	1.38	8.84

Major area, region and country or area	Total fertility rates			Percentage change	
	1980-1985	1985-1990	1990-1995	1980-1985—1985-1990	1985-1990—1990-1995
Netherlands	1.51	1.56	1.70	3.31	8.97
Switzerland	1.53	1.55	1.65	1.31	6.45
Latin America and the Caribbean	3.92	3.40	3.05	-13.27	-10.29
Caribbean	3.18	2.96	2.84	-6.92	-4.05
Bahamas	2.58	2.17	2.01	-15.89	-7.37
Barbados	1.92	1.62	1.80	-15.62	11.11
Cuba	1.85	1.83	1.87	-1.08	2.19
Dominican Republic	4.21	3.75	3.34	-10.93	-10.93
Guadaloupe	2.55	2.45	2.16	-3.92	-11.84
Haiti	5.17	4.99	4.79	-3.48	-4.01
Jamaica	3.55	2.65	2.38	-25.35	-10.19
Martinique	2.14	2.14	1.99	0.00	-7.01
Puerto Rico	2.42	2.22	2.16	-8.26	-2.70
Trinidad and Tobago	3.20	2.95	2.74	-7.81	-7.12
Central America	4.55	3.92	3.48	-13.85	-11.22
Costa Rica	3.50	3.36	3.14	-4.00	-6.55
El Salvador	5.00	4.52	4.04	-9.60	-10.62
Guatemala	6.12	5.77	5.36	-5.72	-7.11
Honduras	6.16	5.55	4.94	-9.90	-10.99
Mexico	4.29	3.60	3.16	-16.08	-12.22
Nicaragua	6.00	5.55	5.04	-7.50	-9.19
Panama	3.46	3.14	2.87	-9.25	-8.60
South America	3.78	3.27	2.91	-13.49	-11.01
Argentina	3.15	2.96	2.79	-6.03	-5.74
Bolivia	5.50	5.00	4.56	-9.09	-8.80
Brazil	3.81	3.20	2.75	-16.01	-14.06
Chile	2.80	2.73	2.66	-2.50	-2.56
Colombia	3.51	2.90	2.67	-17.38	-7.93
Ecuador	4.70	4.10	3.62	-12.77	-11.71
Guyana	3.26	2.77	2.55	-15.03	-7.94
Paraguay	4.82	4.58	4.34	-4.98	-5.24
Peru	4.65	4.00	3.57	-13.98	-10.75
Suriname	3.39	2.97	2.68	-12.39	-9.76
Uruguay	2.57	2.43	2.33	-5.45	-4.12
Venezuela	3.90	3.45	3.12	-11.54	-9.57
Northern America	1.80	1.89	2.04	5.00	7.94
Canada	1.66	1.70	1.78	2.41	4.71
United States of America	1.82	1.92	2.07	5.49	7.81
Oceania	2.62	2.52	2.51	-3.82	-0.40
Australia-New Zealand	1.94	1.89	1.95	-2.58	3.17
Australia	1.93	1.86	1.91	-3.63	2.69
New Zealand	1.96	2.04	2.14	4.08	4.90
Melanesia	5.31	4.95	4.61	-6.78	-6.87
Fiji	3.80	3.20	2.98	-15.79	-6.88
Papua New Guinea	5.58	5.25	4.86	-5.91	-7.43
Solomon Islands	6.38	5.82	5.39	-8.78	-7.39
Micronesia	5.00	4.70	4.40	-6.00	-6.38
Guam	3.10	2.85	2.60	-8.06	-8.77
Polynesia	5.20	4.50	4.00	-13.46	-11.11
French Polynesia	3.82	3.57	3.32	-6.54	-7.00
USSR[d]	2.35	2.43	2.25	3.40	-7.41

Source and notes to follow.

Source: *World Population Prospects: The 1992 Revision* (United Nations publication, Sales No. E.93.XIII.7).

[a]Medium variant; rates are averages for each five-year period.

[b]On 22 May 1990, Democratic Yemen and Yemen merged to form a single State. Since that date, they have been represented as one Member of the United Nations with the name "Yemen".

[c]The former State of Czechoslovakia was dissolved on 31 December 1992 and became the independent States of the Czech Republic and Slovakia on 1 January 1993.

[d]The area of the former State of Yugoslavia currently comprises the independent States of Bosnia and Herzegovina, Croatia, Slovenia, the former Yugoslav Republic of Macedonia and the Federal Republic of Yugoslavia. Unless otherwise indicated, data for Yugoslavia shown in this publication for the period beginning 27 April 1992 refer to the Federal Republic of Yugoslavia in terms of its boundaries as they exist from that date. Data for the period prior to 27 April 1992 refer to the former Socialist Federal Republic of Yugoslavia in terms of its boundaries as they existed prior to that date.

[e]Through accession of the German Democratic Republic to the Federal Republic of Germany with effect from 3 October 1990, the two German States have united to form one sovereign State. As from the date of unification, the Federal Republic of Germany acts in the United Nations under the designation "Germany".

[f]Data for the former Union of Soviet Socialist Republics.

TABLE A.2. PROPORTION OF CURRENTLY MARRIED WOMEN USING A CONTRACEPTIVE METHOD, BY AGE GROUP AND SPECIFIC METHOD, LESS DEVELOPED AND MORE DEVELOPED REGIONS, 1975-1990

Major area, region and country or area	Year	Age group	Any method	Modern method	Sterilization Female	Sterilization Male	Pill	Inject-ables	Intra-uterine device	Condom	Female barriers	Rhythm	With-drawal	Absti-nence	Other methods
Africa															
Eastern Africa															
Burundi	1987	15-49	8.7	1.2	0.1	0.0	0.2	0.5	0.3	0.1	0.0	4.8	0.7	2.0	0.0
Ethiopia	1990	15-49	4.3	2.6	0.2	0.0	1.9	0.0	0.3	0.1	0.0	0.5	0.1	1.1	0.0
Kenya	1977/78	15-50	6.7	4.2	0.8	0.0	2.0	0.6	0.7	0.1	0.0	1.1	0.2	1.1	0.1
	1984	15-49	17.0	9.6	2.6	0.0	3.1	0.5	3.0	0.3	0.1	3.8	0.6	2.7	0.2
	1988/89	15-49	26.9	17.8	4.7	0.0	5.2	3.3	3.7	0.5	0.4	7.5	0.2	::	1.3
Malawi	1984	15-49	6.9	1.1	a	a	0.7	0.1	0.3	0.0	a	0.2	3.5	2.1	
Mauritius	1975	<50b	45.7	29.2	...	0.0	21.0	1.6	1.5	5.1	0.6	13.9	1.5	a	1.0
	1985	15-49	75.4	45.6	4.7	0.0	21.0	6.2	2.3	10.8	0.0	17.1	12.7		
Rwanda	1983	15-50	10.1	0.9	0.0	0.0	0.2	0.4	0.3	0.0	0.0	c	c	9.2	0.1
Uganda	1988/89	15-49	4.9	2.5	0.8	0.0	1.1	0.4	0.2	0.0	0.0	1.6	0.3	::	0.4
Zimbabwe	1984	15-49	38.4	26.6	1.6	0.1	22.6	0.8	0.7	0.7	0.1	0.6	6.5	2.1	2.6
	1988/89	15-49	43.1	36.1	2.3	0.2	31.0	0.3	1.1	1.2	0.0	0.3	5.1	::	1.5
Middle Africa															
Cameroon	1978	15-49	2.4	0.6	...	...	0.2	::	0.2	0.2	0.0	1.1	0.4	::	0.3
Northern Africa															
Algeria	1986/87	15-49	35.5	31.3	1.3	0.0	26.5	0.6	2.1	0.6	0.2	0.9	3.1	0.2	0.4
Egypt	1974/75	15-49	24.9	22.4	a	a	19.9	::	2.5	a	a	a	a	a	2.4
	1980	15-49	24.2	22.7	0.7	0.1	16.5	0.1	4.0	1.1	0.2	0.5	0.4	0.1	0.4
	1981/82	<45d	33.8	30.8	1.1	0.0	20.5	0.2	6.9	1.1	1.0	0.8	a	::	2.3
	1984	<50	29.7	28.7	1.5	0.0	16.5	0.3	8.4	1.3	0.7	0.6	0.3	::	0.1
	1988/89	15-49	36.7	35.4	1.5	0.0	15.3	0.1	15.7	2.4	0.4	0.6	0.5	::	0.2
Morocco	1980	15-49	19.7	16.6	0.8	0.0	13.9	0.0	1.6	0.3	0.3	1.1	1.0	0.0	0.9
	1983/84	15-49	25.5	21.2	1.7	::	16.8	::	2.0	0.4	0.3	1.5	1.6	0.0	1.2
	1987	15-49	35.9	28.9	2.2	0.0	22.9	0.3	2.9	0.5	0.1	2.3	3.1	0.3	1.2
Sudan	1978/79	15-50	4.6	3.7	0.3	0.0	3.1	0.0	0.1	0.1	0.1	0.5	0.1	0.3	0.0
	1989/90	15-49	8.7	5.6	0.8	0.0	3.9	0.1	0.7	0.1	0.0	2.2	0.3	::	0.6
Tunisia	1978	15-49	31.4	25.1	7.5	0.0	6.6	0.3	8.8	1.3	0.6	3.8	1.9	0.0	0.6
	1980	15-49b	27.0	::	::	::	::	::	::	::	::	::	::	::	
	1983	15-49	41.1	34.2	12.5	0.0	5.3	0.4	13.2	1.3	1.5	4.4	1.8	0.0	0.7
	1988	15-49	49.8	40.4	11.5	::	8.8	0.8	17.0	1.3	1.0	6.3	2.4	::	0.7
Southern Africa															
Botswana	1984	15-49	27.8	18.6	1.5	0.0	10.0	1.0	4.8	1.2	0.1	0.3	0.3	8.5	0.1
	1988	15-49	33.0	31.7	4.3	0.3	14.8	5.4	5.6	1.3	0.0	0.2	0.3	0.5	0.3
Lesotho	1977	15-49	5.3	2.4	0.8	0.0	1.2	0.2	0.1	0.1	0.0	0.1	2.5	::	0.2

49

TABLE A.2 (continued)

Major area, region and country or area	Year	Age group	Any method	Modern method	Sterilization Female	Sterilization Male	Pill	Injectables	Intra-uterine device	Condom	Female barriers	Rhythm	Withdrawal	Abstinence	Other methods
Namibia	1989	<50[b]	26.4	26.1	6.0	0.1	6.6	12.5	0.9	..	..	0.0	..	..	0.1
South Africa	1981	<50	48.0	46.0	8.0	0.0	15.0	14.0	6.0	3.0	c	c	3.0	0.0	..
Swaziland	1988	15-49	19.9	17.2	3.1	0.2	5.6	5.6	1.8	0.7	0.2	0.5	1.2	..	1.1
Western Africa															
Benin	1981/82	15-49	9.2	0.5	0.0	0.0	0.2	0.0	0.1	0.1	0.1	1.3	2.5	4.7	0.2
Côte d'Ivoire	1980/81	15-49	2.9	0.5	0.0	0.0	0.4	0.0	0.1	0.0	0.0	0.3	0.1	1.8	0.2
Ghana	1979/80	15-49	9.5	5.5	0.5	0.0	2.4	0.1	0.3	0.6	1.6	0.7	0.2	3.1	0.0
	1988	15-49	12.9	5.2	1.0	0.0	1.8	0.3	0.5	0.3	1.3	6.2	0.9	..	0.6
Liberia	1986	15-49	6.4	5.5	1.1	0.0	3.3	0.3	0.6	0.0	0.2	0.6	0.1	1.5	0.2
Mali	1987	15-49	4.7	1.3	0.1	0.0	0.9	0.1	0.1	0.0	0.1	1.3	0.1	..	0.5
Mauritania	1981	15-49	0.8	0.3	0.2	0.0	0.0	0.0	0.0	0.0	0.1	0.1	0.4	0.0	0.0
Nigeria	1981/82	15-49	4.8	0.6	0.1	..	0.2	0.2	0.1	0.0	..	0.3	0.1	3.7	0.0
	1990	15-49	6.0	3.5	0.3	0.0	1.2	0.7	0.8	0.4	0.1	1.4	0.5	..	0.6
Senegal	1978	15-49	3.8	0.6	0.0	0.0	0.3	0.0	0.2	0.1	0.0	0.4	0.0	2.5	0.3
	1986	15-49	11.3	2.4	0.2	0.0	1.2	0.1	0.7	0.1	0.1	0.9	0.1	6.7	1.3
Togo	1988	15-49	33.9	3.0	0.6	0.0	0.4	0.2	0.8	0.4	0.6	6.4	2.3	21.8	0.2
Asia															
Eastern Asia															
China	1982	15-49	70.6	67.8	17.9	7.1	6.0	..	35.4	1.4	a	a	a	a	2.8
	1988	15-49	72.1	71.2	27.6	7.9	3.4	0.2	29.9	1.9	0.3	0.5	0.1	a	0.3
Hong Kong	1977	15-49	71.9	64.0	18.7	f	23.0	2.2	2.9	12.9	4.3	7.9	a	a	0.7
	1982	15-49	72.3	63.9	19.9	1.2	19.4	2.7	3.5	14.6	2.6	8.1	a	a	0.4
	1987	15-49	80.8	75.0	22.9	0.9	16.4	2.5	4.5	26.0	1.8	5.4	a	a	0.5
Japan	1975	15-49	60.5	59.2	2.8	f	1.8	..	5.2	47.1	2.3	18.1	4.1	..	..
	1977	15-49	60.4	60.2	3.2	f	2.0	..	5.5	47.7	1.8	16.3	3.1	..	1.2
	1979	15-49	62.2	61.5	2.5	f	2.0	..	5.2	50.4	1.4	14.4	3.2	..	1.0
	1981	15-49	55.5	51.0	..	..	..	..	3.6	46.1	a	11.6	2.4	..	4.1
	1984	15-49	57.3	51.0	8.3	1.6	1.3	..	3.5	44.6	0.7	11.7	2.9	..	3.6
	1986	15-49	64.3	59.7	3.3	0.9	1.0	..	3.0	43.2	0.3	9.2	2.8	..	1.8
	1988	15-49	56.3	51.0	5.7	f	1.0	..	3.0	43.2	0.3	9.2	2.8	..	1.8
	1990	15-49	58.0	51.9	..	g	a	3.3	42.9	a	8.9	a	..	5.2	a
Republic of Korea	1976	15-44	44.2	32.9	4.1	4.2	7.8	a	10.5	6.3	a	7.1	a	a	4.2
	1978	15-44	48.8	38.4	10.9	5.6	6.6	a	9.5	5.8	a	a	a	a	10.4
	1979	15-44	54.5	43.1	14.5	5.9	7.2	h	9.6	5.2	a	a	a	a	11.4
	1982	15-44	57.7	47.4	23.0	5.1	5.4	a	6.7	7.2	0.7	a	a	a	10.3
	1985	15-44	70.4	59.4	31.6	8.9	4.3	a	7.4	7.2	a	a	a	a	11.0
	1988	15-44	77.3	70.2	37.2	11.0	2.8	a	6.7	10.2	2.3	a	a	a	7.1

50

TABLE A.2 (continued)

Major area, region and country or area	Year	Age group	Any method	Modern method	Sterilization Female	Sterilization Male	Pill	Inject-ables	Intra-uterine device	Condom	Female barriers	Rhythm	With-drawal	Absti-nence	Other methods
South-eastern Asia															
Indonesia	1976	10-49	18.3	17.3	0.1	0.0	11.6	a	4.1	1.5	..	0.8	0.1	0.1	1.1
	1979	10-49	31.2	24.6	0.4	0.1	16.7	a	6.4	1.0	..	0.5	0.1	0.3	5.9
	1980	10-49	26.8	21.9	a	a	14.3	a	6.7	0.9	a	a	a	a	4.9
	1985	10-49	38.5	36.9	1.2	0.4	15.4	7.4	11.9	0.6	a	a	a	a	1.6
	1987	15-49	47.7	44.0	3.1	0.2	16.1	9.8	13.2	1.6	a	1.2	1.3	a	1.2
Malaysia	1984	15-49	51.4	29.8	7.5	0.2	11.6	0.5	2.2	7.7	0.2	10.0	5.9	2.0	13.4
Philippines	1978	15-49	36.0	15.9	4.6	0.7	4.5	0.2	2.3	3.5	0.1	8.5	9.4	a	2.1
	1983	15-49	30.1	17.8	9.1	f	4.9	0.1	2.5	1.2	a	7.1	4.1	a	1.1
	1986	15-49	43.6	20.6	11.4	f	5.9	0.2	2.4	0.7	a	8.5	8.7	a	5.9
	1988	15-44	36.2	21.6	11.4	f	6.9	0.2	2.4	0.7	a	8.1	5.6	a	0.8
Singapore	1977	15-44	71.3	62.8	21.0	0.9	17.0	..	3.1	20.8	a	a	a	a	8.5
	1982	15-44	74.2	73.0	22.3	0.6	11.6	h	h 24.3	14.2	h	h	h	1.2	
Thailand	1975	15-49	33.1	30.4	6.3	2.1	13.7	1.9	5.9	0.4	0.1	0.9	0.9	0.7	0.3
	1978/79		53.1	49.1	12.9	3.4	22.0	4.6	4.0	2.2	a	a	a	a	4.0
	1979	15-44	48.5	47.5	14.8	3.9	20.6	5.4	2.1	0.7	a	a	a	a	1.0
	1980	15-49	44.5	43.3	11.4	2.1	22.2	3.5	4.1	a	a	a	a	a	1.2
	1981	15-44	59.0	56.3	18.7	4.2	20.2	7.1	4.2	1.9	a	a	a	a	2.7
	1984A	15-44	64.6	62.0	23.5	4.4	19.8	7.6	4.9	1.8	a	a	a	a	2.6
	1984B	15-44	58.9	58.6	18.9	3.3	23.4	7.4	5.6	a	a	a	a	a	0.5
	1987	15-49	65.5	63.6	22.8	5.7	18.6	8.5	6.9	1.1	0.0	0.9	0.9	a	0.1
	1987	15-44	67.5	65.5	22.4	5.5	20.0	9.2	7.2	1.2	0.0	1.0	0.9	a	0.1
Viet Nam	1988	15-49	53.2	37.7	2.7	0.3	0.4	..	33.1	1.2	a	8.1	7.0	..	0.3
Southern Asia															
Bangladesh	1976	<50	7.7	4.8	0.3	0.5	2.8	0.0	0.4	0.8	0.0	1.0	0.5	1.1	0.3
	1979	<50	12.1	9.1	2.4	0.9	3.6	0.3	0.3	1.5	0.1	2.2	0.2	0.8	..
	1981	<50	18.6	11.0	4.0	0.8	3.5	0.4	0.4	1.6	0.3	3.9	1.8	1.2	0.7
	1983	<50	19.1	13.7	6.2	1.2	3.3	0.2	1.0	1.5	0.3	2.4	1.3	0.4	1.4
	1983	<50	27.2	18.1	5.8	2.5	5.4	0.1	1.0	2.7	0.6	5.9	0.9	1.1	1.3
	1985	<50	25.2	18.3	7.8	1.5	5.1	0.5	1.4	1.8	0.2	3.8	0.9	0.5	1.7
	1989A	<50	30.8	23.2	8.5	1.2	9.6	0.6	1.4	1.8	0.1	4.0	1.8	1.0	0.8
	1989B	<50	31.4	24.4	9.0	1.4	9.1	1.1	1.7	1.9	0.2	3.9	1.2	0.5	1.5
India	1980	15-49d	34.1	26.9	21.4	f	0.9	..	0.4	4.2	a	a	a	a	1.5
	1988	15-44d	42.9	38.6	30.8	f	1.1	..	1.7	4.7	0.3	a	a	a	7.1
Nepal	1976	15-49	2.5	2.5	0.1	1.7	0.4	..	0.1	0.2	..	..	a	0.1	..
	1981	15-49	6.8	6.8	2.4	2.9	1.1	0.1	0.1	0.4	..	..	..	..	..
	1986	15-49	13.9	13.9	6.3	5.7	0.8	0.5	0.1	0.6	..	..	..	..	..

TABLE A.2 (continued)

Major area, region and country or area	Year	Age group	Any method	Modern method	Sterilization Female	Sterilization Male	Pill	Inject-ables	Intra-uterine device	Condom	Female barriers	Rhythm	With-drawal	Absti-nence	Other methods
Pakistan	1975	15-49	5.2	3.8	0.9	0.1	1.0	..	0.6	1.0	0.2	0.1	0.1	1.2	0.1
	1979/80	15-49	3.3	..	..	..	..	..	..	..	..	..	0.7	..	..
	1984/85	15-49	7.6	6.4	2.2	0.0	1.2	0.5	0.7	1.7	0.1	0.1	1.2	..	0.4
	1990/91	15-49	11.9	9.0	3.5	0.0	0.7	0.8	1.3	2.7	0.0	1.3	1.5	3.5	0.3
Sri Lanka	1975A	15-49	31.9	18.7	9.2	0.7	1.5	0.3	4.7	2.3	*	8.0	6.6	3.5	0.0
	1975B	15-49	43.4	19.9	8.1	1.0	2.4	0.2	5.9	2.3	0.0	12.2	*	*	4.7
	1977	15-49	48.6	26.9	13.7	1.7	2.4	0.0	5.4	3.7	*	*	*	*	21.7
	1981/82	15-49	42.7	30.2	17.9	3.5	2.2	1.3	2.8	2.5	-	9.2	3.1	*	0.2
	1982	15-49	54.9	30.4	17.0	3.7	2.6	1.4	2.5	3.2	-	13.0	4.7	*	6.8
	1987	15-49	62.0	40.5	24.8	4.9	4.1	2.7	2.1	1.9	0.0	15.0	3.4	3.0	0.1
Western Asia															
Jordan	1976	15-49	25.2	17.3	1.8	0.1	11.9	..	2.0	1.4	0.1	2.1	3.3	0.4	2.0
	1983	15-49	26.0	20.8	3.8	0.0	7.8	0.2	8.3	0.6	0.1	2.9	2.4	..	..
	1985	17-51	26.5	22.3	4.9	0.0	6.0	0.1	10.8	0.4	0.1	3.0	1.2	..	..
	1990	15-49	34.9	26.9	5.6	0.0	4.6	0.0	15.3	0.8	0.6	3.9	4.0	..	0.2
Syrian Arab Republic	1978	15-49	19.8	15.0	0.3	0.1	11.8	0.3	0.6	0.6	1.3	2.8	1.6	0.0	0.4
Turkey	1978	15-49	38.0	13.5	0.5	0.2	6.1	0.3	3.0	3.1	0.3	1.0	16.8	0.1	6.8
	1983	<50	51.0	22.7	1.1	0.0	7.5	0.2	7.4	4.1	2.4	1.2	25.0	..	2.3
	1988	15-49	63.3	31.1	1.7	0.1	6.2	0.1	14.0	7.2	1.8	3.5	25.7	0.1	3.0
Yemen	1979	<50	1.1	1.1	0.1	0.1	0.7	0.0	0.1	0.1	0.0	0.0	0.0	0.0	0.0
Europe															
Eastern Europe															
Bulgaria	1976	18-44	76.0	8.0	1.0	1.0	2.0	..	2.0	2.0	..	4.0	59.0	5.0	1.0
Czechoslovakia	1977	<45	95.0	49.0	3.0	0.0	14.0	18.0	13.0	1.0	7.0	29.0	1.0	9.0	..
Hungary	1977	<40	73.1	51.8	..	..	36.1	..	9.6	4.3	1.8	3.1	17.1	..	1.1
	1986	15-39	73.1	62.3	..	..	39.3	18.6	3.5	0.9	2.1	8.3	..	0.3	..
Poland	1977	<45	75.0	26.0	..	..	7.0	..	2.0	14.0	3.0	30.0	19.0	..	..
Romania	1978	15-44	58.0	5.0	..	..	1.0	..	0.0	3.0	1.0	24.0	26.0	..	3.0
Northern Europe															
Denmark	1975	18-44	63.0	60.0	..	..	22.0	..	9.0	25.0	4.0	1.0	1.0	..	2.0
Finland	1977	<45[j]	80.0	78.0	4.0	1.0	11.0	..	29.0	32.0	1.0	1.0	2.0	0.0	..
Norway	1977	18-44[j]	71.0	65.0	4.0	2.0	13.0	..	28.0	16.0	2.0	3.0	4.0	..	0.0
	1988	..	84.3	73.0	6.9	3.8	23.0	..	23.0	15.6	0.7	4.5	5.2	..	1.5
Sweden	1981	20-44	78.0	71.0	2.0[f]	23.0	..	20.0	25.0	e	*	[a] 7.0	..	..	..

52

TABLE A.2 (continued)

Major area, region and country or area	Year	Age group	Any method	Modern method	Sterilization Female	Sterilization Male	Pill	Inject-ables	Intra-uterine device	Condom	Female barriers	Rhythm	With-drawal	Absti-nence	Other methods
United Kingdom	1975	16-40[b]	76.0	13.0	f	30.0	.6.0	18.0	2.0	1.0	2.0	5.0	1.0	3.0	1.0
	1976	18-39[b]	77.0	74.0	8.0	8.0	32.0	..	8.0	16.0	2.0	1.0	5.0	0.0	0.0
	1983	18-44	83.0	79.0	14.0	14.0	24.0	..	7.0	17.0	3.0	2.0	6.0	..	0.0
	1983	18-39[b]	81.0	79.0	12.0	12.0	29.0	..	9.0	15.0	2.0	1.0	4.0	1.0	1.0
	1986	16-49	81.0	78.0	15.0	16.0	19.0	1.0	8.0	16.0	3.0	2.0	6.0	..	0.0
	1986	18-44[k]	75.0	72.0	11.0	12.0	26.0	..	8.0	13.0	2.0	2.0	4.0	..	1.0
	1989	18-44[k]	72.0	71.0	11.0	12.0	25.0	..	6.0	16.0	1.0	2.0	4.0	..	1.0
Southern Europe															
Italy	1979	18-44	78.0	32.0	1.0	0.0	14.0	.2.0	13.0	2.0	9.0	36.0	..	1.0	
Portugal	1979/80	15-49	66.3	32.8	0.9	0.1	19.1	1.5	3.6	5.6	2.0	4.0	25.6	..	4.0
Spain	1977	15-44[j]	51.0	20.0	..	..	13.0	.1.0	5.0	1.0	6.0	22.0	2.0	1.0	
	1985	18-49	59.4	38.0	4.3	0.3	15.5	a5.7	12.2	a	3.6	15.8	a2.1		
Yugoslavia[p] ...	1976	<45	55.0	12.0	..	..	5.0	..	2.0	2.0	3.0	4.0	36.0	..	3.0
Western Europe															
Austria	1981/82	..	71.4	56.3	1.0	0.3	40.0	..	8.4	4.0	2.6	8.7	5.5	0.6	0.4
Belgium	1975/76	20-44	87.0	47.0	6.0	f	30.0	..	3.0	8.0	0.0	7.0	32.0	..	..
	1982/83	20-44	81.0	63.0	17.0	f	32.0	..	8.0	6.0	0.0	4.0	13.0	..	..
France	1978	20-44	78.7	47.6	4.6	f	26.6	..	10.3	6.1	a	6.4	22.2	..	2.5
	1988	20-44	81.2	66.6	6.7	0.0	29.7	..	25.9	4.3	a	6.4	6.6	..	1.6
Germany, Federal Republic of[q] ...	1985	15-44	77.9	67.6	10.3	2.1	33.7	0.0	14.6	5.7	1.2	4.2	4.2	..	1.7
Netherlands ...	1975	..	75.0	69.0	2.0	2.0	50.0	..	4.0	10.0	1.0	3.0	2.0	0.0	1.0
	1977	16-49[j]	73.0	65.2	12.9	f	40.0	..	4.3	8.0	a	a	a	a	7.8
	1982	18-37	77.0	74.0	8.0	11.0	38.0	-	10.0	7.0	a	a	a	a	3.0
	1985	21-39	76.0	72.0	25.0	f	30.0	-	9.0	8.0	a	a	a	a	4.0
	1988	18-37	76.0	71.0	4.0	11.0	41.0	-	7.0	8.0	a	a	a	a	4.0
Switzerland ...	1980	d ..	71.2	64.9	15.8	f	28.0	..	10.6	8.4	2.1	4.2	1.8	..	0.4
Latin America and the Caribbean															
Caribbean															
Cuba	1987	15-49	70.0	67.0	22.0	..	10.0	..	33.0	2.0	0.0	1.0	1.0	..	0.0
Dominican Republic	1975	15-49	31.7	26.0	11.9	0.1	7.9	0.2	2.8	1.5	1.6	1.2	3.7	..	0.9
	1980	15-49	42.0	35.0	21.0	..	9.0	g	5.0	g	g	a	a	a	6.0
	1983	15-49	45.8	41.7	27.4	0.1	8.6	0.0	3.8	1.5	0.3	1.1	2.5	..	0.5
	1986	15-49	50.0	46.7	32.9	0.1	8.8	0.3	3.0	1.4	0.2	1.4	1.5	..	0.4
Guadeloupe ...	1976	15-44	43.6	30.5	11.5	..	9.7	..	3.4	5.7	0.2	4.9	6.5	..	1.7

53

TABLE A.2 (continued)

Major area, region and country or area	Year	Age group	Any method	Modern method	Sterilization Female	Sterilization Male	Pill	Injectables	Intra-uterine device	Condom	Female barriers	Rhythm	Withdrawal	Abstinence	Other methods
Haiti	1977	15-50	18.9	5.4	0.2	0.1	3.5	..	0.4	1.1	0.1	4.8	4.7	3.4	0.6
	1983	15-49	6.9	3.9	0.7	0.1	2.2	0.2	0.2	0.5	0.0	1.4	1.6	..	0.0
	1987	15-49	6.7	5.0	1.3	0.0	2.3	0.8	0.4	0.2	0.0	1.0	0.3	..	0.6
	1989	15-49	10.2	9.8	2.5	0.0	4.1	1.6	0.6	0.5	0.1	0.4	0.4	..	0.0
Jamaica	1975/76	15-49	38.3	36.2	8.1	0.0	11.8	6.2	2.0	6.6	1.5	0.3	1.4	0.4	0.0
	1979	15-44	54.9	54.2	9.8	0.0	23.8	11.4	2.0	6.5	0.7	0.2	0.5	..	0.0
	1983	15-49	51.4	48.4	10.9	0.0	19.3	7.6	2.0	7.6	1.0	1.1	1.9	..	0.0
	1989	15-49	54.6	51.3	13.6	0.1	19.5	7.6	1.5	8.6	0.4	1.0	2.4	..	0.0
Martinique	1976	15-44	51.3	37.9	11.7	..	17.3	..	2.6	4.6	1.7	4.7	6.2	*	2.6
Puerto Rico	1976	15-49b	64.6	54.3	35.4	2.8	12.7	..	3.4	*	*	*	*	*	10.3
	1982	15-49b	64.1	57.6	38.6	4.0	7.7	..	3.6	3.7	*	4.4	*	*	2.2
	1982	15-44	70.4	62.1	39.7	4.4	9.3	..	4.1	4.6	*	5.5	*	*	2.8
Trinidad and Tobago	1977	15-49	51.6	45.7	4.3	0.2	18.0	1.0	2.2	15.0	5.0	2.3	2.8	0.3	0.5
	1987	15-49	52.7	44.4	8.2	0.2	14.0	0.8	4.4	11.8	5.0	2.6	5.3	0.0	0.4
Central America															
Costa Rica	1976	20-49	64.4	53.5	12.3	1.0	22.5	2.0	5.2	8.8	1.7	5.1	4.6	0.5	0.7
	1978	15-49	63.8	54.9	14.0	0.8	23.3	2.0	4.8	8.7	1.3	4.9	3.5	..	0.5
	1981	15-49	65.2	55.9	17.3	0.5	20.6	2.2	5.7	8.4	1.2	6.2	2.8	..	0.3
	1986	15-44	69.5	58.2	13.9	0.5	20.7	1.0	8.0	13.4	0.7	8.1	3.1	..	0.1
El Salvador	1975	15-49b	19.3	18.0	8.6	f	6.5	0.4	2.0	0.5	..	1.0	m	..	0.3
	1978	15-44	34.4	32.3	17.8	0.2	8.7	0.4	3.3	1.5	0.4	1.7	0.3	..	0.0
	1985	15-44	48.4	45.5	31.8	0.7	7.2	0.8	3.5	1.3	0.2	2.1	0.8	..	0.1
	1985	15-49	47.3	44.5	31.8	0.7	6.6	0.7	3.3	1.2	0.2	1.9	0.8	..	0.1
	1988	15-44	47.1	43.5	29.6	0.6	7.6	0.9	2.0	2.4	0.4	2.4	1.0	..	0.0
Guatemala	1978	15-44	18.1	15.2	5.9	0.4	5.4	1.1	1.3	0.7	0.4	2.6	0.3	..	..
	1983	15-44	25.0	20.6	10.2	0.9	4.7	0.0	2.6	1.2	1.0	3.4	1.0	..	..
	1987	15-44	23.2	19.1	10.4	0.9	3.9	0.5	1.8	1.2	0.4	2.8	1.2	*	0.1
Honduras	1981	15-49	26.9	23.5	8.1	0.1	11.7	0.3	2.4	0.3	0.6	1.6	1.6	..	0.0
	1984	15-44	34.9	30.4	12.1	0.2	12.7	0.3	3.8	0.9	0.4	2.9	1.7	..	..
	1987	15-44	40.6	32.9	12.6	0.2	13.4	0.3	4.3	1.8	0.3	3.5	3.9	..	0.2
Mexico	1976	15-49	30.3	23.3	2.7	0.2	10.8	1.7	5.7	0.8	1.4	3.1	3.6	0.0	0.4
	1978	15-49	40.0	32.8	7.0	0.2	13.8	2.8	6.5	1.0	1.5	3.0	3.3	0.0	1.0
	1979	15-49	38.9	33.0	9.2	f	13.1	2.6	6.1	0.9	1.1	*	*	*	5.9
	1982	15-49	47.7	41.5	13.4	0.3	14.2	5.1	6.6	0.9	1.0	3.8	0.4	0.0	1.9
	1987	15-49	52.7	44.6	18.6	0.8	9.7	2.8	10.2	1.9	0.6	*	*	*	8.1
Nicaragua	1981	15-49	27.0	22.8	7.1	0.1	10.5	1.4	2.3	0.8	0.6	1.0	0.4	..	3.0

54

TABLE A.2 (continued)

Major area, region and country or area	Year	Age group	Any method	Modern method	Sterilization Female	Sterilization Male	Pill	Inject- ables	Intra- uterine device	Condom	Female barriers	Rhythm	With- drawal	Absti- nence	Other methods
Panama	1976	20-49	54.1	46.2	21.2	0.4	17.2	0.7	3.7	1.2	1.8	2.6	3.0	1.4	1.1
	1979	15-44	60.6	56.3	29.7	f	19.0	h	3.7	1.7	2.2	2.9	1.4	..	0.0
	1984	15-44	58.2	54.2	32.4	0.4	11.8	0.8	6.0	1.6	1.2	2.3	1.4	..	0.3
South America															
Bolivia	1983	15-44	26	12	3	0	3	1	4	0	1	14	1	..	..
	1989	15-49	30.3	12.2	4.4	0.0	1.9	0.7	4.8	0.3	0.1	16.1	1.0	..	0.9
Brazil	1986	15-44	65.8	56.7	26.9	0.8	25.2	0.6	1.0	1.7	0.5	4.3	5.0	..	..
Colombia	1976	15-49	42.5	30.4	4.0	0.2	13.3	0.4	8.5	1.7	2.3	5.1	4.7	0.9	1.3
	1978	15-49	46.1	37.3	7.5	..	17.2	h	7.7	1.4	3.5	4.0	..	..	4.7
	1980	15-49	48.5	41.0	10.7	0.2	17.4	h	8.1	h	4.6	4.9	..	..	2.7
	1986	15-49	64.8	52.5	18.3	0.4	16.4	2.4	11.0	1.7	2.3	5.7	5.7	..	0.9
	1990	15-49	66.1	54.7	20.9	0.5	14.1	2.2	12.4	2.9	1.7	6.1	4.8	..	0.5
Ecuador	1979	15-49	33.6	25.7	7.8	0.2	9.5	0.8	4.8	1.0	1.6	4.8	2.3	0.4	0.4
	1982	15-49	39.9	32.9	12.4	0.0	10.3	0.7	6.4	1.1	2.0	4.8	1.5	..	0.7
	1987	15-49	44.3	35.8	15.0	0.0	8.5	0.7	9.8	0.6	1.2	6.1	2.0	..	0.3
	1989	15-49	52.9	41.5	18.3	0.2	8.6	0.4	11.9	1.3	0.8	8.8	2.5	..	0.0
Guyana	1975	15-49	31.4	28.3	8.5	0.1	9.0	0.3	5.6	2.9	1.9	1.0	1.1	0.6	0.4
Paraguay	1977	15-44	28.6	23.3	3.2	f	11.8	0.9	4.0	2.6	0.8	1.9	3.3	..	..
	1979	15-49	36.4	23.5	2.1	0.1	11.9	1.7	5.4	1.5	0.8	4.2	2.4	0.0	6.3
	1987	15-44	44.8	29.0	4.0	0.0	13.5	3.6	5.1	2.3	0.5	5.7	2.9	..	7.2
	1990	15-49	48.4	35.3	7.4	0.0	13.6	5.2	5.7	2.6	0.8	5.3	2.9	..	5.0
Peru	1977/78	15-49	31.4	11.0	2.8	0.0	4.1	1.0	1.3	1.0	0.8	10.9	3.3	2.1	3.9
	1981	15-49	41	17	4	0	5	2	4	1	1	17	4	..	3
	1986	15-49	45.8	23.0	6.1	0.0	6.5	1.3	7.4	0.7	1.0	17.7	3.6	..	1.5
Venezuela	1977	15-44	49.3	37.7	7.6	0.1	15.3	0.2	8.6	4.8	1.1	4.0	4.7	0.0	2.8
Northern America															
Canada	1984	18-49	73.1	69.7	30.6	12.9	11.0	..	5.8	7.9	1.5	2.2	1.0	a	0.4
United States of America	1976	15-44	67.8	60.5	9.5	9.0	22.5	..	6.3	7.3	5.9	3.4	2.0	..	1.7
	1982	15-44	68.0	62.4	17.4	10.4	13.5	..	4.8	9.8	6.5	3.2	1.2	..	1.1
	1988	15-44	74.3	69.1	23.4	12.9	15.1	..	1.5	10.6	5.6	2.1	a	a	3.2
Oceania															
Australia	1986	20-49	76.1	72.2	27.7	10.4	24.0	..	4.9	4.4	0.8	2.0	1.6	..	0.3
New Zealand	1976	..	69.5	61.5	11.4	9.1	28.6	a	4.4	8.0	a	1.5	a	a	8.3

Source and notes to follow.

TABLE A.2 (*continued*)

Source: *World Contraceptive-use Data Diskettes, 1991* (United Nations publication, ST/ESA/SER.R/120).

NOTE: Distribution of percentage methods used may not add up exactly to total in column for "Any method" because of rounding. Figures shown without decimals were rounded to integer.

[a]Included in the category "others".

[b]Ever-married women.

[c]Included in the category "abstinence".

[d]Sample of husbands and wives.

[e]Included in the category "condom".

[f]Included in the category "female sterilization".

[g]Included in the category "intra-uterine device".

[h]Included in the category "female barrier".

[i]Included in the category "injectable".

[j]Women in first marriage only.

[k]All women.

[l]Included in the category "pill".

[m]Included in the category "rhythm".

[n]On 22 May 1990, Democratic Yemen and Yemen merged to form a single State. Since that date, they have been represented as one Member of the United Nations with the name "Yemen".

[o]The former State of Czechoslovakia was dissolved on 31 December 1992 and became the independent States of the Czech Republic and Slovakia on 1 January 1993.

[p]Data for the former Socialist Federal Republic of Yugoslavia.

[q]Data for the former Federal Republic of Germany.

REFERENCES

Andorka, Rudolf (1989). Successes and failures in the field of population policies since 1984. *Population Bulletin of the United Nations* (New York), No. 27, pp. 30-41. Sales No. E.89.XIII.7.

Askew, Ian (1989). Organizing community participation in family planning projects in South Asia. *Studies in Family Planning* (New York), vol. 20, No. 4 (July-August), pp. 185-202.

Basu, Alaka Malwade, and Ramamani Sundar (1988). The domestic servant as family planning innovator: an Indian case study. *Studies in Family Planning* (New York), vol. 19, No. 5 (September-October), pp. 292-298.

Bongaarts, John (1984). A simple method for estimating the contraceptive prevalence required to reach a fertility target. *Studies in Family Planning* (New York), vol. 15, No. 4 (July-August), pp. 184-190.

Bruce, Judith (1990). Fundamental elements of the quality of care: a simple framework. *Studies in Family Planning* (New York), vol. 21, No. 2 (March-April), pp. 61-91.

Bulatao, Rodolfo A. (1991). The Bulatao approach: projecting the demographic impact of the HIV epidemic using standard parameters. In *The AIDS Epidemic and its Demographic Consequences.* Proceedings of the United Nations/World Health Organization Workshop on Modelling the Demographic Impact of the AIDS Epidemic in Pattern II Countries, New York, 13-15 December 1989. New York: United Nations. Sales No. E.91.XIII.5, pp. 90-104.

________, and Ronald D. Lee, eds., with Paula E. Hollerbach and John Bongaarts (1983). *Determinants of Fertility in Developing Countries*, vol. 1, *Supply and Demand for Children.* New York: Academic Press.

Caldwell, John C. (1980). Mass education as a determinant of the timing of fertility decline. *Population and Development Review* (New York), vol. 6, No. 2 (June), pp. 225-255.

________ (1982). *Theory of Fertility Decline.* New York: Academic Press.

Chamratrithirong, Apichat, and Peerasit Kamnuansilpa (1984). How family planning availability affects contraceptive use: the case of Thailand. In *Survey Analysis for the Guidance of Family Planning Programs*, John A. Ross and Regina McNamara, eds. Liège, Belgium: Ordina Editions.

Chandrasekaran C., and Albert I. Hermalin, eds. (1975). *Measuring the Effect of Family Planning Programmes on Fertility.* Dolhain, Belgium: Ordina Editions.

Church, Cathleen A., with assistance of Judith Geller (1989). *Lights! Camera! Action! Promoting Family Planning with TV, Video and Film.* Population Reports, Series J, No. 38. Baltimore, Maryland: The Johns Hopkins University, Population Information Program.

Church, Cathleen A., and Judith S. Geller (1990). *Voluntary Female Sterilization: Number One and Growing.* Population Reports, Series C, No. 10. Baltimore, Maryland: The Johns Hopkins University, Population Information Program.

Cleland, John, and W. Parker Mauldin (1991). The promotion of family planning by financial payments: the case of Bangladesh. *Studies in Family Planning* (New York), vol. 22, No. 1 (January/February), pp. 1-18.

Coale, Ansley J. (1973). The demographic transition reconsidered. In *International Population Conference, Liège, 1973*, vol. 1. Liège, Belgium: International Union for the Scientific Study of Population.

Easterlin, Richard A. (1975). An economic framework for fertility analysis. *Studies in Family Planning* (New York), vol. 6, No. 3 (March), pp. 54-63.

________, Kua Wongboonsin and Mohamed Aly Ahmed (1988). The demand for family planning: a new approach. *Studies in Family Planning* (New York), vol. 19, No. 5 (September-October), pp. 257-269.

Freedman, Ronald (1966). Fertility. In *Proceedings of the World Population Conference, Belgrade, 1966*, vol. 1, *Summary Report.* New York: United Nations. Sales No. E/F.66.XIII, pp. 35-49.

Gordon, Gill, and Tony Klouda (1989). *Preventing a Crisis. AIDS and Family Planning Work.* Rev. ed. London: MacMillan.

Hatcher, Robert A., and others (1989). *Contraceptive Technology.* International ed. Atlanta, Georgia: Printed Matter, Inc.

Havelock, Ronald G., and others (1971). *Planning for Innovation Through Dissemination and Utilization of Knowledge.* Ann Arbor, Michigan: University of Michigan, Centre for Research on the Utilization of Scientific Knowledge.

Hobcraft, John (1991). Child spacing and child mortality. In *Demographic and Health Surveys World Conference, August 5-7, 1991, Washington, D.C., Proceedings*, vol. II. Columbia, Maryland: IRD/Macro International Inc.

_____ (1992). Fertility patterns and child survival: a comparative analysis. *Population Bulletin of the United Nations* (New York), No. 33, pp. 1-31. Sales No. E.92.XIII.4.

In-Joung Whang, ed. (1976). *Management of Family Planning Programs in Asia: Concepts, Issues and Approaches*. Kuala Lumpur: Asian Centre for Development Administration.

Isaacs, Stephen, and Nuray Fincancioglu (1989). Promoting family planning for better health: policy and programme implications. *Population Bulletin of the United Nations* (New York), No. 26. pp. 102-125. Sales No. E.89.XIII.6.

International Union for the Scientific Study of Population (1979). *Patterns of Response to Family Planning Programs*. IUSSP Paper, No. 14. Liège, Belgium.

Jain, Anrudh K. (1989). Fertility reduction and the quality of family planning services. *Studies in Family Planning* (New York), vol. 20, No. 1 (January-February), pp. 1-16.

Jejeebhoy, Shireen J. (1990). FamPlan: the great debate abates. *International Family Planning Perspectives (New York)*, vol. 16, No. 4 (December), pp. 139-142.

Johnson-Acsadi, Gwendolyn, and Maurice Szykman (1984). Selected characteristics of "exposed" women who wanted no more children but were not using contraceptives. In *Survey Analysis for the Guidance of Family Planning Programs*, John A. Ross and Regina McNamara, eds. Liège, Belgium: Ordina Editions, pp. 175-218.

Keller, Alan (1991). Management information systems in maternal and child health/family planning programs: a multi-country analysis. *Studies in Family Planning* (New York), vol. 22, No. 1 (January/February), pp. 19-30.

Krishnan, Vijaya (1991). Female labour force participation and fertility: an aggregate analysis. *Genus* (Rome), vol. 47, No. 1-2 (gennaio-giugno), pp. 177-192.

Laily, Noor, and others (1984). Perception of family planning service availability in rural Malaysia. In *Survey Analysis for the Guidance of Family Planning Programs*, John A. Ross and Regina McNamara, eds. Liège, Belgium: Ordina Editions.

Lande, Robert E., and Richard Blackburn (1989). *Pharmacists and Family Planning*. Population Reports, Series J, No. 37. Baltimore, Maryland: The Johns Hopkins University, Population Information Program.

Lande, Robert E., and Judith S. Geller (1991). *Paying for Family Planning*. Population Reports, Series J, No. 39. Baltimore, Maryland: The Johns Hopkins University, Population Information Program.

Lapham, Robert J., and George B. Simmons, eds. (1987). *Organizing for Effective Family Planning Programs*. Washington, D.C.: National Academy Press.

Lesthaeghe, Ron, ed. (1989). *Reproduction and Social Organization in Sub-Saharan Africa*. Berkeley, California: University of California Press.

Lettenmaier, Cheryl, and others (1988). *Mothers' Lives Matter: Maternal Health in the Community*. Population Report, Series L, No. 7 (September). Baltimore, Maryland: The Johns Hopkins University, Population Information Program.

Liskin, Laurie, and others (1990). *Condoms—Now More Than Ever*. Population Reports, Series H, No. 8. Baltimore, Maryland: The Johns Hopkins University, Population Information Program.

Mauldin, Parker, W. (1991). Estimation procedure. In *Contraceptive Requirements and Demand for Contraceptive Commodities in Developing Countries in the 1990s*. New York: United Nations Population Fund.

_____ , and John Ross (1991). *Family Planning Programs: Efforts and Results, 1982-89*. Research Division Working Paper, No. 34. New York: The Population Council.

Nortman, Dorothy (1978). *Birth Rates and Birth Control Practice: Relations Based on the Computer Models TABRAP and CONVERSE*. New York: The Population Council.

Population Council (1987). *International Conference on Better Health for Women and Children through Family Planning*. New York.

Population Crisis Committee (1992). *Washington Population Update* (January). Washington, D.C.

Program for Appropriate Technology in Health (1991). *Current Trends in Local Production of Contraceptives: Toward Meeting the Commodity Requirements of the Year 2000*. Seattle, Washington.

Ross, John, and Stephen L. Isaacs (1988). Cost, payments and incentives in family planning programs: a review for developing countries. *Studies in Family Planning* (New York), vol. 19, No. 5 (September-October), pp. 270-283.

Sadik, Nafis, ed. (1991). *Population Policies and Programmes: Lessons Learned from Two Decades of Experience*. New York: New York University Press.

Seidman, Myrna, and Marjorie C. Horn, eds. (1991). *Operations Research: Helping Family Planning Programs Work Better*. New York: Wiley-Liss.

Simmons, Ruth, and James F. Phillips (1990). *The Proximate Operational Determinants of Fertility Regulation Behavior*. Research Division Working Paper, No. 15. New York: The Population Council.

Sittitrai, Werasit, Kua Wongboonsin and Pichit Pitaktepsombati (1989). *A Study on Some Organizational Issues in Community Participation in the Context of a Family Planning Programme: The Case of Thailand*. Bangkok: Chulalongkorn University, Institute of Population Studies.

Szykman, Maurice (1982). The concept of demand for family planning and its measurement. *The Role of Surveys in the Analysis of Family Planning Programs*, Albert I. Hermalin and Barbara Entwisle, eds. Liège, Belgium: Ordina Editions.

Trussell, James, and Anne R. Pebley (1984). The potential impact of changes in fertility on infant, child and maternal mortality. *Studies in Family Planning* (New York), vol. 15, No. 6 (November-December), pp. 267-280.

_____ , and Kia I. Reinis (1989). Age at first marriage and age at first birth. *Population Bulletin of the United Nations* (New York), No. 26, pp. 126-185. Sales No. E.89.XIII.6.

United Nations (1975). *Report of the United Nations World Population Conference, 1974, Bucharest, 19-30 August 1974*. Sales No. E.75.XIII.3.

_____ (1979). *Manual IX: The Methodology of Measuring the Impact of Family Planning Programmes on Fertility*. Population Studies, No. 66. Sales No. E.78.XIII.8.

_____ (1984). *Report of the International Conference on Population, 1984, Mexico City, 6-14 August 1984*. Sales No. E.84.XIII.8.

_____ (1985). *Women's Employment and Fertility: A Comparative Study of World Fertility Survey Results for 38 Developing Countries*. Population Studies, No. 96. Sales No. E.85.XIII.5.

_____ (1986). *Manual IX, Addendum: The Methodology of Measuring the Impact of Family Planning Programmes on Fertility*. Population Studies, No. 66/Add.1. Sales No. E.86.XIII.4.

_____ (1987). *Fertility Behaviour in the Context of Development: Evidence from the World Fertility Survey*. Population Studies, No. 100. Sales No. E.86.XIII.5.

_____ (1989a). *Adolescent Reproductive Behaviour*, vol. II, *Evidence from Developing Countries*. Population Studies, No. 109/Add1. Sales No. E.89.XIII.10.

_____ (1989b). *Compendium of Statistics and Indicators on the Situation of Women*. Sales No. E/F.88.XVII.6.

_____ (1990a). *Population and Human Rights: Proceedings of the United Nations Expert Group Meeting, Geneva, 3-6 April 1989*. Sales No. E.91.XIII.8.

_____ (1990b). *Results of the Sixth Population Inquiry among Governments*. Population Policy Paper, No. 31. ST/ESA/SER.R/104.

_____ (1991a). *The AIDS Epidemic and its Demographic Consequences*. Proceedings of the United Nations/World Health Organization Workshop on Modelling the Demographic Impact of the AIDS Epidemic in Pattern II Countries, New York, 13-15 December 1989. Sales No. E.91.XIII.5.

_____ (1991b). *Measuring the Dynamics of Contraceptive Use.* Population Studies, No. 109. Sales No. E.91.XIII.7.

_____ (1991c). *World Population Monitoring, 1991: With Special Emphasis on Age Structure.* Population Studies, No. 126. Sales No. E.92.XIII.2.

United Nations Secretariat (1992). Evolution of population policy since 1984: a global perspective. In *Population Policies and Programmes.* Proceedings of the United Nations Expert Group Meeting, Cairo, 12-16 April 1992. Sales No. E.93.XIII.5.

United Nations, Economic and Social Commission for Asia and the Pacific (n.d.). *Report and Selected Papers of the Regional Project on Pre-testing and Evaluation of Educational Material Used in Family Planning Programmes.* Asian Population Studies Series, No. 27. Bangkok.

_____ (1969). *Assessment of Acceptance and Effectiveness of Family Planning Methods: Report of an Expert Group.* Asian Population Studies Series, No. 4. Bangkok. Sales No. E.69.II.F.15.

_____ (1976). *Measures of Efficiency for Family Planning Evaluation Programmes.* Asian Population Studies Series, No. 30. Bangkok.

United Nations Educational, Scientific and Cultural Organization (1982). *Public Administration and Management: Problems of Adaptation in Different Socio-cultural Contexts.* Paris.

United Nations Fund for Population Activities (1980). *Organizational Determinants of Family Planning Clinic Performance.* Population Development Studies, No. 5. New York.

United Nations Population Fund (1989a). Amsterdam Declaration. A Better Life for Future Generations. In *Report of the International Forum on Population in the Twenty-first Century, Amsterdam, The Netherlands, 6-9 November 1989.* New York.

_____ (1989b). *South Asia Study on Population Policies and Programmes: Nepal.* New York.

_____ (1989c). *South Asia Study of Population Policy and Programmes: Pakistan.* Islamabad.

_____ (1990a). *South Asia Study of Population Policy and Programmes: Bangladesh.* Dhaka.

_____ (1990b). *South Asia Study of Population Policy and Programmes: India.* New Delhi.

_____ (1990c). *South Asia Study of Population Policy and Programmes: Comparative Overview of Bangladesh, India, Nepal and Pakistan.* New York.

_____ (1991a). *Contraceptive Needs and Logistics Management.* New York.

_____ (1991b). *Contraceptive Requirements and Demand for Contraceptive Commodities in Developing Countries in the 1990s.* New York.

_____ (1992a). *Population* (New York), vol. 18, No. 3 (March).

_____ (1992b). *The State of World Population, 1992: A World in Balance.* New York.

Warwick, Donald P. (1988). Culture and the management of family planning programs. *Studies in Family Planning* (New York), vol. 19, No. 1 (January-February), pp. 1-18.

Weinberger, Mary Beth (1991). Recent trends in contraceptive behavior. In *Demographic and Health Surveys World Conference, August 5-7, 1991, Washington, D.C., Proceedings,* vol. I. Columbia, Maryland: IRD/Macro International, Inc.

Westoff, Charles F., and Anne R. Pebley (1984). The measurement of unmet need for family planning in developing countries. In *Survey Analysis for the Guidance of Family Planning Programs,* John A. Ross and Regina McNamara, eds. Liège, Belgium: Ordina Editions.

World Health Organization (1989). *The Health of Youth.* Background document No. A42, Technical discussion/2. Geneva.

_____ (1990). *Research in Human Reproduction: Biennial Report, 1988-1989.* Geneva.

Worth, Dooley (1989). Sexual decision-making and AIDS: why condom promotion among vulnerable women is likely to fail. *Studies in Family Planning* (New York), vol. 20, No. 6 (November-December), pp. 297-307.

Part Three

SOCIETY AND FAMILY PLANNING

IV. SOCIOCULTURAL MILIEU, WOMEN'S STATUS AND FAMILY PLANNING

Marvellous Mhloyi[*]

The relative importance of "status of women" as a fertility determinant is obvious in the proliferation of work in the area. Persistent acknowledgement of the elusiveness of the concept and efforts to clarify the concept notwithstanding, no standard definition exists. This problem is inevitable given the socio-economic, cultural and temporal specificity of the term. In its literary sense, status means position or rank in relation to others (Merriam-Webster, 1979). Hence, status as a gender issue means the relative position of women *vis-à-vis* men. From this perspective, one concept encapsulates status: the lineage system, patriarchy or matriarchy. The former system is the "supremacy of the father in the clan or family, the legal dependence of wives and children, and the reckoning of descent and inheritance in the male line" (Merriam-Webster, 1979). In the latter system, the mother is supreme; the matriarchal system is not of concern in this paper largely because it is limited to very few societies, although understanding this system would greatly illuminate on the interrelations between "status" and fertility decisions and outcomes in patriarchal societies. Implicit in this literary definition are the recurrent concepts of male dominance enhanced by control over resources as elaborated by Cain, Khanam and Nahar (1979).

This literary definition is further complicated by the other definitions of status, such as prestige (Epstein, 1982), power (Cain, Khanam and Nahar, 1979), autonomy (Dyson and Moore, 1983) and rights (Dixon, 1975). Mason (1984) contends that most of these terms and definitions refer in part to gender inequality and in particular to prestige, power or access to resources; they do not, however, include the other macrolevel dimension which refers to women's overall position in society (Safilios-Rothchild, 1985). In the most obvious sense, gender inequality refers to men's situational advantages (Caldwell, 1981).

The objective of this review is not necessarily to assess the adequacy of these definitions; it is to establish a common base for the discussions. However, it appears that the concept of status of women is a misnomer in a number of cases. As argued by Mason (1984), the literature to date reflects two ways through which changes in gender inequality may influence fertility decisions. The first argument is that as "husbands and wives become more equal, the wife's fertility desires will play an increasingly strong role in fertility decisions" (Mason, 1984, p. 71). She cautions that this assumption must not overlook the fact that in some societies, because fertility is considered a female specialization, women may have a larger say in fertility decisions. She also maintains that the assumption that male and female fertility desires are different may not always hold. As Cain, Khanam and Nahar (1979) argue, many treatments of the relation between women's economic status and fertility abstract from the corporate context of the household and thus overlook the fact that regardless of sometimes extreme inequality between sexes, women's welfare and interests are still often closely aligned with the corporate interests of a family as a whole. The second argument she identifies is that "a more egalitarian relationship between the sexes is likely to increase the weight given to the wife's health and well-being as factors in fertility decision making" (Mason, 1984, p. 72). In these cautionary statements, however, she uses similarly confusing terms, "equal" and "egalitarian". Also evident in the literature is a gross oversight of passion between sexes, as well as a judgmental position which perceives men as intentional oppressors of women. Although there are indeed some men that intend to abuse their wives, fertility may not necessarily be the most desired form of abuse; in fact, some men abuse their wives for getting pregnant.

The economic and social disadvantages that women face are inextricably a component of the socialization process in which women themselves are significant players. Thus, inadvertently women unconsciously contribute, to some extent, to their economic and social inequality. Yet, a great number of men may also be suffering from this unconsciousness, which is enhanced by the overall economic and social benefits accruing

---

[*]Department of Sociology, University of Zimbabwe, Harare, Zimbabwe.

from such inequality. Thus, although this discussion focuses on status of women, it is important to point out that policies must not only endeavour to improve the status of women through direct manipulation of the variables that directly refer to them but must also include an intervention that educates both males and females regarding the relevance of gender inequality to the welfare of the corporate family. Although such programmes will be directed to releasing men from the cultural entrapments that foster female subordinance and the advantages accruing from it, they must also endeavour to empower women to break out of the cultural cocoon in which they actively socialize their daughters to be subordinate to their male kin, beginning from the male siblings and goint on to husbands—an intergenerational low-status transfer. If one could only believe in a natural human desire and instinct to survive, it would become clear that an important ingredient for the success of intervention programmes should be effective communication on the disadvantages of sex inequality to family welfare. Including this message in the cultural beliefs and practices of respective groups would persuade both males and females to endeavour to change the status quo to the extent that they, as members of a corporate entity, articulate and work towards the achievement of corporate goals.

The literature in one way or another, suggests a negative causal relation between status of women and fertility by means of contraception. Granted that marriage is the universally sanctioned context, albeit in varying degrees, within which fertility must take place, and that a family is a social entity in which commonality of interest with regard to the well-being of the individual members thereof is most expected, and perhaps experienced, it is misleading to refer simply to status of women from the the socio-economic and cultural milieu within which marriage, roles and obligations are defined. Granted also that roles and obligations differ according to traditional lineage, religious and other social constructs, and that the resultant social systems have gender inequality in some or many aspects of life, areas in which one finds such inequalities between sexes are of interest for different reasons. Some sex differentiation of roles and obligations and the resultant inequality may be necessary for the well-being of the cooperate family.

For instance, in the most traditional socio-economic context, where hunting and gathering are the means of survival, the involvement of males in going into an unknown environment to hunt wild animals and of women in gathering plants and fruits and preparing food is an ideal division of labour which safeguards women from risky situations, particularly when they are pregnant or nursing babies, which is thus far a biological dictate. Fertility in such populations is generally low, approximately four children, as is the case for the Kung hunters and gatherers. The average birth interval in this population is approximately four years. It has been argued that this practice is adaptive to the socio-economic context in which the carrying of heavy loads by a woman with an infant on her back increases the chances of infant mortality. Thus, the long birth intervals and the consequent low levels of fertility form a fertility-maximizing strategy and not necessarily an attempt to limit fertility because of low family size desires. The survival strategies determine fertility. In such contexts the concept of status of women as used in current fertility studies may not necessarily be pertinent. The process of improving the status of women would ideally be undertaken concomitantly with the improvement of the status of men in that society; it is a process of development.

At the other end of the development continuum, represented by the most economically developed countries, other than the biological role of reproduction, roles and obligations need not necessarily be gender-differentiated. However, gender inequality still exists in such countries at varying degrees, depending upon the degree of gender differentiation of roles and obligations in the respective traditional cultures. This is evident in the fact that while some countries provide paternity leave, others only have maternity leave. What is posited here is that with the passage of time, as populations decline because of low levels of fertility and mortality, fertility will increasingly become valued to the extent that reproduction will confer a new form of status. This view implies that at the two extremes of the development continuum, fertility is not necessarily related to low status of women *per se*; the problem is the transitional stage that developing countries are experiencing. As countries move from the most traditional stage, differential provision of options by sex culminates in the gender inequality that is being addressed under different names in fertility studies.

For convenience in utilizing this literature to guide the present discussion, two areas are highlighted: (*a*) that concerning gender relations and power; and (*b*) gender options.

In discussing the relation between socio-economic milieu, status of women and family planning (fertility), the following premises are made:

(a) Fertility is an option largely for two reasons:

(i) For psychosocial satisfaction as determined by the respective socio-economic contexts. In order to achieve this need, patriarchal societies emphasize the importance of sons, which in turn has a positive impact on fertility. Yet, one would argue that one son is adequate to fulfil such an obligation. To the extent that couples consider the hoarding mechanism irrelevant because of low mortality levels even within a context of son preference, fertility will not remain as high as contraceptive use increases;

(ii) As a survival strategy;

(b) Couples try to maximize on their survival and that of their children. However, where there are limited survival options, children are perceived as a survival strategy or as an insurance against life chance risks. In such societies, children are desired for both of the reasons mentioned above;

(c) Family planning is a means to achieve an articulated desired family size (fertility demand). This demand ranges between a family size which is "up to God" and that to which a number is attached. A desired number which is up to God is that which is perceived, often subconsciously, to be consistent with a given context; it is an average fertility in a natural fertility regime (Mhloyi, 1987).

Of the two broad themes in the literature on status of women, that of gender options is more relevant to fertility studies. It should be noted, however, that options available to both males and females as couples in a conjugal union determine the average desired family. To the extent that such options are differentially acquired with a bias towards men, women may desire more children than men. This aspect entails the extent to which men have control over the means of production and valued resources, such as land, income, credit facilities and skills as they are acquired through education and training. Thus, the objective in this paper is to discuss the underlying factors of gender inequality and how such factors impinge upon fertility goals, which in turn determine contraception for fertility limitation. Policy recommendations are derived from such discussion.

A. FACTORS UNDERLYING GENDER INEQUALITY

Although this discussion must focus on the status of women, it is important to reiterate that the definition changes over time within the respective sociocultural milieu as a process of development. On the other hand, development is an international definition which hinges on the international monetary system. Most factors used as indices for status of women are those which enhance success in that international market, hence the overemphasis on education and training, labour force participation, employment, access to credit facilities and income. This section thus discusses how traditional sociocultural contexts determine the differential acquisition of these factors, indeed, other valued resources which confer economic supremacy of males over females.

The lineage system

Although this author has earlier argued that woman's interests are closely aligned with the corporate interests of the family, she has also pointed out the fact that the lineage system determines the family structure. That system determines family governance and assigns roles and obligations, thus governing the calibration of women's relative position *vis-à-vis* men through the control of valued resources. This discussion simply highlights the areas within which patriarchy gives rise to gender inequality, thereby rendering fertility (unregulated) an important option for women.

Ownership of land

In the patriarchal agrarian societies which typify most developing countries, land, the economic base, belongs to the patriarchy. Access to land and control over the produce differ by society, and they in turn determine the relative dependence of women upon fertility. African and Asian examples are used to illustrate this relation.

Cain (1984) undertook a comparative study of some poor, agricultural villages in Bangladesh and southern India. A common characteristic of both societies was the dependence of the elderly upon their children for support; and a major difference was the degree of female dependence upon males. In Bangladesh, the division of labour that had evolved effectively excluded women from all the most important activities which would permit them access to land and control over the produce (Cain, 1984). Women were also not permitted to seek employment in cash agriculture. On the other hand, he observed that women in the Indian villages were permitted to participate in agricultural work where there were activities specific to women. The Indian women could thus provide for themselves by either selling their labour for cash or by producing their own food. Women in Bangladesh were less likely to retain access to and/or ownership of land and to be able to support themselves after the death of their spouses. He therefore concluded that Bangladesh women were more likely to desire sons that would support them in the event their husband died than were Indian women. The consequent effect of this higher demand for sons was that high fertility more profitable for Bangladesh women than Indian women. Apparently (Cain, 1984) observed no practice of family planning in Bangladesh but found significant contraceptive prevalence in the Indian villages.

At a regional level, Dyson and Moore (1983) argue that the status of women in Bangladesh roughly corresponds to that of northern India, and that of the three Indian villages to the southern region of India. Fertility patterns are also comparable and, again, are similarly linked to the status of women.

In most of traditional sub-Saharan Africa, the family was the centre of economic and social life; land was the source of economic survival. Under customary law, the man was the legal custodian of his family and was thus in control of property acquired during marriage. Since men had the rights to land as the head of family, they allocated parcels of land to their wives, who would produce food for children and the entire family, including the extended family members. Tasks in the family were organized on the basis of sex. Women took care of the household and farming activities; thus, they were responsible for food production and its disposal. Men were involved in initial clearing of the grounds, while women were responsible for the seed from its sowing to the granary and subsequently the table. Children assisted their mothers in crop production and animal raising, the success of which was a symbol of wealth for the family, but the accolades were directed to men. Thus, men acquired status and influence in society through their women (Mhloyi, 1988).

Because access to land and thus survival was through men, production of sons was important to men for the continuity of their lineage and to women for the access to land and any other resources that sons could afford to their mother in the event of the death of the husband.

The system of levirate was also designed to assure widows of a male head of household and thus family security. The subordination of women to men was highly institutionalized, and their physical or intellectual products belonged to her husband and his lineage from the day the bride-price was paid (Mhloyi, 1988).

This traditional and rather historic perspective is given simply as a backdrop for the discussion of how and in what form gender inequalities are fostered within these societies today. It still typifies the current "African culture" and partially explains the low levels of family limitation.

Inheritance

In these patriarchies, female economic subordinance is perpetuated through the laws guarding inheritance. In both Africa and Asia, inheritance is largely through the male kin; wives cannot inherit property acquired by the couple in the event of the husband's death; sons also take precedence over daughters. This gender bias is often enforced by religion. For instance, the Muslim law stipulates that a daughter inherits half of what a son inherits. It has been argued that some women within that system opt to relinquish to their brothers the land they might have inherited in order to generate good will (Bertocci, 1981).

Closely linked to woman's subordinance as fostered by religion is the practice of purdah, female seclusion. This seclusion limits a woman's likelihood to engage in innovative behaviour, such as contraception; it also limits the acquisition of other ideas and tastes which are inimical to high fertility and thus enhance contraceptive use.

The process of modernization

The most important modernization factors, which may eventually mitigate against the effect of gender inequality emanating from traditional lineage systems as depicted above, are education (and training) and labour force participation. Access to credit facilities and other valued resources is also important. The differential acquisition of such valued resources by gender reflects in part the traditional roles and obligations as prescribed by the lineage itself and also the historical biases as introduced in the process of development. The following brief discussion highlights the gender inequality in a few variables and shows how such disparities work against family planning.

64

Education

Education of women is the socio-economic variable with the most pervasive impact on fertility. Education affects fertility outcomes by affecting both the supply and the demand for children. On the supply side, education reduces the duration of exposure to conception (assuming most conception is within marriage) by delaying age of entry into marriage and increasing marriage disruption. Education has a depressant effect on infant and child mortality, thereby rendering the hoarding mechanism irrelevant and consequently decreasing the demand for children. Although education has a negative impact on breast-feeding, this impact is counteracted by the positive impact on contraception. Education also reduces the demand for children not only by reducing infant and child mortality but also by exposing women to new ideas and tastes which mitigate against the taste for children. It also affords women skills that enhance their marketability in the modern labour market, thereby enhancing their acquisition of the valued pecuniary remunerations. (For a comprehensive discussion of the effects of education and fertility, see Cochrane, 1979.)

Education therefore has a pervasive impact on fertility; it is, however, differentially acquired by males and females, with a bias towards the former. Although efforts have been made to reduce this bias, the gap still remains. For instance, the World Bank (1988) reported that in 1960 females accounted for 34 per cent of primary-school enrolment, compared with 44 per cent in sub-Saharan Africa. There are, however, differences in the region. On the one end of the spectrum are such countries as Botswana and Swaziland, in which girls account for at least 50 per cent of the enrolment, while the Central African Republic, Chad and Guinea Bissau, fewer than 35 per cent of children enrolled in school were girls. The gender differences in enrolment are also found in Asia; unfortunately, given the economic structural adjustment programmes which most countries have adopted, the divergence between sexes may widen. This is the situation largely because the economic programme often demands a reduction of public spending, with education and health being the most affected. Yet, it has been observed that in the face of limited resources, sons get preference in the acquisition of education; in Asian countries, it is common knowledge that sons receive preferential treatment even in terms of food and health.

The differentials in enrolment, particularly at higher levels, are accentuated by the higher drop-out rates for girls. In sub-Saharan Africa, this drop-out rate is partially explained by teenage pregnancy, but it occurs also because as parents' resources become limited, boys remain in school and girls are advised and/or opt to drop out, on the premise that the sons or brothers are the future heads of families. In addition, girls are also more useful to their mothers at home. This sex-selectivity in educational investment is partially a consequence of family expectations as determined by the existing roles and obligations of the respective sexes. For instance, in some Asian countries, it is not culturally acceptable for parents to receive assistance from daughters (discussions with an Indian colleague).

Female labour force participation

Labour force participation is expected to foster contraceptive use (fertility regulation) in a number of ways. First, it is generally argued that employment of women, particularly employment outside the home, is incompatible with high fertility. This role incompatibility effect might be slightly mitigated by the availability of substitute caregivers for children. Secondly, employment affords women acquisition of the valued monetary power, thereby adding a new dimension to status. Broadening the contribution of women to the welfare of the family enhances women's involvement in decision-making while it erodes the influence of the extended kin group, because the next of kin also benefit from the monetary gains accrued by the working daughter-in-law. Lastly, the interaction of women with colleagues in the labour market fosters the acquisition of new ideas and tastes which are inimical to reproduction. It enhances innovative behaviour as women become more knowledgeable and confident.

Female labour force participation is also desirable as a key to minimize hunger. As Snyder (1990) argues, one in three households in the world—one in two in some areas—has a woman as its sole breadwinner. He also observes that women produce up to 80 per cent of the food in Africa, 60 per cent in Asia and the Pacific and 40 per cent of the food in Latin America; and that women direct their earnings to meet family needs more than males. He adds that women, however, have limited access to resources to increase their productivity as farmers or entrepreneurs.

The gender bias in labour force participation has been documented widely and remains regardless of government efforts to reverse the situation. For instance, in

Bangladesh, where the Government has begun to set up a ministry of women's affairs, has made education more available to women (who have subsequently performed better than their male counterparts) and has made female opportunities broader than those of males. There are complaints that these working women still face discrimination and biased evaluation, compared with their male counterparts. Women still earn less than their male counterparts.

Access to credit facilities

As alluded to earlier, the dependence of females upon males is also enhanced by policies that restrict the access of women to credit facilities. These restrictions range from complete inability of a women to acquire a loan for her own use to acquisition facilitated by the countersigning of applications by a male family member. In most countries, there are simply no credit facilities available for the type of activities in which most females engage. Where such facilities may be available, women do not fully utilize such facilities because they lack the ssary managerial, accounting and other technical skills.

Technological transfer

It has been shown that although women produce most of the food, as agriculture becomes commercialized women become marginalized. A shift from subsistence to cash cropping is often accompanied by improvement in technology and cropping patterns. New technology is often used by males, who will consequently control the cash from the sale of the produce. More often than not extension workers are males, who will supervise females. The cropping patterns sometimes change to the extent that women cease to cultivate crops which traditionally used to be a female preserve and a source of their income. This was the case in Zimbabwe, when cultivation of maize, which is the staple food, was reduced as farmers were diversifying to cultivate cash crops, such as tea, tobacco and cotton. In addition to the erosion of women's income base, this change had a negative impact on the nutrition of the entire family. Several authors have argued that the key to alleviate hunger and poverty in most agricultural-based economies is to increase women's access to new agricultural technology and other input items; they have to be part of the development process (Gladwin and McMillan, 1989; Stamp, 1990).

B. SUMMARY

The foregoing brief discussion was intended to provide the context and justification for policy recommendations with regard to the relation between status of women and fertility. It is apparent from the review that fertility is important for a number of reasons: as a means of any family to replenish itself; as a survival strategy; and as a status symbol. The level of fertility needed for the effective achievement of these goals differs from one society to another and between sexes, depending upon the prescribed rules guarding marriage and the roles and obligations assigned to the male and female members of the family.

With modernization, males and females have differentially acquired the valued resources, skills and training that facilitate success in the international monetary system. Fertility goals and consequently fertility regulation will depend upon the extent to which a couple values children. The value of children, and the ultimate family size, will be enhanced to the extent that females depend upon the male kin and sons, and, consequently, high fertility as the logical option. In turn, family size desires will determine whether family planning is practised. It is also apparent that removing this inequality enhances the status of women, which in turn, has a positive impact on family planning. In turn, family planning enhances the well-being of the entire family by reducing maternal and child mortality and increasing the quality of life as resources available to the households increase. Considering that women are at least 50 per cent of the population, development policies that ignore this significant proportion are not only poorly conceived but retrogressive and myopic. However, efforts to reverse the observed gender inequality must be culturally sensitive. Given a natural human desire to survive, an essential ingredient for the success of intervention programmes should be effective communication on the disadvantages that sex inequality imposes on family welfare. If this message were included in the cultural beliefs and practices of respective groups, both males and females would be persuaded to change the status quo as they work towards the achievement of corporate goals.

C. POLICY RECOMMENDATIONS

The following recommendations are made with regard to policy:

66

1. Granted that the family (through marriage) is the socially sanctioned unit in which most fertility takes place, there must be explicit policies and legislation to protect the basic rights of all its members, irrespective of sex. Such legislation would govern marriage contracts and divorce, and inheritance. This need calls for the integration of traditional and statutory law.

2. Changes in family law must be accompanied by educational campaigns which stress the importance of the family unit, mutual respect, love and corporate interest and integrated inclusive planning. Such campaigns must highlight the importance of such attributes to the welfare of families, which the respective societies purport to value and protect.

3. Efforts must be made to improve the economic contribution of the individual members of the family irrespective of sex. Such efforts would entail:

(a) Equal educational opportunities between males and females;

(b) Equal access to training and acquisition of skills in all economic spheres ranging from agriculture to industries;

(c) Availability of credit facilities for women's activities;

(d) Equal opportunities for labour force participation and enhancement of female labour force participation by providing child care whenever necessary and legislating both paternity and maternity leave to minimize female labour force attrition and delayed promotions resulting from women's absence from work owing to their participation in child-rearing.

(e) Legislation to provide equal pay and taxation for males and females.

4. Given the long traditions that guide the existing legal and economic structures, there is need to design an educational campaign that would include, as part of socialization, the concept of equality between children regardless of sex. Such campaigns must highlight the desirability of every child to feel equally valued by the family and consequently by society to the well-being of which she must contribute. They should foster high self-esteem in girls.

5. Policy must emphasize the importance of family planning not necessarily to limit population growth (although it is an extremely important goal in developing countries), as has been the emphasis, because even the most educated population scientist does not normally consider what his/her next child will contribute to the population growth rate.

Instead, family planning must be emphasized for enhancing maternal and child health and also for affording women the time to participate in other activities which foster the well-being of the family. The advantages of a smaller family size must be emphasized; for example, better chances of providing good nutrition for the family, which in turn fosters children's growth and future productivity; and the importance of investing in fewer children, who can subsequently succeed in the modern labour market and provide the parents with the necessary security. It is the creation of the demand of family planning. This approach has thus far been ignored as expensive and sometimes not necessary. It must be noted, however, that the positive aspects of small family size are not necessarily obvious to the many people that are guided by tradition. Besides, simple marketing dictates demand as a prerequisite of any supply.

6. Given that family planning is a basic human right, women must have the right to abortion as a contraceptive failure backup. It is unfortunate that the so-called "pro-life activists" are self contradictory. Respecting the right to life of an embryo while relegating the survival of sometimes a pregnant 45-year old mother of parity 10, with children ranging from 2 to 20 yesrs to chance is not only trivializing life; it is also insensitive to the potential impact of orphanhood on the living children and truly irresponsible. Such orphanhood may increase the mortality of the living children. Perhaps there is credibility in the phrase on one of the banners carried by some activists in the United States of America, which reads "an embryo has rights until it is born a female". They also tend to question the integrity and morality of woman. Ironically, abortion, unlike family limitation, is deeply rooted in most cultures.

All these recommendations are made with the awareness that in most countries the economic situation may not allow such investments in social services. A case in point is the reduction of spending in social services undertaken as a means to improve the economy; this is one aspect of the structural adjustment programmes that most African countries have recently adopted. Yet, this author would hasten to add that ignoring the social investment is short-sighted.

REFERENCES

Abdullah, Tahrunnesa Ahmed and Sandra A. Zeidenstein (1982). Village Women of Bangladesh: Prospects for Change. Elmsford, New York: Pergamon Press.

Anker, Richard and Catherine Hein (1985). Fertility and employment in the Third World. *POPULI* (New York), vol. 12, No. 2, pp. 29-37.

Anonymous (1984). Interview: Dr. Nafis Sadik on population and women in development—the second decade of women. What roles? *POPLEONE* (Freetown), vol. 1, No. 1 (July), pp. 23-24.

Bertocci, Peter J. (1981). Elusive villages: social structure and community organization in rural East Pakistan. Doctoral dissertation. East Lansing, Michigan: Michigan State University, 1970.

Cain, Mead (1984). *Women's Status and Fertility in Developing Countries: Son Preference and Economic Security*. World Bank Staff Working Papers, No. 682. Population and Development Series, No. 7. Washington, D.C.: The World Bank.

_____, Syeda Rokeya Khanam and Shamsun Nahar (1979). Class, patriarchy, and women's work in Bangladesh. *Population and Development Review* (New York), vol. 5, No. 3 (September), pp. 405-438.

Caldwell, John C. (1981). The mechanisms of demographic change in historical perspective. *Population Studies* (London), vol. 35, No. 1 (March), pp. 5-27.

Cochrane, Susan H. (1979). *Fertility and Education: What Do We Really Know?* World Bank Staff Occasional Papers, No. 26. Baltimore, Maryland: and London: Johns Hopkins University Press

Deen, M. A. (1984). Women and development problems and issues. *POPLEONE* (Freetown), vol. 1, No. 1 (July), pp. 10-13.

Dixon, Ruth B. (1975). *Women's Rights and Fertility*. Reports on Population/Family Planning, No. 17. New York: The Population Council.

Dyson, Tim, and Mick Moore (1983). On kinship structure, female autonomy, and demographic behaviour in India. *Population and Development Review* (New York), vol. 9, No. 1 (March), pp. 35-60.

Epstein, T. Scarlett (1982). A social anthropological approach to women's roles and status in developing countries: the domestic cycle. In *Women's Roles and Population Trends in the Third World*, Richard Anker, Mayra Buvinic and Nadia H Youssef, eds. London: Croom Helm.

Gladwin, C. H., and D. McMillan (1989). Is a turn around in Africa possible without helping African women to farm. *Economic Development and Cultural Change* (Chicago, Illinois), vol. 37, No. 2 (January), pp. 345-369.

Mason, Karen Oppenheim (1984). *The Status of Women: A Review of Its Relationships to Fertility and Mortality*. New York: The Rockefeller Foundation.

Merriam-Webster (1979). *Webster's New Collegiate Dictionary*. Springfield, Massachusetts: G. C. Merriam Company.

Mhloyi, Marvellous (1987). The proximate determinants and their socio-cultural determinants: the case of two rural settings in Zimbabwe. In *The Cultural Roots of African Fertility Regimes: Proceedings of the Ile-Ife Conference, 1987*. Ile-Ife, Nigeria: Obafemi Awolowo University; and Philadelphia: University of Pennsylvania.

_____ (1988). The determinants of fertility in Africa under modernization. In *Proceedings of the African Population Conference, Dakar, 1988*, vol. 1. Liège, Belgium: International Union for the Scientific Study of Population.

_____ (1990). The role and status of women and its impact on fertility in Zimbabwe. Paper prepared for the World Bank.

Rogers, S. G. (1983). Efforts towards women's development in Tanzania: gender rhetoric vs. gender realities. In *Women in Developing Countries: A Policy Focus*, Kathlee A. Staudt and Jane S. Jaquette, eds. New York: Haworth Press.

Sadik, Nafis (1985). Muslim women today. *Populi* (New York), vol. 12, No. 1, pp. 36-51.

Safilios-Rothchild, Constantina (1985). *Socioeconomic Development and the Status of Women in the Third World*. Centre for Policy Studies Working Papers, No. 112. New York: The Population Council.

Snyder, M. (1990). Women: the key to ending hunger. The Hunger Project Papers, No. 8. New York: The Global Hunger Project.

Stamp, Patricia (1990). *Technology, Gender, and Power in Africa*. 2nd ed. Ottawa, Canada: International Development Research Centre.

Thuhane, T. T. (1989). Towards a strategy of linking women. Population growth, poverty alleviation and sustainable development. Unpublished.

United Nations (1975). *Report of the United Nations World Population Conference, Bucharest, 19-30 August 1974*. Sales No. E.75.XIII.3.

Wilson, W. (1985). The community of African women. *Beyond Relief* (Washington, D.C.), vol. 1, No. 2 (July), pp. 1-8.

World Bank (1988). *Education in Sub-Saharan Africa: Policies for Adjustment, Revitalization and Expansion*. World Bank Policy Study. Washington D.C.

V. SOCIAL POLICY AND FERTILITY TRANSITIONS

Thomas W. Merrick[*]

The 1990s bring a new set of challenges for international family planning programmes. Fertility transitions are now under way in a large number of developing countries, and contraceptive prevalence has risen from very low rates to levels that include half or more of married women of reproductive age. One of the key questions for population policy is whether efforts to expand the supply of contraceptives, which played a key role in getting fertility declines under way, will be sufficient to complete the transition to low fertility; or whether greater attention needs to be given to demand factors once transitions have reached an intermediate stage. This question is also relevant for countries still in an earlier stage in the fertility transition, to the extent that they may want to draw on lessons learned from the experience of countries that have moved from incipient to intermediate stages of the transition.

Debate about the relative importance of "supply" and "demand" for family planning has waxed and waned for over two decades. When efforts to expand family planning were just beginning in developing countries during the early 1970s, there was considerable scepticism about whether demand for services would be sufficient to bring about significant change in reproductive behaviour. "Development is the best contraceptive" was a catch phrase at the World Population Conference at Bucharest in 1974. In research on fertility determinants, there was a tendency to dichotomize supply and demand, often with recommendations that fertility might decline faster if either spending on family planning were to be increased or, alternatively, spending were to be shifted from family planning programmes to changing the underlying social structure that generated demand for large families.

Subsequent experience has shown that there was considerable latent demand for family planning and that contraceptive use would increase if high-quality family planning services responded to the needs of potential clients. However, success in family planning involves more than isolated distribution of contraceptives. The programmes that succeeded were those which moved with the social, economic and cultural currents of the societies in which they were organized. Programmes that failed to find these currents had less impact, and in some instances, counter-currents were so strong that movement was impossible. This experience has also shown that the supply and demand dichotomy is too restrictive a framework for addressing linkages between family planning and the socio-economic setting. As Demeny notes: "[H]ow family planning programs are organized and how services are delivered have a significant influence on the capacity of these programs to attract clients. Thus, supply influences demand. Conversely, the ability of even the most determined suppliers of contraceptives to sustain an effective family planning program is a function of the level of demand." And he concludes that "supply—'programme effort'—is not an independent variable: it reflects, *inter alia*, demand" (Demeny, 1992, p. 321).

As supply and demand issues again come into question for countries that have succeeded in supplying latent demand and are moving into the intermediate stages of their fertility transition, it is important that the policy implications of these lessons not be lost by once more dichotomizing "supply" and "demand" for family planning, particularly in extreme positions supporting one to the exclusion of the other. A more useful approach for social policy at intermediate stages of the fertility transition is on the synergies between socio-economic forces, social sector investments, including family planning and reproductive health, and fertility. The right questions are what social sector investments are likely to strengthen the demand for family planning and reproductive health services and how can the design of services be better tailored to the socio-economic structure in which they are expected to be effective? This paper offers some further reflections on these questions.

A. PROGRESS IN UNDERSTANDING LINKAGES BETWEEN FAMILY PLANNING FERTILITY AND SOCIAL SETTING

Over the past two decades, a substantial literature has evolved on fertility and family planning. It is based on

---

*Senior Population Adviser, Population Health and Nutrition Department, The World Bank, Washington, D.C., United States of America.

an equally large volume of data accumulated through such projects such as the World Fertility Survey (WFS), the Contraceptive Prevalence Surveys (CPS) and the current Demographic and Health Surveys (DHS) (Freedman and Blanc, 1992). An advantage of these inquiries is their reliance upon a common set of variables, which has increased international (and, to a lesser extent, intertemporal) comparability. They also make it possible to obtain timely measurement of fertility rates, contraceptive prevalence, unmet need and other programmatically useful information. Because of the wealth of statistical information, debate about fertility is better informed than during the 1970s.

One caveat is that gains in comparability and timeliness in fertility surveys involve trade-offs in the precision of information about individual and household characteristics which could shed additional light on supply and demand issues. Other large-scale survey efforts, such as those measuring level of living and periodic household income and employment, do present a richer array of social and economic measures but do not provide the information on fertility and family planning that one finds in DHS-type surveys. When analysts utilize fertility survey data to study links between socio-economic variables and fertility, they are generally limited to a narrow range of socio-economic measures, while the broader surveys that do provide such information are relatively weak on fertility and family planning information.

Another limitation of household-level inquiries is that they provide little information on how family planning services are obtained and that the information they do provide depends upon how well survey respondents know the characteristics of the service delivery points they use—for example, whether they are "public" or "private", what range of services they actually provide and who else uses them. Survey-based information about costs and the structure of service delivery is very limited. Administrative data may shed some light on this point but are often distorted to reflect favourably on providers. Operations research projects that focus on process variables, such as the quality of client and provider relationships and linkages between programme structure and input and programme performance, are a useful source of additional information but are generally limited in geographical scope, which makes it difficult to utilize their findings in studies that require multiple observations based on a single measure (Gallen and Reinhart, 1986).

Even with these limitations, research flowing from these new sources of information has done much to clarify the linkages between programme effort and socio-economic variables. Several important lines of inquiry have emerged since the Conference at Bucharest in 1974, when the idea first gained prominence that "development" and "family planning" were somehow competing approaches to fertility reduction in developing countries. At that time, there were indeed claims by some that fertility would decline if only contraceptives could be supplied in massive numbers and by others that socio-economic forces so dominated fertility behaviour that family planning programmes would have little effect. A lot has been learned since then, with most of the evidence pointing to synergies rather than competition between supply and demand factors. The literature is by now extensive; here one need only recall its main points.

The first of these research developments is based on recognition that the effects of socio-economic factors on fertility are usually mediated by intermediate or "proximate" determinants of fertility, as elaborated by Bongaarts (1978). This perspective shifts the focus of research on socio-economic determinants of fertility from direct to indirect linkages, taking account of physiological and demographic factors that have more immediate effects on reproductive outcomes: (a) use of contraceptives; (b) intended and involuntary infertility and interruption of pregnancy; and (c) patterns of marriage and cohabitation. Both socio-economic variables and programmes affect these proximate variables, and Bongaarts and his followers have urged that research focus on understanding these channels and their interactions to inform policy and budgetary decisions.

A second line of inquiry that has helped to clarify understanding of the synergies between broader socio-economic forces and programmatic variables in accelerating fertility decline is the series of cross-national studies carried out by Mauldin in collaboration with his colleagues Bernard Berelson, Robert Lapham and John Ross (Mauldin and Ross, 1991). These studies, which examine the effects on fertility of standard measures of progress in socio-economic development in conjunction with a series of programme effort indicators, show that fertility declines most rapidly in countries with high scores on both sets of indicators. Although a great deal of care is needed in drawing conclusions from aggregative cross-national measures, the finding that countries can experience fertility declines under less favourable socio-economic conditions or with lower programme effort suggests that both sets of variables are important. Moreover, interactions between the variables (which complicate the analytical task of distinguishing between the effects of programme input and contextual variables) lend further support to the view that it is the synergies between these variables that are important from a programmatic perspective. To find these synergies, one must focus on specific country experiences.

This approach is borne out by a third and very informative line of research that has evolved in the post-Bucharest era: country-level studies of the fertility transitions currently occurring in many developing countries, particularly in Asia and Latin America and the Caribbean. One example of this type of work is the growing literature on the fertility transition in Bangladesh. That country was once considered an example of a socio-economic setting so unfavourable to fertility decline that it was thought unlikely that family planning programmes could have any impact. Indeed, the failure of a number of early efforts to increase contraceptive use by expanding services seemed to confirm this view (Cleland and Phillips, 1992).

Fortunately, Bangladesh was able to draw on lessons from carefully designed experimental programmes, such as those in the Matlab district, which sought to shape intervention strategies on local, social, economic and cultural conditions. The subsequent success of this experiment and application of its lessons in other parts of the country suggested, first, that programmes had to do more than merely supply contraceptives; and secondly, that when programmes were made more responsive to the actual needs and sensitivities of potential clients, contraceptive use would increase and fertility decline would accelerate. A specific example in the Bangladesh case is the selection of outreach workers: initial efforts to expand outreach services using male health workers and even older female midwives met with little success in the villages; these workers could dispense supplies but were not credible counsellors in dealing with the concerns of potential users, most of whom were reluctant to talk about sexual practices. However, when younger women were recruited from villages and trained in a range of outreach skills, they proved to be very effective change agents (Phillips and others, 1992).

The Bangladesh experience also illustrates how programme effort can be made more effective by attention to key structural variables. In Bangladesh, as in many countries in early stages of the transition to lower fertility, there was latent demand for family planning, but the climate of demand was weak because of women's uncertainties and concerns about change in reproductive behaviour, which, in turn, increased their psychological cost of controlling fertility even if monetary costs were being reduced through programme efforts. It was only when programmes became sensitive to costs in this broader sense (through counselling, education and other initiatives) that latent demand was translated into increased contraception and fertility decline. This success led to word-of-mouth communication about the benefits of family planning among villages and helped expand the demand for services (Cleland and Phillips, 1992).

B. RECENT RESEARCH AND SOCIAL POLICY

Much of the renewed discussion about the relative importance of supply and demand factors in fertility and family planning has focused on whether investments in female education or funding of family planning p rogrammes is the more effective approach to acceleration of fertility decline in developing countries (Summers, 1992). As Cochrane demonstrates, the effects of individual education on fertility are likely to work through multiple channels:

"Education through literacy gives people access to more sources of information and a wider perspective on their own culture. Education is also a socializing process and inculcates social values. Exposure to these values would depend on the years of schooling. Education is widely believed to provide economic skills, and the level of those skills may depend on the grade level attended. Even if education does not provide such skills, jobs are often rationed on the basis of credentials such as education certificates." (Cochrane, 1979)

Because of these linkages, economists seeking to measure the influence of demand factors on fertility rely upon educational attainment as a measure of the cost of child care *vis-à-vis* opportunities to increase income by working outside the home. Another channel of influence on fertility behaviour is through educational opportunities for children, where the logic is that parents may choose to have a smaller number of children in order to be able to provide them with a better education. Education can also influence fertility through its effect on the setting for delivery of family planning programmes by increasing the number of skilled service providers.

That schooling has a powerful effect on reproductive behaviour is undisputed. The relation, however, is far from simple one-way causation. In her recent review of findings from research on linkages between education and fertility, Jejeebhoy (1992) found differing patterns in different stages of development. Her report puts greater emphasis on sociocultural channels than on purely economic ones. In the early stages of development, the primary effect of education is through fertility-enhancing factors, such as decreased breast-feeding. The impact of education on fertility is greatest when it offers women more than a limited role in family decisions and access to resources. She raises a policy concern about relying upon changes in the distribution of educational attainment to reduce fertility even though some fertility decline can be expected because of change in that distribution. Although the proportion of poorly educated women in the developing world is declining, these women still constitute the majority in many countries, and further declines in fertility will depend upon their behaviour. Thus, she notes that fertility is not likely to decline unless family planning programmes are established to help address the unmet need of the less educated women (Jejeebhoy, 1992).

Given these multiple channels of potential influence, it should not be surprising that educational attainment repeatedly turns up as the variable that explains the most variance in regression analyses of the number of children reported by women in survey data. Moreover, when education is pitted against weak measures of "family planning programme input", such as women's perception of the distance to the nearest family planning clinic or community-level measures of the "supply" of services, it would be a surprise if education did not explain most of the variance.

This aspect is, in fact, what is being found in recent studies purporting to show that most, if not all of the recent fertility declines in developing countries are "demand-driven" and that increased access to contraception has had little or no effect on such declines (Subbarao and Raney, 1992; Schultz, 1992; Psacharopoulos and Rosenhouse, 1992; Pritchett, 1992). These studies are based either on international cross-sections with country-level data or on country-level cross-sections with household-level data. Both employ measures of fertility, contraceptive use and educational attainment to test the relative strength of "supply" and "demand" in explaining fertility decline. Most discuss the complex structural relations underlying the linkage between these

variables but revert to the so-called "reduced form" in their statistical tests, with female educational attainment as the operative variable representing demand. Because of the high statistical (and behavioural) association between fertility and contraceptive use, most studies also attempt to "endogenize" contraceptive use by estimating it using exogenous variables that "explain" cross-national or cross-household variation in it. For a variety of reasons, neither household-level nor cross-national studies do very well in explaining contraceptive use in this way (Schultz, 1992).

Cross-national studies have used such indices as the Mauldin and Ross programme effort scores, which do correlate well with contraceptive use but suffer from being highly correlated with demand variables as well (Mauldin and Ross, 1991; Boulier, 1985). Other measures, such as programme expenditures, lack cross-country comparability or are basically weak measures of programme input. Country-level cross-sections do not work much better. An example is a recent study of fertility decline in Indonesia during the 1980s, which is very careful to control for the endogeneity of programme input items that influence fertility behaviour (Gertler and Molyneaux, 1992). Its authors take note of the close connection between fertility decline and increased contraceptive prevalence, but in order to avoid biasing the analysis by regressing fertility on an "outcome" variable, they attempt to measure district-level family planning programme "input" in four ways: (a) monthly mobile family planning team visits; (b) village contraceptive distribution centres; (c) number of health clinics registered in the family planning reporting system; and (d) number of family planning clinic workers. In individual-level regression results, they then report that although contraceptive prevalence accounted for 75 per cent of the fertility decline, educational attainment "accounted" for 87 per cent of the increase in contraceptive use and programme input for only 4-8 per cent of the decline. From a policy perspective, interpreting these findings to suggest that programme input does not affect contraceptive use is misleading. What they have found is that weak measures of programme input do not provide much information about contraceptive use. Had they tried, the authors would also have found that "input" variables for individual educational attainment—the number of schools, the number of teachers and the number of textbooks—would not have explained much of the regional variance in educational attainment, which, from a social investment perspective, is also an "output" variable.

Although much of the debate has centred on the role of formal education as a "demand" variable, the role of informal education, exposure to the mass media and other modernizing variables should not be forgotten in the discussion of forces that strengthen the motivation to control fertility through the use of contraception. Many family planning programmes have used the media to raise consciousness about family planning and to motivate couples to space and limit births. Even non-specific content of mass media messages, particularly those which expose audiences to new values, play an important role in this process. Although these influences are difficult to quantify, they are recognized as playing an important role in building demand for family planning (Gilluly and Moore, 1986; Church, 1989).

From a theoretical perspective, there is not a prima facie case for the primacy of either "supply" (of family planning services) or "demand" (for children, or derived demand for services). Approaches that look at both the supply of and demand for children recognize that family planning programmes can do a lot to reduce the costs of realizing child-bearing aspirations. As Easterlin and Crimmins point out, "Unlike popular views and a number of scholarly theories, the present approach does not assert the primacy of any single determinant of fertility control—motivation, its demand or supply components, or regulation costs. Rather it views the respective roles of these factors as an empirical issue. . .Their volume seeks to elucidate that issue (Easterlin and Crimmins, 1985, p. 10). Their findings emphasize the importance of motivation for control of fertility but note that a variety of social and programme forces influence both motivation and the costs of regulation.

From a policy perspective, the issue is whether analytical work can provide programmatically useful information about the synergistic relations between family planning programmes and individual- and community-level "setting" variables that influence both fertility and programme performance. To the extent that research approaches ignore such synergies, their contribution is likely to be limited. In fact, to the extent that they counterpoise the two sets of variable rather than explore interactions, they may be misleading.

What is often missed is a sequence of changes that, in broad outline, were alluded to earlier in this paper. In the very early stages of the transition process, there is, on average, high fertility and little fertility limitation (with variation related to spacing such practices as breast-feeding and abstinence from intercourse for some time after a birth). There are pockets of family planning practice among more educated women and élite groups, who generally have constituted the largest segment of latent demand potential for expanded services. When organized family planning is initiated, these groups are typically the first to utilize services.

At one time it was argued that once this latent demand was satisfied, further change in reproductive behaviour would not occur without more fundamental socio-economic changes to reduce the incentives for large families. Undeterred by this discouraging advice, family planning advocates mounted information and public education campaigns to attract added clients from among groups with latent demand and sought to increase awareness and motivation to practise family planning among groups that still expressed a preference for large families. As time passed and programme effort expanded, the prevalence of family planning continued to grow. One feature of this expansion was a "demonstration effect" created by the adoption of family planning among groups that were perceived to be improving the level of living through the behaviour changes they adopted (including having fewer children and practising family planning) and that communicated their satisfaction with the services that helped them accomplish these changes (Cleland and Wilson, 1987). Of course, the reverse also happened when services did not meet client needs; hence the growing emphasis on service quality among providers.

If the country in question was also investing in education, cohorts with higher educational attainment replaced their less educated older sisters in the prime child-bearing ages of the society's reproductive population, reinforcing the process of change through a variety of channels that were mentioned earlier. At the same time, family planning was being adopted and fertility was also declining among older, less educated women and among less educated younger women for whom services were being provided. Obviously, motivation counted for the latter groups, but it was being promoted through informal channels rather than added schooling, from which these groups did not benefit.

C. ILLUSTRATIVE CASES

Indonesia is one case in point. Since the late 1960s, the total fertility rate in Indonesia has declined by 40 per cent, from 5.5 to 3.3 births per woman. Contraceptive prevalence has risen from less than 10 to about 50 per cent. Indonesia has one of the most effective national family planning programmes in the world; much of the increase in contraceptive use has been attributed to it. At the same time, Indonesia has invested heavily in education, so that by the late 1980s primary education was virtually universal. It is clear that both supply and demand forces were at work. Yet, as Freedman notes:

"[N]o one has yet developed a methodology for disentangling the changes in the desired number of children which are induced by social change, and those which arise from the direct communication of such ideas by an organized program or in other ways.... It is likely that the overall increase in effective demand was a synergistic joint effect of the broad social changes and the strong family planning program. Given what is at stake and the independent value of both development and the service aspects of the program, it is prudent to consider both as essential parts of the Indonesian population policy." (World Bank, 1992, p. 144)

The experience of Bangladesh also illustrates how programme effort can achieve results in an adverse setting. Much of the Bangladesh family planning programme effort has been directed to less educated, rural women. From 1983 to 1991, the contraceptive prevalence rate for women with secondary education increased by 10 percentage points, from 42 to 52 per cent. At the same time, contraceptive prevalence for women with no schooling increased by 21 percentage points, from 16 to 37 per cent. Correlations between education and contraceptive use would probably be stronger than those for programme input at both dates and yet would completely miss the impact of programme effort in increasing prevalence among uneducated women by much more than among more educated women (Mitra, Lerman and Islam, 1992).

An important synergistic effect made clear by the Bangladesh experience relates to changes in the status of women. The low status of women and the lack of opportunity for women outside the home were seen as major obstacles to change in reproductive behaviour in Bangladesh. By training and employing younger women from villages as outreach workers, the programme was not only more effective in serving the needs of clients but also provided a vehicle for improving the status of the women employed by the programme (Simmons, Mita and Koenig, 1992; Hong and Seltzer, 1992).

Another country illustration is provided by the work of Knodel and his colleagues in Thailand, a country now well advanced in its fertility transition (Knodel, Chamratrithirong and Debavalya, 1987; Knodel, 1992). In addition to reviewing data taken from surveys taken at various points during that transition, their research drew on qualitative information acquired through focus groups designed to provide deeper insight into the process of social change than survey data could show. They emphasize the pervasiveness of the reproductive revolution across a broad spectrum of Thai society and report that the least educated, recently married rural women expressed only slightly higher family size preferences than the best educated urban women. The Thai experience reinforces the point made in reference to Bangladesh, about how social change and programme efforts reinforce each other. After an initial stage in which family planning expanded on the basis of existing latent demand, there follows a period during which increases in birth control practice and changes in the views of couples about the possibility and appropriateness of family limitation may themselves stimulate reductions in desired family size and contribute to further increases in contraceptive use and declines in fertility. Thus, changes in the propensity to transform family size preferences into appropriate behaviour may be more important than changes in the preferences themselves (Knodel, 1992).

In Latin America, where modernization (in terms of urbanization and educational attainment) was more advanced when fertility transitions began, the experience also shows important interactions between programme effort and setting variables. Colombia, now well advanced in its fertility transition, had a total fertility rate in excess of 6.0 births per woman in the mid-1960s. At that time, the fertility rate for women with a complete primary education was 3.9, compared with 7.15 for women with less than completed primary education. Only 16 per cent of girls aged 12-17 were in secondary school (Birdsall, 1979).

Between 1965 and 1990, Colombia mounted one of the most successful efforts to expand family planning services for all segments of its population. Contraceptive use has expanded to all levels of society, as have other social services. By 1990, the proportion of girls aged 12-17 years in secondary school had increased to

56 per cent. Total fertility among women with a second-ary education had fallen to 2.4 births per woman. However, the fertility rate for women with no education had declined to 4.9 and for those with an incomplete primary education to 3.6 births per woman. What this finding demonstrates is that improved educational attainment and expansion of family planning contributed to increased contraceptive use and fertility decline. By providing subsidized services to less educated women, the programme brought the health and welfare benefits of smaller families to groups that would not have had them under a strategy that simply left the process to the market and the hope that improved education of future generations would complete the fertility transition (Population Reference Bureau, 1992).

These processes of change are clearly more complex and richer in social and cultural detail than can be described in a brief synopsis. The point of sketching them is to ask whether analyses of cross-sectional survey compiled at one point during the process are likely to provide much information about them. These analyses will surely show the high correlations between educational attainment, fertility levels, use of contraception and the role of other intermediate variables. But they are unlikely to tell much about how efforts to expand services and motivate potential users affected change over time.

To be effective in accelerating fertility declines in developing countries, the allocation of resources among social sectors needs to be informed by research that will help programmes focus on reinforcing the links between social change, family planning programme effort and reproductive behaviour. Research strategies based on a priori logic in which social change and programme effort influence fertility independently of each other does not provide such guidance. They also ignore promising approaches that enrich understanding of these linkages.

D. CONCLUSIONS AND RECOMMENDATIONS

Debate about the relative importance of "supply" and "demand" factors is not likely to disappear. It is hoped that discussion can again move from stereotypical extremes to understanding that provides effective guidance to social policy. Far from being effective, extreme views are more often misleading. It may be amusing to imagine the zealous supply advocate flying around in a helicopter dropping pills and condoms on villagers and expecting them to have fewer children in response, and equally amusing to imagine the naïve demand advocate designing curricula for more educated couples to perform mind-over-matter exercises with their reproductive systems to enable them to control their fertility without contraceptive methods, but neither stereotype does much to promote understanding of how social policy may affect fertility transitions.

Social policy is concerned with the policies and programmes to bring about positive social changes and with the allocation of resources to activities that affect such changes. In particular, it decides how public sector subsidies should be directed to achieve socially desirable goals, such as increasing educational attainment and enabling individuals to control reproduction so that they can achieve the health and welfare benefits of a smaller family and society can benefit from slower population growth rates. Social policy directed to accelerating the transition to lower fertility has been most effective when informed by understanding of the synergistic relations between measures to increase access to high-quality family planning services and those broader social and economic conditions which affect both the capacity to provide and the motivation to use such services. Furthermore, these relations are more likely to be dynamic than static, so that interaction between "supply" and "demand" factors in shaping family planning behaviour can be expected to shift as societies move through their transition from high to low fertility.

In the early stages in the transition, the direction of fertility policy requires an assessment of how much latent or potential demand for services exists and how it can be translated into actual use of services if they were made available. Supply-oriented strategies focus on that objective. But planners also need to think ahead to how conditions could change as those initial objectives are accomplished and society advances into more mature stages of the fertility transition. Experience has shown that high-quality services generate additional demand for family planning. At the same time, investments in human resource development, particularly female education, will increase motivation for smaller families but have a longer gestation period for effects to occur. Those investments need to be made early in order for that expectation to be met. This need is borne out by the experience of such countries as Indonesia, which put a lot of effort into increasing the supply of family planning in the early stages of its fertility transition but also invested heavily in education, so that increases in educational attainment played an increasingly important reinforcing role as that country moved into the middle stages of the transition.

At the same time, access to contraception will remain an issue for social policy throughout the fertility transition and even after it has been completed. This is particularly the case when family planning is considered in the context of the broader range of health services. Again, the issues are not static. The challenges shift from actuating latent demand to meeting growing levels of stated demand, maintaining quality of services and extending access to poorly served groups. Questions about the division of labour between the public sector and the private market in the financing and provision of such services take on greater significance than they had in those early latent-demand stages when subsidies were directed actualizing that demand. Although some societies may share the view that the public sector should always be the main provider/financier of family planning, issues of resource scarcity and social philosophy may require consideration of alternative approaches that seek to direct public subsidies to underserved groups and towards reduction in bottlenecks that inhibit effective allocation of resources in this sector by the private market.

Here again, policy needs to be informed about the synergistic relations between use of family planning and the larger social context in which contraceptive choices are made. This understanding would be a lot easier if the fertility transition and broader social changes that affect it took place in an even, orderly fashion across all groups in a society. Unfortunately, that does not usually happen. Some groups lead, others follow. The benefits of expanded access to both education and family planning typically accrue to groups in a relatively privileged position—the sons and daughters of the educated are more likely to be in school. Fertility decline and use of contraception also start among more educated groups.

Enlightened social policy seeks, in general, to increase access to education and other social services, including family planning services, for less privileged groups. The experience of such countries as Bangladesh has shown that family planning services and fertility decline can be extended to less educated women and that efforts to do this have social and economic effects that reach well beyond influencing reproductive behaviour. One of the most important of the benefits has been enabling less educated parents to keep their sons and daughters in school longer.

Social policy often has to cope with the reality of allocating scarce public sector resources among apparently competing objectives. It is important to remember that this competition is at the level of public sector decision makers and not at the level of individual behaviour. If, in the process of attempting to inform public sector decision-making about linkages between "supply" and "demand" factors in family planning, research strategies focus only on this competition and fail to capture the real-world synergies that drive reproductive and human resource investment behaviour, they will be of little use for policy.

In the regard, cross-sectional studies at either the cross-national or cross-household level need to be interpreted with a great deal of caution. Both concern outcome measures (total fertility, contraceptive use, educational attainment) that are of great interest to social planners. Although they are relatively inexpensive and often appealing in their intuitive simplicity, they can miss many if not most of the very significant and yet complex changes in reproductive behaviour that have been taking place in the developing countries over the past two decades. They often blur differences between social classes with changes that are occurring within social groups over time. The desire to quantify changes and test for statistical significance of explanatory factors leaves out many of the qualitative aspects of these changes. Well-informed social policy can be guided by indicative findings, but their significance needs to be viewed against more qualitative approaches that sift evidence about changes from a variety of sources, including those which are more sensitive to individual and cultural nuance than questions in sample surveys and vital statistics data.

Lastly, there is need to stop talking as if family planning programmes and female education were mutually exclusive alternative approaches in social policy to accelerate fertility transitions. Both are worthwhile in being cost-effective and in bringing enormous benefits to individuals and societies. Their effects differ in timing but are still reinforcing. The most important contribution of research to policy is in identifying these interrelations and translating findings about them into concrete recommendations about where most effectively to target the subsidies that will increase the access of women and men in developing countries to both.

REFERENCES

Birdsall, Nancy (1979). *Fertility Declines in a Developing Economy: The Case of Colombia.* Population and Human Resources Department Working Paper. Washington, D.C.: The World Bank.

Bongaarts, John (1978). A framework for analyzing the proximate determinants of fertility. *Population and Development Review* (New York), vol. 4, No. 1 (March), pp. 105-132.

_____ , W. Parker Mauldin and James F. Phillips (1990). The demographic impact of family planning programs. *Studies in Family Planning* (New York), vol. 31, No. 6 (November/December), pp. 299-310.

Boulier, Brian (1985). Family planning programs and contraceptive availability: their effects on contraceptive use and fertility. The Effects of Family Planning Programs on Fertility in the Developing World, Nancy Birdsall, ed. World Bank Staff Working Papers, No. 677. Washington, D.C.: The World Bank.

Church, Cathleen A., with assistance of Judith Geller (1989). *Lights! Camera! Action! Promoting Family Planning with TV, Video, and Film.* Population Reports, Series J, No. 38. Baltimore, Maryland: The Johns Hopkins University, Population Information Program.

Cleland, John, and Christopher Wilson (1987). Demand theories of the fertility transition: an iconoclastic view. *Population Studies* (London), vol. 41, No. 1 (March), pp. 5-30.

_____ , and James Phillips (1992). The determinants of reproductive changes in Bangladesh. Discussion draft. Washington, D.C.: The World Bank.

Cochrane, Susan H. (1979). *Fertility and Education: What Do We Really Know?* World Bank Occasional Papers, No. 26. Baltimore, Maryland; and London: The Johns Hopkins University Press.

Demeny, Paul (1992). Policies seeking a reduction of high fertility: a case for the demand side. *Population and Development Review* (New York), vol. 18, No. 2 (June), pp. 321-332.

Easterlin, Richard A., and Eileen M. Crimmins (1985). *The Fertility Revolution: A Supply-Demand Analysis.* Chicago, Illinois: The University of Chicago Press.

Freedman, Ronald, and Ann K. Blanc (1992). Fertility transition: an update. *International Family Planning Perspectives* (New York), volume 18, No. 2 (June), pp. 44-50.

Gallen, Moira, and Ward Reinhart (1986). *Operations Research: Lessons for Policy and Programs.* Population Reports, Series J, No. 31. Baltimore, Maryland: The Johns Hopkins University, Population Information Program.

Gertler, Paul J., and John W. Molyneaux (1992). Economic opportunities, program inputs and fertility decline in Indonesia. Prepared for a World Bank review of population policies in Asia. Santa Monica, California: Rand Corporation.

Gilluly, Richard H., and Sidney H. Moore (1986). *Radio—Spreading the Word on Family Planning.* Population Reports, Series J, No. 32. Baltimore, Maryland: The Johns Hopkins University, Population Information Program.

Hong, Sawon, and Judith Seltzer (1992). The impact of family planning on women's lives: a conceptual framework and research agenda. Discussion draft. Washington, D.C.: United States Agency for International Development.

Jejeebhoy, Shireen (1992). Women's education, fertility and the proximate determinants of fertility. Paper prepared for the United Nations Expert Group Meeting on Population and Women, Gaborone, Botswana, 22-26 June 1992.

Knodel, John (1992). Fertility decline and children's education in Thailand: some macro and micro effects. Research Division Working Papers, No 40. New York: The Population Council.

_____ , Aphichat Chamratrithirong and Nibhon Debavalya (1987). *Thailand's Reproductive Revolution.* Madison, Wisconsin: The University of Wisconsin Press.

Mauldin, Parker W., and John A. Ross. (1991). Family planning programs: efforts and results, 1982-89. *Studies in Family Planning* (New York), vol. 22, No. 6 (November/December), pp. 350-367.

Mitra, S. N., Charles Lerman and Shahidul Islam (1992). *Bangladesh Contraceptive Prevalence Survey 1991: Key Findings.* Dhaka: Mitra & Associates.

Phillips, James F., and others (1992). *Worker-client Exchanges and Contraceptive Use in Rural Bangladesh.* Research Division Working Papers, No. 32. New York: The Pulation Council.

Population Reference Bureau (1992). *Fertility and Family Planning in Latin America: Challenges of the 1990s.* Washington, D.C.

Pritchett, Lant (1992). Fertility, population growth and economic performance. Draft working paper. Washington, D.C.: The World Bank.

Psacharopoulos, George, and Sandra Rosenhouse (1992). Population growth, education and employment in Latin America: with an illustration from Bolivia. Paper presented at the United Nations Expert Group Meeting on Population Growth and Economic Structure, Paris, 16-20 November.

Schultz, T. Paul (1992). Modern economic growth and fertility: is aggregate evidence credible? New Haven, Connecticut: Yale University.

Simmons, Ruth, Rezina Mita and Michael A. Koenig (1992). Employment in family planning and women's status in Bangladesh. *Studies in Family Planning* (New York), vol. 23, No. 2 (March/April), pp. 97-109.

Subbarao, Kalanidhi, and Laura Raney (1992). *Social Gains from Female Education: A Cross-national Study.* World Bank Discussion Papers, No. 194. Washington, D.C.: The World Bank.

Summers, Lawrence (1992). The most influential investment. *Scientific American* (New York), vol. 267, No. 2 (August), p. 120.

World Bank (1992). The World Bank and Indonesia's population program. In *Population and the World Bank: Implications from Eight Case Studies.* Operations Evaluations Department Report, No. 10021. Washington, D.C.

77

Part Four

**REVIEW OF EXISTING FAMILY PLANNING PROGRAMMES:
LESSONS LEARNED**

VI. REVIEW OF EXISTING FAMILY PLANNING POLICIES AND PROGRAMMES: LESSONS LEARNED

W. Parker Mauldin[*] and Steven W. Sinding[**]

The objective of this paper is to give a broad overview of the characteristics, strengths and weaknesses of family planning programmes and their impact on contraceptive prevalence and fertility in developing countries, taking into consideration the social and economic conditions in each country. Illustrative examples of important programme initiatives are cited. The last section summarizes the major lessons that have been learned from three decades of organizing and implementing family planning programmes.

Mortality rates began to decline quite rapidly a little more than four decades ago, leading to high rates of population growth. The causes of mortality decline are not firmly established, although there is substantial evidence that both socio-economic development and public-health technology played important roles, each contributing about 50 per cent of the overall mortality decline (Preston, 1980).

Rapid population growth was welcome in many countries and was viewed as a sign of vigour for a number of years. Historically, population size has been regarded as an important determinant of national power—the larger the population, the greater the power potential of a country. However, technological advances have, to a large extent, invalidated this thesis (Choucri, 1974).

The primary response of Governments to rapidly increasing population has been the adoption of population policies designed to reduce rates of fertility and thereby to reduce rates of population growth. An Indian analysis of the impact of population growth on economic development led to the adoption of a population policy in 1952, but, as Raina (1966) notes, ". . .the family planning program should not be concerned in the limited sense of birth control or merely spacing of children. The purpose was ultimately to promote, as far as possible, the growth of the family as a unit of society in a manner

designed to facilitate the fulfilment of those conditions necessary for welfare". However, another decade and a half elapsed before a sizeable number of countries adopted policies to reduce rates of population growth.

A. EASTERN AND SOUTH-EASTERN ASIA[1]

Eastern and South-eastern Asia[2], which are refered to here as Eastern Asia for convenience, had a population of about 850 million in 1950; by 1990, the population had doubled to 1,700 million. It had a gross national product (GNP) per capita of only $156 in 1960, but this figure increased by a factor of four to $675 in 1990 (table 3). Several countries or areas in that region have a per capita GNP of thousands of dollars, aside from Hong Kong and Singapore, in which it is more than $11,000. In each of these cases, there have been dramatic increases in income since 1960, often increases of 10-fold or more. Adult literacy increased from 55 to 72 per cent from 1960 to 1985, and enrolment in primary plus secondary schools from 50 to 76 per cent (figure 1). Life expectancy increased from 49 in 1960-1965 to 67 in 1985-1990, and the infant mortality rate (IMR) dropped during the same period from 119 to 43 (table 4 and figure 3). Thus, there have been major improvements in these socio-economic indicators. (See tables 3 and 4 for comparative data on selected socio-economic indices, by region, and table 5 for data on contraceptive prevalence and strength of family planning programmes, by region).

During the 1960s, many of the countries or areas in Eastern Asia adopted policies to reduce their rates of population growth and gradually developed well-organized and vigorous family planning programmes. The region is well advanced in its transition to low fertility. In 1960-1965, the average number of children born to a woman was 5.9; in 1985-1990, it was 2.75, a decrease of 53 per cent, or a decrease of 83 per cent towards

[*]Consultant to Population Sciences, The Rockefeller Foundation, New York, United States of America.
**Director, Population Sciences, The Rockefeller Foundation, New York, United States of America.

TABLE 3. ADULT LITERACY AND PRIMARY- PLUS SECONDARY-SCHOOL ENROLMENT,
1960 AND 1985; AND PERCENTAGE OF MALES IN THE NON-AGRICULTURAL,
LABOUR FORCE AND GROSS NATIONAL PRODUCT PER CAPITA, 1960 AND 1990

	Percentage literate		Percentage primary- plus secondary-school enrolment		Percentage males aged 15-64 in non-agricultural labour force		Gross national product per capita	
	1960	1985	1960	1985	1960	1990	1960	1990
Africa	18	46	24	49	22	35	466	477
Eastern Africa	14	50	27	49	15	29	275	215
Middle Africa	24	53	28	60	22	46	430	464
Southern Africa	56	72	46	75	56	58	1 442	2 421
Western Africa	12	38	14	38	22	33	438	355
Arab States	18	45	34	65	32	68	621	1 765
Asia	35	60	44	65	28	37	160	531
Eastern and South-eastern Asia	55	72	50	76	29	37	156	675
Eastern Asia	67	69	60	78	30	35	124	607
South-eastern Asia	53	78	45	74	23	46	278	924
Southern Asia	26	42	26	47	27	37	165	437
Latin America and the Caribbean	66	82	58	79	42	69	1 053	2 144
Caribbean	67	84	64	82	43	71	1 275	1 380
Central America	61	81	50	72	35	59	878	2 182
South America	67	83	59	83	44	73	1 086	2 212
Least developed countries	18	40	16	40	14	32	172	211

Source: The Population Council data bank.

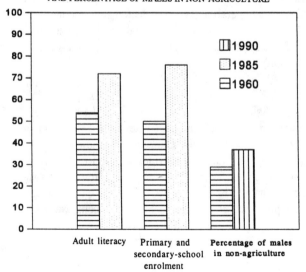

FIGURE I. EASTERN AND SOUTH-EASTERN ASIA: ADULT
LITERACY, PRIMARY- PLUS SECONDARY-SCHOOL ENROLMENT
AND PERCENTAGE OF MALES IN NON-AGRICULTURE

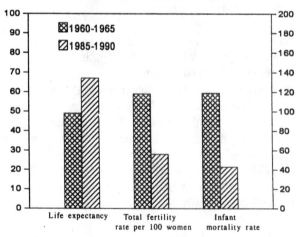

FIGURE II. EASTERN AND SOUTH-EASTERN ASIA: LIFE
EXPECTANCY, TOTAL FERTILITY RATES AND INFANT MORTALITY
RATES, 1960-1965 AND 1985-1990

NOTE: left scale: life expectancy, total fertilty rate per 10 women;
right scale, infant mortality rate

TABLE 4. LIFE EXPECTANCY, INFANT MORTALITY AND TOTAL FERTILITY RATES, BY REGION, 1960-1965 AND 1980-1985

	Life expectancy		Infant mortality rate		Total fertility	
	1960-1965	1985-1990	1960-1965	1985-1990	1960-1965	1985-1990
Africa	41	51	165	109	6.7	6.6
Eastern Africa	41	50	157	114	6.9	6.8
Central Africa	40	50	163	98	6.0	6.2
Southern Africa	49	60	131	76	6.5	4.7
Western Africa	40	49	181	112	6.9	6.9
Arab States	46	59	160	79	7.1	5.6
Asia	48	63	134	74	5.9	3.5
Eastern and South-eastern Asia	49	67	119	43	5.9	2.8
Eastern Asia	50	69	118	32	5.9	2.4
South-eastern Asia	47	62	121	63	5.9	3.7
Southern Asia	45	57	157	102	6.0	4.7
Latin America and the Caribbean	57	67	100	54	6.0	3.6
Caribbean	59	69	97	44	5.4	2.9
Central America	57	68	94	47	6.8	3.9
South America	57	66	104	59	5.8	3.5
Least developed countries	40	50	167	122	6.6	6.2

Source: The Population Council data bank.

TABLE 5. FAMILY PLANNING PROGRAMME EFFORT SCORES, 1972, 1982 AND 1989; AND
CONTRACEPTIVE PREVALENCE, 1990, BY REGION

	Family planning programme effort						Contraceptive Prevalence 1990
	1972	1982	1989	1972	1982	1989	
	(unit weights)			(weight by # F_{15-49})[a]			
Africa	3	14	35	4	13	38	12
Eastern Africa	4	15	36	5	15	37	9
Central Africa	2	11	28	5	11	31	11
Southern Africa	0	20	47	0	19	59	52
Western Africa	3	12	33	4	13	38	7
Arab States	7	18	27	14	24	38	26
Asia	37	46	53	65	70	75	56
Eastern and South-eastern Asia	42	48	52	72	77	80	69
Eastern Asia	49	55	57	81	83	85	74
South-eastern Asia	39	42	48	44	58	65	54
Southern Asia	27	41	56	53	59	68	39
Latin America and the Caribbean	32	39	52	17	47	49	63
Caribbean	47	49	59	43	49	57	50
Central America	35	41	61	19	59	73	55
South America	30	39	52	17	47	49	63
Least developed countries	3	15	33	5	24	41	16

Source: The Population Council data bank.
[a] Weight by number of women aged 15-49 years.

or below. In Singapore, the total fertility rate (TFR) decreased from 4.93 in 1960-1965 to 1.8 in 1985-1990, and its population policy has shifted from efforts to decrease population growth in the 1970s to its current policy of increasing growth. Hong Kong, the Republic of Korea and Taiwan Province of China have below-replacement fertility, and Thailand reduced its TFR from more than 6.0 in 1960-1965 to about 2.1 in the late 1980s.

Since the 1960s, several other countries in the region have adopted policies to lower fertility, including the large countries of China and Viet Nam. The combined population of countries that now seek to lower fertility is more than 1.5 billion, or about 92 per cent of the population of developing countries in that region.

Countries or areas with family planning programmes that are rated as "strong" include China, Hong Kong, the Republic of Korea, Taiwan Province of China, Thailand and Viet Nam; in addition, the Philippines has a "moderately strong" family planning programme (Mauldin and Ross, 1991).

The family planning programmes have varied considerably in organizational structure and in their modes of operation. Indonesia has had:

". . . continuing strong government support from the President and through him the whole administrative structure. Because of this, plus its effective leadership, BKKBN (the National Family Planning Coordinating Board) has successfully engaged support from many ministries and agencies, including health, education, religion, home and defense." (World Bank, 1992).

BKKBN is a coordinating agency and does not deliver family planning services itself, although it is very much involved in information, education and communications (IEC), and in "motivation". BKKBN has been successful in working with religious leaders, asking for their advice, and keeping them informed about planned activities.

In most countries throughout the world, ministries of health have primary responsibility for family planning programmes, but in the Republic of Korea and Taiwan Province of China, for example, family planning was the responsibility of newly created units within the ministries of health. Thus, those countries or areas had

vertical family planning programmes, which were very successful. Both used research extensively, trying out new approaches in relatively small areas and applying what was learned to the national programme.

Other lessons learned from the experiences in this region are discussed below.

Carefully designed and well-executed family planning demonstration programmes have important influences on population policies and on the adoption of elements in national programmes (Freedman and Takeshita, 1969; Cernada, 1970; Bang, 1966; Phillips, 1988).

As Freedman and Berelson point out, "...any method that extends acceptability through its intrinsic attractiveness is obviously a valuable adjunct, and particularly when it is able to generate its own programmatic activity or delivery system expansion...." (1976, p. 12). This double advantage of new methods—their acceptability and their appeal to administrators—led to the introduction of additional methods in many programmes.

A case in point is the Republic of Korea (Kim, Ross and Worth, 1972), which had a programme at the health-centre level before the introduction of intra-uterine device (IUD) technology. A programme and policy were established in late 1961, and during the next two years the programme provided vasectomy with about 20,000 procedures per year, a very low acceptance rate. It also distributed large quantities of foam, spermicides and condoms. These contraceptives were distributed quite liberally, partially for publicity purposes, to establish that the new programme was under way. However, the numbers of acceptors were quite moderate.

Then in 1964, with the introduction of IUD, the Government (not just the Ministry of Health and Social Affairs but the Economic Planning Board and the highest levels of government) saw the intrinsic potential of the new method. It decided to establish a comprehensive IUD programme and quickly expanded the national programme by training and assigning 1,473 fieldworkers at the *myun* or township level.

In the first year, more than 100,000 IUDs were inserted; in the second year, 225,000; and in the third year, 380,000, thus approximately doubling the number each year. In 1967, there was a deliberate reduction to about 300,000 to ensure quality of care. Thus, in four years about 1.0 million out of 3.8 million married women of reproductive age (MWRA), or more than 25 per cent, accepted the use of IUDs. An even more impressive figure is that by late 1969 one third of all MWRA had tried IUD.

In the present authors' view, any reasonably objective observer would credit these results to the introduction of a new technology in a strong family planning programme. IUD had a strong appeal to individuals and to the Government—stimulating it to increase greatly the numbers of programme personnel and also service points (largely through an arrangement with private physicians using a coupon system with a small reimbursement). At that time, per capita income was extremely low; and, again, few observers would argue that in such a short time span there would have been sufficient socio-economic progress to produce similar results.

As the programme history in the Republic of Korea continued, there was further evidence of the importance of technology. The pill was introduced in 1968 for IUD drop-outs only and then in 1969 for everyone. It produced yet another programme expansion, with distribution extended down to village depots and mother's clubs. Thus, in this second phase it exemplified the observation of Freedman and Berelson.

The number of acceptances of pills was quite large, as Kim, Ross and Worth (1972) document, with continued substantial percentages using IUD. Simultaneously, some 150,000 couples per month were using conventional contraceptives, mainly condoms.

Simplified sterilization procedures were introduced in the mid-1970s. This procedure in turn led to many more service points, as laparoscopic equipment (through donors) was dispersed widely throughout the country. A steady growth in the number of sterilizations followed. The simplified technology included both laparoscopes and minilaparotomy, permitting out-patient sterilization with local anaesthesia and at many more locations than before. The response was appreciable and when added to that for the other methods resulted in very rapid increases in the proportions of couples adopting and using contraception. Another boost was given to the number of sterilizations around 1982 when incentives for acceptances were greatly increased (Mauldin and Ross, 1989).

In the following discussion, little attention has been given to the dramatic success of China in lowering fertility, because of its unique political system and the authors' belief that lessons learned from that programme probably are not exportable to countries with very different political systems.

B. Southern Asia[3]

The population of Southern Asia was 481 million in 1950 and currently is more than 2.5 times that number, or 1,200 million. Its people are poor; their per capita GNP was only $165 in 1960 and $437 in 1990. The Islamic Republic of Iran is the only country in the region with a per capita GNP above $500 (it was estimated to be $12,490 in 1990). Adult literacy has increased appreciably from its low level of 26 in 1960 but, at 42 per cent in 1985, remains considerably below the 50 per cent mark. Primary- plus secondary-school enrolment parallels the adult literacy rates; 26 per cent in 1960; and 47 per cent in 1985. There has been some shift in the labour force from agriculture to non-agriculture, but almost two thirds of males aged 15-64 in the labour force are in the agricultural sector (figure 3). Life expectancy is quite low at 57 years, although this represents an increase of 12 years from the period 1960-1965. Infant mortality has decreased by more than one third, from 157 in 1960-1965 to the still high figure of just over 100 in 1985-1990 (figure 4).

There have been significant improvements in a number of socio-economic indicators during the past three decades, but the peoples of the region remain poor, large proportions are illiterate and school enrolment ratios are low. Infant mortality remains high and life expectancy low. This is a region with more than twice the population of sub-Saharan Africa, and its peoples are as illiterate, unschooled and poor as those of Africa.

All but one of the countries in Southern Asia say that their rates of population growth are too high, and all but one of these countries have adopted policies to reduce rates of population growth. Afghanistan reports that its rate of growth is too high but has not taken steps to lessen the rate of growth. Bhutan states that its rate of population growth is satisfactory and no intervention is needed. Despite their poverty and low standing on socio-economic indicators, Bangladesh and India have developed "strong" family planning programmes; the use of contraception has increased to a level of about 40 per cent in Bangladesh and 45 per cent in India. Fertility fell by more than one child per woman from

85

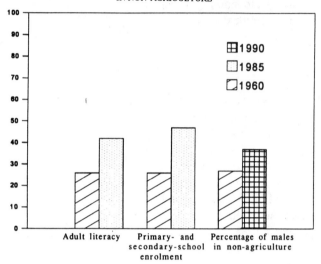

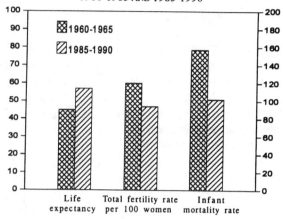

NOTE: Left scale: life expectancy, total fertilty rate per 10 women;
right scale: infant mortality rate.

1960-1965 to 1985-1990, but is about 4.8 in Bangladesh and 4.0 in India.

Sri Lanka is also poor in economic terms, although less so than Bangladesh and India; their per capita GNPs are 470, 350 and 310, respectively. However, Sri Lanka has a higher life expectancy (70), lower IMR (28), higher adult literacy (87), higher primary- plus secondary-school enrolment (83) and significantly lower TFR (2.67). In the region as a whole fertility decreased from 6.0 to 4.7 children between 1960-1965 and 1985-1990, a decline of 22 per cent. The demographic transition has begun, but the pace of decline of fertility in the future is uncertain.

For the most part, ministries of health (or of health and population welfare) have responsibility for population activities in countries in Southern Asia. Pakistan is the exception. Pakistan has had a policy to reduce rates of population growth since 1960, but accomplishments of the programme to date have been disappointing. Changes in political leadership and lack of high-level support for the family planning programme during the 1970s and 1980s are cited as the principal barriers to the development of a strong programme. There have been several changes in the administrative structure of the programme. It has variously been the primary responsibility of the Ministry of Health, the Planning Commission and currently the Ministry of Population Welfare. There is currently a renewed emphasis on family planning in Pakistan, and ambitious plans have

been developed to increase contraceptive prevalence from 12 per cent in 1990 to about 30 per cent by the end of this decade.

C. LATIN AMERICA AND THE CARIBBEAN[4]

The population of Latin America and the Caribbean grew at an average annual rate of 2.5 per cent from 1950 to 1990, increasing from 165 million to 448 million. At the beginning of this period, the growth rate was about 2.75 per cent per annum, but it has decreased to a current level of about 2 per cent per annum. Its per capita GNP is much higher than that of developing countries in other major areas, averaging just over $1,000 in 1960 and $2,144 in 1990. It also ranks higher on many other socio-economic indices than do other less developed regions of the world. In 1985-1990, life expectancy was about 67 years, IMR was 54, the adult literacy rate was 82 and the enrolment ratio in primary plus secondary schools was 79. A large majority of males in the labour force were in non-agriculture, 69 per cent (figures 5 and 6).

There are relatively small differences in adult literacy and life expectancy between the Caribbean, Central America and South American. Adult literacy varies from 81 to 84 per cent; life expectancy from 66 to 69 years. There are larger differences in primary- plus secondary-school enrolment, with Central America ranking lowest at 72 per cent. Central America also has

FIGURE V. LATIN AMERICA: ADULT LITERACY, PRIMARY-PLUS SECONDARY-SCHOOL ENROLMENT AND PERCENTAGE OF MALES IN NON-AGRICULTURE

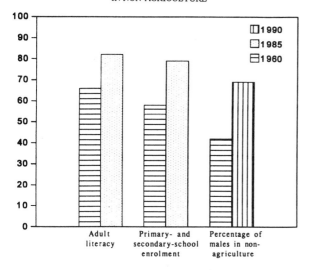

FIGURE VI. LATIN AMERICA: LIFE EXPECTANCY, TOTAL FERTILITY RATES AND INFANT MORTALITY RATES, 1960-1965 AND 1985-1990

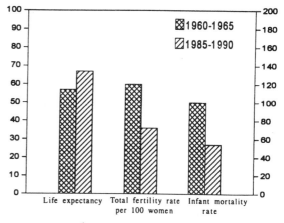

NOTE: Left scale: life expectancy, total fertility rate per 10 women; Right scale: infant mortality rate.

the lowest proportion of males in non-agricultural employment, 59 per cent, compared with 71 and 73 per cent for the Caribbean and South America. The Caribbean ranks lowest on per capita income, $1,380, compared with about $2,200 for Central and South America.

Countries containing more than half the population of Latin America and the Caribbean consider that their fertility rates are satisfactory and that no intervention is appropriate (United Nations, 1992); however, each of these countries provides direct support for contraception, except Argentina, which provides indirect support. Twelve countries in the major area, with about 37 per cent of the population, say that their fertility rates are too high and have adopted policies to reduce them. Most of their family planning programmes are scored as "moderately strong", although El Salvador and Mexico are ranked as "strong" and Haiti as "weak."

TFR in Latin America and the Caribbean is 3.57, a decrease of 2.39, or 40 per cent, from 5.96 in 1960. TFR is lowest in the Caribbean (2.9) and highest in Central America (3.9), with South America having a rate of 3.5. Bolivia has the highest fertility rate in the region, 6.06; and Cuba the lowest, 1.83.

The primary impetus to adoption of policies to reduce fertility in Latin America and the Caribbean has come from the medical profession, whereas in other major areas, and also in Mexico, the major stimulus has come from economists. Physicians in Latin America have

been greatly concerned about the large number of septic abortion cases and the number of hospital beds that they occupy. Politicians were slow to react, to some considerable extent because of concerns about the opposition of the official Catholic Church to "artificial" methods of contraception. Private family planning associations, particularly Profamilia in Colombia, as well as the Association of Medical Faculties (ASCOFAME), also in Colombia, have played a very important role in advancing the cause of family planning, and also in the provision of services (Ott, 1977). Mexico has a strong social security system; and it, as well as the Ministry of Health, has provided contraceptive services to its members and their families. Contraceptive prevalence is relatively high throughout most of the major area, averaging about 60 per cent. It is very low in Haiti (11 per cent) and low in Guatemala (26 per cent) and Bolivia (31 per cent).

Brazil, the largest country in the major area, with a population of more than 150 million, reduced TFR by 2.69 children per woman, from 6.15 in 1960-1965 to 3.46 in 1985-1990. Its per capita GNP was lower than the average for the area in 1960 but at an estimated $2,680 in 1990 is well above that average. Much of the fertility decline during the past three decades can be attributed to improving socio-economic conditions, although some analysts argue that the plight of the poor has worsened and the poor have adopted family planning and a reduced number of children as a strategy for survival (Berquo, 1980).

D. THE ARAB STATE[5]

The group of Arab States is the smallest in terms of population, 219 million, but it extends over a large area. Two thirds of the population are in Africa and one third in Western Asia. There are a number of quite small, mostly oil-rich, countries in this grouping; Egypt has the largest population (52 million), twice as much as Algeria, Morocco and the Sudan, each of which has a population of 25 million. Data on per capita GNP are not available for a number of these countries, including the Libyan Arab Jamahiriya, the Sudan, Iraq, Kuwait, Lebanon and Oman; their populations are about 30 per cent of the total of the group. Therefore, the averages cited below must be considered rough approximations.

Per capita GNP grew from about $620 in 1960 to $1,765 in 1990, much higher than in Africa and in each of the Asian regions, but somewhat lower than in Latin America and the Carribean. Income per capita is appreciably higher in the Western Asian countries than in the African countries. The adult literacy rate was only 18 in 1960 but increased to 45 in 1985, and the primary-plus secondary-school enrolment ratios almost doubled, rising from 34 in 1960 to 65 in 1985. The male labour force shifted from about two thirds in agriculture in 1960 to about two thirds in non-agriculture in the late 1980s (figures 7). Life expectancy increased from 46 years in 1960-1965 to 59 in 1985-1990, and infant mortality fell from 160 in 1960-1965 to 79 in 1985-1990 (figure 8).

FIGURE VII. ARAB STATES: ADULT LITERACY, PRIMARY-PLUS SECONDARY-SCHOOL ENROLMENT AND PERCENTAGE OF MALES IN NON-AGRICULTURE

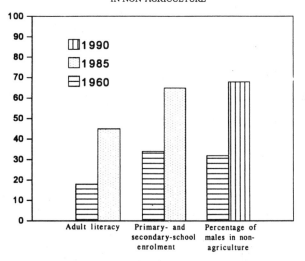

FIGURE VIII. ARAB STATES: LIFE EXPECTANCY, TOTAL FERTILITY RATES AND INFANT MORTALITY RATES, 1960-1965 AND 1985-1990

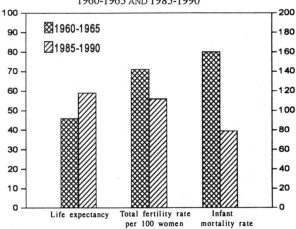

NOTE: Left scale: life expectancy, total fertility rate per 10 women; Right scale: infant mortality rate.

Countries with more than 60 per cent of the population of the group have population policies designed to reduce their rates of fertility, and more than 25 per cent of the people live in countries where fertility rates are considered to be satisfactory, with no intervention needed. Oman and Saudi Arabia, which have TFRs of more than 7.0, say their rates are satisfactory and that intervention to maintain them at this high level is appropriate. Kuwait, with TFR only slightly below 4.0, says its rate is satisfactory but that it is appropriate to intervene to raise the rate.

The average family planning programme in the Arabs States is weak; only Tunisia has a programme that is

rated as strong. Egypt, Lebanon and Morocco, each of which seeks to lower its fertility, are rated as having moderately strong family planning programmes. Algeria has a score only trivially below the cutting point of "moderately strong". However, for the region as a whole, the average programme effort score was only 14 in 1972, 24 in 1982 and 38 in 1989 (figures weighted by the number of MWRA in each country). Using unit weights, the corresponding figures are appreciably lower, 7, 18 and 27, respectively. The family planning programme effort scores are appreciably lower in the Arab countries in Western Asia than in those in Africa. Contraceptive prevalence varies from close to zero for several of the States in the Persian Gulf area to a high of

88

54 in Tunisia, 48 in Egypt, 44 in Algeria and 42 in Morocco. For the region as a whole, contraceptive prevalence averages a rather low 20 per cent.

TFR for the region has fallen by 1.5 children per woman, or 21 per cent, from 7.12 to 5.6, from 1960-1965 to 1985-1990. Thus, both fertility and the natural rate of increase remain high. Only Lebanon, among countries with 1 million or more population, has TFR of fewer than 4.0, and its rate is relatively high at 3.8. The rate of natural increase is 2.8 per cent per annum; accordingly, even if fertility were to decrease substantially in the near future, the population would continue to grow rapidly.

The ministries of health are responsible for the family planning programmes in almost all the countries in the region; however, Egypt is an important exception. Its National Population Council has responsibility for overall planning, and the Ministry of Health is the primary governmental service agency. Egypt has a large number of health outlets, including small hospitals in rural areas, but attendance by medical personnel assigned to the large number of rural health units has been uneven in the past. Pharmacies and non-governmental organizations have played important roles in making contraceptive supplies readily available.

Tunisia developed a strong family planning programme at a relatively early date and has had continuing high level political support for its population programme. It is one of the few countries with a predominantly Muslim population that has legalized abortion. Tunisia reduced TFR from 7.1 in 1960-1965 to 4.4 in the late 1980s, a reduction of almost 40 per cent.

E. SUB-SAHARAN AFRICA

The population of sub-Saharan Africa trebled from 1950 to 1992; and it is increasing at a rate that, if continued, would result in another trebling in about 36 years. Eastern Africa, with a per capita GNP of only $215, is the poorest region in Africa; per capita income has decreased since 1960, when it was $275. Middle and Western Africa rank marginally higher. But overall per capita income has not improved since 1960. (Southern Africa was the most prosperous region in 1960, with a per capita income of $1,442, which increased to more than $2,400 in 1990.) The median incomes in the various regions of sub-Saharan Africa are appreciably lower than these average figures because of a highly skewed income distribution.

Adult literacy has increased appreciably in sub-Saharan Africa during the past 25 years, but at 38 per cent is quite low in Western Africa; it is about 50 per cent in Eastern and Middle Africa and 72 per cent in Southern Africa (figure 9). Primary- plus secondary-school enrolment rates mimic adult literacy rates, in both trends and levels. Outside of Southern Africa, the labour force is overwhelmingly agricultural, despite an appreciable increase in non-agricultural employment during the past quarter century (figure 10).

FIGURE IX. SUB-SAHARAN AFRICA: ADULT LITERACY, PRIMARY-PLUS SECONDARY-SCHOOL ENROLMENT AND PERCENTAGE OF MALES IN NON-AGRICULTURE

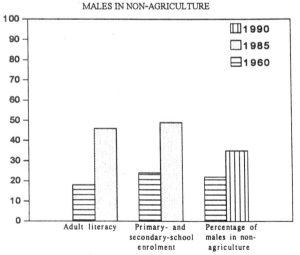

FIGURE X. SUB-SAHARAN AFRICA: LIFE EXPECTANCY, TOTAL FERTILITY RATES AND INFANT MORTALITY RATES, 1960-1965 AND 1985-1990

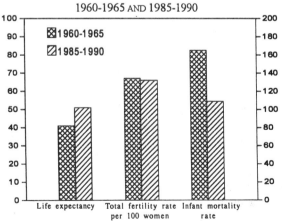

NOTE: Left scale: life expectancy, total fertility rate per 10 women; Right scale: infant mortality rate.

Life expectancy at birth increased about 10 years from 1960-1965 to 1985-1990 in each of the regions but is only 50 years in each region except Southern Africa, where it is 60 years. IMR was more than 150 in 1960-1965, except in Southern Africa, and is currently about 100, again except in Southern Africa where the rate is about 75.

Population policies have been slow to evolve, although currently more than half the people of sub-Saharan Africa live in countries that consider their rates of population growth too high and seek to lower growth. An additional 16 per cent are in countries that consider their rates of population growth to be satisfactory but also intervene to lower their growth rates. The countries in this latter group have rates of natural increase above 3 per cent. Almost one fourth of the people live in countries where rates of population increase, on average, 2.94 per cent per annum, and TFRs are 6.3, but the Governments of these countries say their rate of population growth is satisfactory and that no intervention is appropriate.

Only Botswana has a family planning programme that is rated as "strong", and several countries, including Kenya, South Africa and Zimbabwe, have programmes that are rated as "moderately strong". All other countries in sub-Saharan Africa have programmes that are rated as "weak" or "very weak". Fertility has declined significantly in Botswana, Kenya, South Africa and Zimbabwe, although TFR remains at more than 5.0, except in South Africa. Kenya adopted an anti-natalist population policy in the late 1960s, but its family planning programme was not strongly implemented until the early 1980s. It has had major improvements in adult literacy, primary- plus secondary-school enrolment and infant mortality. To the best of the authors' knowledge, there has not been a reasonably definitive study that assesses the relative contributions of improvements in socio-economic factors and of family planning programmes to the recent decline in fertility, but informed observers credit a substantial part of the drop in Kenyan fertility to the strengthened family planning programme. The situation in Zimbabwe is much the same as in Kenya, with the socio-economic indices being significantly higher in Zimbabwe than in Kenya, but with both countries ranking well above the other countries of the region (except South Africa). The two countries are also similar in the strength of their family planning programmes, each being rated as "moderately strong".

An interesting variation of service delivery called "market-based distribution" was first developed at Ibadan, Nigeria, and has been carried out in other areas of Nigeria and also in Ghana. Market traders, mostly women, are recruited and trained as agents to sell contraceptives, such as condoms and pills, and selected medications. At the close of training they are given a supply of contraceptives, a case to hold them a sign advertising their services and a certificate indicating that they are trained (Bertrand, 1991; Ladipo and others, 1990).

The Africa Operations Research/Technical Assistance Project has developed a methodology for examining the supply side of family planning programmes —situation analysis studies (Fisher, 1992). These studies visit a representative sample of service delivery points (SDPs); studies usually include 100-300 SDPs per country. They maternal and child health and family planning (MCH/FP) staff and clients, observe client-provider interactions and inspect SDPs to determine what supplies and equipment are on hand. These studies are completed in from six to eight weeks of fieldwork using from three to five teams of field researchers made up of nurses, social scientists and supervisors.

Situation analysis studies have uncovered a similar pattern of service delivery in several African countries. Results indicate that approximately 20 per cent of SDPs serve 75 per cent of the clients. For example, in Zimbabwe, 14 per cent of SDPs serve 75 per cent of clients; and in Nigeria, 19 per cent of SDPs serve 75 per cent of clients (figure 11). Although there are some differences, this general pattern appears in all types of facilities, that

FIGURE XI. NIGERIA: PERCENTAGE OF 152 SERVICE DELIVERY POINTS THAT PROVIDED SERVICES TO 47,588 NEW CLIENTS IN 1991

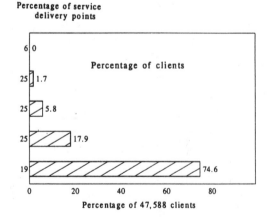

90

is, hospitals and MCH/FP clinics. Analysis to date suggests that clinics that serve a large number of clients are more likely to have: a larger proportion of staff trained in family planning; more types of contraceptives available; IUD services; progesterone-only pills available; signs announcing family planning services and family planning posters; cleanliness in the examination area; a source of water; blood pressure gauges and an examination table.

These studies provide a rapid assessment of many aspects of service delivery. The studies cited underscore the weakness of many programmes, and also the great variability in the effectiveness of different service points. They also provide suggestions to programme managers as to what aspects of the programme need strengthening.

Although fertility remains high in sub-Saharan Africa, and socio-economic variables in general are low, many countries now seek to lower their rates of growth; and as family planning programmes are strengthened,

there is expectation that fertility will fall in a number of other countries during the next decade or two.

F. LEAST DEVELOPED COUNTRIES[6]

The least developed countries are concentrated in sub-Saharan Africa, where there are 22 countries with a population of 1 million or more in this category; the total population of this group of countries is more than 450 million. (The Asia and the Pacific region includes 7 such countries; the Americas only 1, Haiti; and sub-Saharan Africa, 16). Adult literacy is only 39 per cent and primary- plus secondary-school enrolment is 38. Two thirds of the labour force is in agriculture. TFRs in these countries have remained almost constant during the past 25 years and average about 6.1. Per capita income was only $172 in 1960 and improved quite modestly to $211 in 1990 (figures 12). Life expectancy among the least developed countries is only about 50 years, and IMR is more than 120 (figure 13).

FIGURE XII. LEAST DEVELOPED COUNTRIES: ADULT LITERACY, PRIMARY-PLUS SECONDARY-SCHOOL ENROLMENT AND PERCENTAGE OF MALES IN NON-AGRICULTURE

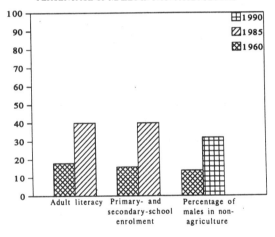

FIGURE XIII. LEAST DEVELOPED COUNTRIES: LIFE EXPECTANCY, TOTAL FERTILITY RATES AND INFANT MORTALITY RATES, 1960-1965 AND 1985-1990

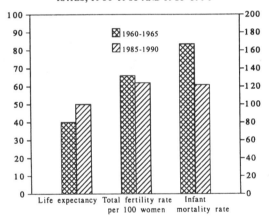

NOTE: Left scale: life expectancy, total fertility rate per 10 women; Right scale: infant mortality rate.

Despite these depressing statistics, which all too accurately reflect the conditions under which the vast majority of people in those countries live, more than 40 per cent of the countries, containing 60 per cent of the population of the entire group, say that their rates of population growth are too high and that intervention to lower rates is appropriate. However, their family

planning programmes are weak, except in Bangladesh and Botswana, whose programmes are strong, and Nepal, whose programme is rated as moderately strong.

Bangladesh is among the most disadvantaged countries in the world. It is very poor; adult literacy and school enrolment rates are low; life expectancy is only

50 years, and IMR is more than 100. Yet TFR fell from about 6.7 in 1960-1965 to 4.8 in the late 1980s, a decline of more than 25 per cent. Bangladesh is an outstanding example of a large, very densely populated, very poor and disadvantaged country that has had continuing high-level political support for its population policies and p rogrammes. In the mid-1970s, Bangladesh developed a broad, multifaceted, strong family planning programme. It has encouraged non-governmental organizations to develop and support their own family planning programmes. The so-called "menstrual regulation" method of uterine aspiration is widely used. Incentives, or compensatory payments, have been offered to clients, service personnel, and (until 1988) to recruiters or motivators, for the acceptance of sterilization and IUDs. Many population projects in Bangladesh have taken a multisectoral approach, using women's programmes, agricultural outreach, community development programmes, communication and broadcasting media and other channels to foster demand for family planning and enhance the availability of services. Eight ministries have been involved in implementing components of the projects, and the National Population Control Council was formed in late 1989 to coordinate their activities (Jain and Nag, 1992).

More than 100 million persons among the least developed countries live in countries that classify their rates of population growth as satisfactory, with no intervention considered appropriate. In these countries, rates of population growth average 2.5 per cent, TFR is 5.4 and IMRs are more than 100. Per capita income is very low, $189.

Prospects for rapid declines in fertility among the least developed countries are poor, except for a small number of countries. The pace of socio-economic improvement has been very slow, and family planning programmes for the most part are weak. Bangladesh and Botswana illustrate what government policies and programmes can accomplish. There is little evidence to suggest that other countries in this group will follow those examples.

G. COSTS AND INCENTIVES

There are many different monetary policies with regard to contraceptives throughout the world. They range from high user charges in some countries, to free contraceptives in many, to monetary incentives and disincentives in others (Ross and Isaacs, 1988; Cleland and Robinson, 1992). A larger number of countries in Southern Asia offer incentives, or compensatory payments, for the adoption of contraception than do countries in any other region—or in all other regions combined. Several countries pay clients for having a sterilization and a few also do so for an IUD insertion (see table 6). A few developing countries charge for all contraceptives, a few charge for some methods but not for others and some provide all methods free of charge. Incentive payments are also offered to service providers for both sterilizations and IUD insertions in a number of countries, and to recruiters in a few countries. Community incentives have been offered in a few instances. These incentives have been offered to mothers' clubs, villages or a local administrative area. Lastly, incentives and disincentives are sometimes offered to the population at large, or to those employed in a given factory or commercial company, with benefits being tied to the *nth* child: salary level; tax exemptions; maternity leaves; eligibility for preferred housing; schools; etc. (David, 1987; Ross and Isaacs, 1988).

China does not offer monetary incentives for the use of contraceptives, although it does bring strong pressure on couples not to have more than one child (in the case of cities) or two (in rural areas), and enacts fines and other penalties for exceeding this number. (In the comparisons given below, China is excluded because of the uniqueness of its family planning programme.) There are about 213 million users of contraceptives in developing countries, and about 75 million users of sterilization and IUDs in the developing countries that provide incentives for use of these methods. Thus, 35 per cent of all users of contraceptives in developing countries use methods for which incentives are paid to clients and/or service providers and/or recruiters. Among the persons that have been sterilized for contraceptive purposes, 71 per cent are in countries that pay incentives for sterilization. Among IUD users, the comparable figure is 52 per cent.

It is difficult to assess the effectiveness of incentive programmes. For example, among the 14 developing countries with contraceptive prevalence rates of 60 per cent or more, about half offer incentives and half do not. Similarly, among developing countries with a population of 40 million or more, about half do and half do not offer incentives. Among countries that have the highest percentage of sterilized couples of reproductive age the story is the same—half do and half do not offer

TABLE 6. DEVELOPING COUNTRIES IN WHICH PAYMENTS ARE GIVEN FOR STERILIZATION AND INTRA-UTERINE DEVICE INSERTION

Major area and country	Clients		Payment to service personnel		Recruiters	
	Sterilization	Intra-uterine device	Sterilization	Intra-uterine device	Sterilization	Intra-uterine device
Africa						
Ethiopia	–	–	x	–	–	x
Lesotho	–	–	–	–	x	–
Sierra Leone	–	–	–	–	–	–
Southern Asia						
Bangladesh	x	x	x	x	–	–
India	x	x	–	–	–	–
Nepal	x	–	x	x	x	–
Pakistan	x	–	x	–	x	–
Sri Lanka	x	–	x	–	–	–
Other Asia						
Indonesia	–	–	x	x	–	–
Republic of Korea	x	–	x	x	x	–
Philippines	–	–	–	–	x	x
Taiwan Province of China	–	–	–	x	x	x
Viet Nam	x	x	–	–	–	–
Latin America and the Caribbean						
Colombia	–	–	x	–	–	–
Dominican Republic.	–	–	x	x	–	–
Dominican Rep. (Profamilia) ...	–	–	x	x	x	x
Paraguay	–	–	x	–	x	–

Source: The Population Council data bank.

incentives. For countries with 10 per cent or more married women of reproductive age using IUDs, only two of nine countries offer incentives. Countries that offer incentives do not differ appreciably from countries that do not on such variables as school enrolment, literacy, life expectancy or percentage of the labour force in agriculture, nor do they differ on levels of contraceptive prevalence. Countries that offer incentives rank somewhat lower on per capita GNP and somewhat higher on IMRs than other countries.

The International Population Conference in 1984 considered incentives and made the following recommendation for further implementation of the World Population Plan of Action:

"Legislation and policies concerning the family and programmes of incentives and disincentives should be neither coercive nor discriminatory and should be consistent with internationally recognized human rights as well as with changing individual and cultural values." (United Nations, 1984, p. 25)

An ethical aspect of cash payments is whether they are so large that they "coerce" the disadvantaged, primarily the poor, into actions that otherwise they would not take. A frequently used argument in favour of payments is that there are costs associated with undergoing voluntary sterilization, for example, costs of travel, food, child care and loss of earnings because of time lost from work. Those costs are sufficiently high that the poorest of the poor often cannot afford them and consequently do not have access to a desired method of contraception in the absence of adequate monetary payments.

In Bangladesh, for example, sterilization clients are paid 175 taka (Tk), about $5.25. This is a relatively trivial sum for persons in the upper middle and upper income classes, but it amounts to several days' wages for an unskilled labourer. Does this amount "coerce" the poor into having a sterilization without adequate knowledge of the consequences of the operation? Studies show that even the poor that elect to have a sterilization say they do not want more children and that they know that having a sterilization means that they cannot have more children.

Recruiters were paid Tk 45 for accompanying a sterilization client to a clinic until 1988, when such payments were discontinued. Usually the "recruiter" was a family member or a government worker; and there is a need for this service, particularly for women in a society where they almost never travel alone. However, these payments led to the creation of self-employed recruiters, who sought out potential clients, almost exclusively men, in places where men were likely to be looking for work. There is some evidence that those recruiters put as much pressure as they could on potential clients to have a sterilization as soon as possible, "today" and did not provide their clients with adequate information about what was involved and about alternative contraceptive methods. In principle, counselling at the clinic corrects deficiencies of the recruiter, and in fact this was usually the case. However, it was decided to discontinue payments to recruiters in order to avoid the possible negative influence of some of the recruiters. On the basis of a number of studies carried out in Bangladesh and discussions with a wide variety of persons in Bangladesh, it was concluded that coercion is very rare or non-existent (Cleland and Mauldin, 1991).

H. EXPERIMENTAL AND DEMONSTRATION STUDIES

Experimental and demonstration studies, and operations research, have been carried out in all regions of the world, and have contributed greatly to policy formation and programme implementation. There have been hundreds of such studies (Mauldin and Ross, 1966; Cuca and Pierce, 1977; Forrest and Ross, 1978; Ross and Forrest, 1978; Ross and Lloyd, 1992), although there have been very, very few with good experimental design, particularly during the past 15 years or so. In 1976, Freedman and Berelson (1976) took note that such pilot, experimental or demonstration projects had been numerous and varied; there were about 40 of some substance and quality, plus probably a few hundred smaller efforts; and they included special efforts of a health, informational, incentive, local-agent, commercial and "intensive" character. Space and time limitations permit a brief description of only a small number of

demonstration or experimental studies, which are illustrative of the more prominent studies.

J. TAIWAN PROVINCE OF CHINA: THE TAICHUNG STUDY

In 1962, the new IUDs, the Lippes loop and Margulies coil, were first introduced into Taiwan Province of China and created new era for the family planning programme (Hsu and Chow, 1966).

The Taichung family planning programme was a unique, large-scale experimental effort to make family planning available quickly to the entire population of an Asian city and to observe the effects systematically (Freedman and Takeshita, 1969). The following materials relating to the Taichung programme are also taken from Freedman and Takeshita.

The principal objectives of the Taichung study were to answer the following major questions:

1. To what extent can the practice of family planning be increased by a massive information and service campaign of short duration?

2. Is it necessary to approach both husbands and wives in an educational programme, or is it enough to approach the wife alone?

3. Can family planning ideas be spread cheaply and quickly by written communication, through the mails?

4. Can direct communication to systematically spaced subgroups of a population indirectly affect a much larger population by diffusion from the initial focuses of direct contact?

5. Does a new method of contraception, IUD, have distinctive advantages in terms of acceptance and diffusion?

6. If there is a significant adoption of family planning, will it accelerate the decline of fertility already begun at Taichung and in Taiwan Province of China?

Four "treatments", ranging from much to little effort, were directed to approximately 36,000 married couples with the wife aged 20-39 years, at Taichung. These treatments were allocated among 2,389 lins, a neighbourhood unit containing about 20 households.

Everything: husband and wife

This treatment entailed personal visits to husbands and wives by trained health workers, mailings of information to newlyweds and to couples with two or more living children and meetings in the neighbourhoods that mixed entertainment and information about family planning, using slides, film strips, flip-charts etc.

Everything: wife only

This treatment was the same as "Everything: husband and wife" except that husbands were not contacted.

Mailings

There were no personal visits (unless requested) or meetings in the neighbourhood; instead, a series of letters and pamphlets were sent to newlyweds and to couples with two or more children. The mailings provided general information on methods, rationale and location of clinics, and included a return mail form for requesting more information or a personal visit from a field worker.

Nothing

No effort was made to reach couples directly. However, posters were distributed throughout the city, and some meetings were held at the *li* level, a neighbourhood unit containing about 350 households.

The city was divided into three sectors, each subject to a different density of effort. For example, in the heavy-density sector each of the "Everything" treatments was allocated to 25 per cent of the *lins*; in the medium-density sector, 17 per cent; and in the light-density sector, 10 per cent.

The intensive experimental programme ran from February to October 1963. By March 1964, acceptances reached 5,453. Some educational efforts were carried out in 1964, and an offer of free IUDs was made in early 1965. By July 1965, there had been 10,776 acceptors of contraception. Among the many findings were:

(*a*) Contacting both the husband and wife had no discernible greater effect than contacting just the wife;

(*b*) Personal contacts increased acceptance;

(*c*) Use of letters did not prove effective;

(*d*) Heavy density of effort led to higher acceptance rates.

This major study led to an island-wide programme that has been extremely successful.

K. REPUBLIC OF KOREA: THE KOYANG/KIMPO STUDIES

Koyang was the experimental area and Kimpo the control; the national family planning programme, which was just beginning, offered services in Kimpo, but there was no accelerated effort there. The action-research field programme was organized and conducted in steps as follows: (*a*) reconnaissance and training (April-July 1962); (*b*) baseline survey of fertility and attitude towards family planning (September 1962); (*c*) education and service programme (from October 1962 to September 1964); and (*d*) after-survey (September 1964) (Bang, 1966).

The purpose of the project was to assess the impact of the intensive Koyang programme as compared with the milder national programme carried out in the Kimpo area. In Koyang, fieldworkers visited each home, group meetings were held and contraceptive supplies were given free of charge. The experiment demonstrated that substantial proportions of rural women would adopt contraception, with about equal proportions being sterilized (or naturally sterile) in the two areas; however, more than twice as many adopted non-surgical contraception in Koyang as in Kimpo. The principal policy finding was that a well-planned family planning programme would result in large proportions of rural women adopting contraception.

L. THAILAND: THE PHOTHARAM STUDY

In August 1964, the Family Health Research Project was initiated in the rural area of Photharam, where fewer than 1 per cent of MWRA had even the vaguest knowledge of contraception. Information about and supplies of contraceptives—IUDs, oral pills, condom and foam tablets—were offered. After six months, 20 per cent of MWRA were using contraceptives (Winich, Hawley and Peng, 1966).

According to Peng:

"Each of the households in the sample was visited by

95

a trained midwife interviewer and an interview was held with one married woman in each household who was 20 to 45 years of age and whose husband was living. . . .

"The action program offers contraceptive information and supplies through six clinics housed in local health installations widely spaced over the district. Two medical teams, each composed of a doctor and two nurses, staff the clinics, spending one to four afternoons per week in each. Their work is supplemented by seven field workers who, through home visits, carry an educational program to the people. The educational program is elaborated with general village meetings and meetings with variously selected groups. Since literacy is low and mass media virtually absent in the district, communication is necessarily by word of mouth." (1965, p. 1).

The early positive results of this study were instrumental in the adoption of a national family planning programme in Thailand.

L. TURKEY: THE ETIMESGUT STUDY

In Etimesgut District, Turkey, within the pattern of the Turkish National Health Services, an integrated health/family planning programme was launched in 1966, using auxiliary nurse-midwives and general practitioners as the primary change agents. Indications of the success of the programme are a decline in total fertility during the period 1969-1973, a significant increase in use of effective contraceptives and a significant decline in infant mortality during 1969-1973 (Fisek, 1974). The district 65,000 inhabitants, 56 per cent of whom were in rural villages and the remainder in towns of 10,000-20,000 population. Medical and paramedical personnel scheduled visits for antenatal care, delivery, post-partum care, child care and family planning. TFR declined from 4.9 in 1967 to 3.3 in 1974, and infant mortality fell from 142 to 93.

M. INDIA: THE ERNAKULAM STUDIES

In 1970, the District Collector in Ernakulam District of Kerala State, India, decided to hold a massive vasectomy camp; and he undertook personal and direct responsibility for the camp. Appeals for assistance in the campaign went to the private sector, voluntary agencies

and local leaders. The entire governmental sector was notified about the camp and they were asked to participate fully. Responsibility for the various components of the campaign was delegated to committees at various levels and operational plans for promoting the campaign, motivating the people and operating the camp were prepared. At this camp, 15,005 vasectomies were performed, setting an all-India record (Soni, 1971). A second camp was held in July 1971, at which 62,913 vasectomies and 505 tubectomies were performed.

Compensation payments at both camps were substantially larger and more varied than the normal cash payment of 21 Indian rupees (Rs) approved by the central Government. Persons that were sterilized received up to Rs 86 at the first camp and up to Rs 114 at the second camp. The camps were promoted as family planning festivals; and the camp site was decorated with lights, pictures, banners and large illuminated red triangles. At the first camp, there were 40 operating booths at the main camp site; for the second camp there were 50 operating booths, with 100 doctors performing the operations.

The results were remarkable, and similar camps were established in other areas under different supervision. In some of these camps, however, less care was taken to ensure high-quality medical care and deaths were reported, bringing an end to the idea of massive sterilization camps.

N. BANGLADESH: THE MATLAB STUDY

Matlab Thana is an administrative division of 280,000 people in a rural area of Bangladesh. Its population density is 2,000 people per square mile. Transport is difficult, mostly by boat, and incomes are low. Fishing and farming are the main activities.

Between 1975 and 1981 the International Centre for Diarrhoeal Disease Research, Bangladesh, conducted two experiments in Matlab Thana to measure the effects of availability, access and quality of family planning services on contraceptive use. Before 1975, family planning services were based in a Government-run centre in Matlab town. A small staff provided a conventional range of contraceptives and IUD insertions but made little attempt to reach out to the villagers, except for two brief house-to-house campaigns conducted nationally. Throughout Bangladesh, an unmet need for contraception clearly existed. A national survey in 1968 no more children and that 13 per cent would consider using contraception, but that only 1.9 per cent were currently using a method.

Contraceptive Distribution Programme

The first of two experiments, the Contraceptive Distribution Programme, from 1975 to 1978, tested the effect of house-to-house distribution of oral contraceptives and, one year later, of condoms. Female workers were given six half-days of training on the proper use of the condom and the pill, and information on adverse symptoms, expected side-effects and simple treatments for them. These workers were mostly elderly, widowed and illiterate women, with almost no personal experience of contraceptives. Beginning in October 1975, they visited each household in the project area of 150 villages. During a visit of 5-10 minutes, women were told about the benefits of spacing and limiting births, the proper use of the pill and possible side-effects. Those that were interested were given a six-month supply of pills. For 30 months, workers were responsible for recruiting users, resupplying them with pills and advising on side-effects.

The impact of the programme was great but short-lived. Contraceptive use in the project area jumped from 1.1 to 17.9 per cent in three months but declined to 11 per cent after two years. During the same period, the rate of contraceptive use outside the project area increased from 2.9 to 3.8 per cent. After a year, 34 per cent of married women in the project area had accepted contraception but only 42 per cent of those women were continuing to use it. Some 10-14 months into the programme, fertility had declined by 11-17 per cent, but this effect lasted only one year. The limited impact of the project was attributed to poor management of side-effects, inadequate training of staff, insufficient information provided to clients, the narrow range of contraceptive methods offered (which discouraged method-switching) and too little supervision.

Family Planning-Health Services Project

In October 1977, a second experiment, the Family Planning-Health Services Project, also tested house-to-house distribution of contraception, but with much better quality of services. Female village workers were recruited locally and received seven weeks of pre-service training and weekly in-service training sessions. They had to be literate, married with children, have

contraceptive experience and come from respected families. The 80 workers (one per 1,000 people in the experimental area) received technical supervision and medical backup from four clinics staffed by qualified women paramedics, and administrative supervision from a male senior health assistant.

The project provided comprehensive services for the special needs of each current and prospective client. The methods offered included not only pills and condoms but also foam tablets and injectables. In addition, women were referred to centres where tubectomy, IUD insertion and menstrual regulation could be performed, and where their husbands could get a vasectomy. All households were visited once a fortnight, regardless of whether couples were using contraceptives. Side-effects were managed through reassurance, frequent method-switching and medical referral for treatment. Workers also provided aspirin, vitamins and iron tablets, thereby gaining access to households that had previously rejected family planning.

In the first three months, contraceptive use in the project area rose from 7 to 21 per cent. Unlike the trend in the earlier project, however, the rate continued to climb slowly to 34 per cent. Continuation rates were dramatically improved: after a year, 39 per cent of eligible women in the project had accepted contraception and 81 per cent of those women were continuing to use it. During the first two project years, fertility declined by from 22 to 25 per cent, compared with villages outside the project area. After a three-year plateau at 34 per cent, contraceptive use began to rise again and at last report was about 60 per cent—almost exclusively based on modern methods, with the injectable Depo-Provera accounting for almost half of contraceptive use. (In the rest of the country in 1983, modern methods accounted for only 14 per cent of contraceptive use.) Tetanus toxoid and oral rehydration therapy have been added to the Matlab project service package but these services do not seem to have been responsible for the increase in contraceptive use.

Replicability

The Family Planning-Health Services Project has been highly effective in increasing contraceptive use in field conditions typical of rural Bangladesh. But it may be hard to replicate on a larger scale because this project was able to draw on extra resources unavailable to the national family planning programme. For example, although fieldworkers in the project receive salaries equivalent to workers in the national programme, their supervisors' salaries are much higher. The project also used costly speedboats to move supervisors and research staff around the area, and management was decentralized to an extent rarely found in national programmes. The managerial and organizational structure that guaranteed close, supportive supervision, worker accountability, continuous training, good record-keeping and continuous feedback to workers should receive much of the credit for project success.

The Government of Bangladesh and the International Centre subsequently embarked on an extension project to transfer some of the management techniques of the Matlab project to government health and family planning workers in several *thanas* in northern Bengal and to measure the impact of these changes on fertility, mortality and contraceptive use. The project was developed to test the results of minimal changes in the national programme structure, with no special input other than for training, organization-building and research.

O. KENYA: CHOGORIA

The Chogoria Hospital Community Health Department provides integrated MCH/FP and curative services in the catchment area of Embu District, Kenya. As reported by Goldberg, McNeil and Spitz:

"The catchment area has an extensive network of family health educators (FHEs) and voluntary community health workers (CHWs), providing family planning and other community health services. Since its inception, the CHD has been distributing family planning methods to women living throughout its catchment area. Family planning services are available both through community-based distribution (CBD) and from integrated-service clinics." (1989, p. 18).

This is neither a demonstration nor an experimental project; rather, it is an unusually successful community-based programme in the provision of family planning services in one area in Kenya. A Community Health Survey was conducted in 1985, and contraceptive prevalence was estimated to be 43 per cent, compared with 17 per cent for all of Kenya one year earlier. Similarly, TFR in the Chogoria area was 5.2, compared with 7.7 in Kenya. Factors thought to be important in the achieve-

ment of this relatively high contraceptive prevalence are: (*a*) an integrated health/family planning programme; (*b*) community involvement in the delivery of services; (*c*) a large network of volunteer workers; (*d*) the widespread availability of contraceptive methods; and (*e*) the rapport the hospital has gained with the people.

P. LESSONS LEARNED

Family planning programmes must do many things in order to be effective (Mauldin and Ross, 1991); therefore, there are many aspects of family planning programmes that could usefully be listed, described and analysed. The authors have chosen to select about a dozen components that have been shown to be important in successful programmes.

Political commitment

Continuing high-level political commitment is very helpful to implementation of family planning programmes (e.g., Bangladesh, China, Indonesia and Kenya). But while it is very helpful, such commitment is not essential; a number of countries or areas have developed strong and successful programmes without overt political support at the highest levels (e.g., the Republic of Korea, Taiwan Province of China, Thailand, Costa Rica and Colombia); and Hong Kong developed a strong programme without ever having adopted a formal policy and without official support. In general, the less conducive the social setting is to economic development and the adoption of family planning, the more important is political commitment. Several Latin American countries have experienced rapid increases in contraceptive prevalence and rapid decreases in fertility without strong political commitment because of the strong desire among their highly literate and low-mortality populations to limit family size.

Leadership

Strong leadership and supervision are important elements in strong and effective family planning programmes, e.g., Indonesia, Taiwan Province of China and Colombia.

Administrative structure

Successful family planning programmes have been developed with quite different administrative structures.

The two principal administrative approaches are: (a) responsibility for planning and implementation of the programme in the Ministry of Health, for example, Cuba and Thailand; (b) a national coordinating board for planning and coordinating the family planning programme, with the Ministry of Health being the primary service delivery agency, for example, Indonesia, Egypt, Kenya and China (in China, however, the State Family Planning Commission also provides a large proportion of family planning services). There are many variations on these two basic approaches. As Berelson noted in 1964, any reasonable organization will work—if it is highly placed enough in the political hierarchy and can attract a first-class director.

Civil bureaucracy

Involvement of the civil bureaucracy adds strength to a family planning programme, particularly in countries where the civil bureaucracy is well organized and reaches into all villages and cities, for example, China and Indonesia. The negative side of this approach is that civil authorities sometimes become overzealous, resulting in undue pressure and even coercion.

Contraceptive availability

The essential requirement of every programme is to ensure that contraceptive services shall be close at hand and accessible for the mass of the population. Unquestionably, the rural populations of most developing countries would use contraception more than they do now if only it were readily available to them (Ross, Rich and Molzan, 1989). Strategies for providing contraceptive services include making them available at the village level, establishing programme outlets at a high density so as to reduce travel time, creating more than one source of supply, authorizing paramedical personnel and midwives to distribute condoms and pills, and stressing high quality of services. Programmes following these principles include those in Colombia, Mexico, the Republic of Korea, Taiwan Province of China and Thailand.

The needs and preferences of individual clients vary over time, and shifting from one method of fertility control to another is typical and for the most part should not be discouraged. Data on continuation rates of specific methods of contraception underestimate the period of use of contraception of an individual or couple. Continued use of contraception by individuals is increased if a number of methods are readily available at affordable prices.

It is important to shift the method mix towards high-continuation methods, both because their use effectiveness tends to be higher than other methods and because the percentage of couples who must be recruited each year declines rapidly as continuation rates increase. Sterilization has the longest continuation of any method; Norplant, which is new and available in only a few countries, has the next best continuation rate, followed very closely by the better IUDs and then the pill.

As Freedman and Berelson state concerning some Asian countries or areas:

"The impact of a new technology upon program uptake is illustrated by a few country programs where a method new to that society was introduced. . . . In Taiwan [Province of China] each new method seemed to add another layer of use to the existing practice, presumably by attracting a new clientele; in South Korea the pill was partly introduced through newly established Mothers' Clubs; in Thailand the large increase in pill use at the end of the 1960s resulted from the administrative decision to allow pill distribution by nurse/midwife field workers without [a] doctor's prescription; in Hong Kong, with relatively easy logistics, there was a deliberate programmatic decision to substitute the pill for the IUD as the method of choice more readily administered, especially to younger women for spacing purposes, and in India the condom added another layer of use to that achieved by the other two methods." (1976, p. 12).

Jain (1989) estimated that the widespread addition of one contraceptive method to the choice of methods in a country would be associated with an increase of about 12 percentage points in the practice of contraception. This increase in contraceptive prevalence, according to the empirical relation between contraceptive prevalence and TFR, would, on average, lead to reduction of 0.8 point in TFR.

Modes of service delivery

There are many channels for delivery of family planning services—hospitals (including post-partum programmes), clinics, home-visiting workers, mobile teams, pharmacies, shops, outlets in industrial companies, community-based distribution (CBD), social marketing etc. The proliferation of types of delivery channels is an outgrowth of efforts to supplement the health infrastructure and also to give clients alternative sources of supply. The key finding is that ready availability of contraceptive methods attracts additional users; thus, in many settings alternative modes of distribution increase use.

Many sample surveys obtain information on sources of supply of contraceptive services and commodities, and information is available on sources of supply for more than 80 per cent of contraceptive users in each region except sub-Saharan Africa, where information is available for 55-60 per cent of all users. Almost all users in Eastern Asia, and three fourths of users in Southern Asia obtain their contraceptive supplies from public sources. The corresponding figures are just under one half in sub-Saharan Africa, a little more than one third in Latin America and the Caribbean and just under 30 per cent in Northern Africa and Western Asia. There does not appear to be any significant shift to the private sector as programmes mature. There have been relatively small shifts towards the private sector for 6 countries, no appreciable change over time for 10 countries and relatively large increasing dependency upon the public sector in 6 countries. Recently, Indonesia instituted a programme designed to increase the role of the private sector, and early reports indicate that this effort is succeeding.

Community-based distribution and social marketing

Community-based distribution programmes recruit local personnel, typically women, to go from door to door offering condoms (and sometimes pills) at subsidized prices. The "distributor" often is permitted to keep a portion of the funds collected. A variation on this system is that a local agent keeps a supply of selected contraceptives in her home and sells them to villagers that come to her home. Social marketing programmes utilize existing commercial outlets, such as small stores, to sell contraceptives at reduced (and subsidized) prices. Community-based distribution and social marketing programmes have been initiated and developed in many countries—70 locations in 40 countries. In general, programmes appear to have been more effective where the CBD worker is able to go to the doorstep, that is, where there is active outreach. Other successful programmes have required that the initial prescription and contraceptive supply be given in a fixed health

facility by more senior personnel, with follow-up by CBD workers at their own homes, from local mothers' clubs or from local "depots". In other programmes, CBD workers have made one or more rounds of home visits to introduce services and give initial supplies, subsequently requiring adoptors to obtain resupplies by going to the home of the CBD worker or to a nearby depot (Ross and others, 1987).

According to Sherris, Ravenholt and Blackburn:

"Contraceptive social marketing programs in 13 countries are now selling condoms, pills, and other family planning supplies at subsidized prices through retail stores. More than a decade of experience has shown that, if contraceptive social marketing (CSM) programs are well-managed, well-publicized, and well-adapted to local conditions, they can reach about 5 to 15 per cent of all couples of reproductive age. In three countries—Bangladesh, Colombia, and Egypt—these programs serve at least 30 per cent of current family planning users. Thus CSM programs can play an important role in meeting family planning needs, along with other family planning programs and conventional commercial sales. In addition, CSM programs are often more cost-effective than other delivery systems." (1985, p. 1).

It should be added, however, that descriptions of contraceptive social marketing programs rarely permit an evaluation of their impact on contraceptive prevalence in a country, or a large area of a country, and cost-effectiveness is not adequately addressed.

Experimental and demonstration studies

An important lesson learned is that national programmes can benefit from special studies. These studies have been carried out to determine the feasibility of introducing family planning into a country; and when results have been positive, policies have been formulated and programmes implemented throughout the country. These experimental and demonstration studies have been used to determine the acceptability of different methods of contraception and the use of paramedical personnel for IUD insertions, prescription of pills etc. The basic lesson learned is that the way to determine whether a given "idea" is workable is to try it in some area before deciding whether it should be introduced throughout the country.

Non-governmental organizations

The non-governmental sector has been particularly important in stimulating Governments to develop population policies and implement programmes. The Planned Parenthood Federation of Korea has developed a close and unique role with the Government, carrying out the IEC functions of the national programme. Private associations have delivered a significant proportion of family planning services in a number of Latin American countries, as well as in Bangladesh, where a large number of non-governmental organizations account for more than 20 per cent of all contraceptive use. In Colombia, the Association of Medical Schools historically and the Profamilia organization in more recent years have contributed greatly to the introduction of family planning and the provision of services.

Incentives or payments

It has been learned that monetary payments for use of specific methods of contraception affect the timing of adoption of a contraceptive method and that increasing the amount of compensation typically leads to an increase in acceptance, particularly among men. Beyond that, however, it is not clear whether monetary payments increase the level of contraceptive prevalence. An unanswerable but intriguing question is: if the same amount of funds spent on payments for the adoption of a contraceptive method had been spent on strengthening other aspects of the programme, such as training, improved supervision, IEC or logistics, would the contraceptive prevalence rate be lower than it is in countries where payments have been made, or would it be as high or higher than it currently is?

An ethical aspect of cash payments is whether they are so large that they "coerce" the disadvantaged, primarily the poor, into actions that otherwise they would not take. As mentioned above, a frequently used argument in favour of payments is that there are costs associated with undergoing voluntary sterilization, for example, costs of travel, food and child care, and loss of earnings because of time lost from work. Those costs are sufficiently high that the poorest of the poor often cannot afford them and consequently do not have access to a desired method of contraception in the absence of adequate monetary payments. In brief, ethical considerations must be taken into consideration when incentives or payments for the adoption of fertility regulation are contemplated.

Q. INFORMATION, EDUCATION AND COMMUNICATION

All family planning programmes use information, education and communication extensively, although the nature of the IEC programmes varies enormously. At the simplest level, as in the Khanna study in India in the late 1950s, communication is person to person—from fieldworkers to prospective clients. More sophisticated programmes use mass media extensively, particularly radio and television. Special campaigns have shown impressive increases in the number of family planning acceptors (Church, 1989; Piotrow and Meyer, 1991; Ross, Rich and Molzan, 1989). However, it is difficult to assess the effectiveness of continuing IEC programmes and activities because many other "efforts" of family planning programmes are under way at the same time. Experience has shown that IEC messages are more effective if they are continuously present in the environment. Furthermore, campaigns reach more people if various types of media, such as radio, television, posters, pamphlets and newspapers, are used. Radio messages are often particularly effective, because radio reaches a wide audience in many developing countries (Ross, Rich and Molzan, 1989).

Costs[7]

Total expenditures on family planning in developing countries in 1990 are estimated to be from $4 billion to 5 billion. Donors provided $971 million, of which $169 million was loans. Individual clients are thought to have spent about the same amount as the donors, with Governments of developing countries contributing the remainder, at least half of the total. For the 18 major donors, population assistance constituted 1.2 per cent of official development assistance in 1990, about the same during the 1980s but lower than the proportion for the 1970s, which was just under 2 per cent of the total. Government expenditures are difficult to estimate because many of their family planning programmes are integrated with broader health services, and buildings and other facilities are shared.

The public sector provides most contraceptive supplies and services, particularly in Asia. The private sector is especially strong in Latin America and the Caribbean, and covers about half of all users. Worldwide, there has not been much movement from the public to the private sector during the past two decades, although Indonesia has embarked upon a much publicized programme to encourage greatly increased reliance upon the private sector.

Many public sector programmes in Asia provide contraception free of charge, such as Bangladesh, China, India and Indonesia (where there is a small charge for sterilization and Norplant). Similarly, contraceptives are given without charge in Colombia, Costa Rica, Ecuador, El Salvador and Mexico; and are provided without charge, except a small fee for sterilization, in the Dominican Republic, Honduras and Panama. In Africa, there is a small charge for most contraceptive methods in a number of countries (e.g., Benin, Botswana, Ethiopia, Ghana, Nigeria and Zaire), but there is no charge for contraceptives in Burundi, Cameroon, Kenya, Mali, Mauritania, Mauritius, Mozambique, Rwanda, Zambia and Zimbabwe. Virtually all programmes seek to make contraceptive methods available to clients either without charge or at a price that is easily affordable.

R. CONCLUSIONS

"Proposition 1. Debate on the question of whether family planning programmes can have a fertility effect is essentially a thing of the past.

"The weight of the evidence is affirmative, and after twenty-five years of experience attention has turned elsewhere, to 'second generation' issues: the relationship between programme strength, social setting and fertility change; and to the manner in which programmes can function in different environments." (Phillips and Ross, 1992, p. 325).

There is an extensive body of literature that assesses the impact of family planning programmes on contraceptive prevalence and fertility (Forrest and Ross, 1978; Ross and Forrest, 1978; Lapham and Mauldin, 1987; Ross and Lloyd, 1992); and studies range from relatively small experimental/demonstration programmes to national and cross-national studies. For example, Schultz (1992) estimates that more than half the fertility decline in Thailand is attributable to family planning programmes. Bongaarts, Mauldin and Phillips (1990) estimate that family planning programmes have already produced a population reduction of 412 million to 1990, and this impact will increase rapidly in the future.

The literature includes many examples of very rapid increases in contraceptive prevalence as family planning programmes become well organized and accessible to a large majority of the population. There are many examples of increases of contraceptive prevalence of 2 percentage points per annum for a full decade and a corresponding decrease in fertility.

At times there has been controversy as to whether socio-economic development or family planning is more important. The authors believe that this has become a largely academic question as research has repeatedly shown that both contribute to declining fertility and that the more each of them is present, the faster fertility will decline. Socio-economic development is obviously the more important because it sets the parameters within which programmes function, but no matter how rapid socio-economic development is, the transition from high to low fertility will be greatly aided by well-organized family planning programmes, as the past decade has clearly demonstrated.

NOTES

[1] The countries and areas included in the regional divisions used in this chapter do not in all cases conform to those included in the geographical regions established by the Population Division of the Department for Economic and Social Information and Policy Analysis of the United Nations Secretariat.

[2] Including Cambodia, China, Democratic People's Republic of Korea, East Timor, Hong Kong, Indonesia, Lao People's Democratic Republic, Malaysia, Mongolia, Myanmar, Philippines, Republic of Korea, Singapore, Thailand and Viet Nam.

[3] Including Afghanistan, Bangladesh, Bhutan, India, Iran (Islamic Republic of), Nepal, Pakistan, Sri Lanka.

[4] Including the Caribbean, Central and South America.

[5] Including Algeria, Egypt, Iraq, Jordan, Kuwait, Lebanon, the Libyan Arab Jamahiriya, Mauritania, Morocco. Oman, Saudi Arabia, Somalia, the Sudan, the Syrian Arab Republic, Tunisia, the United Arab Emirates and Yemen.

[6] Each of the countries classified as least developed is also included in discussion of regional groups of countries. Howver, it was decided that it would be desirable to examine family planning programmes and socio-economic setting of the least developed countries as a group. The Population Council data bank does not include most countries of fewer than 1 million population. The least developed countries, as defined by the United Nations, that are included in this analysis are: Afghanistan, Bangladesh, Benin, Bhutan, Botswana, Burkina Faso, Burundi, Central African Republic, Chad, Ethiopia, Gambia, Guinea, Buinea-Biseau, Haiti, Lao People's Democratic Republic, Lesotho, Liberia, Malawi, Mali, Mauritania, Mozambique, Myanmar, Nepal, Niger, Rwanda, Sierra Leone, Somalia, Sudan, Togo, Uganda, United Republic of Tanzania and Yemen.

[7] Estimates of total costs, by sector, are taken from World Bank (1992).

REFERENCES

Bang, Sook (1966). The Koyang study: results of two action programs. *Studies in Family Planning* (New York), vol. 1, No. 11 (April), pp. 5-12.

Berquó, Elsa S. (1980). Algumas indacações sobre a recente queda de fecundidade no Brasil. In *Teresopolis: VI Reunião do Grupo de Trablho sobre o Processo de Reprodução da População*. Santiago, Chile: Consejo Latinoamericano de Ciencias Sociales.

Bertrand, J. T. (1991). Recent essons from operations research on service delivery mechanisms. In *Operations Research: Helping Family Planning Programs Work Better*, Myrna Seidman and Marjorie C. Horn, eds. New York: Wiley-Liss.

Bongaarts, John, W. Parker Mauldin and James E. Phillips (1990). The demographic impact of family planning programs. *Studies in Family Planning* (New York), vol. 21, No. 6 (November-December), pp. 299-310.

Cernada, George P., ed. (1970). *Taiwan Family Planning Reader*. Taichung, Taiwan Province of China: The Chinese Center for International Training in Family Planning.

Choucri, Nazli (1974). *Population Dynamics and International Violence*. New York: Lexington Books.

Church, Cathleen A., with assistance of Judith Geller (1989). *Lights! Camera! Action! Promoting Family Planning with TV, Video and Film*. Population Reports, Series J, No. 38. Baltimore, Maryland: The Johns Hopkins University, Population Information Program.

Cleland, John, and and W. Parker Mauldin (1991). The promotion of family planning by financial payments: the case of Bangladesh. *Studies in Family Planning* (New York), vol. 22, No. 1 (January-February), pp. 1-18.

Cleland, John, and Warren Robinson (1992). The use of payments and benefits to influence reproductive behaviour. In *Family Planning Programmes and Fertility*, James F. Phillips and John A. Ross, eds. Oxford, United Kingdom: Clarendon Press; and New York: Oxford University Press.

Cuca, Roberto C., and Catherine S. Pierce (1977). *Experiments in Family Planning: Lessons from the Developing World*. Baltimore, Maryland: The Johns Hopkins University Press.

David, Henry P. (1987). Incentives and disincentives in family planning programs. In *Organizing for Effective Family Planning Programs*, Robert J. Lapham and George B. Simmons, eds. Washington, D.: National Academy Press.

Fisek, Nusret H. (1974). An integrated health/family planning program in Etimesgut District, Turkey. *Studies in Family Planning* (New York), vol. 5, No. 7 (July), pp. 210-220.

Fisher, A. (1992). The African pattern of family planning service delivery: the majority of clients are survey by a minority of clinics. Paper presented at Operations Research Day, 13 November 1992, Proceedings. New York: The Population Council.

Forrest, Jacqueline D., and John A. Ross (1978). Fertility effects of family planning programs: a methodological review. *Social Biology* (Port Angeles, Washington), vol. 25, No. 2, pp. 145-163.

Freedman, Ronald, and Bernard Berelson (1976). The record of family planning programs. *Studies in Family Planning* (New York), vol. 7, No. 1 (January), pp. 3-40.

Freedman, Ronald, and John Y. Takeshita (1969). *Family Planning in Taiwan: An Experiment in Social Change*. Princeton, New Jersey: Princeton University Press. The volume refers to Taiwan Province of China.

Goldberg, Howard I., Malcolm McNeil and Alison Spitz (1989). Contraceptive use and fertility decline in Chogoria, Kenya. *Studies in Family Planning* (New York), vol. 20, No. 1 (January-February), pp. 17-25.

Hsu, T. C., and L. P. Chow (1966). Taiwan, Republic of China. In *Family Planning and Population Programs: A Review of World Developments*, Bernard Berelson and others, eds. Chicago, Illinois: The University of Chicago Press. This article refers to Taiwan Province of China.

Jain, Anrudh K. (1989). Fertility reduction and the quality of family planning. *Studies in Family Planning* (New York), vol. 20, No. 1 (January-February), pp. 1-16.

_____, and Moni Nag (1992). South Asia. In *Population Trends and Issues in the Developing Countries: Regional Reports*, Susan Greenhalgh and others. Research Division Working Papers, No. 35. New York: The Population Council.

Kim, Taek Il, John A. Ross and George C. Worth (1972). *The Korean National Family Planning Program*. New York: The Population Council. This volume refers to the Republic of Korea.

Ladipo, O. A., and others (1990). Family planning in traditional markets in Nigeria. *Studies in Family Planning* (New York), vol. 21, No. 6 (November/December), pp. 311-321.

Lapham, Robert J., and W. Parker Mauldin (1987). The effects of family planing on fertility: research findings. In *Organizing for Effective Family Planning Programs*, Robert J. Lapham and George B. Simmons, eds. Washington, D.C.: National Academy Press.

Mauldin, W. Parker, and John A. Ross (1966). Family planning experiments: a review of design. In *Proceedings of the American Statistical Association, Social Statistics Section*. Washington, D.C.

_____ (1989). Historical perspectives on the introduction of contraceptive technology. In *Demographic and Programmatic Consequences of Contraceptive Innovations*, Sheldon J. Segal, Amy O. Tsui and Susan M. Rogers, eds. New York: Plenum Press.

_____ (1991). Family planning programs: efforts and results, 1982-89. *Studies in Family Planning* (New York), vol. 22, No. 6 (November/December), pp. 350-367.

Ott, Emiline Royco (1977). Population policy formation in Colombia: the role of ASCOFAME. *Studies in Family Planning* (New York), vol. 8, No. 1 (January), pp. 2-10.

Peng, J. Y. (1965). Thailand: family growth in Pho-tharam district. *Studies in Family Planning* (New York), vol. 1, No. 8 (October), pp. 1-2.

Phillips, James F. (1988). Translating pilot project success into national policy development: two projects in Bangladesh. *Asia-Pacific Population Journal* (Bangkok), vol. 2, No. 2 (June), pp. 3-28.

_____, and John A. Ross (1992). Family planning programmes and fertility effects: an overview. In *Family Planning Programmes and Fertility*, James F. Phillips and John A. Ross, eds. Oxford, United Kingdom: Clarendon Press; and New York: Oxford University Press.

Piotrow, Phyllis T., and Rita C. Meyer (1991). Promoting family planning: findings from operations research and program research. In *Operations Research Helping Family Planning Programs Work Better*, Myrna Seidman and Marjorie C. Horn, eds. New York: Wiley-Liss.

Preston, Samuel (1978). Mortality, morbidity and development. *Population Bulletin of the United Nations Economic Commission for Western Asia* (Beirut), No. 15 (December), pp. 63-78.

_____ (1980). Causes and consequences of mortality decline in developing countries during the twentieth century. In *Population and Economic Change in Developing Countries*, Richard A. Easterlin, ed. Chicago: University of Chicago Press.

Raina, B. L. (1966). India. In *Family Planning and Population Programs: A Review of World Developments*, Bernard Berelson and others, eds. Chicago, Illinois: The University of Chicago Press.

Ross, John A., and Jacqueline Darroch Forrest (1978). The demographic assessment of family planning programs: a bibliographic essay. *Population Index* (Princeton, New Jersey), vol. 44, No. 1 (January), pp. 8-27.

Ross, John A., and Stephen Isaacs (1988). Costs, payments, and incentives in family planning programmes: a review for developing countries. *Studies in Family Planning* (New York), vol. 19, No. 5 (September-October), pp. 270-283.

Ross, John A., and others (1987). Community-based distribution. In *Organizing for Effective Family Planning Programs*, Robert J. Lapham and George B. Simmons, eds. Washington, D.C.: National Academy Press.

Ross, John A., and Cynthia B. Lloyd (1992). Methods for measuring the fertility impact of family planning programmes: the experience of the last decade. In *Family Planning Programmes and Fertility*, James F. Phillips and John A. Ross, eds. Oxford, United Kingdom: Clarendon Press; and New York: Oxford University Press.

Ross, John A., Marjorie Rich and Janet P. Molzan (1989). *Management Strategies for Family Planning Programs*. New York: Columbia University, Center for Population and Family Health, School of Public Health.

Schultz, T. Paul (1992). Assessing family planning cost-effectiveness: applicability of individual demand-programme supply framework. In *Family Planning Programmes and Fertility*, James F. Phillips and John A. Ross, eds. Oxford, United Kingdom: Clarendon Press; and New York: Oxford University Press.

Sherris, Jacqueline D., Betty Butler Ravenholt and Richard Blackburn (1985). *Contraceptive Social Marketing: Lessons from Experience*. Population Reports, Series J, No. 30. Baltimore, Maryland: The Johns Hopkins University, Population Information Program.

Soni, Vena (1971). *The Ernakulam Camps*. New Delhi: The Ford Foundation.

United Nations (1984). *Report of the International Conference on Population, 1984, Mexico City, 6-14 August 1984*. Sales No. E.84.XIII.8.

_____ (1992). *World Population Monitoring, 1991: With Special Emphasis on Age Structure*. Population Studies, No. 126. Sales No. E.92.XIII.2.

Winich, Asavasena, Amos H. Hawley and J. Y. Peng (1966). Thailand. In *Family Planning and Population Programs: A Review of World Developments*, Bernard Berelson and others, eds. Chicago, Illinois: The University of Chicago Press.

World Bank (1992). *Effective Family Planning Programs*. Washington, D.C.

Part Five

ISSUES RELATING TO IMPLEMENTATION OF FAMILY PLANNING PROGRAMMES

VII. QUALITY OF FAMILY WELFARE SERVICES AND HUMAN RESOURCE DEVELOPMENT

J. P. Gupta and Helen H. Simon*

Realizing the problem of overpopulation, several developing countries introduced family planning measures into their national development programmes. Only recently, however, have both developed and developing countries realized that to reduce population growth rate, it is imperative to consider the factors beyond the jurisdiction of the health department, which have been termed "beyond family planning measures", such as age at marriage, female literacy, women's status, social security and socio-economic development.

In most of the countries, the family planning p rogramme is female-oriented, as the methods available and promoted are mostly female methods—intra-uterine device (IUD), pill, hormone injectables, Norplant implants, female condom and female sterilization. For males, the condom is widely promoted not only for family planning but also for prevention and control of the acquired immunodeficiency syndrome (AIDS), but male sterilization is not popular. Even though male methods, such as various vaccines, pills and implants in vas, are being developed, none of them are available for use as they are still in the experimental stage.

The Third All-India Survey on Family Planning Practices in India found that non-availability of services and lack of awareness of various methods were mentioned by about one sixth of the respondents, almost all of them living in rural areas. Inaccessibility of services was more frequently mentioned in the eastern and northern zones, while it was not considered as a problem in the western and southern zones. On the other hand, lack of awareness of the various methods was one of the problems for 15 per cent of such respondents in the western zone. A rural-urban breakdown of the data shows that the method-related reasons mentioned by more than half the respondents, including fear of the operation and one's inability to work hard after the operation, were more frequently mentioned in rural than in urban areas. Method-specific problems or religious or family opposition to family planning were more fre-

quently mentioned in the eastern zone than in other zones (Operations Research Group, 1990).

Even though availability of services, choice of methods, physical accessibility, cost of service, waiting time, sociocultural factors, normative approach of planning, inadequate programme management, and inadequate realization of "beyond family planning" measures are all important factors to consider in improvement of programme performance, quality of services has emerged as the most important factor to be improved if any impact on the objectives of the family planning programmes in the countries is to be achieved. It was found that a programme can achieve better demographic results when it concentrates on a small number of annual acceptors and provides them with good care to enhance satisfaction and thus to improve continuation rates, rather than trying to recruit a large number of acceptors at one time and not take care of them (Jain, 1989). Only recently, this dimension has assumed importance and some literature is available on quality of services. Different techniques are being evolved for quality assurance to ensure that the services provided shall be of the right quality and at a reasonable cost.

A. QUALITY OF SERVICES

Definition, concept and relativity

Very few systematic studies with guidelines to define and measure quality of services are available. The three issues—namely, quality, cost and availability of services—are difficult to consider separately. Quality has sometimes been counted as synonymous with the availability or accessibility of contraceptives. Only a judgement can determine whether quality is good or bad, satisfactory or unsatisfactory. Early family planning literature discussed quality largely with regard to clinical operations. This approach neglected the other

*National Institute of Health and Family Welfare, New Delhi, India.

dimensions of care, including interpersonal communication, as is explained in below.

Quality: different connotations to different people

Quality is defined here in terms of the way individual couples or clients are treated by the system providing the services. Bruce (1990) evolved a working definition of quality of services that incorporates the following six elements: (a) choice of contraceptive methods; (b) information given to users; (c) provider competence; (d) client/provider relations; (e) recontact and follow-up mechanisms; and (f) appropriate constellation of services.

If quality of services is going to rank with quantity of services as an indicator of programme performance, the "classical" clinical dimensions of quality of care and the subjective interpersonal aspects must be brought together in a simple and generally agreed upon framework (Donabedian, 1988).

The service providers may have a different perspective of what needs to be done to improve the quality of their services. Their views and perceptions also need due consideration if the emphasis on quality of care is to be translated into action. To some extent, one needs to tackle the widespread alienation of the service providers from the recipients but an improvement in the timeliness and quantity as well as the quality of services might also require additional expenditure and investment to offset the impact of inflation.

The concept of quality is relative. In many developing countries, the question of accessibility of services is likely to be a priority concern and emphasis can shift to the quality of services after basic accessibility is assured. Perhaps, it is best to focus on quality even as accessibility is being improved because the utilization of services is a function of both (Visaria and Visaria, 1991).

Quality of family welfare services in different countries

The quality of family welfare services in Latin America was surveyed, taking into account the six elements. Free selection of contraceptive method is restricted in most Latin American family planning programmes because access is limited to a few methods, owing to (a) inadequate information provided to users; (b) high prices charged for some methods; and (c) some methods being inappropriate for particular clients or population (Diaz and Halbe, 1990).

Family planning programme performance in four counties in rural China were studied from the point of view of both quality and achievements of demographic goals; and differences in family planning service, quality and performance were analysed. Two of the counties have set up new institutions for family planning service delivery. The "three in one" centre is a new type of institution for delivering family planning services in rural China; it integrates three types of services formerly provided by separate institutions: clinical contraceptive services; information, education and communication (IEC) services; and provision of supplies. These centres were created to improve both availability and quality of services in the community. Two counties (one with and one without the new centre) in a high family planning performance province are compared with two counties (one with and one without the new centre) in a lower performance province. Quality is measured by variables related to provider competence, information, services and availability and accessibility of clinical services. Demographic performance is measured by crude birth rates, contraceptive prevalence rates, planned birth rates and rates of one-child pledgers. This analysis found that although availability and access to services have been improved in the counties that have set up the three in one centres, quality remains low even though demographic performance has improved to some extent (Kaufman and others, 1989).

In Indonesia, a system of community health centres staffed by a doctor, a dentist, a midwife, a nurse etc. were developed in response to the needs of rural community. These centres provide programmes of family planning, health education, maternal and child health (MCH) care, immunization, dental care and nutritional improvement. At the village level, health care is provided at integrated service posts staffed by volunteers trained to treat common health problems with single means, such as oral rehydration in diarrhoea. These measures have led to a reduction in infant and maternal mortality. Even though the quality of care still needs to be improved, the policy of the Indonesian Government is to work towards increasing both the quantity and quality of health-care services in health centres and hospitals. Standards and quality are fairly consistent in the Government-run community and village centres (Jacobalis, 1989).

In Malaysia, contraceptive prevalence rose from 8 per cent at the beginning of the programme to 52 per cent in 1985 and total fertility declined from 5.3 to 3.8. The programme maintains quality service to its clients through its integration into total health services and through incorporation of family planning training into the curricula of medical and nursing schools and provision of continuous training to its staff. Another way in which quality of service is assured is to provide a wide selection of safe, effective and acceptable contraceptives at a free or subsidized rate and to make them easily accessible (e.g., phasing out the 50 mcg oestrogen oral contraceptive in 1986 and introducing a safer oral contraceptive with 30 mcg of noestrogen and a progesterone (Malaysia, 1990).

Sri Lanka has adopted a "cafeteria approach" to family planning. The client is given option of selecting any method from wide range of methods, and advice and counselling are provided by health workers at all levels to help the client make a decision.

The experience of the researchers in Africa has been that it is not the demand for family planning services but rather the way the services are delivered that accounts for the low numbers of acceptors in that major area. For example, in Kenya, improvements in the quality of sterilization services and an increase in the number of institutions that can provide minilaparotomy under local anaesthesia have led to increased acceptance of sterilization. The Kenya Situation Analysis Study found a rating of "moderate" for the Kenya national family planning programme and a "moderate-high" rating in terms of quality of care (Miller and others, 1990).

A study carried out in the states of Gujarat, Rajasthan and Uttar Pradesh by the Indian Council of Medical Research (ICMR) and the Operations Research Group in India, showed that the lack of knowledge of services available and the distances to primary health centres were mainly responsible for inaccessibility. The clients and patients in this study judged the governmental services to be less adequate than those offered by private and non-governmental facilities (ICMR, 1986).

A survey of households in two districts of Gujarat State, India, Baruch and Panchmahal, found relatively high levels of client satisfaction with available family planning services. In general, the survey failed to observe an association between contraceptive prevalence and service quality (Visaria and Visaria, 1991).

A study of contraceptive use dynamics was conducted for target populations in Orissa (India), and found that overall, counselling, quality and follow-up are poor (Khan, Patel and Chandrasekar, 1990). In a study to evaluate the quality of family welfare services provided to the target population residing in rural areas, a total of 398 primary health centres from 199 districts were covered in collaboration with state health directorates. The study found that quality of services related to the family planning component of the programme was better than that for the MCH component. However, family planning services were comparatively less accessible to communities located away from the primary centre headquarters and subcentres. Furthermore, accessibility is greatly limited for spacing methods, compared with sterilization, as is evident from a large number of villages with no IUD acceptor during the study period of one year. The quality of sterilization offered through camps was generally satisfactory, although some aspects, such as proper screening, stand-by transport and change of clothes, needed to be further studied and improved by some states (ICMR, 1991).

A study of MCH and family planning user perspectives and service constraints in rural Bangladesh found constraints on female workers' delivery of family planning and MCH services due to staffing density, work motivation, workers' technical competence, MCH supplies, supervision, availability and quality of care at subcentres (Simmons and others, 1988).

Choice of methods

Choice of methods refers to both the number of methods offered on a consistent basis and their intrinsic variability. In principle, a programme should offer enough methods efficiently to serve significant subgroups, such as those wishing to delay child-bearing, to space pregnancies and, lastly, to terminate child-bearing. It is important to define the minimum and optimum numbers of methods that programmes should offer and to develop management capabilities that will assist users in switching easily among available methods.

Range of available contraceptive methods

In most of the countries, among all family planning methods, female methods are given more emphasis. The family planning programmes in such countries or areas as Colombia, El Salvador, Indonesia, the Philippines, Singapore, Taiwan Province of China, Thailand and Tunisia could very well be termed "female-oriented" because mainly female methods were advocated and adopted. This situation is also found in some of the developed countries, such as Sweden, where out of 1,578 sterilizations performed in 1968, only 5 were male operations. In India, however, up to 1977, male sterilization was the most important contraceptive (Khan and Dastidar, 1985). For example, in 1976/77, vasectomies accounted for 75 per cent of all sterilizations and for 50 per cent of all methods. In the post-1977 period, the trend slowly changed; and since that time female sterilization has outnumbered male sterilizations. The 1989/90 service statistics show that the percentage of tubectomies to total sterilizations was as high as 91.8 per cent (India, 1991). Some of the reasons for promoting and stressing female family planning methods could be male dominance in decision-making at different levels and in family planning research, socio-economic dependence of women, fear of physical injury in accepting vasectomy and prevailing myths among males about this method. The Government of India established four centres of excellence in India in four regions, northern, eastern, western and southern in 1988, in collaboration with the United Nations Population Fund (UNFPA), the Association for Voluntary Surgical Contraception (AVSC) and the National Institute of Health and Family Welfare (NIHFW) to train the medical personnel in the country in standards of voluntary surgical contraception. No-scalpel vasectomy is being popularized through these centres in a medical college, and at the National Institute of Health and Family Welfare at New Delhi by conducting training programmes for medical personnel.

Choice of contraceptive methods in different countries

Annex table A.3 shows the percentage distribution of current contraceptive users, by method, in selected developing and developed countries. The trend in contraceptive practice shows that the percentage of pill users among total contraceptive users has more often decreased than increased in recent years. The most dramatic drops was recorded in Puerto Rico and the United States of America. Excluding Jordan, countries where prevalence of the pill has dropped substantially have a high overall level of contraceptive use; and except for Finland and Jordan, there are countries where at least 20 per cent of couples currently use sterilization. In Finland and Jordan, the switch-over was primarily from the pill to IUD. In addition, smaller decreases in

pill prevalence are seen in some other countries, most of which have shown considerable increase in the acceptance of sterilization. In China, Egypt, Hungary, Indonesia, Jordan and Tunisia, IUD accounts for 25-41 per cent of contraceptive practice. Although IUD is important in a substantial number of countries, it accounts for less than 10 per cent of contraceptive use in roughly 60 per cent of the countries covered in table A.3. In only a few countries has the prevalence of IUD declined, and China is in this group. Other countries with a decline of more than 2 per cent in proportion of couples using IUD include the Republic of Korea and Sri Lanka, which has shown an increase in the acceptance of sterilization. In Asia, there are several countries or areas where the condom is used by a large number of couples. Hong Kong has shown an increase of condom use by couples in recent years, but some of the developed countries, including Hungary, have shown a substantial decrease.

Effect of multiple methods on contraceptive prevalence

Jain (1989) shows in a study of the relation between contraceptive prevalence and the availability score for 72 countries, that the addition of a method to the choice of methods available in a country would be associated with an increase of about 12 percentage points in the practice of contraception. The overall contraceptive use-pattern for five countries or areas, namely, Hong Kong, India, the Republic of Korea, Taiwan Province of China and Thailand, also shows the same effect of adding a method to family planning programme (Freedman and Berelson, 1976). Jain (1989) found that a little less than two methods were effectively available per country and countries with more methods available had markedly higher contraceptive prevalence.

Acceptance and continuation of contraceptive methods

Acceptability and continuation of a method depend upon the attitude of the couple towards the method, their tolerance and knowledge of its side-effects, which indicates the type of services available at first visit as well as follow-up and the strategies used to promote a method. The acceptance and continuation rates depend upon each other and are affected by a host of other factors. Even though the couples' desire or motivation to regulate their fertility is one of the important factors, accessibility of the services, low cost and quality of services are some of the other important factors determining acceptability and continuation rates.

110

Effect of multiple methods on continuation

Discontinuation rates are usually defined in terms of a particular method without considering the need for switching among various methods. If this need for switching is recognized and multiple methods are available, then the total experience of the clients with different methods should be taken into account, instead of that for only one method, thus improving the continuation of contraceptive use and reducing the need to recruit "new" acceptors into the programme. Annex table A.4 shows 12-month use-failure and continuation rates from a review of recent prospective and retrospective follow-up studies of acceptors (United Nations, 1991).

It is not possible to assign accurate values to annual discontinuation rates for different methods. A majority of discontinuation of methods of first year is attributable to side-effects. The most comprehensive study (Kreager, 1977) found that in the range of studies of first-year continuation rates, 4-34 per cent of IUD acceptors had the devices removed for medical reasons or due to untolerated side-effects and 8-50 per cent of pill acceptors discontinued use for the same reasons. In a study

conducted by NIHFW, New Delhi, in the State of Rajasthan, 76 per cent of IUD acceptors had the device removed due to medical reasons and 80 per cent of the pill acceptors discontinued the pill for the same reason (Bhatnagar and others, 1988). Bardhan and Dubey (1983), in another study conducted by NIHWF in the State of Rajasthan, report that 73 per cent of IUD acceptors had the device removed due to medical reasons. In general, IUD is the most studied method, with average discontinuation rates of 25-30 per cent per annum. Pills and condoms both have much higher discontinuation rates of 50-60 per cent per annum. The reasons for switching of method given in tables 7 and 8 in respect of India and Sri Lanka indicate that in a large number of cases, the reasons could be attributed to the method. In a recent study of acceptors of oral contraceptives, IUD and condoms in five Indonesian family planning clinics, clients were asked 18 months after initial contact whether they had received the methods they requested, whether they were still using contraceptives and if not, when they had discontinued. Of those that had not received the method requested, 85 per cent had discontinued within one year, whereas of those that had received the method requested, only 25

TABLE 7. REASONS FOR SHIFTING OR DISCONTINUING FAMILY PLANNING METHODS,
INDIA
(Percentage)

| Reason | Past users of | | | |
	Intra-uterine device	Pills	Oral contra-ceptives	Traditional methods
Shifted to permanent method	12	27	10	32
Felt risky	12	6	3	15
Method failed	4	7	6	15
No sexual satisfaction	1	12	0	4
Created menstrual problem	29	0	9	0
Affected health	17	3	22	0
Got dislocated	4	0	0	0
Caused nausea	0	0	15	0
Put on weight	0	0	3	0
Caused heat in the body	0	0	5	0
Wanted to have a child	11	25	10	17
No privacy	0	3	0	0
Inconvenient	0	3	0	3
It did not suit	5	6	6	6
Others	5	8	11	10
TOTAL (thousands)	1 858	2 471	684	2 334

Source: Operations Research Group, *Family Planning Practices in India: Third All-India Survey*, vol. II (Baroda, Ministry of Health and Family Welfare, 1990).

TABLE 8. PERCENTAGE DISTRIBUTION OF RESPONDENTS SWITCHING FROM ONE TYPE OF CONTRACEPTIVE TO ANOTHER, BY REASON FOR DISCONTINUING, FIRST METHOD, SRI LANKA

	Types of switching from					
Reason	Pill to rhythm/ withdrawal (N= 93)	Intra-uterine device to rhythm/ withdrawal (N=38)	Rhythm to pill (N=41)	Withdrawal to pill (N=32)	Rhythm to pill (N=53)	Withdrawal to intra-uterine device (N=41)
Desire to try other method	9	0	44	47	43	27
Side-effects	50	24	2	3	2	2
Intention to have a child	17	10	29	22	26	37
Recommended time was up	8	5	0	0	0	0
Impossible to conceive	0	3	0	0	4	0
Less satisfying sex	0	0	0	3	2	2
Dislike for method	0	0	7	6	2	2
Method failure	1	5	15	19	11	20
Other	15	53	2	0	9	10

Source: Ken T. Thomas and others, "Contraceptive method-switching in Sri Lanka: patterns and implications", *International Family Planning Perspectives* (New York), vol. 14, No. 2 (June 1988), pp. 54-60.

per cent had discontinued within one year. Thus, it is important to note that regardless of the method, women that had not received their chosen method had lower continuation rates (Pariani, Hern and Van Assdol, 1987).

Informed choice

It has been said that a small number of acceptors with a total or high continuation rate contribute more to programme performance than a large number of initial acceptors with a high discontinuation rate (Jain, 1989). To achieve this objective, clients need to be informed adequately on: (*a*) methods available; (*b*) distinctive factors of available methods; (*c*) how to use the methods; (*d*) side-effects of various methods; (*e*) misconceptions about methods; (*f*) requirements of self-administered methods; (*g*) limitations of methods; (*h*) risk and complications; and (*i*) required follow-up.

Client information levels and programme performance

Knowledge about contraceptive methods

Acceptance of family planning methods is directly influenced by knowledge of contraceptives among the eligible couples. The World Fertility Survey (WFS) found that a very high proportion of women—three out of four in every country—knew of at least one modern method (Sadik, 1981). In Bangladesh, about 83 per cent

of women knew of at least one modern method; the corresponding percentages for Fiji, Indonesia, Jordan, Malaysia and Pakistan were 100, 78, 97, 93 and 76 per cent, respectively (Khan and Dastidar, 1985). These data show more about awareness than actual knowledge of the methods among women. In a recent national family planning survey in India, it was observed that at the national level, from 89 to 95 per cent of the currently married persons had heard about two permanent methods. The percentages for the condom, IUD and oral pills were 66, 60 and 55, respectively. The study also found that no more than 52 per cent had actual knowledge about tubectomy. The corresponding percentages were 38, 31, 51 and 39 for vasectomy, IUD, condom and pill, respectively (Operations Research Group, 1990). Table 9 shows the level of knowledge, ever-use and current use of contraception further supports the loss of clientele, which occurs for several reasons and which perhaps could be minimized by taking several steps, including providing appropriate information before a person adopts a family planning method and then continues with the chosen method or switches to another method.

Misconceptions

Many women have misconceptions of various types about contraceptive methods, which discourage them from adopting those methods. These misconceptions are reported to be prevalent among women in many coun-

TABLE 9. LEVELS OF KNOWLEDGE, EVER-USE AND CURRENT USE OF CONTRACEPTION IN DEVELOPING COUNTRIES[a]

Region and country or area	Year of survey	Age range to which estimates refer	Percentage of ever-married or currently married[b] women that knew of any contraceptive method	Percentage of currently married[b] women who		
				Knew of a source of family planning information or supplies	Had ever used contraception	Were currently using any method
Africa						
Eastern Africa						
Burundi	1987[c]	15-49	78	70	30	9
Kenya	1984	15-49	84	52[d]	33	17
Malawi	1984	15-49	4[e]	..	..	7[d]
Mauritius	1985	15-49	..	..	..	75
Rwanda	1983	15-50	72	..	18[f]	10
Zimbabwe	1984	15-49	90	71[f]	66[f]	38
Middle Africa						
Cameroon	1978	15-49	34	..	11	2
Northern Africa						
Egypt	1984	Under 50	85	81[f]	48[f]	30
Morocco	1987[c]	15-49	98	94	59	36
Sudan (Northern)	1978/79	15-49	51	23	13	5
Tunisia	1983	15-49	97	92	60[f]	41
Southern Africa						
Botswana	1984	15-49	80	73	54	28
Lesotho	1977	15-49	65	27	23	5
South Africa	1981/82	Under 50	..	..	..	48[g]
Western Africa						
Benin	1982	15-49	40	..	34	9[h]
Côte d'Ivoire	1980/81	15-49	85	..	71	3
Ghana	1979	15-49	69	43	40	10
Liberia	1986	15-49	70	44	19	6
Mali	1987[c]	15-49	43	30	19	5
Mauritania[i]	1981	15-49	8	..	2	1
Nigeria	1981/82	15-49	34	..	13[f]	5
Senegal	1986	15-49	92	50[j]	38	12
Sierra Leone	1969/70	15-49	78[k]	..	6[k]	..
Latin America and the Caribbean						
Caribbean						
Antigua	1981	15-44	93[d]	..	..	39
Barbados	1980-81	15-49	97[d]	..	74	46
Dominica	1981	15-44	90[d]	..	..	49
Dominican Republic	1986	15-49	99[l]	99	73	50
Grenada	1985	15-44	92[d]	69[d,m]	..	31
Guadeloupe	1976	15-49	..	..	62[f]	44
Haiti	1983	15-49	87	63	19[f]	7[n]
Jamaica	1983	15-44	100[o]	..	76	52
Martinique	1976	15-49	..	..	66[f]	51
Montserrat	1984	15-44	99[d,o]	94[d,m]	..	53
Puerto Rico	1982	15-44	..	..	..	70
Saint Kitts and Nevis	1984	15-44	99[d,o]	90[d,m]	..	41
Saint Lucia	1981	15-44	92[d]	..	..	43
Saint Vincent and the Grenadines .	1981	15-44	98[d]	..	..	42
Trinidad and Tobago	1987[c]	15-49	99	98	83	53

TABLE 9 *(continued)*

Region and country or area	Year of survey	Age range to which estimates refer	Percentage of ever-married or currently married[b] women that knew of any contraceptive method	Percentage of currently married[b] women who		
				Knew of a source of family planning information or supplies	Had ever used contraception	Were currently using any method
Central America						
Costa Rica	1986	15-44	99[o]	980[p]	..	70
El Salvador	1985	15-49	93	75	61	47
Guatemala	1987[c]	15-44	72	66	34	23
Honduras	1984	15-44	93[p]	76[p]	..	35
Mexico	1987[c]	15-49	91[o]	..	..	53
Nicaragua	1981	15-49	77[d]	..	44	27
Panama	1984	15-44	96[o]	72[q]	..	58[n]
South America						
Bolivia	1983	15-44	57	..	35	26
Brazil	1986	15-44	100	92[j]	86	66
Colombia	1986	15-49	99	99	83	65
Ecuador	1987[c]	15-49	90[d]	88	63	44
Guyana	1975	15-49	95	..	56	31
Paraguay	1987	15-44	96[d,n]	91[q]	..	45
Peru	1986[c]	15-49	89	86	65	46
Venezuela	1977	15-44	98	68	70	49
Asia and Oceania						
Eastern Asia						
China	1985	15-49	..	..	..	74
Hong Kong	1982	15-49	99[r]	..	90	72
Republic of Korea	1985	15-44	100[s]	94[j,s]	84	70
South-eastern Asia						
Indonesia	1987[c]	15-49	94	93	65	48
Malaysia (peninsular)	1984	15-49	99	94	77	51
Philippines	1983	15-44	94[t]	77[t]	..	45
Singapore	1982	15-44	100	95[s,u]	..	74
Thailand	1987[c]	15-49	100	99	84	66
Southern Asia						
Afghanistan	1977/73	15-44	4	..	..	2
Bangladesh	1985	<50	100	..	32	25
India	1980	15-49	95[v]	..	39	34
Nepal	1986	15-49	56	34[p]	16	14
Pakistan	1984	15-49	61	20[r,w]	12	8
Sri Lanka	1987[c]	15-49	99	98	74	62
Western Asia						
Iraq	1974	15-49	..	..	38[f,x]	14
Jordan[y]	1985	19-51[z]	97[o]	..	42	26
Lebanon	1971	15-49	91[o]	..	67	53
Syrian Arab Republic	1978	15-49	78	..	34	20
Turkey	1983	15-49	94	..	71	51
Yemen	1979	<50	25	..	3	1
Oceania						
Fiji	1974	15-49	100	..	69	41

Sources and notes to follow

TABLE 9 *(continued)*

Source: Levels and Trends of Contraceptive Use as Assessed in 1988, Population Studies, No. 110 (United Nations publication, Sales No. E.89.XIII.4), table 2.

[a]Estimates based on the most recent surveys available.

[b]Including consensual unions.

[c]Preliminary or provisional.

[d]For all women of ages specified.

[e]Percentage that knew of the pill, the most widely known modern method; 14 per cent knew of traditional medicine.

[f]For ever-married women.

[g]Estimate of the Population Division of the Department of International Economic and Social Affairs of the United Nations Secretariat, based on separate surveys of major ethnic groups.

[h]Excluding from the count of contraceptive users women abstaining post-partum.

[i]Percentage that knew of a source for sterilization, the most widely known modern method; 62 percent knew of a source for folk methods.

[j]For currently married women and single women with children.

[k]Percentage that knew of a modern method.

[l]Percentage that knew of source for the pill, the most widely known method.

[m]Excluding douche, abstinence and folk methods.

[n]Percentage that knew of the pill.

[o]For 1981.

[p]For 1979.

[q]For 1977.

[r]For 1976.

[s]For 1978, ages 15-49.

[t]Percentage that knew of a government clinic.

[u]Percentage that knew of vasectomy the most widely known method.

[v]Women that had ever used contraception are assumed to know a supply source.

[w]Including breast-feeding.

[x]Excluding the West Bank.

[y]Interviews in 1985 with husbands of women surveyed two years earlier, when they were aged 15-49.

tries, for example, India, Indonesia, Mexico and Sri Lanka. Women in Indonesia did not accept IUD because they were afraid of weakness, bleeding, cancer and the possibility of its piercing through the uterine wall (Suyono and others, 1981). In Mexico, IUD was avoided due to fear of side-effects as changes in menstrual period, cramps and unbearable pain (Folch-Lyon, de la Macorra and Schearer, 1981). In India, 32 per cent of women did not accept IUD as they believed that it has serious repercussions on the health of women and that the severity of side-effects ranged from excessive bleeding and weakness to cancer (Khan and Prasad, 1983).

In Mexico, there was widespread belief that the pill caused nervousness and cancer. Such perceived after-effects and misconceptions might prevent women from adopting pills (Folch-Lyon, de la Mocorra and Schearer, 1981). Like IUD and pills, the fear that tubectomy could cause weakness, abdominal pain, weight gain and at times even death was found to deter women to opt for this particular method. The proportion of such women in India was reported to be about 22 per cent of the women of reproductive age. Almost same proportion of men perceived serious after-effects with vasectomy, such as impotency, physical weakness or death. Hence they were not in favour of husbands accepting vasectomy (Khan and Prasad, 1983).

Access to source of information

Various communication channels, such as interpersonal communication and mass media, are used to provide family planning information in various countries. Advertisements in newspapers were used to disseminate information about contraception in India, the Islamic Republic of Iran, Japan, the Republic of Korea, Sri Lanka, Taiwan Province of China and Thailand; and in countries in Africa and western hemisphere. Studies in these countries or areas clearly showed that such advertisements did help disseminate the information, but because there are more literate men than women and males have more opportunity to read newspapers, the ads had more impact on males than females (Sweeney, 1977).

Radio is also extensively used for disseminating information about family planning methods. A review of research findings from 15 countries or areas, including Bangladesh, India, Pakistan, the Republic of Korea and Taiwan Province of China in Asia; Kenya and

Nigeria in Africa; Colombia, Costa Rica, the Dominican Republic, El Salvador and Honduras in Latin America and the Caribbean; and the Islamic Republic of Iran and Morocco in the Middle East, showed the effectiveness of radio in teaching the masses. These messages also reach more males than females (Sweeney, 1977).

Technical competence

The beneficiaries cannot judge the technical skills of the health personnel. Therefore, the providers are usually evaluated more by the amount of time they spend with them and their caring attitude than by their technical skills. The beneficiaries bear the consequences of deficient technical skills of the providers in the form of unnecessary pain, infection, other serious side-effects or, in some circumstances, death.

Clinical incompetence of providers is often one of the important factors associated with poor programme performance. A multicentric study conducted by ICMR in three rural areas of three states of India—namely, Gujarat, Rajasthan and Uttar Pradesh—showed that family planning performance in Gujarat was relatively better than that of Rajasthan and Uttar Pradesh. This situation was owing to functionaries being more experienced and well equipped with professional training in MCH and family planning services in Gujarat, compared with functionaries in Uttar Pradesh and Rajasthan, who were academically better than their counterparts in Gujarat (Visaria and Visaria, 1991).

Competency-based training

The training programme should place relatively less emphasis on formal classroom study and more on "learning by doing" on the job under supervision at a site where the health functionaries are expected to work.

Training in clinical techniques to develop skills (in IUD insertion, implant insertions and removal, and sterilization operations) should be imparted under supervision. In the Islamic Republic of Iran, auxiliary midwives with one month of training in IUD insertion, including a minimum of 30 IUDs inserted under supervision, had similar rates of removal for medical reasons, expulsion without reinsertions, accidental pregnancies and removal for personal reasons as did the medical doctors. The midwives had a slightly lower rate of "removal for personal reasons", which may indicate their superior communication skills (Zeighami and others, 1976).

Monitoring and data collection/quality assurance

The client case audit systems are designed to assure that client care is being performed according to the standards set for a particular service. This task requires reviewing medical records to ascertain whether services are being provided according to criteria specified in the established standards. An audit process should be developed for sterilization, IUD insertions, oral contraceptives etc. and should be specific to the organizational needs.

The final report of the audit should be sent to providers of services, administrators and other appropriate persons so that remedial measures can be initiated to improve the quality of client care. The Government of India, under the project of Centres of Excellence, has initiated Quality Assurance of Family Welfare services in the country and NIHFW was given the responsibility of monitoring and evaluating these services.

Interpersonal relations

"Interpersonal relations" is defined as the affective content of the client-provider transaction. The client-provider contact should be characterized by two-way communication. The desired outcome of this transaction, from the point of view of the provider, may be that the client develops a belief in the competence of the provider, trust of a personal nature and a willingness to make contact again or even recommend the services to others. The counsellors provide, in effect, a guarantee of the technology by their presence and manner of communication (Simmons and others, 1988).

Client's feelings

Workers' ability to respond sympathetically on an individual basis to clients can be undermined if they are working under the pressure of targets to attain demographic goals. An experiment undertaken in 1983/84 in the district of Rajasthan State (India) found that the target orientation was not conducive to systematic programme operations. An innovative experiment was implemented in which workers analysed client data and classified their clients into four groups, each requiring a distinctive approach. Although this approach did not directly correct the demographic ideology underlying the programme, managers encouraged workers to understand more about a client's individual outlook (Giridhar and Satia, 1986).

Similarly concerned over the impact of targeting systems and worker performance, some experiments were undertaken within the extension area of Bangladesh to see if a new record-keeping system could improve the client orientation of workers. It was judged, however, that unless the target system was revised, the reorientation of staff could have only limited effects (Koblinsky and others, 1987, cited in Bruce, 1990).

Continuity and follow-up

Supporting continuity of use among all clients may remain a desired goal, but priorities for specific follow up must be set. Indiscriminate revisiting may waste time and undermine workers' morale. Distinctions should perhaps be made between the needs of a couple stating that they want more children, a long-term established user of a provider-dependent method and a young, new user of a self-administered method. The concept of new clients could be extended to include all those that are within their first year of use with a new method (not those that only made an initial visit). These persons might benefit from orally and visually reinforced educational messages and receive specific follow-up methods early in the method adoption process. Programmes should also focus on assisting clients in more effective self-care over the long term.

Appropriate constellation of services

A woman's needs over the course of her lifetime are biologically as well as psychologically integrated. For the most part, services segment these needs, sometimes in an extreme and detrimental way. Pregnant women, recently delivered mothers, fully lactating women and sexually active adolescents are denied contraceptive information for different reasons. Contradictions abound in programming approach. The appropriate constellation of services is one that responds to a client's rhythms and health concepts, rather than inflexible medical demarcations of where a "need" begins and where it ends.

Even within fairly limited geographical locations, contrasting configurations of services, depending upon clients' needs and managers' resources and imagination, may be acceptable and even desirable.

Experiments in expanding the constellation of services extend from the integration of conventional reproductive health services (MCH/FP) with less

regularly offered, but vital, adjuncts, such as the diagnosis and treatment of reproductive tract infections and sexually transmitted diseases, to programmes with an explicit social purpose. The latter category includes programmes that use health services for women as their base but view the empowerment of women as an overall goal.

Post-partum services

The definition of the appropriate services for mother and child in the immediate post-partum period has seemingly already been answered through the nominal integration of MCH services and the International Post-partum Programme (1968-1970). That programme found that women who had just delivered a baby might be interested in hearing information about contraception but that almost half of the contraceptive acceptors in the sample outside the United States of America took up contraception between the first and the twenty-fourth month post-partum, with a sharp peak at about six months (less than 3 months, 9 per cent; 4-12 months, 49 per cent; 13-30 months, 27 per cent; 30 months, 15 per cent) (Zatuchni, 1970).

Coverage, quality and sustainability are the core programmatic issues that face post-partum family planning programmes in the 1990s. The four elements most critical to high-quality post-partum services which need to be addressed to are: (*a*) clearly stated operational policies; (*b*) development of systems capable of sustaining family planning services; (*c*) documentation of the cost/benefit ratio of improved post-partum care and efforts to ensure financial sustainability; and (*d*) collaboration among users, providers and the international reproductive health community (Townsend and Ojeda, 1985, as cited in Bruce, 1990).

Concept of accessibility

There is some overlap between the concept of quality developed by Bruce (1990) and the concept of accessibility suggested by Hermalin and Entwisle (1985), which consists of six components, including range of services offered at each outlet, particularly the specific contraceptive methods available at the outlet; and the quality of services provided, including such elements as waiting time, training and competence of staff, privacy and courtesy accorded the client and hours of operation. Two elements in the Hermalin and

Entwisle framework are similar to three elements—choice, provider competence and constellation of services—in Bruce's framework. Hermalin and Entwisle focus more on accessibility of services and include other components, such as actual distance, travel time and cost of services.

Physical accessibility

Information available on this aspect indicates that despite vast family planning infrastructure, the physical accessibility of contraceptives in several developing countries is constrained by such factors as the distance of the nearest clinic or sources of supplies, long waiting time, non-availability of contraceptives on time, non-suitability of clinic hours and absence of trained female staff, especially physicians, and at times the non-function of the extension staff.

The problem of physical inaccessibility is more serious in rural than urban areas. According to WFS data, in almost all of the 36 countries examined, family planning methods are available within an hour's travel in urban areas (Khan and Dastidar, 1985). In rural areas of Costa Rica and Thailand, methods are generally available within an hour's travel. However, there are many countries, such as Brazil, Guatemala, Honduras and Tunisia, where distance and cost of travel are serious constraints for women for getting supplies and other services. Similar observations were made for Senegal, the Sudan and other African countries. In these countries, contraceptives are still available only in urban areas. For example in Kenya, outlets tend to be far apart and, on average, the land area per clinic is 1,127 square kilometres. Analysis of WFS data clearly demonstrates that travel cost and distance constitute a serious hindrance to the acceptance of family planning in developing countries.

Similar observations were reported even from rural India, where according to a recent study only about 18 per cent of the rural couples had ever used the services provided by the government outlets. The major reasons for not utilizing these services were long distance, lack of communication facilities, long waiting time and sometimes indifferent behaviour of the clinic staff (Khan, Dastidar and Bairathi, 1983; Mehta and others, 1983). Yet another microlevel study showed that although there are primary health centres in rural areas, females could not avail themselves the facilities simply because the staff assigned to the clinics rarely reported on duty (Khan and others, 1983). Similar findings were reported from other studies in India (Khan and others, 1983; Misra and others, 1982; Sundaram, 1983), Yemen (Myntti, 1979) and Java (Hull, 1979).

In several countries, the private sector has not responded favourably to the marketing of contraceptives in rural areas due to the belief that this market is very limited. Thus, they have concentrated their efforts largely in urban areas (Business International, 1978). A study on social marketing of condoms in India also arrived at similar conclusions: it observed that in urban India, 29.4 per cent of retailers were stocking condoms, but in rural India, only 8.1 per cent were doing so.

Waiting time is frequently mentioned in the literature as an important factor discouraging women from seeking medical as well as family planning services. However, not many studies could point out precisely the length of time women had to wait to get these services at the clinic. The few available studies indicate that the waiting time was as high as 3 hours in hospitals and family planning clinics in El Salvador and about 1 hour and 12 minutes in a primary health centre in India (Khan, Prasad and Quaisen, 1984). Yet another study of six clinics in the Dominican Republic indicates that the average waiting time ranged from 56 to 130 minutes (Mundigo and Stycos, 1973). Similar observations elsewhere have also been reported (Scrimshaw, 1977).

Development of new contraceptives

A review of the ongoing research for the development of new contraceptives indicates that in the next 10 years, the new or improved contraceptives which will be available for use will be only female-oriented, as can be seen from table 10.

It is an irony that in family planning much greater emphasis is laid on female methods without much consideration about their after-effects on the health of women. Some claim that a double standard is used: inadequately tested contraceptive methods are liberally provided to women; whereas more stringent requirements are used for men (Hammer, 1982). One can only hope that this worst fear does not turn out to be true, for the survival and well-being of the family and the society at large depends as much upon women as upon men.

118

TABLE 10. CONTRACEPTIVES LIKELY TO BECOME AVAILABLE BY 1990 AND BETWEEN 1990 AND 2000

Products likely to become available	
By 1990	Between 1990-2000
For men	
None	Pills and injectables
	Vaccines
For women	
Improvements in :	Pills: once a month post-coital
Intra-uterine device	menses-indroducing abortifacient
Injectable contraceptives	IUD releasing non-steroidal drugs
Barrier methods	Vaccines
Kits and devices for determining the fertile period	
Implants	
Vaginal rings	
Suppositories or injections to induce menses	
Post-coital pills	
Non-surgical sterilization	

Source: C. C. Standley, "New leads in technology for fertility regulation", paper presented at the World Health Organization Seminar on Operations Research in Family Planning, Lima, 20-21 June 1984 (Geneva).

    IUD = intra-uterine device.

B. ORGANIZATION OF PROGRAMMES: NEED FOR INTEGRATION AND INVOLVEMENT OF NON-GOVERNMENTAL AGENCIES

The close relation of MCH and family planning is well recognized. There is little doubt that the antenatal and postnatal periods are the most suitable for educating mothers and other members of the family about the need of family planning. Moreover, along with the curative and preventive health services, it is easy for a family planning worker to talk about family planning more freely with the clients. With this understanding, the family planning services in India were integrated with MCH and other preventive and curative services. Various studies, however, have pointed out the advantages as well as the shortcomings of the integration of MCH and family planning.

It would be naïve to counsel the total abandonment of surveillance and discipline. Health workers can be best helped by the continuous search for opportunities for improvement of various processes.

A few steps to improve the quality are outlined below:

(*a*) Leaders must take the lead in quality improvement;

(*b*) Investment in quality improvement must be substantial;

(*c*) Respect for the health-care worker must be re-established;

(*d*) Dialogue between clients and providers of health care must be open and must be carefully maintained;

(*e*) Modern technical, theoretical tools for improving processes must be put to use in health-care settings.

(*f*) Health-care institutions must "organise for quality";

(*g*) Investment needs to be made in quality improvement by refining managerial techniques requiring new structures which are not currently found in health maintaining organizations.

The multidimensional approach with an increased emphasis on interdepartmental integration and coordination of activities is consistent with the viewpoint that family planning is part of a wider effort to improve the quality of life.

Most Governments in the Asia and the Pacific region foresee a closer link between family planning and health provision. Family planning fieldworkers are increasingly being trained to play an active role in immunization, nutrition and oral rehydration schemes. In parallel, health personnel are being encouraged to give greater emphasis to family planning. Furthermore, several

119

Governments have recently taken specific action to encourage the participation of non-governmental organizations in the national family planning efforts. Regardless of the organizational superstructure, it is field delivery characteristics at the grass-roots level that largely determine programme effectiveness.

C. CONTINUOUS IMPROVEMENT AS IDEAL HEALTH CARE

In modern health care, there are two approaches to the problem of improving quality—two theories of quality that describe the climate in which care is delivered. One will serve well; the other probably will not.

One theory used by supervisors and managers relies upon inspection to improve quality. The experts call this mode "quality by inspection". This theory has proved that relying upon inspection to improve quality is at best inefficient and a formula for failure.

What Japan had discovered was primarily a new, more cogent and more valid way to focus on quality. This theory can be called the "theory of continuous improvement". The modern quality improvement expert cares far more about learning and cooperating with the typical worker than about censoring the truly deficient, which is the basis of the theory of "quality by inspection".

Quality improvement has little chance of success in health-care institutions without the understanding, participation and the leadership of individual doctors. Flawless care requires not just sound decisions but sound support for those decisions.

In summation, it is apparent that many dimensions rather than consideration of those dimensions related to technical and clinical aspects of family planning programme, services and care need to be taken care into account. This point has been amply illustrated by Bruce's work related to quality of family planning services (1990). Quality assurance in health services has become an area of great concern, and methods and techniques for measuring quality of services are being developed. Setting of standards, measurement of performance, medical audit and statistical quality control are some of the methods of quality assurance applied in certain situations. There is now a need to consider application of such methods and techniques in relation to quality of family planning services.

D. HUMAN RESOURCE DEVELOPMENT

Family planning/population stabilization programmes often get into complexities in view of the manner in which people are viewed either as resources or as liabilities. The Green and White Revolution in India has demonstrated the infinite possibilities of people acting as agents of exploitation of natural resources of which technological advances and transfer of technology are important mechanisms. The Malthusian school of thought, however, believes in the opposite view. The scenarios in developing countries often present an example of the latter viewpoint when the supply of services, qualitative and quantitative falls short of the demand. These viewpoints represent one set of relations between people and family planning/population stabilization programmes.

The other set of relations refers to stock of manpower that generates demand through IEC efforts and also provides the services for family planning/ population stabilization programmes. The protagonists of the theory that "development is the best contraceptive" believe that population will be able to see the reasoning and therefore will adopt family planning measures either from an individual and family perspective or from a national perspective. The higher the development stage of the country, the greater is the understanding of population problems and issues above the level of individual and family perspective. The strategies of meeting the demands, therefore, will differ according to the way people perceive the problem, either as a national or as an individual and family problem. More often, the efforts in expended programmes in developing countries to make people view the population problem from a national perspective have failed, as people could not raise their perceptions above the level of individual and family concerns. These subtle differences in operational strategies, therefore, must be clearly understood by those responsible for providing services.

The providers of services fall into two groups. There are situations where family planning programmes are vertical programmes having only an appendage type of linking with health services. In the other scenario, providers function in integrated health and family planning programmes. In either situation, the role of such factors as age at marriage, literacy and more particularly female literacy, employment and status of women—"beyond family planning measures" as compared with the contraceptive services—is considered more important from the long-term perspective and sustainable impact. In this framework, the providers of services have to broaden their vision and horizon and develop strategies accordingly.

Health, more particularly MCH with which the family planning programme is integrated in many situations, is a labour-intensive industry, with manpower consuming about 60-80 per cent of the budgets. The success of family planning programmes and services therefore depends to a large extent upon the human resource capital of the health and family planning sector. In view of the importance of "beyond family planning measures", the human resources capital in such departments/ ministries and sectors as education, social welfare, women, and child and youth, will also play a crucial role in achieving success of family planning efforts.

It is has been amply realized that the success of a programme depends upon appropriate utilization of the services, an important component of which is that provision of services and resources, in terms of manpower with optimal mix, money, material, drugs, supplies and equipment, must be commensurate and available at the right place for the right purpose. The key factor for ensuring this constellation of services is manpower in the sectors mentioned above, ranging from grass-root workers to supervisors, administrators, planners and policy makers belonging to several disciplines, functioning in integrated manner in team spirit within a given political administrative and social environment which is conducive for the manpower to function. For these services to be effective and efficient in order to make an impact, the entire range of manpower development processes, consisting of three major dimensions—planning, production and management —will need to be given adequate consideration. Quite beyond the entry of personnel with appropriate qualifications and experience for various positions in the health and other related sectors, the processes related to induction training, promotional training and continuing education with defined periodicity will have to be given due consideration. In addition to these factors, continuous monitoring and evaluation of manpower systems need to be incorporated into the organizational structures in the departments and ministries mentioned above. Adequate consideration must be given to preparation of training curricula, materials and aids relevant to needs and consistent with linguistic and cultural requirements, training of trainers, qualitative improvement of training infrastructures, conducive environments for training, availability of appropriate library and documentation services, proper pre- and post-training and follow-up

evaluation, balance between imparting knowledge, developing skills and inculcating appropriate attitudes and other factors. Often the training efforts are centred around imparting knowledge, and competency-based training is almost neglected even though at the service delivery point it is the most crucial variable in so far as improvement in quality of service is concerned. Innovations in educational systems and processes are badly needed, yet hardly any attention is given towards this need. Linking training processes with job requirements and promotional opportunities, dissemination of materials and continuous contact of trainees with training institutions through such mechanisms as newsletters and bulletins are vital for continuous improvement of human capital concerned with providing family planning services. All these measures are likely to be more effective if attempts are simultaneously made to bring organizational development processes into operation in the organization at several levels. The role of studies and researches in education and training processes and health manpower development systems thus cannot be overemphasized. A substantial number of these dimensions have been incorporated for implementation in National Training Project covering eight states in India and the macro-strategy for training of health and family welfare personnel formulated by NIHFW.

From the considerations mentioned above, it is reasonably clear that for effective and efficient delivery of services, more particularly, improving quality of services a crucial variable is the quality of manpower delivering such services. Henceforth, in any attempt to improve the quality of services in a family planning/population stabilization programme, this variable needs to be given more importance. Care must be taken that such attempts are as necessary for paramedical and other health and health-related sector personnel as they are for medical manpower. Simultaneously, efforts will need to be made with regard to initiation and continuation of organizational development processes in relation to organizational structure at various levels. Such efforts, to be meaningful, require networking of several persons, institutions and agencies, vertically and horizontally, within countries and between countries, at least in the countries with more or less similar level of development and sociocultural settings within geographical regions. International agencies, such as the United Nations Children's Fund (UNICEF), UNFPA and the World Health Organization (WHO), have a stake in these processes and therefore must play crucial roles in an interlinked and complementary manner.

ANNEX

Contraceptive use by method; use-failure and continuation

TABLE A.3. PERCENTAGE DISTRIBUTION OF CURRENT CONTRACEPTIVE USERS, BY METHOD USED

A. Developing countries

Major area, region and country or area	Year (1)	Total (2)	Total clinic and supply[a] (3)	Sterilization Female (4)	Sterilization Male (5)	Pill (6)	Injectables (7)	Intra-uterine device (8)	Condom (9)	Vaginal methods (10)	Rhythm (11)	Withdrawal (12)	Absti-nence (13)	Douche (14)	Other or not stated (15)
Africa															
Eastern Africa															
Burundi	1987[c]	100	14	1	0	2	6	3	1	0	55	8	23	..	1
Kenya	1977/78	100	64	13	1	30	8	10	2	1	16	2	16	0	2
	1984	100	56	15	0[d]	18	3	18	2	1	22	4	16	0	1
Malawi	1984	100	11	[d]	[d]	10	1	4	0	[d]	[d]	3	51[d]	——30——	
Mauritius	1975	100[e]	64	..	..	46	4	3	11	[d]	30	3	[d]	..	2
	1985	100	60	6	0	28	8	3	15[f]	1	23	17	..	..	0
Rwanda	1983	100	8	0	0	2	4	3	0	0	–	91	–	0	1
Zimbabwe	1984	100	69	4	0	59	2	2	2	0	2	17	5	..	7
Middle Africa															
Cameroon	1978	100	24	..	..	10	–	6	8	0	47	16	..	1	12
Northern Africa															
Egypt	1974/75	100[g]	90	..	..	80	–	10	4	2		——10——	..		0
	1984	100[g]	97	5	0	56	1	28	1	0	2	1	0	1	4
Morocco	1980	100	84	4	0	71	0	8	1	0	6	5	1	1	3
	1987[c]	100	81	6	0	64	1	8	3	2	6	9	6	0	1
Sudan (Northern)	1978/79	100	83	6	1	68	1	2	4	2	10	2	..	0	2
Tunisia	1978	100	79	24	0	21	1	28	3	2	12	6	0	..	2
	1983	100	83	30	0	13	1	32	3	4	11	4			
Southern Africa															
Botswana	1984	100	67	5	0	36	4	17	4	0	1	1	31	..	0
Lesotho	1977	100	48	15	0	23	4	2	2	1	2	47	..	0	4
South Africa[h]	1981/82	100	94	16	0	30	30	12	6		——7——				

122

TABLE A.3 (continued)

Major area, region and country or area	Year (1)	Total (2)	Total clinic and supply[a] (3)	Sterilization — Female (4)	Sterilization — Male (5)	Pill (6)	Injectables (7)	Intra-uterine device (8)	Condom (9)	Vaginal methods (10)	Rhythm (11)	Withdrawal (12)	Abstinence (13)	Douche (14)	Other or not stated (15)
Western Africa															
Benin	1982	100[i]	5	0	0	1	0	1	1	1	27	27	51	2	0
Cote d'Ivoire	1980/81	100	17	0	0	14	0	2	0	0	3	3	62	5	2
Ghana	1979	100	58	5	0	25	1	3	7	17	2	2	32	0	0
Liberia	1986	100	88	17	0	52	5	9	2	3	9	2	..	..	3
Mali	1987[g]	100	28	2	0	20	2	2	2	0	28	2	33	0	11
Nigeria	1981/82	100	12	1	0	5	3	1	0	0	6	2	80	1	1
Senegal	1978	100	15	1	..	8	1	4	2	0	10	..	67	1	8
	1986	100	21	2	0	11	1	6	1	1	8	1	59	..	12
Asia															
Eastern Asia															
China	1982	100	96	25	10	8	..	50	2	1		——4——			
	1985	100	99	36	12	7	..	41	3	0	——1——				
Hong Kong	1972	100	87	——23——		36	3	10	7	8	6		——7——		
	1982	100	88	28	2	27	4	5	20	4	11		——1——		
Republic of Korea	1974	100	77	5	8	24	1	23	15	1	13	8	1	1	0
	1985	100	84	45	13	..[d]	11	10			——16——				0
South Asia															
Southern Asia															
Bangladesh	1976	100	62	4	6	36	—	5	10	0	13	7	15	1	2
	1985	100	73	31	6	20	2	6	7	1	15	4	2	..	7
India	1970	100	69	19	26	2	—	5	18	1		——29——			
	1980	100	80	——63——		3	—	1	12	—		——20——			
Nepal	1976	100	98	4	67	15	—	2	9	..	..	..	2	..	0
	1986	100	100	45	41	6	4	1	4	..	..	..	..	..	0
Pakistan	1975	100	72	18	1	18	—	12	19	3	2	2	22	..	2
	1984/85	100	85	29	0	16	7	9	22	1	1	9	..	..	5
Sri Lanka	1975	100	59	29	2	5	1	15	7	0	25	5	11	0	0
	1987[c]	100	65	40	8	7	4	3	3	0	24	5	5	0	0
Western Asia															
Iraq	1974	100[g]	89	4	—	60	4	4	10	7	5	3	..	..	3
Jordan	1972	100[n]	78[p]	——4——		63	—	4	5	2	10	14	3	5	6[s]
	1985	100	84	18	0	23	0	41	2	0	11	5	..	..	..

TABLE A.3 (continued)

Major area, region and country or area	Year (1)	Total (2)	Total clinic and supply[a] (3)	Sterilization Female (4)	Sterilization Male (5)	Pill (6)	Injectables (7)	Intrauterine device (8)	Condom (9)	Vaginal methods (10)	Rhythm (11)	Withdrawal (12)	Abstinence (13)	Douche (14)	Other or not stated (15)
Southeastern Asia															
Indonesia	1976	100	94	1	0	63	–	22	8	:	4	0	1	:	6
	1987	100	92	6	0	34	20	28	3	1	0	0	:	:	7
Malaysia (Peninsular)	1974	100	72	10	1	49	1	2	8	0	10	6	5	:	7
	1984	100n	58	15	0	23	1	4	15	0	19	11	4 ——8——		26
Philippines	1978	100	45	13	2	13	0	6	10	0	24	26	5	0	0
	1986	100	47	24	1	14	0	5	3	0	19	21	4	:	8
Singapore	1973	100	87	——18——		36	–	5	28		——12——				
	1982	100	80	30	1	16	–	°	33	–	——19——			2	
Thailand	1978/79	100	92	24	6	41	9	8	4	–			——8——		
	1987c	100m	97	33	8	30	14	11	2	0	1	1		0	
Lebanon	1971	100m	43p	2	0	26	–	2	13	:	13	53	0	:	..
Syrian Arab Republic	1978	100	76	2	0	59	2	3	3	7	14	8	:	1	..
Turkey	1968	100n	70p	:	:	7	–	5	14	4	:	56	:	37	..
	1983	100	45	2	:	15	0	15	8	5	2	49	:	3	1
Latin America and the Caribbean															
Antigua	1981	100	95	——22——		41	12	12	5	3	3	2	:	:	0
Barbados	1980/81	100j	96	31	1	35	5	9	11	5	3	2 ——4——		:	0
Dominica	1981	100	96	——30——		34	20	4	7	1	2	1	4		0
Dominican Republic	1975	100	82	38	0	25	1	9	5	5	4	12	:	:	1
	1986	100	93	66	0	18	0	6	5	1	3	3	:	2	1
Grenada	1985	100	88	7	–	25	9	8	26	12	2	9	:	:	–
Guadeloupe	1976	100	71	27	–	22	–	8	13	1	11	14	–	:	1k
Haiti	1977	100	28	1	1	18	–	2	6	1	26	25	18	3	1
	1983	100k	57	10	1	32	3	3	7	0	20	23	:	3	..
Jamaica	1975/76	100	94	21	0	31	16	5	17	4	1	4	1	0	0
	1983	100	94	21	0	38	15	4	15	2	2	4	:	:	0
Martinique	1976	100	75	25	–	33	–	5	8	3	9	12	:	2	3k
Montserrat	1984	100	99	——3——		58	6	21	6	4	——1——		:	:	..
Puerto Rico	1968	100	84	57	2	19	–	3	3	d	3	7	:	——6——	:
	1982	100	90	60	6	12	–	6	6	:			:		
Saint Kitts and Nevis	1984	100	91	——6——		48	6	9	14	7	7	——16——		:	0
Saint Lucia	1981	100	94	——25——		49	5	2	9	3	2 ——9——			2	:
Saint Vincent and the Grenadines	1981	100	95	——28——		31	7	6	20	3	2	1	:	:	1

124

TABLE A.3 (continued)

Major area, region and country or area	Year (1)	Total (2)	Total clinic and supply[a] (3)	Sterilization Female (4)	Sterilization Male (5)	Pill (6)	Injectables (7)	Intra-uterine device (8)	Condom (9)	Vaginal methods (10)	Rhythm (11)	Withdrawal (12)	Abstinence (13)	Douche (14)	Other or not stated (15)
Trinidad and Tobago	1977	100	89	8	0	35	2	4	29	10	5	5	1	1	0
	1987[c]	100	84	16	0	27	2	8	22	9	5	10	0	——1——	
Central America															
Cost Rica	1976	100[l]	84	21	1	36	2	8	13	3	8	7	4	..	1
	1986	100[l]	82	21	1	29	2	12	19	1	11	4	0	——7——	
El Salvador	1975	100[m]	93	——45——	[d]	34	2	10	3	..	4	——5——	..	..	2
	1985	100	91	67	[d]	14	[d]	7	3	0	4	—	—	—	—
Guatemala	1978	100[k]	84	33	2	30	6	7	4	2	14	2	..	..	0
	1987[c]	100	82	45	4	17	2	8	5	2	12	5	..	..	0
Honduras	1981	100	88	30	1	44	1	9	1	2	6	6	..	..	0
	1984	100	85	35	1	36	1	11	3	1	8	5	..	..	0
Mexico	1976	100	77	9	1	36	6	19	2	5	10	12	..	1	..
	1987[c]	100	85	35	2	18	5	20	4	1	————15————				0
Nicaragua	1981	100	84	26	0	39	5	9	3	2	4	1	3	1	1
Tropical South America															
Bolivia	1983	100	42	12	0	12	4	15	0	4	54	4	..	..	0
Brazil	1986	100	86	41	1	38	1	2	3	1	7	8	..	..	..
Colombia	1984	100[k]	93	56	1	20	1	10	3	2	4	2	..	..	..
	1976	100	72	9	0	31	1	20	4	5	12	11	2	1	2
Educator	1986	100	81	28	1	25	4	17	3	4	9	9	..	..	1
	1979	100	77	23	1	28	3	14	3	5	14	7	1	1	0
Guyana	1987[c]	100	81	34	0	19	2	22	1	3	14	5	..	..	1
	1975	100	90	27	0	29	1	18	9	6	3	4	2	0	1
Paraguay	1977	100[k]	81	——11——		41	3	14	9	3	7	12	..	..	..
	1987	100	65	9	0	30	8	11	5	1	13	5	..	..	16
Peru	1977/78	100	35	9	0	13	3	4	3	3	35	11	7	11	2
	1986[c]	100	50	14	0	14	3	16	2	2	39	8	..	..	3
Venezuela	1977	100	76	15	0	31	0	17	10	2	8	10	..	5	1
Oceania															
Fiji	1974	100	86	39	0	20	1	12	15	0	6	7	1	..	1

125

TABLE A.3 (continued)

B. Developed countries

Major area, region and country or area	Year (1)	Total (2)	Total clinic and supply[a] (3)	Sterilization — Female (4)	Male (5)	Pill (6)	Injectables (7)	Intra-uterine device (8)	Condom (9)	Vaginal methods (10)	Rhythm (11)	Withdrawal (12)	Abstinence (13)	Douche (14)	Other or not stated (15)
Eastern Asia															
Japan	1975	100[n]	99[p]	5 (F+M)		3	—	9	78	4[q]	30	7	..	1	0
	1986	100[n]	92[p]	13	2	2	—	5	69	1	18	5	..	..	5
Europe															
Eastern Europe															
Bulgaria	1976	100	10	1	1	3	—	2	3	0	5	79	7	:	1
Czechoslovakia	1970	100	37	0	0	4	—	14	19	:	3	52	:	:	8
	1977	100	52	3	0	15	—	19	14	1	7	31	1	:	9
Hungary	1977	100	71	2	:	49	—	13	5	2	5	23	1	:	1
	1986	100	85	:	:	54	—	25	5	1	3	11	0	:	0
Poland	1972	100[e]	22	:	:	4	—	1	17	0	33	38	:	0	8
	1977	100[e]	35	:	:	10	—	2	19	4	41	25	:	:	0
Romania	1977	100[e]	9	:	:	1	—	:	6	2	41	44	0	:	6
Northern Europe															
Denmark	1970	100[e]	:	:	:	37	—	4	30	9	2	7	:	:	11
	1975	100[e]	95	:	:	5	—	14	39	7	1	2	:	:	3
Finland	1971	100	70	0	0	26	—	4	40	0	1	21	:	:	8
	1977	100	97	5	1	14	—	36	40	1	1	3	:	:	:
Norway	1977	100	92	6	3	18	—	39	23	3	4	5	0	:	:
Sweden	1981	100	92	4 (F+M)		30	—	26	32 (condom + vaginal)		9 (rhythm–douche)				0
United Kingdom															
England and Wales	1975	100[n]	91[p]	17 (F+M)		39	—	8	24	3	1	7	1	:	4
Great Britain	1983	100[n]	98[p]	15	15	36	—	11	19	2	1	5	1	:	1
Southern Europe															
Italy	1979	100	42	1	:	18	—	3	17	3	11	46	0	:	1
Portugal	1980	100	49	1	0	29	2	5	8	3	6	39	:	:	5
Spain	1977	100	39	0	:	26	—	1	10	2	12	44	:	1	2
	1985	100	64	7	1	26	d	10	21	2[d]	6	27	3	:	4

126

TABLE A.3 (continued)

Major area region and country or area	Year (1)	Total (2)	Total clinic and supply[a] (3)	Sterilization Female (4)	Male (5)	Pill (6)	Injec-tables (7)	Intra-uterine device (8)	Condom (9)	Vaginal methods (10)	Rhythm (11)	With-drawal (12)	Absti-nence (13)	Douche (14)	Other or not stated (15)
Yugoslavia	1970	100[e]	17	..	..	9	—	2	6	0	3	73	..	..	8
	1976	100[e]	22	..	..	9	—	3	4	6	8	65	..	..	5
Western Europe															
Austria	1981/82	100	79	1	0	56	—	12	6	4	12	8	1	..	1
Belgium (Flemish population)	1975/76	100	57	——7——		35	—	4	9	0	8	37[f]	0	..	0
	1982/83	100	78	——21——		39	—	10	8	0	5	16[f]	0	0	0
France	1972	100	32	0	0	17	—	2	12	1	14	52	..	..	2
	1985	100	62	5	..	34	—	13	8	2	9	29	..	..	..
Germany, Federal Republic of	1985	100	87	13	3	43	0	19	7	2	5	5	..	..	2[s]
Netherlands	1977	100[f]	94	——19——		60	—	6	9	[d]	2	1	——6——		1
	1985	100	95	7	12	55	—	12	9	3	6	2	..	..	1
Switzerland	1980	100	91	——22——		39	—	15	12	3	6	2			1
Americas															
Northern America															
Canada	1976	100	86	30	..	39	—	6	6	5	6	3	..	..	4
	1984	100	95	42	18	15	—	8	11	2	3	1		1	
United States of America	1973	100	91	12	11	36	—	10	14	8	4	2		1	2
	1982	100	92	26	15	20	—	7	14	10	5	2		0	1
Oceania															
New Zealand	1976	100[j]	88[l]	16	13	41	..	6	12	..	2	————12————			

Source: Levels and Trends of Contraceptive Use as Assessed in 1988, Population Studies, No. 110 (United Nations publication, Sales No. E.89.XIII.4), table 10.

NOTE: Except as noted separately, figures are based on current contraceptive users among married women of the ages shown for each country and date in table 4 (if two dates are shown) or tables 2 and 3 (if one date is shown). Data are confined to countries where at least 2 per cent of married women of reproductive age were using contraception. Many surveys did not ask specifically about use of abstinence or douche, and some did not ask about sterilization. These methods may have been included in the "Other" category if they were mentioned by the respondent. Methods about which information was not given in the source tabulation are indicated in the table by two dots (..). Where information about the use of injectables was not available, it has been assumed that use of that method is negligible and it is indicated by an em dash (—). A zero (0) indicates that the source showed fewer than 0.5 per cent to be using a specific method. Figures in the table may not add to 100 per cent because of rounding.

[a] Methods in columns (4)-(10). Particular clinic and supply methods may be excluded when these are not distinguished in source from non-supply methods.

[b] Including spermicides, diaphragm, cervical cap, contraceptive sponge.

[c] Preliminary or provisional.

[d] Combined with "Other".

[e] Excluding sterilization.

[f] Including 2 per cent using rhythm and a supply method (usually condom) in combination.

[g] Adjusted from source to exclude breast-feeding.

[h] Estimates of the Population Division of the Department of International Economic and Social Affairs of the United Nations Secretariat based on surveys of various ethnic groups in 1976, 1981, 1982.

127

Table A.3 (*continued*)

[i]Women that have not resumed sexual relations since the last birth are not counted as users of contraception.
[j]Percentages do not add to 100 because women using a combination of methods are shown under each method.
[k]Combined with vaginal methods, rhythm and withdrawal.
[l]Calculated assuming that clinic and supply methods are not used in combination with other clinic and supply methods.
[m]Including women using a combination of methods.
[n]Users among all women.
[o]Excluding douche, abstinence and folk methods.
[p]For ages 20-44.
[q]Based on users ever in a union.
[r]Percentage using foam.
[s]Including practice of rhythm and withdrawal in combination.
[t]Standardized on the age distribution of women interviewed in 1985.

TABLE A.4. TWELVE-MONTH CONTRACEPTIVE USE-FAILURE AND CONTINUATION RATES: REVIEW OF RECENT PROSPECTIVE AND RETROSPECTIVE FOLLOW-UP STUDIES OF ACCEPTORS

Country	Year or period	Sample size	Prospective/ retrospective	Method/ subpopulation	Use-failure	Continu-ation	Loss to follow-up (percentage)
				A. Intra-uterine device			
1. Developed countries	1980	..	P	..	3.5	..	..
			R	..	..	..	..
2. Developing countries	1960s	..	P	Minimum	1.5	59.8	..
			R	Maximum	6.0	75.5	..
				Average	2.0-3.0	..	..
3. Developing countries and United States of America	1970s	..	P	..	0.5-5.0	50.0-85	..
Bangladesh	..	121	P	TCu 220C	0.0	58.4	..
Chile (a)	..	821	P	TCu 200	2.5	..	..
Chile (b)	..	471	P	TCu 200	2.7	82.9	..
Chile (c)	..	200	P	TCu 200	2.1	73.3	..
Colombia	..	775	P	TCu 200	2.5	78.6	..
Iran (Islamic Rep. of)	..	719	P	TCu 200	2.6	71.5	..
Republic of Korea	..	1050	P	TCu 200	1.0	68.7	..
Thailand	..	1996	P	TCu 200	1.0	81.9	..
United States of America	..	978	P	TCu 200	1.8	83.2	..
4. Bangladesh	..	999	P	..	..	80	..

TABLE A.4 (continued)

Country	Year or period	Sample size	Prospective/ retrospective	Method/ subpopulation	Use-failure	Continu-ation	Loss to follow-up (percentage)
5. China	1982	892	P	TCu 380Ag	0.2	85.9	..
		887	P	TCu 220Ag	0.8	90.8	..
		983	P	Mahua Ring	3.5	83.4	..
6. Colombia	1971-1972	600	R	TCu 200	3.5	65.7	4
		426	R	Dalkon Shield	4.8	61.2	..
		600	R	Lippes Loop	4.9	63.4	..
7. Ecuador	1981-1982	283	P	TCu 200	2.4	87.9	..
8. Egypt Assiut	1980-1981	100	P	TCu 380Ag	1.0	86.5	6
9. India Bombay	..	1 624	R	..	0.08	..	..
10. Iran (Islamic Rep. of)	1975	232	R	..	0.5	75.2	9
11. Italy	1980-1984	98	P	IUD Post-coital	2.7	85	7
12. Japan	1970s	..	P	..	3.0-3.7	71.8-89.6	..
13. Malaysia	1980s	1 725	P	ML CU250	2.5	74	6
				TCu 220C	1.7	73	7
				Cu7	4.9	69	8
14. Netherlands	1978-1984	160	P	ML Cu250	0.60	..	0
		140	P	ML Cu375	0.75	..	..
		150	P	MLAG Cu250	0.62	..	..
15. Nigeria Ibadan	1965-1968	628	R	LL3C	3.3	86.5	10
	1968-1970	529	R	M-211	1.4	84.3	6
16. Nigeria	1983	100	P	After MR	0 —	78	..
		100	P	Interval	0	80	..
17. Sudan	..	67	P	Lippes Loop	0.0	70.2	35
		69	P	Cu7	0.0	73.0	40

TABLE A.4 (continued)

Country	Year or period	Sample size	Prospective/ retrospective	Method/ subpopulation	Use-failure	Continu-ation	Loss to follow-up (percentage)
18. United States of America	1970-1975	3 536	P	TCu 380A	0.7	73.0	18
		1 850	P	TCu 220C	0.8	..	..
					0.8	73.6	20
		9 838	P	TCu 220	0.9	..	..
					2.6	72.9	17
					3.1	..	..
B. Oral contraceptives							
1. Bangladesh	1978	390	P	..	..	41	22
2. Brazil	..	930	P	..	1	41.6	21
3. Brazil Rio Grande do Norte	1977	931	P	Source: Programme	..	47.0	..
		1 112	R	All sources	..	53.7	..
						54.7	63
4. Sri Lanka	1978-1980	201	P	OC: standard dose	..	61.1	13
		181	P	OC: low dose	..	42-75	..
						33-51	..
5. WHO sites: Bangkok Thailand Bombay, India Singapore Szegad, Hungary	..	925	P	..	1.27	48.4	..
6. Developing countries	1960s	..	..	..	..	..	..
India (Bombay)		324	P	..	..	..	..
Sri Lanka		651	P	..	..	53.1	..
Turkey		2 158	P	..	..	75.7	..
						12.3	..
C. Barrier methods and spermicides							
1. Developed and developing countries Bangladesh(a)	1970s	150	P	Neo Sampoon	6.5	..	..

TABLE A.4 (continued)

Country	Year or period	Sample size	Prospective/ retrospective	Method/ subpopulation	Use-failure	Continu-ation	Loss to follow-up (percentage)
Bangladesh(b)							
Taiwan Province of China							
Yugoslavia		698	P	Neo Sampoon	11.1	..	..
2. Ghana (Accra)	1982	99	P	Neo Sampoon	9.6	62.4	19
		101	P	Ortho VT	11.3	48.6	22
		100	P	Emko VT	12.5	38.5	23
3. United Kingdom							
London, England	1980-1982	126	P	Sponge	24.5	44.7	<1
		123	P	Diaphragm	10.9	52.0	0
4. United States	1981-1985	463	P	Cervical cap	8.1	89.7	18
5. Yugoslavia	1980-1981	225	P	F. Tabs	12.8	71.6	1.2
		225	P	Songe	10.4	72.9	0.6

D. Periodic abstinence

Country	Year or period	Sample size	Prospective/ retrospective	Method/ subpopulation	Use-failure	Continu-ation	Loss to follow-up (percentage)
1. Developed and developing countries							
Australia	..	1 132	..	..	..	..	..
			P	Billings	26.4	..	..
				Symtothermal	14.3	..	..
Colombia	..	..	P	Billings	24.2	39.9	..
				Symtothermal	19.8	46.9	..
United States of America							
Los Angeles, California	..	838	P	Billings	24.8	30.3	..
				Symtothermal	9.4	35.3	..
WHO sites:							
Total	..	..	P	Billings	22.3	..	..
Dublin, Ireland	..	..	P	Billings	17.7	..	..
Auckland, New Zealand	..	..	P	Billings	31.0	..	..
Manila, Philippines	..	..	P	Billings	17.9	..	..
San Miguel, El Salvador	..	..	P	Billings	33.2	..	..

TABLE A.4 (continued)

Country	Year or period	Sample size	Prospective/ retrospective	Method/ subpopulation	Use-failure	Continu-ation	Loss to follow-up (percentage)
2. Developed and developing countries	1970s	..	P	Cerv.muc. Symtothermal	5.7-26.7 3.3-19.8	26.3-99.5 23.7-62.4	.. ..
3. Chile	1981-1983	660	P	..	16.8	..	..
4. India Tamil Nadu	..	1 000	P	Billings	0.4	99.5	..
5. Philippines	1971	142	R	BBT: First BBT: all Calen: first Calen: all	24 40 27 38	32 41 47 52	.. ..
6. United States of America San Diego, California	1979-1980	148	P	Fertility awareness	13.2	..	..

E. Injectables

Country	Year or period	Sample size	Prospective/ retrospective	Method/ subpopulation	Use-failure	Continu-ation	Loss to follow-up (percentage)
1. WHO sites: 10 centres	.. ..	832 846	P P	NET-EN DMPA	3.6 0.7	.. ..	.. ..
2. Bangladesh	..	2 000	P	DMPA	0	56	..
3. Bangladesh	..	913	P	NET-EN	0.2	62.7	9
4. India	1981-1982	1 207 1 181	P P	NET-EN/2m NET-EN/3m	0.0 1.1	31.4 32.5	.. ..
5. Mexico Rural	1979-1981	5 792	P	NET-EN	0.2	43.0	16
6. Pakistan	..	2 147	P	NET-EN	0.0	21.7	19
7. South Africa Stellenbosch	..	10 875	P	3-monthly 6-monthly	0.11 0.49	32 28	53 66

TABLE A.4 (continued)

Country	Year or period	Sample size	Prospective/ retrospective	Method/ subpopulation	Use-failure	Continu-ation	Loss to follow-up (percentage)
8. Thailand	1978	624	R	DMPA	0.003	59.1	38
F. Implants and vaginal rings							
1. Brazil, Chile, Dominican Republic, Finland, United States of America	1980s	189	P	Norplant	0.0	78 79	..
2. Brazil, Chile, Dominican Republic, Finland, Jamaica	1977-1981	990	P	Norplant	0.4	77.1	1
3. Chile	1980s	458	P	Norplant	0.0	..	..
4. China	..	108	P	Low dose Vaginal ring	3.7	71.2	0
5. Colombia	1982-1984	389	P	Norplant	0.0	91.6	5
6. Ecuador	1981-1982	283	P	Norplant	0.0	87.4	..
7. Egypt Assiut	1980-1981	250	P	Norplant	0.8	89.6	7
8. India	..	876	P	Implant D	3.9	86.4	..
9. Thailand	1982	704	P	Norplant	0.3	88.4	21

Source: Measuring the Dynamics of Contraceptive Use, Proceedings of the United Nations Expert Group Meeting, New York, 5-7 December 1988, Population Studies, No. 106 (United Nations publication, Sales No. E.91.XIII.7).

NOTE: DMPA = depot-medroxy progesterone acetate; IUD = intra-uterine device; NET-EN = nonethisterone enanthate; OC = oral contraceptive.

133

Amin, Ruhol, and others (1987). Family planning in Bangladesh, 1969-1983. *International Family Planning Perspectives* (New York), vol. 13, No. 1 (March), pp. 16-20.

Bardhan, A., and D. C. Dubey (1983). Psychosocial factors involving continuation/ discontinuation of IUD and oral pill in the State of Rajasthan. Mimeographed.

Bhatnagar, S., and others (1988). A field study of IUD acceptors in the State of Uttar Pradesh. New Delhi: National Institute of Health and Family Welfare. Mimeographed.

Bruce, Judith (1990). Fundamental elements of the quality of care: a simple framework. *Studies in Family Planning* (New York), vol. 21, No. 2 (March-April), pp. 61-91.

Business International (1978). International fact finding study: private sector marketing of contraceptives in eight developing countries. Study prepared for The Population Council, New York.

Chen, Pi-chao (1984). China's other revolution: findings from the One in 1,000 Fertility Survey. *International Family Planning Perspectives* (New York), vol. 10, No. 2 (June), pp. 48-57.

Diaz, J., and H. Halbe (1990). Quality of care in family planning clinical services in Latin America. *Profamilia* (Bogotá, Colombia), vol. 6, No. 16 (December), pp. 16-30.

Donabedian, Avedis (1988). The quality of care. How can it be assessed? *Journal of the American Medical Association* (Chicago, Illinois), vol. 260, pp. 1743-1748.

Dwyer, Joseph C., and Jeanne M. Haws (1990). Is permanent contraception acceptable in sub-Saharan Africa? *Studies in Family Planning* (New York), vol. 21, No. 6 (November/ December), pp. 322-326.

Folch-Lyon, Evelyn, Luis de la Macorra and S. Bruce Schearer (1981). Focus group and survey research on family planning in Mexico. *Studies in Family Planning* (New York), vol. 12, No. 12 (December), pp. 409-432.

Freedman, Ronald, and Bernard Berelson (1976). The record of family planning programs. *Studies in Family Planning* (New York), vol. 7, No. 1 (January), pp. 3-40.

Giridhar, G., and J. K. Satia (1986). Planning for service delivery at health centres: an experiment. *Asian and Pacific Population Journal* (Bangkok), vol. 1, No. 2 (June), pp. 39-56.

Hammer, Vicki (1982). The status of women and family planning. Paper presented at the Meeting of WHO and Federation of Indian Gynaecologists and Obstetricians, San Francisco, October.

Henshaw, Stanley K. (1987). Induced abortion: a worldwide perspective. *International Family Planning Perspectives* (New York), vol. 13, No. 1 (March), pp. 12-15.

Hermalin, Albert I., and Barbara Entwisle (1985). Future directions in the analysis of contraceptive availability. *International Population Conference, Florence, 1985*, vol. 3. Liège, Belgium: International Union for the Scientific Study of Population, pp. 445-458.

Hull, Valerie J. (1979). Women, doctors and family health care: some lessons from rural Java. *Studies in Family Planning* (New York), vol. 10, No. 11/12 (November-December), pp. 315-32

India, Ministry of Health and Family Welfare (1991). *Year Book of Family Welfare Programmes in India, 1989-90*. New Delhi: Department of Family Welfare.

Indian Council of Medical Research (1986). Role of health delivery services in acceptance of family planning (Phase I) a multicentric study. New Delhi.

_____ (1991). Evaluation of quality of maternal and child health (MCH) and family planning (FP). A report. Mimeographed.

Jacobalis, S. (1989). Basic issues related to quantity and quality of health care, and quality assurance in Indonesia. *Australian Clinical Review* (Carlton, Victoria), vol. 9, No. 3-4, pp. 149-154.

Jain, Anrudh K. (1989). Fertility reduction and the quality of family planning services. *Studies in Family Planning* (New York), vol. 20, No. 1 (January-February), pp. 1-16.

Kaufmann, J., and others (1989). The relationship between service quality and demographic outcome in four rural Chinese counties. Paper presented at the International Union for the Scientific Study of Population Seminar on the Role of Family Planning Programs as a Fertility Determinant, Tunis, 26-30 June 1989.

Khan, M. E., and S. K. Dastidar (1985). *Women's Perspective in Family Planning Programmes*. Baroda, India: Operations Research Group.

Khan, M. E., and C. V. S. Prasad (1983a). Family planning practices in India: the Second All-India Survey. Baroda, India: Operations Research Group. Mimeographed.

_____ (1983b). Social marketing of Nirodh. Retailers' views and their problems. New Delhi: Operations Research Group.

Khan, M. E., S. K. Ghosh Dastidar and Shashi Bairathi (1985). Not wanting children yet not practising family planning. *Journal of Family Welfare* (Bombay), vol. 32, No. 2 (December), pp. 3-17.

Khan, M. E., B. C. Patel, and R. Chandrasekar (1990). Contraceptive use dynamics of couples availing of services from Government Family Planning Clinics: a case study of Orisssa. *Journal of Family Welfare* (Bombay), vol. 36, No. 3, pp. 18-38.

Khan, M. E., C. V. S. Prasad and Neshat Quaisen (1984). Reasons for under-utilization of health services. A case study of a PHC in a tribal area of Bihar. Indian Council of Medical Research and Ford Foundation Workshop on Child Health and Nutrition and Family Planning. New Delhi: Indian Council of Medical Research.

Khan, M. E., and others (1983). Role of health delivery services in acceptance of family planning. New Delhi: Indian Council of Medical Research. Mimeographed.

Koblinsky, M. A., and others (1987). Work routines of field workers. Determinants of service, quantity and quality in Bangladesh. Paper presented at the Annual Meeting of the American Public Health Association, New Orleans, 19-22 October.

Kreager, Phillip (1977). *Family Planning Drops-Outs Reconsidered: A Critical Review of Research and Research Findings*. London: International Planned Parenthood Federation.

Lightbourne, Robert E. (1985). Desired number of births and prospects for fertility decline in 40 countries. *International Family Planning Perspectives* (New York), vol. 11, No. 2 (June), pp. 34-39.

Malaysia (1990). The strategy of quality services delivery in population programmes. Country paper presented at the International Council of Management Programmes International Conference, Kuala Lumpur, Malaysia, 12-16 November.

Mehta, Suman, and others (1983). Role of health delivery services in acceptance of family planning. New Delhi: Indian Council of Medical Research. Mimeographed.

Miller, R. A., and others (1990). The situation analysis study of the family planning programme in Kenya. Unpublished.

Misra, B. D., and others (1982). *Organisation for Change: A Systems Analysis of Family Planning in Rural India*. New Delhi: Radint Publications; and Ann Arbor, Michigan: University of Michigan, Center for South and Southeast Asian Studies.

Mundigo, Axel, and Mayone Stycos (1975). Information and education on perspective. The Dominican Republic family planning programme. In *The Clinic and the Information Flow: Educating the Family Planning Client in Four Latin American Countries*, J. Mayon Stycos, ed. London: Lexington Books.

Myntti, Cynthia (1979). Population process in rural Yemen: temporary emigration, breast feeding and contraception. *Studies in Family Planning* (New York), vol. 10, No. 10 (October), pp. 282-289.

Nortman, Dorothy L., and Ellen Hofstatter (1978). *Population and Family Planning Programs*. 9th ed. New York: The Population Council.

Operations Research Group (1990). *Family Planning Practices in India: Third All India Survey*, vol. II. Baroda, India: Ministry of Health and Family Welfare Operations Research Group.

Pariani, S. D. M. Herr and Maurice D. Van Arsdol (1987). Continued contraceptive use in five family planning clinics in Sunabaya, Indonesia. Paper presented at the Annual Meeting of the American Public Health Association, New Orleans, 19-22 October.

Sadik, Nafis (1981). Use of family planning services. In *World Fertility Survey Conference, 1980: Record of Proceedings*, vol. 2. Voorburg, Netherlands: International Statistical Institute.

Scrimshaw, Susan C. (1977). Cultural values and behaviour related to population change. Paper presented for the project on Cultural Values and Population Policy. Chapel Hill: University of North Carolina, Institute of Society, Ethics and the Life Sciences. Mimeographed.

Simmons, Ruth, and others (1988). Beyond supply: the importance of female family planning workers in rural Bangladesh. *Studies in Family Planning* (New York), vol. 19, No. 1 (January-February), pp. 29-38.

Stycos, J. Mayone (1984). Sterilization in Latin America: its past and its future. *International Family Planning Perspectives* (New York), vol. 10, No. 2 (June), pp. 58-68.

Sundaram, E. B. (1983). Women's accessibility to health, family planning and other welfare services. A case study of sex discrimination, Bangalore. Paper presented at the Indian Council of Medical Research Workshop, November.

Suyono, Haryono, and others (1981). Family planning attitudes in urban Indonesia: findings from focus research group. *Studies in Family Planning* (New York), vol. 12, No. 12 (December), pp. 433-442.

Sweeney, William O. (1977). *Media Communications in Population/Family Planning Programs: A Review*. Population Reports, Series J, No. 16. Baltimore, Maryland: The Johns Hopkins University, Population Information Program.

Thomas, Ken T., and others (1988). Contraceptive method switching in Sri Lanka: patterns and implications. *International Family Planning Perspectives* (New York), vol. 14, No. 2 (June), pp. 54-60.

Townsend, John W., and Gabriel Ojeda (1985). Final narrative report: community distribution of contraceptives in rural areas. Joint report of the Population Council and Profamilia, Bogotá, Colombia.

United Nations (1975). *Report of the United Nations World Population Conference, 1974, Bucharest, 19-30 August 1974*. Sales No. E.75.XIII.3.

_____ (1984). *Report of the International Conference on Population, 1984, Mexico City, 6-14 August 1984*. Sales No. E.84.XIII.8.

_____ (1989). *Concise Report on the World Population Situation in 1989, with a Special Report on Population Trends and Policies in the Least Developed Countries*. Sales No. E.90.XIII.32.

_____ (1989). *Levels and Trends of Contraceptive Use as Assessed in 1989*. Population Studies, No. 110. Sales No. E.89.XIII.4.

_____ (1991). *Measuring the Dynamics of Contraceptive Use*. Proceeding of the United Nations Expert Group Meeting, New York, 5-7 December 1988. Population Studies No. 106. Sales No. E.91.XIII.7.

_____, Economic and Social Commission for Asia and the Pacific (1987). *Population Policies and Programmes: Current Status and Future Directions*. Asian Population Studies Series No. 84. Bangkok: ESCAP.

Visaria, L., and P. Visaria (1991). Quality of services and family planning in Gujarat State, India: an exploratory analysis. Working paper No. 34. Paper presented at the ICOMP International Conference on the Strategy of Quality Service Delivery in Population Programmes, Kuala Lumpur, Malaysia Nov. 12-16, 1990.

Way, Ann A., Anne R. Cross and Sushil Kumar (1987). Family planning in Botswana, Kenya and Zimbabwe. *International Family Planning Perspectives* (New York), vol. 13, No. 1 (March), pp. 7-11.

Westinghouse Population Center (1974). *Contraceptive Distribution in the Commercial Sector of Selected Developing Countries: Summary Report*. Columbia, Maryland.

Willson, Peters D. (1984). The 1984 International Conference on Population: what will be the issues? *International Family Planning Perspectives* (New York), vol. 10, No. 2 (June), pp. 43-47.

Zatuchni, Gerald I. (1970). *Overview of Program: Two Year Experience in Postpartum Family Planning*. New York: The Population Council and McGraw Hill.

Zeighami, Elaine, and others (1976). Effectiveness of the Iranian auxilliary midwife in IUD insertion. *Studies in Family Planning* (New York), vol. 7, No. 9 (September), pp. 261-263.

VIII. FAMILY PLANNING SERVICES AND UNREACHED POPULATION GROUPS

*Peter Sumbung**

In the last half of the twentieth century, many Governments, especially in Asian countries, have changed from a pronatalist to an antinatalist population policy. Stimuli for the developing countries of today to call for fertility declines arise largely from convictions that current high rates of population growth retard economic development. Indeed, there are reasons to believe that family planning has contributed to the decline in fertility observed since the 1960s. In this regard, a number of countries, such as China, Indonesia, Singapore and Thailand, are considered to be very successful, whereas some are rated medium or very low in their achievement. The pace of fertility decline in the future will depend upon the pace of improvements in family planning programmes (aside from infant mortality decline, enhancement of female education etc.).

Indicators of the success of a family planning programme can be measured by the magnitude of fertility decline between two points of time. According to Crowley, Cornelius and Sinding (1987), and Bongaarts (1987), contraceptive prevalence (as an indicator of programme performance) is preferable to fertility as the dependent variable because prevalence is more causally linked to programme proximate determinants unrelated to family planning programmes.

The success of a family planning programme depends upon its "strength" or its "weakness" (Lapham and Mauldin, 1984). As mentioned above, China, Indonesia, Singapore and Thailand are among the countries whose programme has been considered "strong". Indicators of the strength of a programme include four dimensions of effort: (*a*) policies and stage-setting activities; (*b*) service and service-related activities; (*c*) record-keeping and evaluation; and (*d*) availability of contraceptive methods.

When a new programme is introduced into a country, as administrators strive to make the full range of safe family planning services widely and easily accessible, the family planning programme often faces significant and complex challenges. These obstacles include problems arising from the fact that a certain group of people—the so-called "unreached population"—have disadvantages or difficulties in communicating that result in difficulties concerning availability of communication media or information, which in turn result in difficulties in the areas of family planning or health services, information with regard to agriculture, fishery, husbandry or even financial problems.

Despite the overall success of a family planning programme in a country (Indonesia, for example) cultural and religious values impose a major barrier for family planning practices (Warwick, 1986). Most Indonesians are Muslim and hold traditional cultural values. Both Islamic and cultural traditions support the dominant role of the husband in decisions regarding family life. Thus, the husband's approval plays an important role in the decision to practise contraception.

It is true that family planning programmes should not be homogenous—they should use different approaches with different subgroups of the population. Every population is differentiated by education, age and family size; and programmes tailored to specific subgroups do better.

Disparity in all those aspects not only can be attributed to geographical areas but also can be related to the existing conditions in terms of gender differences and groups that are inaccessible due either to geographical location or problems of certain age groups or the minority. These groups are categorized as the "unreached population".

---

*Vice Chairman, National Family Planning Coordinating Board, Jakarta, Indonesia.

Much of the difficulty in developing a theory of unreached population derives from the lack of success in establishing links between the estimates, composition and trends in the unreached population, on the one hand; and their demographic significance and social covariates, as well as their current usage pattern and situation for family planning, on the other. Estimates of the total unreached population for family planning and its composition need some definition at the outset. The relation of total unreached population to urban or rural residence and to education and other factors, such as age and number of children, must be considered. It is not obvious whether unreached people should be expected to increase or to decline since both the demand and the supply of family planning have been increasing so rapidly in many countries.

The unreached population is of significance not only because of its demographic role in shaping interregional differences in rates of population growth but also for its programmatic interests.

This paper is directed to exploring the so-called "unreached population" in so far as disparity in family planning services may be attributed to gender issues and inaccessibility of groups due either to geographical location or age and other minorities. Its findings refer to the large unreached groups in developing countries, which, if reached would be likely to result in fertility decline.

The first section discusses some indicators of the success of a family planning programme and reviews some existing opinion about disparity of family planning services. Previous empirical literature is critically reviewed in section B. In section C, an attempt is made to identify the conditions under which such differences seem most likely to occur. Lastly, after a discussion of programme implications, there is a brief presentation of research needed.

A. LITERATURE REVIEW

According to Sumarsono, Pandi and Kantner (1990), although women in Indonesia have traditionally married at young ages and divorce rates have been relatively high by Asian standards, the Indonesian National Contraceptive Prevalence Survey of 1987 found that age at marriage had been increasing

and the proportion of women married more than once was declining. The mean age at first marriage for women increased from 19.1 years in 1976 to 21.2 in 1985. Between 1976 and 1987, the proportions of currently married women that had married more than once declined from 15 to 7 per cent for ages 15-24, from 28 to 15 per cent for ages 25-34 and from 37 to 29 per cent for ages 35-49. In addition, from 1980 to 1987 the percentage of women aged 15-49 that had never married increased from 21.5 to 26.4 per cent. Despite these changes, marriage is still nearly universal in Indonesia (in 1987, more than 98 per cent of women over age 40 had been married at least once), and Indonesian women still married at relatively young ages.

According to a World Bank report (1990), public sectors in Indonesia have been able to contribute to one of the most impressive demographic transitions in the developing world. However, the Government of Indonesia faces new challenges in its family planning programme: to attract a substantial number of new acceptors (including a growing number of young people); to improve contraceptive continuation rates; and to increase the proportion of more effective contraceptive methods. Further declines in fertility are needed in order to accomplish set goals of continued slowing of population growth. However, achievement of the necessary fertility decline to realize these projections will be more difficult than in the past because it will require a more substantial expansion of contraceptive usage than any increase thus far achieved. Also, the couples that still need to be brought into the programme have higher family size preferences and are harder to reach. Among those are the urban poor, those living in outlying rural areas and those with a low level of education.

In a study of programme and non-programme factors associated with fertility in 73 developing countries, Mauldin and Lapham (1987) found that adequacy of supervision, accessibility of services; use of mass media for information, education and communication (IEC) efforts; and use of evaluation data were among the important programme factors associated with fertility decline.

In a survey of 250 men in the Sudan in 1982, Mustafa and Mumford (1984) found that 60 per cent of men with wives of reproductive age wished to use family planning services, whereas 20 per cent of couples were currently using an effective method. Nevertheless, the men in the study expressed a desire to have a large family. The authors observed that in the Sudan, most family decisions were usually made by the husbands, and family planning was not an exception.

In another survey in the Sudan in 1985, Khalifa (1988) found that the decision not to practise family planning was determined by men. Furthermore, husbands had taken the responsibility for providing contraceptive methods when family planning was practised.

In a Nigerian village, Mott and Mott (1985) found a high level of agreement between matched husband and wife pairs with regard to family planning attitudes and behaviour, which could reflect, in part, small variance in society where contraceptive practice is not very high.

A survey of male Nigerian students by Adamchak and Adebayo (1987) reports male disapproval of contraceptive adoption by women without prior consent of the husband, although a desire for family planning information and service was expressed.

In a study of characteristics of new contraceptive acceptors in Zimbabwe, male attitudes are hypothesized to be a major facilitating or inhibiting factor in female contraceptive use and 80 per cent of acceptors reported prior partner's approval (Dow and others, 1986). The Zimbabwe Reproductive Health Survey in 1984 (Zimbabwe, 1985) found that 42 per cent of the Zimbabwean women ever in a union believed that men have the sole responsibility for deciding whether a couple should use family planning.

In a study on family planning knowledge, attitudes and practices (KAP) of men in Zimbabwe, involving 711 currently married men aged 20 years or over, Mbizvo and Adamchak (1989) found that although male knowledge of family planning was high, significantly high numbers of those ever using a method were found older, more educated urban residents and men with five or more children. The dominant reason for practising family planning was for spacing.

Apparently, knowledge, approval and use of family planning do not lead to limiting the number of children.

Joesoef, Baughman and Utomo (1988) interviewed 9,072 eligible women in five cities in Indonesia. The authors found that in all cities, husband's approval was the most important determinant of contraceptive use, followed by number of living children and wife's education. Because most of the family planning programmes in Indonesia are designed to serve primarily women, the finding of husband's approval as the most important determinant has major pro-gramme implications.

Green (1990) states that despite increased research and activities focusing on male involvement in family planning, much more could be done, particularly among providers. She further says that programmes for males have not received the attention they deserve. In a personal communication in 1991, Jeffrey Spieler of the United Nations Agency for International Development stated that although attempts are being made to focus more on male involvement, there is frequently more lip service than actual work and a need exists to turn language into action.

B. Unreached population

The role of men

In family and community

The issue of male involvement in family planning has increasingly received considerable attention in many parts of the world. In many developing countries, men play a dominant role in decision-making with regard to fertility and family planning and have generally been assumed to be the obstacle in these programmes.

According to some experts, this is a major limitation facing family planning programme promotion and population policy development is that they neglected men in studying the circumstances that govern a couple's contraceptive behaviour. In the developing countries, great efforts have been made in recent years to expand public programmes to provide a means of reducing fertility. Both research and services in this area, however, have been dominated by findings derived almost exclusively from women.

In general, policies and programmes based on such findings have not had a high level of success in increasing contraceptive prevalence and simultaneously reducing overall fertility in developing countries. Most countries in Africa (Mbizvo and Adamchak, 1989) and in Western Asia still have low contraceptive prevalence and high fertility. Men's initiative could assume an especially prominent role in the individual couple's family planning effort.

In many developing countries, it was found that most family decisions were made by the husband. With regard to men's attitude to family planning, there is some controversy. According to Mustafa and Mumford (1984), although a relatively large number of men in the Sudan wished to use family planning services (60 per cent), in fact, only 20 per cent were currently using an effective method and they still expressed a desire for a large family. Moreover, when family planning was practised, husbands had taken over the responsibility for providing contraceptive methods (Khalifa, 1988). So strong is the husband's position that even when respondents in Nigeria expressed a desire for family planning information and for targeting men, they were also reported to disapprove of contraceptive adoption by women without prior consent of the husband (Adamchak and Adebayo, 1987).

In many parts of the world, the man's attitude was hypothesized to be a major facilitating or inhibiting factor in female contraceptive use (Dow and others, 1986). In a most explicit case, women sometimes believe that men have the sole responsibility for deciding whether a couple should use family planning. Men also indicate that women should be responsible for obtaining family planning information and have contraceptives supplied, but men should have the decision to pursue family planning and to determine the number of children. Further, although the knowledge, approval and use of family planning were high among men, this situation does not lead to limiting the number of children, because family planning is practised primarily for spacing (Mbizvo and Adamchak, 1989).

From a study of condom use among Haitian men (Boulos, Boulos and Nichols, 1991), it was strikingly concluded that although the condom was universally known to men, it was used by almost none of them in 1986. This extremely low use of condoms was not due to supply constraints or to general opposition to family planning but rather to a general lack of interest among males to practise contraception themselves. The overwhelming majority felt that the responsibility for practising family planning should be borne by the woman.

In Indonesia, it was found that the husband's approval of contraceptive use was the most important determinant (Joesoef, Baughman and Utomo, 1988). A considerable number of women were not using contraception because of the husband's disapproval. This finding has major implications for family planning programmes in Indonesia.

It is clear from this review that the failure to understand sociocultural factors and the role of men in inhibiting or promoting contraceptive adoption could substantially affect promoting of family planning programmes and programme success in different societies.

Condom service delivery programmes need a strong IEC component to assure better compliance, which will lead to higher continuation rates.

Evidence indicates that men have considerable knowledge and use of family planning and considerable control over the decision-making process. When contraception was practised, the vast majority practised it for spacing only. Thus, the fertility level was still high, in part because couples, or the male partners, still desire a large family. The role of men in fertility and family planning is becoming increasingly important in the context of raising contraceptive prevalence and reducing the level of fertility.

From this brief discussion on the role of men in family planning, the author concludes that recognizing the need to involve men, programmes should relate the role of men as decision makers and the use of the so-called "male methods" in family planning.

Family planning acceptance among indigenous minority groups

Levels of contraceptive use have increased substantially throughout the developing countries in the past decade, largely because of the greater availability of contraceptive information and services. Much of this increase, however, has occurred in urban areas with largely modernized populations. Providing services to rural populations and indigenous groups has proved considerably more difficult and contraceptive use among these populations has remained low.

There is a growing regional interest in focusing on these hard-to-reach groups. Among them are the urban poor, men, those living in remote areas or on an island, special groups of unmet need of family planning, other minorities and certain indigenous groups. The strategies that have succeeded in increasing contraceptive use among the majority population have not had the same effect in indigenous communities. Family planning professionals need to better understand the barriers to acceptance of family planning services in these communities before undertaking widespread promotional activities. Research on the sources of resistance to family planning needs to be carried out.

Each country is divided into distinct sociocultural groups. In general, urban-dwellers are people of mixed modern Western heritage or descent that have adopted Western dress and the national language. In contrast, indigenous groups maintain their traditional dress and customs and speak any of the numerous local dialects. Although estimates of indigenous populations vary widely because of problems of definition and data collection, a commonly accepted estimate is very small. The largest linguistic group represents approximately one fifteenth of the entire world population and is scattered from Northern America to South America and from Andaman in the Indian Ocean to Australia.

Maternal and child health indicators among this population are consistently lower than those among urban-dwellers, as are the rates of utilization of general health services. Among indigenous women, the total fertility rate for the period 1983-1987 were

very high, compared with the average for urban women. Although contraceptive use among urban women has increased substantially during the past decade (from 22 to 51 per cent of women of reproductive age), levels of use have remained extremely low among indigenous women.

Results of prior studies (Ward, Bertrand and Puac, 1992) offer some explanations for these wide fertility differentials. For example, one study found that contraceptive prevalence was related to the physical accessibility of contraceptive services among Ladino women but not among Mayan women. Another study showed that the direct monetary cost of services did not constitute a barrier to their use. Moreover, several other studies concluded that underutilization among Mayans is attributable, in part, to sociocultural factors. Although religion and their desire for a large family have often been cited as reasons for the limited use of contraceptives among Mayans, information on their beliefs, attitudes and values with regard to reproduction has been extremely limited.

Factors affecting fertility differ widely between Mayans and Ladinos: an earlier age at marriage, lower educational attainment and generally lower socio-economic status undoubtedly contribute to the comparatively low level of contraceptive use among Mayans.

Although current programme efforts in Guatemala—for example, encouraging later marriage and female education—are attempting to lessen the effects of these factors, such effects are not easily changed. There is also a strong need for more acceptable family planning service delivery and for culturally sensitive promotional strategies.

Finding out why an indigenous population, rural or urban poor, men or other certain groups do not practise family planning and how service can better meet their needs requires in-depth examining of the sociocultural factor influencing their reproductive behaviour.

The results of research on how the attitudes and opinions among one indigenous group affect their utilization of family planning are described below.

People in remote areas

Although there has been a growing reach of mass media, television, video, film etc., and despite the fact that their aggregate impact on family planning behaviour has been so substantial, a significant number of people living in remote areas, across seas or on the other side of the mountains have, in fact, a disadvantaged situation, especially in terms of the extent to which services can be rendered. Their geographical location results in a considerable interregional differences in use of family planning as well as that of other programmes. Examples of this situation are the 1,000-island Indonesia, the Philippines and Maldives.

Turning to the level of contraceptive use in remote areas, it can be seen that every advantage for an effort to promote family planning is balanced by many limitations. However, the author believes that increasing satellite transmission, for example, will give rural people better access to television, but this access will be possible only if they have receivers and electricity, or solar or petrol-powered generators.

Young adults and sexuality

Age at first marriage

In the past few years, there has been an overall trend to later marriage throughout the world. In Indonesia, owing to the passage of a national marriage law, the average age at first marriage is slowly rising. In remote areas, however, it is still generally under the national average. In the urban areas, although most teenage child-bearing takes place within marriage, however loosely defined, there are indications that more out-of-wedlock births are occurring, particularly among the youths in urban areas.

While the 1980 census found that 30 per cent of women aged 15-49 had married before age 20, by 1987 this percentage had dropped to 19 (Indonesian, 1989). This decline is also indicated by the trend in median age at first marriage, 16.5 years for women aged 45-49 and 19.6 for women aged 20-29. However, socio-economic differences in age at first marriage persist. Urban women married two years later than rural women, and the median age at first marriage

of those with secondary or higher education was 5.5 years older than that of women without education.

As opportunities for education grow for young people, the time between menarche and marriage will also increase, leaving young women exposed to the risk of premarital pregnancy for a longer period. For a schoolgirl, an unplanned pregnancy carried to term virtually guarantees that she will drop out of school.

Although adolescent child-bearing within marriage is traditional and culturally acceptable in many parts of the world, there have been some disturbing signs that premarital sexual activity and the number of unintended adolescent pregnancies are increasing.

In Botswana, for example, the percentage of women aged 15-19 years with children rose from 15 per cent in 1971 to 24 per cent in 1988 (Lesetedi and others, 1989).

Results from the Zimbabwe Reproductive Health Survey in 1984 (Boohene and Dow, 1987) indicate that one third of Zimbabwean women had their first child before age 18. Increased newspaper coverage episodes of "baby dumping"—the abandonment of newborns and infants—has made the Zimbabwean public aware of the problem of unintended pregnancy.

Premarital sexual activity

In Indonesia, as in most developing countries, premarital pregnancy was believed to be non-existent, at least until recently. Indonesian culture is influenced by the philosophy and teaching of religion, which rigidly defines social expectations and relationships, especially those between men and women. The conduct of unmarried youth, in particular, was strictly enforced. In keeping with these beliefs, pregnancy outside of marriage brought disgrace to families, especially for those living in rural areas. Because of many factors, including the continuing cultural prohibitions of premarital sex, the Indonesian family planning programme does not provide contraceptive services for single women and men.

Since the early 1980s, however, attitudes regarding sexual activity seem to have changed (Hull, 1987). It is widely believed that sexual activity among unmarried men and women has increased, resulting in an increase in premarital pregnancy and induced abortion.

The incidence of sexual activity before marriage provides an indication of the extent of erosion in traditional practices and in family control of young women's behaviour in urban areas. Pregnancy and childbirth outside marriage and the traditional family support systems have also become a matter of increasing concern in may developing countries, especially in the public-health community. The results suggest that premarital sexual relations have become more common over time, as a developing society has undergone marked social change, and that premarital sexual activity appears to be more common among women from non-traditional backgrounds. Relatively few sexually active unmarried women attempt to avoid pregnancy by using a contraceptive method, although premarital contraceptive use is more common in younger cohorts and among more educated women. Much of the contraceptive use, however, is of less effective methods.

Many traditional values and sexual practices have changed during the course of modernization, and it is unlikely that traditional premarital sexual behaviour would be an exception. In fact, previous studies have pointed to a gradual erosion of the traditional sexual norms. This change in the norms may be a consequence of that transformation taking place in the institution of marriage itself and, in particular, the transition from family arranged to individual choice marriages.

In recent years, there has been much interest in teenage fertility in a number of developing countries, including concern about the early initiation of child-bearing and the level of unintended pregnancy and premarital conception (Darabi, Philiber and Rosenfield, 1979; Edmunds and Paxman, 1984; Morris and others, 1986; Senderowitz and Paxman, 1985). The interest is linked to evidence that women who have their first birth at a young age have shorter birth intervals, more unintended pregnancies and more births outside marriage than do women that begin child-bearing at later ages (Senderowitz and Paxman, 1985). Also associated with adolescent child-bearing are low income, low educational levels and disadvantaged social and economic positions later in life

(Liskin, 1985; Senderowitz and Paxman, 1985). Such social and economic consequences are especially devastating in all societies, where opportunities to advance socio-economically are already extremely limited.

The Ministry of Health in Zimbabwe, for example, has recognized the importance of addressing adolescent health issues and has supported efforts to improve health and education programmes targeted at this group. In 1978, the Youth Advisory Service was established as part of the Zimbabwe National Family Planning Council (ZNFPC). This service provides family life education upon request to students in primary and secondary schools. In 1985, the Youth Service decided to document the scope of the problem of unwanted adolescent pregnancy in Zimbabwe.

ZNFPC and the Youth Advisory Services should redouble their efforts to reach young men and women before they initiate sexual activity, in order to give them the information they need to make responsible sexual and contraceptive choices. Those women that do not know about family planning and those that may decide to initiate sex but do not think contraceptive methods are easy to obtain remain unreached groups.

Data from the Zimbabwe study (Boohene and Dow, 1987) suggest that information about family planning, particularly about condoms, may reach boys at an earlier age than girls, but that girls learn about a wider range of contraceptives. Young men should be reached even earlier than young women, because they initiate sex two years earlier, on average, than do young women.

Condoms are the method of choice among sexually active young men, and their use should be promoted by family planning service providers because of their protection against the transmission of sexually transmitted diseases (STDs), including the acquired immunodeficiency syndrome (AIDS). Unlike young men, however, single young women prefer the pill to the condom. With increasing concern about the spread of STDs and AIDS, greater efforts need to be directed towards promoting condom use among young women as well.

Because attitudes towards family planning are positive among both male and females, there is every indication that young people in Zimbabwe that choose to become premaritally sexually active would increasingly use family planning if it were provided with contraceptive information and services.

In addition to socio-economic considerations, there is a growing concern about the health consequences of adolescent pregnancy. Evidence from surveys confirms that babies born to adolescent women have a lower probability of surviving infancy and childhood than do babies borne by older women (Rustein, 1983). According to Molina and Romero (1985), studies in Latin American populations have shown an association of early age at pregnancy with increased rates on infant mortality and health risks to the mother.

Concern about adolescent pregnancy in Chile, specifically, has been expressed by various writers in recent years (Molina and Romero, 1985; Viel, 1986). Viel and Campos (n.d.) point out that whereas overall fertility rates have declined in recent decades, little progress has been made with the rate among those aged 15-19, and the proportion of out-of-wedlock births among young women has been increasing.

Between 1960 and 1980, the total fertility rate for Chile declined significantly—from 4.7 to 2.4 children per woman. However, there was no dramatic drop in age-specific rates among those aged 15-19. In 1960, the age-specific fertility rate among women aged 15-19 was 72.6 per 1,000 women; by 1980, it had declined slightly to 61.5, and in 1984, it was 64.0. These fairly stable rates contrast sharply with declines between 1960 and 1984 of 47 and 56 per cent among women aged 25-29 and 30-34, respectively (Viel and Campos, n.d.; Taucher, 1986). During this period, the more significant change among young women under age 20 occurred outside marriage. Since that time, the proportion has steadily increased to 55 per cent in 1984 (Viel, 1986).

The proportion of young males that have experienced premarital sexual activity differs from one country to the another, and sometimes the level of premarital sexual activity among females in different countries also varies. The difference observed may be attributable to the difference levels of economic development of specific countries involved or to social and cultural factors, because there is great variation in both of these dimensions throughout Latin America.

Chile is more developed and its population has a correspondingly higher level of education attainment. One effect of higher educational levels can be the postponement of sexual activity resulting from higher aspirations and the availability of more alternatives to early marriage and child-bearing (Singh and Wulf, 1991). At the same time, increasing educational levels can cause the age at marriage to rise to where it is difficult for young people to desist from sexual activity prior to marriage (Liskin, 1985). This situation may explain the large increase in premarital sexual activity among Santiaguans from ages 15-19 to ages 20-24 and, consequently, the higher age at first premarital intercourse than in the other Latin American countries. At the same time, there may also be cultural factors influencing differences in adolescent sexual activity.

In the discussion of this problem of premarital sexual activity, it is worth quoting one description by a participant in the most recent London Workshop on Effective Family Planning Programmes in February 1992. He describes how the language used in family planning reflects the rationale behind the programmes and that the orientation towards quality services can begin with a look at how goals are expressed. Whereas the emphasis has traditionally been on married couples, targets, acceptors and promotion, one should also think instead about sexually active individuals, clients served and education. Quality of care implies recognizing the needs of individuals, whether married or not, and addressing both reproductive health problems (infection and infertility) and sexual health problems.

Problem of abortion

The problem of abortion in most developing countries and in certain parts of the developed countries has been primarily categorized and continuously presented as one affecting unmarried, adolescent students.

In Indonesia, in which abortion is strictly prohibited, data have been unavailable, because almost all induced abortions are unregistered and are performed illegally. In a study conducted in five sample areas at Shanghai, Wu and others (1992) found that the abortion rate among single women aged 15-19 had increased from 5 to 56 procedures per 1,000 women. Further, observations and interviews on the gynaecology ward and the case histories collected allow different inferences, such as:

(*a*) Women seeking abortions are not a homogenous group;

(*b*) The reasons for a woman's decision to terminate pregnancy appear to be complex and varied;

(*c*) Pathways to securing treatment are diverse and dangerous;

(*d*) Women may lack knowledge or the ability to seek and secure a legal abortion;

(*e*) Women are unwilling to admit to illegal abortion until they are gravely ill; and

(*f*) Hospital care is being provided in a crisis atmosphere, with no long-term strategy for more effective management, in the face of a worsening situation.

Reliable qualitative data are essential to illuminate the nature and experiences of women that have terminated a pregnancy. Once the cloud obscuring the phenomenon of abortion has been lifted and real women that make their way through pluralistic health systems in search of abortion care are recognized, more enduring issues can be addressed. The usefulness of such contextual data may include the ability to develop innovative, group-specific education and prevention programmes, effective ways to assist women in securing safe care, and improvements in the way health-care providers dispense abortion services to women in need. Surely the seriousness of the problem and the need for appropriate solutions demand reliable documents.

Couples of certain ages as target groups

Women of different ages

Every population is differentiated by education, age and family size. It is rational that family planning should use different approaches with different subgroups of the population and that programmes tailored to specific subgroups become more successful.

Many pregnancies and births occur among women aged 20-34. These women have the highest rates and they make up the largest numbers of married or cohabiting women. They must be reached if a programme is successfully to provide pregnancy services, raise contraceptive prevalence and reduce excessive fertility.

In Indonesia, age-specific fertility rates have fallen over the years (Ross, Rich and Molzan, 1989). Very large declines have occurred at ages 20-24, 25-29 and 30-34. In the early years of the programme, most acceptors were older women that were using contraception primarily to limit their fertility. Only later did a demand for contraception grow among younger women. They had a greater impact on reducing national fertility trends because of their high age-specific fertility and their large numbers.

Each age group shows a different pattern of use. In new programmes, older women at firat accept at higher rates and continue using contraception for longer time periods than younger women. As family planning knowledge spreads, there is usually an increase in the number and proportion of younger users, who typically wish to space and therefore want to use temporary methods. Older women, who wish to stop child-bearing entirely, generally want more effective methods.

Thus, communications messages need to be somewhat different from one age group to the next. Both services and communications must reflect the diversity in the population. The messages should also be continuous, as well as diverse, to address the changing concerns of couples as they move into new life situations.

A time dimension also operates, in that the numbers of young couples to be served will increase for many years to come.

Unmet need for contraception

According to the World Bank, the future challenge for family planning programmes will be to meet the needs of those not currently being served, as well as to improve the quality of existing services. One particular problem highlighted in Indonesia that has implications for programme potential is the fact that not all women that have implied a need for family planning intend to use contraception in the future.

The use and non-use of contraception reflect the motivation to control fertility and the propensity to contracept among those who are motivated. Women can be motivated to control fertility either because they wish to have no additional children or because they wish to postpone the next birth. Not all those motivated to control fertility, however, are using or even intend to use contraception.

Those women wishing to control their fertility but not currently using contraception are referred to as having an "unmet need" for family planning. According to the 1991 Indonesia Demographic and Health Survey (Indonesia, 1992), by this definition approximately 20 per cent of the married women in Indonesia have an unmet need to limit their fertility and another 20 per cent have an unmet need to space their births. Of those women that want to have no more children and stated that their need for contraception is unmet, the higher need is for women with no schooling (33 per cent, compared with only 11 per cent among the highest educational level).

According to Palmore and others (1990), unmet needs for family planning as target groups are basically classified into two categories: (a) manifest unmet need; and (b) latent unmet need. The manifest unmet need can further be broken down into the following subgroups:

(a) Those that are married, of reproductive age and fecund, and stating that they do not desire to have additional child, but that are currently not using any modern contraceptive methods, either for females or or for males;

(b) Those expressing a desire to space births but are not currently using any contraceptive method;

(c) Those that are currently pregnant, but the pregnancy is unwanted and contraceptives were not used prior to the pregnancy;

(d) Those that are currently pregnant, but the pregnancy occurred in an unsuitable or unintended time. Yet, contraceptives were not used prior to the pregnancy.

Latent unmet need can be classified into the following subgroups, which include those not currently using any contraceptive method and simply exclude those from the manifest unmet need groups:

(a) Those desiring to have more children, but the number of children desired is more than two;

(b) Those wanting to postpone their next births (second child), where the interval between the two births is less than three years;

(c) Those that are currently pregnant or amenorrhoeic, when the pregnancy is in fact intended and desired, and the child would be the third birth or beyond;

(d) Those that are currently pregnant for the second birth or amenorrhoeic after a second birth, in which the interval between the second pregnancy and the birth of the first child is less than two years.

Current situation of unmet need in Indonesia

Manifest unmet need

Compared with that of 1987, the manifest unmet need for family planning in Indonesia has increased 1.4 per cent, that is, from 14.4 in 1987 to 15.8 in 1991 (Indonesia, 1992). Most of this result has been attributed to the increase in the group of the manifest unmet need for spacing, that is, 7.1 per cent in 1987 versus 8.3 in 1991. (The percentages of manifest unmet need for limiting in 1987 and 1991 are 7.3 and 7.5, respectively.)

Further analysis of this manifest unmet need for spacing will show that this group belongs to those that are not currently pregnant and are amenorrhoeic, and intend to space their next birth yet do not desire to use any method. Those numbers are 4.3 per cent in 1987 and 5.8 per cent in 1991; whereas those resulting from mistimed pregnancy have declined considerably. The numbers were 2.7 in 1987 and 2.1 in 1991.

Latent unmet need

The group with latent unmet need is, in fact, of great value both for evaluating programmes and for ascertaining the market potential and priorities for future effort. This is specially true for the Indonesian family planning programme, which intends to change people's attitude towards their reproductive goals, with the concept of "two children is enough" and "the minimal three years of interval between the first and the second child".

The latent unmet need group in Indonesia increased from 9.6 per cent in 1987 to 13.7 in 1991. For 1987, among this group 1.7 per cent were for limiting and 8.0 per cent for spacing. The unmet need for limiting, however, has decreased considerably, falling to 6.6 per cent in 1991.

Total unmet need: latent and manifest unmet need combined

Total unmet need in Indonesia in 1987 amounted to 24.1 per cent (Indonesia, 1992). Based on method of

calculation, this total can be broken down into 8.7 per cent manifest need and 15.7 per cent latent unmet need. Classified by spacing or limiting category, the figure is 8.7 per cent for spacing and 15.3 per cent for limiting (Palmore and others, 1990). In 1991, the total became 29.5 per cent, for a 5.4 increase. For the manifest and latent classifications, the respective figures are 15.8 and 13.7 per cent. With regard to spacing and limiting, the figures are 15.4 and 14.5 per cent, respectively.

Programmatic aspect of unmet need

The following points can be made with respect to the programmatic aspect of unmet need:

(a) The proportion of unmet need as a whole has increased, especially for those in the latent category. This situation implies that every effort should be made to increase people's awareness of the importance of reproductive health behaviour and that the concept of small family norm needs to be more intensified and directed;

(b) Looking at the social and demographic factors, it appears that those in young age groups and those in high-parity groups are more likely to obtain family planning methods;

(c) Those with to low economic status tend to experience an unmet need for family planning more than those with higher status. With this in mind, efforts are made to provide cheaper and easier ways of providing contraceptive services;

(d) Those with a low sociocultural level, on either the part of the women themselves or that of the husband, either before or after their marriage, tend to be unwilling to use contraceptive methods;

(e) Also, from this analysis, health status and healthful behaviour, as well as access to family planning services, have great impact on the status of both the met and the unmet need for family planning;

(f) Further analysis shows that the most important intervention exerted would be the accessibility to family planning services, information through mass media, home visit etc. Recent recruitment of graduates for fieldworkers may contribute significantly to those intervention activities (Hardjanto, 1991).

C. DISCUSSION

It is necessary to understand not only the overall family planning services performance but also the factors related to that performance, in order to enhance the prospects of family planning. The quality and quantity of family planning services in a national setting are influenced by socio-economic conditions; resource allocation for the national family planning policy, especially with regard to equity as a principle of family planning facilities depends upon the availability and accessibility of family services; and the service-seeking behaviour of the population, which in turn is influenced by many factors such as social mobilization and perceived quality of services. The effects of utilization of family planning services on maternal health hinge partially on the socio-economic conditions, the effectiveness of the interventions offered and the quality of care, including the availability of contraception and proper equipment.

Estimating the demand for family planning as well as the magnitude of the unreached population is clearly an important objective of every national population programme. Reliable information on levels of contraceptive practice and unmet need for family planning is essential for effective programme management and is useful for forecasting fertility trends. Periodic surveys also generate the data needed to determine changes in demand and supply of family planning.

It has not been clearly studied whether the size of unreached population in the world is smaller or greater than many observers have speculated. Nor have its trend and its social context, as well as its covariates, composition and demographic significance been clearly understood.

The role of men in fertility and family planning in developing countries is becoming increasingly important in the effort to raise contraceptive prevalence and reduce the fertility level. Although male knowledge of family planning was found to be high in many developing countries, use of contraceptives does not lead to limiting the number of children.

As the role of men in family planning is receiving greater attention in literature, male motivation awareness programmes are beginning to emerge in developing countries. For example, Zimbabwe instituted a male motivation campaign in 1989 (Mbizvo and Adamchak, 1991). It is imperative that the need for male KAP research need be met for family planning programme planning, implementation and evaluation.

It is clear from this brief review that failure to understand sociocultural factors and the role of men in inhibiting or promoting contraceptive adoption could substantially affect family planning promotion programmes and programme success in different developing societies. In an effort to redress this lack of attention to males, KAP studies should be carried out in the respective countries. Data to be collected should include knowledge of family planning methods, reasons for practising family planning, approval and ever-use of family planning; and items addressing couple communication, decision-making and family size.

Effective family planning programmes produce optimal results if the environmental and socio-economic conditions of the country are supportive. Such conditions determine the performance or failure of the programmes and the ultimate outcome.

The availability of a wide choice of contraceptives for men and women is likely to increase the chance that the couple will find a contraceptive option that meets their particular requirements. Thus, both adoption and continuation of methods are also likely to be enhanced.

The process of development of a new contraceptive method—or variant of an existing method—and its eventual incorporation into a national family planning service involves a long sequence of biomedical and initial field trials, as is the case with any new drug.

D. IMPLICATIONS FOR PROGRAMME DESIGN

Several policy implications emerge from this discussion and some previous studies. In reference to the unreached population in the world for family planning, there are four groups which should be made targets for programme concern. Those segments of population are most important from the programme point of view, for they are most vulnerable and difficult to reach.

The role of men

Family planning knowledge, attitudes and practices of men

The challenge of future research may be to demonstrate how men from all socio-economic levels can be included in IEC programming that will have a positive impact. Insights about the husband's attitudes and behaviour concerning issues related to fertility and family planning, particularly in developing countries, would be very valuable. Without this information, one would not know the extent of the negative or fatalistic attitudes of husbands towards fertility control and contraceptive use or have information related to the wife's apparent problem in regulating their future fertility.

These groups will be harder to reach than those with unmet need for family planning. To achieve greater husband involvement in family planning, the International Planned Parenthood Federation formulated three areas of improvement—husband's knowledge, support and acceptance of family planning. Improvement in knowledge and support of family planning may be accomplished by developing and implementing programmes that involve husbands in sharing contraceptive responsibility and educating them on the risk of pregnancy or delivery, the importance of birth-spacing and its impact on the lives of existing and future children and the economic aspect of raising children. The programme can be incorporated into the existing training courses either in the family planning clinics or in the office setting, but the husband should be the focus of the programme.

Indigenous groups

It is well known from some studies, one of which is a study of Maya-Quinche communities in Guatemala in 1990 (Ward, Bertrand and Puac, 1992), that in most indigenous populations and in some rural or more isolated areas, social pressure against family planning is a substantial barrier to its use. Community leaders, religious leaders and husbands exert considerable influence on family planning decisions and usually oppose the use of contraceptives.

In addition, factors affecting fertility differ widely among different ethnic groups. An earlier age at marriage, lower educational attainment and generally lower socio-economic status undoubtedly contribute to the low level of contraceptive use. Although current programme efforts in many countries—for example, the 1974 Marriage Law in Indonesia, which encourages later marriage and female education—are attempting to lessen the effects of these factors, such effects are not easily changed. There is therefore a strong need for more acceptable family planning service delivery and for culturally sensitive promotional strategies.

Ascertaining why a certain indigenous group does not practise family planning and how services can better meet their needs requires an in-depth examination of the sociocultural factors influencing their reproductive behaviour. As Hammouda (1987) concludes, "Within the family, the community and the nation, economic pressures are highlighting the problem of excessive population growth. Family planning and population education programmes for both men and women decision makers need to be promoted" (1987, p. 22). Until current male attitudes change, fertility regulation—and ultimately the potential for fertility decline—probably will be quite limited. From their study on a survey in Jamaica in 1985, Warren and others (1992) suggest that programme policy makers may want to concentrate on younger men (under age 30) with regard to family planning, because their attitudes are less rigid. Health education courses introduced into both male and female schools can stress the health benefits of both breast-feeding and child-spacing. How programme officials address these issues will be important for the future success of the family planning programme in developing countries.

Lastly, research in this area is necessary. To avoid the cultural conflicts that have hindered family planning programmes in many areas, it will be important to study the traditions, norms, customs and taboos of the people. A family planning programme that improves and takes advantage of some traditional methods is more likely to be accepted by the population than an exclusively foreign one.

Groups with unmet need for family planning

Effort should be directed to serving the couples that still need to be brought into the programme—those that have higher family size preferences and are harder to reach. Among these are the urban poor, those living in outlying areas and those with low levels of education, as well as those that have difficulties using contraceptives correctly. To maintain the momentum of the fertility transition, these groups should be targeted and their use of family planning should be facilitated.

Adolescents

There is an urgent need to identify appropriate strategies to sensitize and inform people—particularly policy makers, as well as parents, teachers and family planning programme personnel—about the increasing earlier initiation of sexual intercourse among adolescents and of the variety of repercussions.

To improve communication among parents, teachers and youths, and to combat general ignorance about reproductive health and contraception, there is a real need for the preparation and dissemination, in simple, easily understood language, of concise information on reproductive biology and contraception among adolescents and among their parents, guardians and other relatives. In addition, family life education or population education, which is just being introduced into some secondary schools in some countries (for example, Nigeria) needs to be extended into other secondary schools and into teacher-training colleges throughout the country. Out-of-school youth could benefit from family life education if it were included in apprenticeship programme operated by the Nigeria Directorate of Employment, as well as in the youth programmes of voluntary organizations nationwide.

Despite encouraging declarations of the Governments' intent in national population policy, access to contraceptive methods remains problematic. To remove some of the constraints of their effective use, including ignorance of available methods, fear of side-effects, the partner's disapproval and the monetary cost of family planning commodities, there is a need for a special contraceptive service for adolescents, which is confidential, readily accessible and offered either at affordable price or for free.

The need for family planning counselling services to motivate adolescents to use contraceptives effectively cannot be overemphasized. The apparent indifferent attitude towards contraception among young people, particularly among males, needs to be effectively countered by mounting a national campaign similar to the ongoing campaigns against the spread of AIDS and against cigarette smoking. Such a campaign should strive to make adolescents aware of the probable grave consequences of premarital or indiscriminate sexual intercourse.

Despite the controversy surrounding the issue of abortion, the practical realities of the situation demand a revision of the current laws on abortion, if only as a health measure to protect the life and health of women.

E. RESEARCH NEEDED

Male contraceptive methods

In response to this expanding demands for male contraceptive research and in recognition of the fact that male participation can only be effectively mobi-

lized and managed through a worldwide collaborative effort, family planning programmes should carry out research on developing appropriate technologies and generate information in selected areas of male reproductive health as a high priority. Examples of such methods are given below.

Traditional method: withdrawal

Although the withdrawal method has the advantages of no side-effects or complications and is always available, it has one of the highest typical first-year failure rates. As a contraceptive method, it is appropriate for breast-feeding women and assures a return to fertility after discontinuation. It is, however, dependent upon the man's ability to withdraw before ejaculation and interrupts the sexual pleasure of both man and woman.

Natural family planning

As a contraceptive method, natural family planning has a high failure rate because it requires regular menstrual cycles and periods of abstinence, dependent upon cooperation between the man and woman and upon the woman's ability to interpret signs of ovulation. In addition, discontinuation rates are very high.

A "male pill"

Currently, the male partner has only a narrow choice if he wishes to participate in family planning, namely, the choice between the condom and vasectomy or withdrawal. For men to have the full range of choices that women have—that is, barrier methods, sterilization and antifertility pills—there is a clear need for a safe, fully reversible method based on hormonal or chemical antifertility agents.

New techniques of male sterilization

It is known that there are two main factors which limit the acceptability of vasectomy. One is the necessity of a skin incision, which is unacceptable in some cultures; the other is the general lack of reversibility. Although vasectomy accounts for 9 per cent of all contraception methods used by married couples in Eastern Asian countries, and for 6 per cent in the rest of Asia, it accounts for less than 1 per cent in Indonesia. The so-called "no-scalpel technique" developed in China, which offers psychological reassurance for men by replacing the traditional incisions of a scalpel with a tiny puncture, is being applied with a slight modification in two provinces in Indonesia by two surgeons. The efficacy and safety of the procedure, as well as its long-term effect, are yet to be studied. A newer bypass procedure by injecting silicone beneath the skin is also being conducted in some countries (including Indonesia). It is hoped that this procedure will be accepted by all religious and cultural groups.

Hormonal agents directed to suppressing sperm production have just been completed in some countries (including Indonesia), but this method needs further study because the need for weekly injections may make it less appealing in some cultures.

REFERENCES

Adamchak, Donald J., and Akinwumi Adebayo (1987). Male fertility attitudes: a neglected dimension in Nigerian fertility research. *Social Biology* (Port Angeles, Washington), vol. 34, No. 1-2 (Spring-Summer), pp. 57-67.

Blanc, Ann K., and Naomi Rutenberg (1990). *Assessment of the Quality of Data on Age at First Sexual Intercourse, Age at First Marriage, and Age at First Birth.* Demographic and Health Survey Methodological Report, No. 1. Columbia, Maryland: Institute for Resource Development/Macro Systems, Inc.

Bongaarts, John (1987). The proximate determinants of exceptionally high fertility. *Population and Development Review* (New York), vol. 13, No. 1 (March), pp. 133-139.

_____ (1990). *The Measurement of Wanted Fertility.* Research Division Working paper, No. 10. New York: The Population Council.

_____ , and Robert Potter (1983). *Fertility, Biology and Behaviour: An Analysis of the Proximate Determinants.* New York: Academic Press.

Boohene, Esther, and Thomas E. Dow, Jr. (1987). Contraceptive prevalence and family planning program effort in Zimbabwe. *International Family Planning Perspectives* (New York), vol. 13, No. 1 (March), pp. 1-7.

Boulos, Michaelle L, Reginald Boulos and Douglas J. Nichols (1991). Perceptions and practices relating to condom use among urban men in Haiti. *Studies in Family Planning* (New York), vol. 22, No. 5 (September-October), pp. 318-325.

Bradley, Jan, Nsama Sikazwe and Joan Healy (1991). Improving abortion care in Zambia. *Studies in Family Planning* (New York), vol. 22, No. 6 (November/December), pp. 391-395.

Bruce, Judith (1990). Fundamental elements of the quality of care: a simple frame work. *Studies in Family Planning* (New York), vol. 21, No. 2 (March/April), pp. 61-91.

Chowdhury, A. U., and James F. Phillips (1985). Socioeconomic status differentials among currently married women of reproductive age: family planning—health service project, 1974 Matlab census. *Journal of Family Welfare* (Bombay), vol. 31, No. 4, pp. 3-11.

Crowley, John G., Richard M. Cornelius and Steven W. Sinding (1987). A new methodology for evaluating family planning programs. Paper presented at the Annual Meeting of the Population Association of America, Chicago, Illinois, 30 April-2 May 1987.

Darabi, Katherine F., Susan Gustavus Philliber and Allan Rosenfield (1979). A perspective on adolescent fertility in developing countries. *Studies in Family Planning* (New York), vol. 10, No. 10 (October), pp. 300-303.

Dow, Thomas and others (1986). Characteristics of new contraceptive acceptors in Zimbabwe. *Studies in Family Planning* (New York), vol. 17, No. 2 (March-April), pp. 107-113.

Edmunds, M., and John Paxman (1984). Early pregnancy and childbearing in Guatemala, Brazil, Nigeria and Indonesia: addressing the consequences. Pathpaper, No. 11. Boston: Pathfinder Fund.

Fennelly, Katherine, Vasantha Kandiah and Vilma Ortiz (1989). The cross-cultural study of fertility among Hispanic adolescents in the Americas. *Studies in Family Planning* (New York), vol. 20, No. 2 (March-April), pp. 96-101.

Finger, William R. (1992). Getting more men involved. *Network: Family Planning International* (Durham, North Carolina), vol. 13, No. 1 (August), pp. 4-6.

Freedman, Ronald, and Ann K. Blanc (1992). Fertility transition: an update. *International Family Planning Perspectives* (New York), vol. 18, No. 2 (June), pp. 42-44.

Gorosh, Martin (1978). Improving management through evaluation: techniques and strategies for family planning programs. *Studies in Family Planning* (New York), vol. 9, No. 6 (June), pp. 163-168.

Green, C. P. (1990). Male involvement programs in family planning: lessons learned and implications for AIDS prevention. Draft. Geneva: World Health Organization, Global Programme on AIDS.

Hammouda, A. (1987). Contraceptive use, fertility differentials and family planning issues in Jordan. Paper presented at the Symposium on the Jordan Husband's Fertility Survey, Amman, June.

Hardjanto, Rohadi (1991). Manifest and latent unmet need keluarga berencana di Indonesia. Studi Lanjuntan Data SDKI.

Herold, Joan M., Maria Solange Valenzuela and Leo Morris (1992). Premarital sexual activity and contraceptive use in Santiago, Chile. *Studies in Family Planning* (New York), vol. 23, No. 2 (March/April), pp. 128-136.

Hull, Terence H. (1983). Cultural influences on fertility decision styles. In *Determinants of Fertility in Developing Countries*, vol. 2, *Fertility Regulation and Institutional Influences*, Rodolfo A. Bulatao and Ronald D. Lee, eds., with Paula E. Hollerbach and John Bongaarts. New York: Academic Press.

_____ (1987). Fertility decline in Indonesia: an institutionalist interpretation. Paper presented at the Annual Meeting of the Population Association of America, Chicago, Illinois, 30 April-2 May.

Indonesia (1989). *National Contraceptive Prevalence Survey, 1987.* Jakarta: Central Bureau of Statistics and National Family Planning Coordinating Board; and Columbia, Maryland: Institute for Resource Development/Westinghouse.

_____ (1992). *Indonesia Demographic and Health Survey, 1991.* Jakarta: Central Bureau of Statistics, National Family Planning Coordinating Board; and Ministry of Health; and Columbia, Maryland: Institute for Resource Development/ Macro International, Inc.

Joesoef, Mohamed R., Andrew L. Baughman and Budi Utomo (1988). Husband's approval of contraceptive use in metropolitan Indonesia: program implications. *Studies in Family Planning* (New York), vol. 19, No. 3 (May-June), pp. 162-168.

Jain, Anrudh K. (1989). Fertility reduction and the quality of family planning service. *Studies in Family Planning* (New York), vol. 20, No. 1 (January-February), pp. 1-16.

Kenya, Ministry of Economic Planning and Development (1980). *Kenya Fertility Survey, 1977-1978. First Report*, vol. I. Nairobi: Central Bureau of Statistics.

Khalifa, Mona A. (1988). Attitude of urban Sudanese men toward family planning. *Studies in Family Planning* (New York), vol. 19, No. 4 (July-August), pp. 236-243.

Lapham, Robert J., and W. Parker Mauldin (1984). Family planning program effort and birthrate decline in developing countries. *International Family Planning Perspectives* (New York), vol. 10, No. 4 (December), pp. 109-118.

_____ (1985). Contraceptive prevalence: the influence of organized family planning programs. *Studies in Family Planning* (New York), vol. 16, No. 3 (May-June), pp. 117-137.

Lesetedi, Lesetedinyana T., and others (1989). *Botswana Family Health Survey II, 1988*. Gaborone: Ministry of Finance and Development Planning; and Columbia, Maryland: Institute for Resource Development/Macro Systems, Inc.

Liskin, Laurie, and others (1985). *Youth in the 1980s: Social and Health Concerns*. Population Reports, Series M, No. 9. Baltimore, Maryland: The Johns Hopkins University, Population Information Program.

Makinwa-Adebusoye, Paulina (1992). Sexual behavior, reproductive knowledge and contraceptive use among young urban Nigerians. *International Family Planning Perspectives* (New York), vol. 18, No. 2 (June), pp. 59-66.

Mauldin, W. Parker, and Robert Lapham (1987). The measurement of family planning inputs. In *Organizing for Effective Family Planning Programs*, Robert J. Lapham and George B. Simmons, eds. Washington, D.C.: National Academy Press.

Mauldin, W. Parker, and Sheldon Segal (1988). *World Trends in Contraceptive Use, By Method, and Their Relationship to Fertility*. Center for Policy Studies Working Paper, No. 139. New York: The Population Council.

Mbizvo, Michael T., and Donald J. Adamchak (1989). Condom use and acceptance: a survey of male Zimbabweans. *Central African Journal of Medicine* (Harare), vol. 35, No. 11, pp. 519-523.

Molina, R., and M. I. Romero (1985). *Adolescent Pregnancy: the Chilean Experience*. The Health of Adolescents and Youth in the Americas. Scientific Publication, No. 489. Washington, D.C.: Pan American Health Organization.

Morris, Leo, and others (1986). A sexual experience and contraceptive use among young adults in Mexico City. Paper presented at the meeting for the U.S.-Mexico Border Public Health Conference, Monterrey, Mexico, April.

Mott, Frank L., and Susan H. Mott (1985). Household fertility decisions in West Africa: a comparison of male and female survey results. *Studies in Family Planning* (New York), vol. 16, No. 2 (March-April), pp. 88-99.

Mustafa, Mutasim A. B., and Stephen D. Mumford (1984). Male attitudes toward family planning in Khartoum, Sudan. *Journal of Biosocial Science* (Cambridge, United Kingdom), vol. 16, No. 4, pp. 437-450.

Palmore, James A., and Mercedes B. Concepción (1981). Desired family size and contraceptive use. In *World Fertility Survey Conference, 1980: Record of Proceedings*, vol. 2. Voorburg, Netherlands: International Statistical Institute.

Palmore, James A., and others (1990). Manifest and latent unmet need for family planning in Indonesia. In *Secondary Analysis of the 1987 National Indonesian Contraceptive Prevalence Survey*. Jakarta: National Family Planning Coordinating Board; and Honolulu, Hawaii: East-West Population Institute.

Pick de Weiss, Susan, and others (1991). Sex, contraception and pregnancy among adolescents in Mexico City. *Studies in Family Planning* (New York), vol. 22, No. 2 (March/April), pp. 74-82.

The Population Council (1990). Botswana 1988: results from the Demographic and Health Survey. *Studies in Family Planning* (New York), vol. 21, No. 5 (September/October), pp. 293-297.

Ross, John A., Marjorie Rich and Janet P. Molzan (1989). *Management Strategies for Family Planning Programs*. New York: Columbia University, Center for Population and Family Health, School of Public Health.

Rustein, Shea Oscar (1983). *Infant and Child Mortality: Levels, Trends and Demographic Differentials*. World Fertility Survey Comparative Studies, No. 4. Voorburg, Netherlands: International Statistical Institute.

Senderowitz, Judith, and John M. Paxman (1985). *Adolescent Fertility Worldwide Concerns*. Population Bulletin, vol. 40, No. 2. Washington, D.C.: Population Reference Bureau.

Singh, Susheela, and Deidre Wulf (1991). Estimating abortion levels in Brazil, Colombia and Peru, using hospital admissions and fertility survey data. *International Family Planning Perspectives* (New York), vol. 17, No. 1 (March), pp. 8-13.

Sumarsono, Sudibyo Alimoeso, Srihartati P. Pandi and Andrew Kantner (1990). *Analysis of the 1987 National Indonesia Contraceptive Prevalence Survey: Implications for Program evaluation and Policy Formulation. Secondary Analysis of the 1987 National Indonesia Contraceptive Prevalence Survey*. Jakarta: National Family Planning Coordinating Board; and Honolulu, Hawaii: East-West Population Institute.

Suyono, Haryono, and others (1988). Strategic Planning and Management of Population Programmes: Indonesia Case Study. Jakarta: National Family Planning Coordinating Board. Unpublished manuscript.

Taucher, Erica (1986). Fertility and maternal infant health. *Asociación Chilena de Protección de la Familia* (Santiago, Chile), vol. 22, No. 12 (July-December), pp. 26-46.

Thornton, Arland, and Donald Camburn (1989). Religious participation and adolescent sexual behaviour and attitudes. *Journal of Marriage and the Family* (Minneapolis, Minnesota), vol. 51, pp. 641-653.

Turner, R. (1992). Family planning program effort has increased during the 1980s, with East Asia ranked highest. *International Family Planning Perspectives* (New York), vol. 18, No. 2 (June), pp. 73-74.

United Nations (1990). *Global Population Policy Data Base, 1989*. Population Policy Paper, No. 28. ST/ESA.SER.R/99.

_____ (1993). *World Population Prospects: The 1992 Revision*. Sales No. 93.XIII.7.

Viel, Benjamin (1986). Embarazo en la adolescencia. In *Memoria de I Reunion Internacional sobre Salud Sexual y Reproductiva de los Adolescentes y Jovenes*, A. Monroy deVelazco and J. Martinez Manauto, eds. Mexico, D.F.: Centro de Orientación para Adolescentes.

_____, and Waldo Campos (n.d.). Principales indices: biodemográficos de Chile entre 1965 y 1987. Unpublished manuscript.

Ward, Victoria M., Jane T. Bertrand and Francisco Puac (1992). Exploring sociocultural barriers to family planning among Mayans in Guatemala. *International Family Planning Perspectives* (New York), vol. 18, No. 2 (June), pp. 59-65.

Warren, Charles W., and others (1988). Fertility and family planning among young adults in Jamaica. *International Family Planning Perspectives* (New York), vol. 14, No. 4 (December), pp. 137-141.

Warwick, Donald P. (1986). The Indonesian family planning program: government influence and client choice. *Population and Development Review* (New York), vol. 12, No. 3 (September), pp. 453-490.

World Bank (1984) *World Development Report, 1984*. New York: Oxford University Press.

_____ (1989). *World Development Report, 1989*. New York: Oxford University Press.

_____ (1990). *Indonesia: Family Planning Perspectives in the 1990s*. Washington, D.C.

Wu, Z. C. and others (1992). Induced abortion among unmarried women in Shanghai, China. *International Family Planning Perspectives* (New York), vol. 18, No. 2 (June), pp. 51-53.

Zimbabwe (1985). *Zimbabwe Reproductive Health Survey, 1984*. Harare: Ministry of Finance, Economic Planning and Development, National Family Planning Council; and Columbia, Maryland: Westinghouse Public Applied Systems.

_____ (1989). *Zimbabwe Demographic and Health Survey, 1988: Preliminary Report*. Harare: Central Statistical Office; and Columbia, Maryland: Institute for Resource Development/Macro Systems, Inc.

IX. ADOLESCENT FERTILITY AND ADOLESCENT REPRODUCTIVE HEALTH

Asha A. Mohamud[*]

A. OVERVIEW: CURRENT TRENDS IN ADOLESCENT FERTILITY AND ADOLESCENT REPRODUCTIVE HEALTH IN DEVELOPING COUNTRIES

Child-bearing at an adolescent age continues to be a major impediment to improving the status of women. Worldwide, nearly 15 million adolescent women give birth each year; more than 80 per cent of them are in developing countries. The true number of pregnancies to adolescent women is unknown because of a lack of statistics on abortion and miscarriage, but it is undoubtedly higher. In Africa, 65 per cent of women have given birth by age 20, compared with 50 per cent in Latin America and the Caribbean and 54 per cent in Asia (World Assembly of Youth, 1990). As table 11 illustrates, in some developing countries more than 20 per cent of adolescent women aged 15-19 give birth each year.

TABLE 11. BIRTHS TO ADOLESCENT MOTHERS WORLDWIDE, SELECTED COUNTRIES, 1990

Country	Percentage of population aged 10-19	Percentage of women under age 20 giving birth each year[a]
Bangladesh	24	26
Brazil	21	8
Cameroon	22	17
Egypt	21	9
El Salvador	26	15
Ethiopia	23	20
India	22	9
Jamaica	22	11
Kenya	24	14
Netherlands	13	1
Philippines	22	5
Senegal	23	16
United States of America	13	5

Source: Kimberly A. Crews and Carl Haub, *Teen Mothers: Global Patterns* (Population Reference Bureau, Washington, D.C., 1989).

[a]This percentage does not include the total number of young women under age 20 who actually become pregnant, which is unknown because of a lack of data on miscarriage and on induced abortion, a significant factor in many countries even where it is illegal. In the United States of America, where abortion is legal, roughly 10 per cent of teenage women become pregnant each year; 10 per cent of the pregnancies end in miscarriage and 40 per cent are terminated by abortion. Similarly, in Brazil, even though abortion is illegal, there is estimated to be one abortion to every four births to adolescent mothers.

Adolescent sexual behaviour and its outcomes are not isolated issues. They are firmly rooted in and fixed to social attitudes, socio-economic issues; modern influences, such as the media; and levels of specific policy and programme interventions.

Historically, marriage often preceded the onset of menarche and births to teenagers were expected and desired within marriage. However, as countries have become more industrialized and urbanized, the norms concerning early marriage, premarital chastity and marital fidelity have become less salient. The age of puberty is decreasing and as girls aspire for higher educational attainment, the age of marriage is increasing. Consequently, more and more young people face a long "period of risk" of pre-marital sex and early child-bearing taking place outside marriage. Unfortunately, a large number of adolescents in developing countries decide to be more sexually active without access to preventive measures, such as condoms or family planning devices, and thus face undesired consequences, including unwanted pregnancies, sexually transmitted diseases (STDs), including the acquired immunodeficiency syndrome (AIDS), and the social consequences of both.

Dramatic effect of urbanization on patterns of adolescent fertility

The percentage of the developing world population living in urban areas has almost doubled over the past 40 years, growing from 17 per cent in 1950 to 32 in 1988. A significant portion of this urban migration has been youth and young families leaving a traditional agrarian life in search of economic opportunities. In 1984, 36 per cent of youth aged 15-24 in developing

---

[*]Director, International Center on Adolescent Fertility, Washington, D.C., United States of America.

countries lived in urban areas, compared with 31 per cent of the population of the developing world as a whole. By the year 2000, projections indicate that 77 per cent of youth aged 15-24 in Latin America, 47 per cent in Africa and Eastern Asia, and 42 per cent in Southern Asia will live in cities (Barker, 1989).

In general, urbanization has led to a breakdown of the traditional rites of passage for adolescents. In rural areas, youth typically passed from childhood to adulthood with clearly prescribed rites and behaviour with regard to sexuality. Adolescence as a social construct did not exist; young people typically passed from childhood to adulthood and early marriage. In urban areas, on the other hand, marriage typically comes later and higher nutrition leads to lower ages at menarche. These trends, coupled with increased school enrolment, have led to a growing gap between the age of puberty and the age of marriage.

This "biosocial gap", as it is called, means that sexual activity and initial child-bearing occur more frequently outside marriage and without family guidance. In the United States of America, for example, more than two thirds of births to adolescent mothers currently occur outside marriage, compared with one third in 1970 (Simons, 1992). Similarly in developing countries, particularly in urban areas in Africa and Latin America, child-bearing among adolescent women appears to be taking place increasingly outside marriage (United Nations, 1989). In Latin America and the Caribbean, for example, between 30 and 50 per cent of births to adolescent mothers are conceived outside wedlock or a consensual union (World Assembly of Youth, 1990).

Increased school enrolment and postponement of child-bearing

Between 1960 and 1980, women's secondary-school enrolment more than trebled in Africa and nearly doubled in Asia, although it still lags behind that of young men, as table 12 illustrates. Increasing school enrolment rates, which in turn have led to rising ages at marriage, provide increased incentives for young women to postpone child-bearing. This rapid social change has also been accompanied by a loosening of rules governing sexual behaviour. This social change, however, has not been accompanied by an adequate increase in the level of formal sex education and family planning services available to young people in developing countries. Studies in Africa, Asia and, to a lesser extent,

Latin America, show that young people are not receiving adequate sex education and are therefore turning to their misinformed peers for information. This absence of information and family planning services, as described at length below, coupled with increased incentives to postpone child-bearing—mainly education and later age at marriage—has led to an apparent increase in the number of unsafe abortions occurring annually among young women in developing countries.

TABLE 12. SECONDARY-SCHOOL GROSS ENROLMENT RATIOS, SELECTED COUNTRIES, AROUND 1987

Major area and country	Male	Female
Africa		
Kenya	27	19
Nigeria	52	18
Sierra Leone	29	15
Asia		
Bangladesh	24	11
China	50	37
India	50	27
Indonesia	47	35
Thailand	31	28
Latin America		
Chile	72	76
Colombia	55	56
Guatemala	22	19
Honduras	29	36
Mexico	54	53
Nicaragua	29	58
Peru	68	61

Source: Interagency Commission for the World Conference on Education for All, "Meeting basic learning needs: a vision for the 1990s", background document prepared for the World Conference on Education for All, Jomtien, Thailand, 5-9 March 1990; New York, 1990.

NOTE: The gross enrolment ratio for secondary education relates total enrolment regardless of age to the population that, according to national regulations, should be enrolled at this level of education.

Unwanted births and unsafe abortion

There is ample evidence that much of this early child-bearing—whether within or outside marriage—is unwanted. In surveys with young women in Latin America and the Caribbean, between 20 and 60 per cent report that their most recent births were unwanted (Singh and Wulf, 1990). Similarly, in sub-Saharan Africa, recent survey data for unmarried women from

153

eight countries found that for five of the eight countries between 50 and 75 per cent of first pregnancies were reported as unintended (DHS and Population Reference Bureau, 1992).

Alarming rates of unsafe abortion among adolescent women also attest to the issue of unwanted pregnancies. Estimates of clandestine abortions obtained by women of all ages in developing countries range from 10 million to 22 million; extrapolating from those figures, a recent study by the Center for Population Options (CPO) estimates that adolescent women in developing countries may have between 1.0 million and 4.4 million abortions per annum (Hirsch and Barker, 1992).

Data from 27 studies, primarily hospital-based and in urban areas, found that adolescent women under age 20 accounted for approximately 60 per cent of women presenting with abortion-related complications (Hirsch and Barker, 1992). Because of the unsafe conditions under which these abortions are performed, they can be life-threatening to the young women. Scattered studies and qualitative evidence from numerous developing countries demonstrate that adolescents constitute both a high percentage of abortion-related complications and a significant percentage of the estimated 100,000-200,000 deaths that occur each year in developing countries as a result of botched abortions in developing countries (Hirsch and Barker, 1992).

Various studies on adolescents and abortion in developing countries show that the typical young woman seeking an abortion is likely to be in her late teens or early twenties, but she could be as young as 10 or 11. The younger she is, the more likely it becomes that her abortion will occur after the first trimester with a non-medical provider or that it will be self-induced—all factors that increase the risk of complications and/or death. Adolescents in developing countries frequently turn to traditional healers, chemists, shopkeepers or other non-medical personnel for abortion, or self-induce abortion using a variety of unsafe methods, including drinking quinine, alcohol, detergent or toxic teas, or swallowing large doses of over-the-counter substances, such as prostaglandin.

In addition to being more likely to seek abortions from a non-medical provider, adolescents seek an abortion later in their pregnancy and are slower to seek medical help once complications develop. These delays lead to higher rates of complication, costlier courses of treatment and longer hospital stays. Complications include haemorrhage, septicemia, anaemia, cervical and vaginal lacerations, pelvic abscess, perforation of the uterus or bowels, tetanus and secondary sterility. In many cases, these complications lead to death. Treatment of these complications—in addition to the personal cost to young women—strains poorly stocked hospitals and overburdened public-health budgets.

High-risk births

In addition to the risks associated with unsafe abortion, adolescent women that carry a pregnancy to term face a number of medical risks associated with childbirth. Women under age 20 tend to suffer more pregnancy and delivery complications, including toxae-mia, iron-deficiency anaemia, premature delivery, prolonged labour, hypertensive disorders of pregnancy, cervical trauma, pre-eclampsia and death than do women bearing children at age 20 or later. In addition, the children born to young mothers also suffer an increased risk of mortality and morbidity. Babies born to teenage mothers are only half as likely to be born healthy as those born to physically mature women.

In spite of the complications associated with early child-bearing, much of the current research has demonstrated that adequate prenatal care for pregnant teenage mothers can considerably reduce the risk of maternal and child mortality. There is a growing body of work which suggests that provided young women are well-nourished and have access to adequate prenatal care—which is unfortunately not likely for most adolescent women in developing countries—the health risks to young mothers and their offspring are minimal and virtually equal to those of mothers over age 20. Indeed, most research now suggests that the health risks associated with child-bearing for adolescent mothers are more a factor of socio-economic status and social factors related to their status as adolescents rather than an inherent factor of age (WHO, 1989).

Support for prenatal and postnatal care, however, is often non-existent for low-income adolescent mothers. Due to the shame associated with adolescent pregnancy, young women are often slow to acknowledge their pregnancy and slow to seek prenatal care if it happens to be available. One study from Colombia, for example, found that a majority of 10,000 adolescent mothers studied did not have strong support from either their family or their mate. The majority of the young women interviewed were from low-income families and were malnourished, which led to low levels of protein and haemoglobin (Contreras, 1990).

Wanted births

Although a large number of births to adolescent women are unwanted, it is clear that some—perhaps many—births to adolescent mothers are wanted. They are wanted because having a child—aside from being a powerful part of womanhood—gives a sense of purpose. It represents entrance into womanhood and status for young women, who in many societies otherwise have no status. For many young women in developing countries, bearing a child, even outside marriage, can represent a rational choice for addressing feelings of isolation and low self-esteem and status. In cases where age at first marriage continues to be low and fertility is high, births to adolescent mothers are wanted to fulfil family obligations and prove fertility.

For adolescent women that carry a pregnancy to term, there is a need to provide intensive social services. Adolescent mothers need help in coping with their own adolescent development and continuing their education and vocational training while at the same time learning to be a parent. Intensive day-care and parent training programmes are often needed if the child is to have opportunities for healthy development.

High social costs of adolescent child-bearing

In an urban environment, adolescent child-bearing hinders possibilities for educational and vocational attainment. In many countries, pregnancy means automatic expulsion from school. In Kenya, for example, a 1988 study found that 8,000 teenage girls were forced to drop out of primary school because of pregnancy; another study estimated that each year 10 per cent of secondary-school girls drop out due to pregnancy. Similarly, in the United Republic of Tanzania, nearly 19,000 primary- and secondary-school students were expelled from school due to pregnancy in 1982 (Hirsch, 1992). In other settings, pregnancy leads to school drop-out because adolescent mothers need to work to provide for themselves and their child. In some countries, there is also social stigma associated with out-of-wedlock pregnancy. In Rwanda, a study of 510 adolescent mothers found that 10 per cent were disowned by their families (Hirsch, 1992).

Resistance to discussion of adolescent sexuality and fertility

Although many more people currently realize the need to address sexuality and unwanted child-bearing among adolescents, considerable resistance remains which derives from long-standing myths held by many influential persons. Such myths are not supported by what has been learned through sound research. Some common myths identified by Friedman (1992) in a paper on adolescent reproductive health, presented at the International Planned Parenthood Federation (IPPF) Family Planning Congress at Delhi, India, are:

Myth 1. Young people are generally sexually promiscuous. In fact, where sexual behaviour before or outside marriage is relatively common, young people tend to be less promiscuous than adults. They are likely to be more faithful to an individual partner, even if, over time, they change partners. Having multiple sexual partners is very uncommon for young people;

Myth 2. If young people are given information and services about sexuality, contraception and the prevention of STDs and AIDS, they will become promiscuous. All the evidence, however, suggests the contrary. The more sound information young people have, the more responsibly they behave;

Myth 3. Young people have very different value systems than do their parents. Again, the evidence suggests the opposite. Although it is true that patterns of behaviour are beginning to change, research suggests that most young people hold similar values as their parents on deep-seated subjects. The difference tends to be more about relatively superficial subjects, such as music and dress;

Myth 4. If young people are given sound instructions about human biology and the reproductive system, told that sexual intercourse before marriage is immoral, and told of the dangers to their society of overpopulation, they will delay the beginning of sexual relations and will effectively prevent pregnancy when they do begin to have sex. Unfortunately, while these factors are important, alone they are not effective in changing behaviour. Young people have many questions about their feelings, relationships and sexual reactions that need to be answered. They also need specific information about how to obtain and/or use contraceptives or prophylactic methods. They need to ask those questions of knowledgeable people or they are likely to use other sources which may endanger their health and perhaps be life-threatening;

Myth 5. Most adults have sufficient knowledge and skills to help the young understand sexuality and prevention of pregnancy and STDs. In fact, very few people (especially in developing countries) have had education about sexual subjects and perhaps even fewer have had training in the area of interactive discussion with young people, which the most effective way of having an impact on behaviour.

All these myths and discomfort of the adult population with his changing social environment make the provision of sex education and family planning services to adolescents an extremely sensitive and controversial issue. On the other hand, for young women with valid psychological reasons for wanting a child, preventing early pregnancies requires offering alternatives to child-bearing that give meaning and status. In any case, there is much to be done to reach the point where low-income young people, especially young women, in developing countries will have a choice over when to begin their child-bearing.

Sex education and family life education: residual questions about effectiveness

In the past 10 years, there has been widespread recognition on the part of policy makers and service providers of the information gap that exists regarding sexuality and family life among adolescents. Numerous studies in Africa, for example, have shown that with the passing of many traditional sources of information—for example, elders and rites of passage—youth are turning to their equally misinformed peers for information (Barker and Rich, 1992). Similarly, studies in Latin America and the Caribbean have found that adolescents often turn to their peers or family members due to a perceived lack of sources of information.

In the face of this information gap, the United Nations Population Fund (UNFPA) and the United Nations Educational, Scientific and Cultural Organization (UNESCO), in particular, have promoted the widespread presentation of sex education or family life education—training that combines sexuality education with information on family roles and family life. Despite the widespread interest and implementation of family life and sex education curricula in many developing countries, there have been a number of questions about the quality of the information provided. Some youth-serving organizations have charged that these education programmes are frequently overloaded with population education, which, while important, is sometimes substituted for information on sexuality, family planning and AIDS and STD prevention. Others have questioned how effective teachers—who are generally relied upon to present family life education—are in presenting material that they themselves may feel uncomfortable discussing. In other cases, sex education is laden with moralizing and may effectively exclude youth that are already sexually active by focusing exclusively on abstinence from sexual activity.

Indeed, some survey data underline these questions. A recent study in Kenya found that although 65.5 per cent of youth aged 12-19 said they had received some information on reproductive health (many in school), fewer than 8 per cent could correctly identify a woman's fertile period (Ajayi and others, 1989). Similarly, at Mexico City, where 93 per cent of young men and 85 per cent of young women reported having received sex education, 74 per cent of young women could not correctly identify their fertile period (Morris and others, 1987).

Significant barriers to provision of family planning services

For a variety of reasons, family planning agencies and health-care systems in many developing countries have been reluctant to provide adolescents with family planning services. Although a number of governmental and non-governmental organizations—including the affiliates of IPPF—have initiated special eproductive health service projects for adolescents during the past 10 years, family planning continues to be denied either explicitly or implicitly to adolescents in many countries. Indeed, neither the health-care professionals nor the family planning agencies have been trained to deal with the sensitive issues of sexuality. They therefore hold many myths and misconceptions and lack any ethical guidance from their institutions. Consequently, due to a lack of access and societal barriers, adolescent contraceptive use is extremely low in most developing countries, as highlighted below and in table 13).

Few Latin American teenagers report using contraception at first intercourse. In one study of youth aged

TABLE 13. ADOLESCENT CONTRACEPTIVE USE, SELECTED COUNTRIES

Major area and country	Percentage of women under age 20 giving birth per annum	Percentage of married women aged 15-19 using contraception	Percentage of women currently married, ages 15-19
Africa			
Cameroon	17	2.6	47.7
Côte d'Ivoire	22	1.9	54.0
Egypt	9	5.6	95.5[a]
Ghana	14	4.9	26.8
Kenya	14	2.2	25.6
Mauritius	4	54.7	..
Morocco	5	16.7	..
Mozambique	20	..	..
Nigeria	13	4.5	40.6
Senegal	16	9.4	56.5
Zimbabwe	11	24.9	42.8
Asia			
Bangladesh	26	9.1	66.8
China	1	..	..
India	9	..	..
Indonesia	8	26.0	19.0
Nepal	13	0.3	..
Philippines	5	17.6	..
Sri Lanka	4	20.2	7.3
Thailand	5	43.0	16.4
Latin America and the Caribbean			
Brazil	8	47.7	15.0
Chile	6	..	..
Cuba	9	..	..
Ecuador	9	15.3	17.5
El Salvador	15	21.7	30.0
Guatemala	5	9.3	18.7
Jamaica	11	51.0	..
Mexico	8	28.9	..
Peru	8	22.9	12.9
Trinidad and Tobago	8	42.4	20.3

Source: Adolescent Reproductive Behaviour: Evidence from Developing Countries, Population Studies, No. 109/Add.1 (United Nations publication Sales No. E.89.XIII.10).

[a] Currently married women aged 15-44.

15-24, the rate of use ranged from a low of 7 per cent among those at Quito, Ecuador, to a high of 30 per cent at São Paulo, Brazil (Singh and Wulf, 1990; and Morris, 1988).

Of those teenagers using birth control, many rely upon withdrawal and the rhythm method, which have high failure rates. In Brazil, for example, 75 per cent of those that used birth control at first intercourse used rhythm or withdrawal (Morris, 1988).

In Africa, although sexual activity among unmarried teenagers is high, contraceptive use remains low. In a recent study in Kenya, 11 per cent of sexually active teenagers reported using contraceptives (Ajayi and others, 1989).

Contraceptive use, low for married women of all ages in sub-Saharan Africa, is equally low among married adolescents. Percentages of married teenagers that have ever used contraception range from a high of 13 per cent in Ghana to a low of 1 per cent in Benin and Nigeria (Hirsch, 1990).

Statistics on contraceptive use rates for unmarried teenagers in Asia are hard to find. Contraceptive use

157

rates for married adolescents aged 15-19 in Bangladesh, Fiji, Indonesia and the Philippines are approximately half of those for all married women. Even in Thailand, where contraceptive use rates are relatively high for the region, only 43 per cent of married women aged 15-19 used any method, compared with 65.5 per cent of all women surveyed (United Nations, 1989).

One barrier to contraceptive use by teenagers is sheer lack of access. A recent survey of more than 100 programmes working in adolescent reproductive health carried out by the International Center for Adolescent Fertility (ICAF), a part of CPO, found that although 87 per cent of the programmes surveyed provide sexuality education, only 64 per cent provide adolescents with family planning services. In 82 per cent of the African programmes and 83 per cent of the Asian programmes that provide contraceptive services, they are available only to married couples over age 20 (Barker, Hirsch and Neidell, 1990).

Although family planning access is low for adolescents, it has expanded dramatically for adult women over the past 10-20 years. Increased contraceptive use among adult women coupled with such factors as increased economic opportunities and higher school enrolment rates for girls has meant that in many areas of the world, birth rates of adult women are declining. Birth rates of adolescents, however, are largely staying the same—with slight increases in some countries and slight decreases in others.

Adolescents at high risk for HIV/AIDS and other sexually transmitted diseases

In addition to the issue of premature child-bearing, anecdotal evidence from countries throughout the world shows that adolescents are at high risk of contracting STDs, including AIDS. The World Health Organization (WHO) estimates that 1 in 20 teenagers contracts STD each year. WHO also estimates that 20 per cent of persons with AIDS are in their twenties, which, given the latency period of the virus, 8-10 years, means that many of those contracted the disease while in their teens.

The following statistics highlight the trend concerning the human immunodeficiency virus (HIV) among adolescents:

In the United States of America, 691 cases of AIDS among adolescents (ages 13-19) had been reported to the Centers for Disease Control as of 31 May 1991. A greater percentage of adolescents than adults with AIDS are females (26 versus 10 per cent), are Black or Hispanic (56 versus 44 per cent) and were infected with HIV through heterosexual contact (14 versus 5 per cent).

Although similar statistics are not available for Africa, the number of pregnant women that are HIV-positive is a good indication of the incidence of the virus among women of child-bearing age. At Balantyre, Malawi; Lusaka, Zambia; and Kigali, Rwanda, recent studies of pregnant women show seropositivity rates between 22 and 30 per cent. Given that births to adolescent women constitute 20 per cent of all births in sub-Saharan Africa, many of these young HIV-positive mothers are likely to be adolescents.

Limited studies have found HIV-positive levels between 2 and 10 per cent for street youth, both male and female in Brazil, the Dominican Republic, Kenya, Mexico and the United States of America.

In Thailand, one source reports that 6 per cent of the 10,000 HIV-positive people in the country are teenage female prostitutes (aged 15-20 years).

High-risk factors for AIDS among adolescents

During the past decade, adolescents reported higher levels of sexual activity at earlier ages, experienced millions of pregnancies and abortions and suffered persistently high rates of STDs. Adolescents that initiate sexual intercourse at younger ages are more likely to have multiple partners, thus increasing their chances of becoming infected with STDs, including HIV. STDs, such as gonorrhoea and syphilis, also increase the likelihood of HIV transmission through anal, oral or vaginal intercourse.

In the United States, adolescent women are initiating sexual intercourse at an increasingly early age. Between 1970 and 1988, the proportion of adolescent women aged 15-19 that reported having had premarital sexual intercourse increased from 28.6 to 51.5 per cent. The largest increase occurred among those aged 15 years (from 4.5 to 25.6 per cent).

In Africa, women marry very young, which, combined with the practice of polygamy, increases their exposure to STDs and HIV through the husband's multiple partners. In Kenya, Nigeria and Sierra Leone, limited testing for other STDs found that between 16 and 36 per cent of youth had one or more STD.

At Yurimanuas, Peru, 92 per cent of surveyed secondary-school boys had had sexual intercourse and 23 per cent of those young men had been infected with STD, according to a study conducted in 1989 (Macieira, 1991).

Recent interviews with 35 street girls at La Paz, Bolivia, conducted by Fundación San Gabriel, found that 72 per cent of the girls had been pregnant, 19 per cent had sought unsafe abortion and 100 per cent had a sexually transmitted disease at the time of the study (Fundación San Gabriel, 1991).

Similarly, at a family planning clinic in New Zealand, 40 per cent of women with chlamydia infections were younger than 20 years (Macieira, 1991).

Several studies conducted in the United States have shown that sexually active teenagers are much less likely to use condoms after drinking alcohol or using drugs. The use of crack cocaine, for example, is associated with high levels of sexual activity and risk-taking.

Other sociocultural and economic factors also predispose adolescents to the risk of acquiring an STDs, including AIDS. These factors include homelessness, involvement with "sugar daddies" or sexual exploitation, initiating first sexual intercourse with prostitutes and female genital mutilation, which is practised in more than 20 countries in Africa and in a few in Asia (Biddle, 1991; and Macieira, 1991).

New programme models for expansion of reproductive health services for youth

Despite these troubling statistics on STDs and adolescent child-bearing, there has been a tremendous expansion in programmes working in adolescent reproductive health during the past 10 years. A recent survey by CPO of 103 organizations in more than 30 developing countries found that these programmes are working with a variety of programme models ranging from peer education, separate family planning clinics for adolescents, integrated or multi-service youth centres offering reproductive health services in addition to other services and school-based health programmes (Barker, Hirsch and Neidell, 1990).

These programmes provide important models for the expansion of services in adolescent reproductive health

care, a task that must be a priority for family planning, health and population programmes in the next 10 years. Indeed, as the birth rates of adult women continue to fall in the remaining years in the twentieth century, the attention of the international health and family planning community must turn to adolescents.

The data on adolescent reproductive health are clear. Governments and private service providers can pay now for improved sex education and reproductive health services for youth or pay later in terms of school drop-out rates, hospital costs associated with abortion complications and STDs and societal costs related to the spread of AIDS within the youth population.

B. PROGRAMME RESPONSES AND PROGRAMME MODELS

As previously mentioned, there has been a tremendous expansion in both the number and types of programmes in adolescent reproductive health in developing countries during the past 10 years. Unfortunately, these services (with the possible exception of sex education) continue to reach only a small portion of youth as the data on contraceptive use and condom use attest. The most common programme models currently operating in adolescent reproductive health are described below.

Sex education and family life education

Sex education or family life education is part of virtually every programme working in the prevention of early pregnancies and the spread of HIV/AIDS and other STDs among adolescents. Whether it takes the form of informal group discussions, individual counselling or formal courses, there are as many different kinds of sex education as there are philosophies and values related to sexuality.

Sex education can range from simple discussions of human reproduction to in-depth discussions and activities that involve values, feelings, decision-making and goal-setting. A recent CPO survey of 103 adolescent reproductive health programmes found that the following types of sex education were provided by these programmes (programmes could respond in more than one category): (*a*) 87 per cent included reproductive anatomy and conception; (*b*) 49 per cent included basic demographic concepts; (*c*) 66 per cent included communication skills and activities related to self-esteem;

(d) 55 per cent said they provided information on goal-setting and decision-making; and (e) 64 per cent included discussions of female and male roles.

In recent years, there has been an attempt on the part of many programmes and organizations working in adolescent reproductive health to move to a broader concept of sex education to include life planning and to combine the presentation of information with reflection about values, sex roles and thinking about the future. Part of this trend towards a new type of sex education comes from questions about the effectiveness of traditional sex education courses that focus on the biology of reproduction.

Peer programmes

A growing number of programmes in adolescent reproductive health throughout the world have recently begun to realize the impact of peers on the sexual behaviour of adolescents and the usefulness of peer education programmes and peer distribution of non-medical contraceptives. These programmes are based on the simple premise that teenagers talk to each other more than to anyone else about issues related to sexuality. Indeed, research throughout the world indicates that when teenagers have few other sources to turn to for information about sexuality and family planning, they turn to their peers.

An increasing number of programmes throughout the developing world are coming to realize this fact. Data from a recent ICAF publication (Barker, Hirsch and Neidell, 1990) show that about half of the 103 programmes surveyed in Asia and Latin America and about one fourth of the programmes in Africa featured peer education programmes. Overall, 13 per cent of the programmes also promoted peer distribution of non-medical or non-clinical contraceptives.

Essentially, peer programmes are attractive for two simple reasons: (a) adolescents that promote contraceptive use and responsible sexuality serve as a powerful model for their peers; and (b) they legitimize contraceptive use among sexually active young people.

In addition, adolescent distribution of contraceptives facilitates access. Whether in large cities where young people are embarrassed to go into a pharmacy or in towns where they risk community disapproval, peer distribution can help young people surmount these barriers to contraceptive use.

Peer distribution programmes have shown great promise for replication. The Multidimensional Approach to Adolescent Fertility Management, a peer programme at the University of Ibadan in Nigeria, is being studied by a number of other youth-serving programmes in Africa. The peer programme model has also been successfully implemented in Brazil, Ethiopia, Guatemala, Kenya, Mexico, the Philippines and Sierra Leone, among other countries.

Clinic- and hospital-based services

Clinic-based or hospital-based programmes also provide important sources of adolescent reproductive health services for adolescents. In most cases, family planning agencies have recognized the need to provide clinic services with special hours, separate entrances or in some cases completely different facilities for adolescent clients. The reason is that adolescent women are often reluctant to use services that also serve adult women. Separate adolescent reproductive health clinics are most common in Latin America. Hospital-based services in reproductive health for adolescents typically reach adolescent mothers, frequently at the time of birth, for prenatal care or when a pregnancy is detected. These projects take advantage of this window of opportunity to present adolescent women with options in family planning services to prevent or postpone subsequent pregnancies.

School-based clinics and school-based health services: experience from the United States for developing countries

School-based clinics (SBCs) and school-linked clinics (SLCs) are comprehensive health-care centres that provide a wide range of health and social services to adolescents at or near where they spend much of their day—school. They are designed to overcome barriers to adolescent health care use, including concerns over confidentiality, lack of transportation, inconvenient appointment times, cost, lack of insurance coverage and general apprehension or disinterest among adolescents about discussing personal health problems. SLCs differ from the conventional model of SBCs in that they often are free-standing adolescent health clinics serving youth from more than one school and youth that are not in school.

In the United States, CPO runs a support centre for SBCs and SLCs, which provides information exchange,

160

networking and technical assistance in feasibility studies, fund-raising and evaluation. Recent surveys conducted by CPO found that the number of SBCs and SLCs had increased significantly in the United States from 31 in 1984 to 150 in 1989. By 1991, 306 SBCs and 21 SLCs operating in 33 states and Puerto Rico had been identified.

Most SBCs and SLCs offer a wide range of medical and non-medical services but few provide contraceptive services. Over 90 per cent of clinics offer assessment and referrals to community health-care providers and private physicians, general primary health care, diagnosis and treatment of minor injuries, and routine sports physicals. Over two thirds of the clinics perform routine lab tests, including pregnancy tests; prescribe and dispense medications, manage chronic illnesses, give immunizations and make referrals for prenatal care. More than half diagnose and treat STDs and perform gynaecological examinations.

Over 60 per cent of SBCs provide counselling, referrals or follow-up for family planning methods during the school year, but only 28 per cent write prescriptions for birth control pills and fewer than 20 per cent dispense any kind of contraceptive on site. SLCs are somewhat more likely to provide family planing services than SBCs. Nearly half of SLCs write prescriptions for contraceptives or dispense birth control pills, and slightly under than half make condoms and foam available in the clinic. As can be expected, SBCs are more likely to face resistance from the school system to dispense contraceptives to adolescents than are SLCs.

SBCs and SLCs predominantly serve students that do not have access to other sources of health care and are primarily funded by state and federal sources. City and county governments and school districts may also contribute a portion of operating costs while private foundations contribute less than 3 per cent of their funds.

If supported and used effectively, SBCs and SLCs can help adolescents delay first intercourse and increase effective contraceptive use. For example:

(*a*) At Baltimore, Maryland, in a programme providing counselling on two school campuses with medical care nearby, girls enrolled in the programme postponed first sexual intercourse seven months longer than girls that were not enroled (Zabin and others, 1986);

(*b*) One study of six clinics found that there were no greater levels of increased frequency of sexual activity in schools with clinics that made contraceptives available to students (Kirby, Waszak and Ziegler, 1991);

(*c*) According to this same study, in two of the six schools, greater percentages of sexually active students used effective contraception at last intercourse than did students in non-clinic schools (Kirby, Waszak and Ziegler, 1991).

(*d*) Students are more likely to seek contraceptive counselling and referrals from SBCs that dispense or prescribe contraceptives than they are from clinics that do not (Kirby and Waszak, 1989).

Although SBCs and SLCs in developing countries are neither well developed nor well funded, such clinics do exist and, in Africa, for example, provide limited primary health-care services. Rehabilitating and investing in such clinics as sources of general and reproductive health services may prove to be an effective strategy to expand family planning services and health for youth.

Multi-service centre programmes

A multi-service centre programme is a holistic approach to youth development offering a variety of health, educational and recreational services for teenagers at a specific locally accessible location. Recreational services help lure young people to the centre, thus in turn linking them into the medical and educational programmes, while sexually active youth get access to family planning services in an unobtrusive manner. Multi-service programmes therefore address the physical, emotional and social well-being of the adolescents by offering a variety of activities and services identified according to the perceived needs and interests, the available resources and the level of awareness and motivation of the youth-serving agencies.

The three main categories of services offered are health services, educational activities and recreational activities:

(*a*) Health services usually include general physical and gynaecological exams, pregnancy testing, family planning counselling and psychological services, and may include prenatal care and dental services;

161

(b) Educational activities may be focused on sexuality, nutrition, substance abuse, job training, tutoring, family communication and sometimes legal counselling;

(c) While there are no limits as to what can be offered in the recreational department, the most common activities include ball sports, martial arts, drama, dance, puppet shows, studio arts and crafts-making.

Despite the wide variety of issue areas addressed by multi-service programmes, reproductive health is usually a top priority followed by drug abuse and accident prevention. Some multi-purpose centres provide unique services for certain groups of adolescents, such as teenage mothers or handicapped youth. Other specific examples are given below.

At Guatemala City, a teenage hotline is run by volunteers together with home visits, art contests and a production of a newsletter in the Asociación Pro-Bienestar de la Familia de Guatemala (APROFAM) El Camino programme (affiliated with IPPF). In New York City, the Door Programme encourages teenagers to study on their premises through the "homework club" by providing access to a computer bulletin board.

Multi-service centres are often staffed by counsellors and/or social workers, medical personnel and young promoters. Through structured activities, teenagers learn how to plan their life, care for their health, work in groups, recruit and educate other teenagers and promote adolescent health and well-being by reaching out to parents and the community to establish trust and open communication lines.

The above-mentioned Door Programme in New York is one of the first recognized multi-service programmes, followed by the Centro de Orientación para Adolescentes (CORA) at Mexico City. Another notable programme is APLAFA in Panama (also affiliated with IPPF).

Many youth-serving authorities believe that multi-service programmes offer one of the best approaches to improving adolescent reproductive health while others raise questions about its cost effectiveness compared with the peer counselling and contraceptive distribution approach.

Secondary prevention programmes

Secondary prevention refers to the prevention of repeat pregnancies among adolescent women. Such programmes typically include prenatal care and family planning services to prevent or space subsequent births. Additional services often include tutoring or assistance in continuing education, day care, counselling and vocational training. Programmes in Africa and Latin America have had tremendous success in reaching adolescent mothers, including reinserting them into the school system in some cases.

Lessons learned by these programmes

Due to the complexity of the adolescent reproductive health and fertility issue, programmes working with youth face many challenges, including convincing adults that today's teenagers can decide for themselves, keeping the programmes flexible enough to respond to the changing needs of the adolescents and their communities and dealing with inadequate evaluations of the youth programmes themselves. Despite these difficulties, the following generalizations can be made about prog-rammes working on adolescent reproductive health.

In general, youth will not make use of "normal" adult family planning or health clinics unless special provisions are made to ensure their privacy and to attract them. Those from a low-income background do not generally perceive family planning as an urgent need, and thus programmes that feature other services to attract youth are usually more successful (multi-service approach).

Peer programmes—or programmes in which youth serve as transmitters of information and occasionally as distributors of non-medical contraceptives—can be an extremely effective way to reach youth. In areas where sex education is not widely available—and even in places where it is—young people report they most frequently turn to their peers for information about sexuality and family planning. When armed with accurate information about sexuality, fertility, family and general health, teenagers can be excellent "health outreach workers" to their peers.

Programmes that promote only abstinence usually will not work as effectively as programmes offering options, specifically family planning services for youth that decide to be sexually active. None the less, effective educational and support programmes can support youth that make the decision not to be sexually active and can do so effectively.

162

Programmes that use fear tactics, moralization or shaming of sexually active adolescents and those that have already resorted to abortion will alienate a large proportion of youth and may not be effective in reaching their objectives.

The use of contraception by sexually active youth is highly correlated with level of education, having received information on sex education, positive peer attitudes towards contraceptives, positive influence from parents (especially mothers) regarding family planning use and a sense of self-efficacy.

Information from one channel alone is generally not enough to change attitudes about sexual behaviour. Studies have found that AIDS prevention programmes, for example, are more effective when consistent messages come from teachers, parents, media and peers. There is a difficulty of conflicting messages being given to adolescents—media and peers say "yes" to sexual activity, while parents and teachers say "no."

Programmes are more effective when they remove as many barriers as possible—inappropriate schedules, price, location, clinic staff that are insensitive to youth needs etc. Youth seem to respond better to services and are more likely to use services when they are conveniently located, such as in a school, across the street from a school, in a hospital (for teenage mothers giving birth) or on the street corners or other locations where youth normally aggregate. Programmes need to reach adolescents at an early age before they become sexually active, must provide services over an extended period of time and must be integrated.

Role models, young staff or young people can be an important element in programmes reaching adolescents. This effort can include peers talking about their experiences (persons with AIDS, for example, in AIDS prevention or young mothers talking about how they coped with unwanted pregnancy and its consequences). Programmes also must involve young people in the planning and implementation process. Such involvement can have a dramatic impact in terms of self-esteem for those young people—especially young women—that participate and helps ensure that programmes shall be designed with the actual needs of youth involved.

Young people are less likely to face the consequences of unprotected sexual activity if they have something constructive and meaningful to do. Programmes are most effective when they combine basic education, vocational training and other activities that provide hope for the future with access to family planning.

C. An Agenda for Action: Strategies and Recommendations

Much remains to be done adequately to address the needs and problems mentioned in this paper. The author's recommendations for future action in adolescent reproductive health are given below.

Improvement of access to reproductive health services and information for young people

Family planning providers, public-health systems and youth-serving organizations should focus their efforts on providing young people with reproductive health services, including family planning, counselling, AIDS/STD prevention and treatment and safe abortion services. Improvements in access require concerted training and advocacy efforts to overcome deep-seated adult discomfort with adolescent sexuality in many developing countries. Even in those countries where widespread contraceptive distribution to unmarried adolescents may not be feasible in the current political climate, it may still be possible to provide more accurate information which will allow young people to make their own reproductive health decisions.

Creation of a climate conducive to adolescent family planning and condom use

Even in the few countries where services and information are widely available to young people, a variety of cultural factors prevent young people from taking full advantage of these services. Sexual abuse of young women, stereotypes that cast men in the role of aggressor and women as chaste and passive or, alternatively, oversexed and dangerous are just a few of the barriers to frank discussions of sexuality and equality in relationships. Conflicting messages from parents, the media and social leaders may also discourage family planning use while encouraging sexual activity and exploitative relationships. Equality for young women and men, a worthy goal in itself, is also necessary to promote contraceptive use among adolescents. Programmes must also promote life options and activities that give a sense of hope for the future in order to encourage adolescent contraceptive use.

Additional research on adolescent reproductive. health issues, including abortion

Although the existing data provide an excellent starting-point, much more is needed. Specifically, research is needed on factors that influence adolescent sexual activity and contraceptive use, country-specific data on maternal mortality and morbidity associated with unsafe abortion among adolescents and operations research on programmes to reach adolescents with reproductive health services. When possible, the research should include information on the social costs of high rates of unwanted pregnancies, with the goal of informing the public and assisting advocacy efforts.

Improvement of efforts in sex education and family life education

Improvement of sex education programmes should principally involve developing additional curricula which focus on changing attitudes and behaviour and not just on providing information. Improving sex education programmes will also require better training for teachers and other youth-serving professionals that provide sex education. In many cases, this training must involve helping these professionals become comfortable with their own sexuality before they become sex educators. Sex education curricula also need to include accurate and frank information on contraceptives and answer the questions—without censorship—that young people ask.

Support of sex education efforts and reproductive health services with mass communication

Governments and youth professionals should counter-act the influences from the mass telecommunications which cross cultural boundaries with accurate and coordinated information from multiple media channels, including audio-visual, print and folk media.

Increased involvement of youth

Part of youth participation involves listening to them to obtain a better understanding of the type of information and services they want and relying upon input from youth themselves to make this determination. Increased involvement of youth also means expanded reliance upon peer programmes, in which youth serve as transmitters of information and in some cases as distributors of condoms. Improving and expanding peer programmes may require paying peer promoters, as some programmes have done, as well as efforts to make the job of "peer promoter" an attractive position to youth.

Involvement of broad sectors of society to forge coalitions on behalf of adolescent reproductive health

Too often, advocates in the family planning field focus narrowly on the end goal of promoting contraceptive use and hence isolate themselves from groups with related concerns. Rather than focusing exclusively on adolescents and family planning/reproductive health, advocates should make themselves part of a broader movement for adolescent health, allying themselves with church leaders, feminist organizations, education officials, medical professionals and young people themselves.

REFERENCES

Ajayi, Ayo A., and others (1989). *Adolescent Sexuality and Fertility in Kenya: A Survey of Knowledge, Perceptions, and Attitudes*. Boston, Massachusetts: Pathfinder International.

Barker, Gary (1989). *Executive Summary: Youth in the Developing World*. Washington, D.C.: Population Resource Centre.

_____ , and Susan Rich (1990). *Adolescent Fertility in Kenya and Nigeria: Final Report for a Study Tour Conducted June-July 1990*. Washington, D.C.: Center for Population Options and Population Crisis Committee.

_____ (1992). Influences on adolescent sexuality in Nigeria and Kenya: findings from recent focus group discussions. *Studies in Family Planning* (New York), vol. 23, No. 3 (May/June), pp. 199-210.

Barker, Gary, Jennifer S. Hirsch and Shara Neidell (1990). *Serving the Future: An Update on Adolescent Pregnancy Prevention Programs in Developing Countries*. Washington, D.C.: Center for Population Options, International Center on Adolescent Fertility.

Biddle, Christina (1991). *The Facts: Adolescents, AIDS and HIV*. Washington, D.C.: Center for Population Options.

Contreras, D. (1990). Manejo de la adolescente embarazada. *Revista Colombiana de Obstetricia y Ginecología* (Bogotá), vol. 41, No. 1 (enero-marzo).

Crews, Kimberly A., and Carl Haub (1989). *Teen Mothers, Global Patterns*. Washington, D.C.: Population Reference Bureau.

Demographic and Health Surveys and Population Reference Bureau (1991). *Adolescent Women in Sub-Saharan Africa: A Chartbook on Marriage and Childbearing*. Washington, D.C.: Population Reference Bureau.

Ecuador, Centro para Estudios para la Paternidad Responsable (1989). *Encuesta de información y experiencia reproductiva de los jóvenes ecuatorianos en Quito y Guayaquil*. Quito.

Ferrando, Delicia, Susheela Singh and Deirdre Wulf (1989). *Adolescentes de hoy, padres de mañana: Perú*. New York: The Alan Guttmacher Institute.

Friedman, Herbert (1992). A global overview of adolescent reproductive health. Paper presented at the International Planned Parenthood Federation Family Planning Congress, New Delhi, India.

Fundación San Gabriel (1991). Background study on street and working children. Untitled draft. La Paz, Bolivia.

Gyepi-Garbrah, Benjamin (1985a). *Adolescent Fertility in Sub-Sahara Africa: An Overview.* Boston, Massachusetts: Pathfinder International.
_____ (1985b). *Adolescent Fertility in Liberia.* Boston, Massachusetts: Pathfinder International.
_____ (1985c). *Adolescent Fertility in Nigeria.* Boston, Massachusetts: Pathfinder International.
_____ (1985d). *Adolescent Fertility in Sierra Leone.* Boston, Massachusetts: Pathfinder International.
Henriques, Maria Helena, and others (1989). *Adolescentes de hoje, Pais do Amanhã: Brasil.* New York: The Alan Guttmacher Institute.
Henshaw, Stanley (1990). Induced abortion: a world review. *Family Planning Perspectives* (New York), vol. 22, No. 2 (March-April), pp. 76-89.
Hirsch, Jennifer (1992). *The Facts: Teenage Pregnancy in Africa.* Washington, D.C.: Center for Population Options, International Center on Adolescent Fertility.
Hirsch, Jennifer, and Gary Barker (1992). Adolescents and Abortion in Developing Countries: A Preventable Tragedy. Washington, D.C.: Center for Population Options, International Center on Adolescent Fertility.
Hirsch, Jennifer, and Jennifer Hincks (1990a). *The Facts: Young Women and AIDS: A Worldwide perspective.* Washington, D.C.: Center for Population Options.
_____ (1990b). The Facts: Teenage Pregnancy and Sexually Transmitted Diseases in Latin America. Washington, D.C.: Center for Population Options, International Center on Adolescent Fertility.
Kirby, Douglas, Cynthia Waszak and Julie Ziegler (1991). Six school-based clinics: their reproductive health services and impact on sexual behaviour. *Family Planning Perspectives* (New York), vol. 23, No. 1 (January-February), pp. 6-16.
_____ , and Cynthia S. Waszak, with Julie Siegler (1989). *An Assessment of Six School-Based Clinics: Services, Impact and Potential*, Patricia Donovan, ed. Washington, D.C.: Center for Population Options.
Jacobson, Jodi L. (1990). *The Global Politics of Abortion.* Worldwatch Paper, No. 97. Washington, D.C.: Worldwatch Institute.
Ladipo, Oladapo A., and others (1983). Sexual behaviour, contraceptive practice, and reproductive health among the young unmarried population in Ibadan, Nigeria: final report. Ibadan: University College Hospital; Arlington, Virginia: Family Health International; and Boston, Massachusetts: The Pathfinder Fund.
Macieira, Marjorie (1991). It won't happen to me: STD and adolescents. *Passages* (Washington, D.C.), vol. 11, No. 1 (July).
_____ (1993). Multi-service programs. In *Model Programs for Youth.* Washington, D.C.: Center for Population Options.
Mohamud, Asha (1992). AIDS among adolescents in developing countries. Paper presented at the Human Sexuality and AIDS Training Seminar, Margaret Sanger Center, New York, June.
Monterroso, and others (1988). *Encuesta sobre salud y educación sexual de jovenes, Departamento de Guatemala—areas urbanas, reporte final.* Guatemala City: Asociación Guatemalteca de Educación Sexual; and United States Centers for Disease Control, Division of Reproductive Health.
Morris, Leo (1988). Young adults in Latin America and the Caribbean: their sexual experience and contraceptive use. *International Family Planning Perspectives* (New York), vol. 14, No. 4 (December), pp. 153-158.
_____ (1989). Sexual experience and use of contraception among young adults in Latin America. International Conference on Adolescent Fertility in Latin America and the Caribbean, Oaxaca, Mexico, 6-9 November.

_____ , and others (1987). *Young Adult Reproductive Health Survey in Two Delegations of Mexico City: English Language Report.* Mexico City: Academia Mexicana de Investigaciones en Demografía Médica, Centro de Orientación para Adolescentes; Family Health International; and United States Centers for Disease Control, Division of Reproductive Health.
Prada, Elena, Susheela Singh and Deirdre Wulf (1988). *Adolescentes de hoy, padres de mañana: Colombia.* New York: The Alan Guttmacher Institute.
Programa de Salud y Políticas Sociales (1990). Sexualidad y embarazo en los jovenes. Santiago, Chile: Universidad Academia de Humanismo Cristiano.
Riessman, Janet (1991). School-based and school-linked centers fact sheet, based on Cynthia Waszak and Shara Seidell. *School-Based and School-Linked Clinics: Update 1991.* Washington, D.C.: Center for Population Options.
Remez, Lisa (1989). Special report: adolescent fertility in Latin America and the Caribbean: examining the problems and solutions. *International Family Planning Perspectives* (New York), vol. 15, No. 4 (December), pp. 144-48.
Senderowitz, Judith, and John M. Paxman (1985). *Adolescent Fertility: Worldwide Concerns.* Population Bulletin, vol. 40, No. 2. Washington, D.C.: Population Reference Bureau.
Simons, Janet (1992). *The Adolescent and Young Adult Fact Book.* Washington, D.C.: Children's Defense Fund.
Singh, Susheela, and Deirdre Wulf (1990). *Today's Adolescents, Tomorrow's Parents: A Portrait of the Americas.* New York: The Alan Guttmacher Institute.
Tietze, Christopher, and Stanley K. Henshaw (1986). *Induced Abortion: A World Review, 1986.* 6th ed. New York: The Alan Guttmacher Institute.
United Nations (1989). *Adolescent Reproductive Behaviour*, vol. II, *Evidence from Developing Countries.* Population Studies, No.109/Add.1. Sales No. E.89.XIII.10.
_____ (1990). *Patterns of First Marriage: Timing and Prevalence.* Sales No. E.91.XIII.6.
United Nations Fund for Population Activities. Maternal deaths: how many and why? *Population* (New York), vol. 17, No. 7 (July).
Universidad de Chile, Departamento de Salud Pública (1989). *Encuesta sobre salud reproductiva en adultos jovenes, Chile 88.* Santiago, Chile.
Valenzuela, G., and others (1989). *Encuesta de salud reproductiva en adultos jovenes, Santiago, 1988.* Santiago, Chile: Universidad de Chile, Departamento de Salud Pública, Division de Ciencias Médicas Occidente; and United States Centers for Disease Control, Division of Reproductive Health.
World Assembly of Youth and Population Reference Bureau (1990). *The World's Youth Data Sheet, 1990.* Washington, D.C.: Population Reference Bureau.
World Conference on Education for All (1990). *Meeting Basic Learning Needs: A Vision for the 1990s.* World Conference on Education for All, Jontien, Thailand, 5-9 March 1990. New York: Interagency Commission for the World Conference on Education for All.
World Health Organization (1989). The risk to women of pregnancy and childbearing in adolescence. Geneva.
Zabin Laurie S., and others (1986). Evaluation of a pregnancy prevention program for urban teenagers. *Family Planning Perspectives* (New York), vol. 18, No. 3 (May-June), pp. 119-126.

X. DIFFUSION OF INNOVATIVE BEHAVIOUR AND INFORMATION, EDUCATION AND COMMUNICATION ACTIVITIES

Tirbani P. Jagdeo[*]

Two basic strategies underie the thrust of family planning programmes throughout the world—that to generate a demand for family planning and that to supply the services generated by the demand. Information, education and communication (IEC) programmes are at the heart of these demand creation efforts. Experience has shown that effective IEC design needs to be as complex and as discriminating as the social structures within which contraceptive decisions are made, because family planning involves more than just the adoption of new behaviour. It involves the adoption of behaviour that confronts the preferences of the social support and social control centres of family planning acceptors—their concept of status, their religious values and the power hierarchies within their households and communities.

The power of these social control and social support structures varies across society. In some societies, contraceptive decision-making is the prerogative of individuals; in others, of couples; and in still others, of families and wider kinship units mediated by the mores and expectations of tribal, racial and ethnic affiliation. The relevance of social structure to the design and execution of IEC programmes is recognized everywhere. Yet, in the actual design and management of family planning programmes, insufficient attention is paid to understanding and managing the context in which contraceptive decisions are made.

A. NEED FOR INFORMATION, EDUCATION AND COMMUNICATION

The evidence points to a general recognition of the value of IEC as a tool for motivating behaviour change with respect to family planning and an ongoing need for IEC work. The Review and Appraisal of the World Population Plan of Action states that despite greater government support for access to and knowledge of family planning, "data from the World Fertility Survey for developing countries indicate, that of women who wanted no more children and were exposed to the risk of pregnancy, on average over half were not using contraception".

Size of unmet need

Data from the recently completed Demographic and Health Surveys (DHS) provide quantitative confirmation of this need (Mauldin, 1991) and some rather impressive indications of a latent demand for family planning. These data show that in the late 1980s, contraceptive use was below 15 per cent among married women of reproductive age (MWRA) in 13 sub-Saharan African countries and more than 40 per cent in only 2 countries. Surveys in Southern Asia show similarly low user rates of about 8 per cent in Pakistan, 15 per cent in Nepal and 31 per cent in Bangladesh.

These low rates of contraceptive use are at odds with women's fertility preferences. Thapa and others (1991) examine fertility preferences among women exposed to pregnancy and not using a contraceptive method 0-23 months after their last birth in 25 countries in Africa, Asia, and Latin America and the Caribbean. These data show that in Botswana, Egypt, Kenya, Morocco, Tunisia and Zimbabwe, one third of the women interviewed 13-18 months after their last pregnancy wanted "no more children". The desire to space births was proportionately higher in all the African countries studied except Uganda, where child-spacing and child limitation desires were relatively low. In the nine Latin American and Caribbean countries studied, child limitation preferences ranged from 33 per cent in Guatemala to over 50 per cent in Brazil, Mexico and Ecuador, and over 70 per cent in Bolivia and Peru. Similar preferences for child limitation and birth-spacing were observed in Indonesia, Sri Lanka and Thailand. These figures attest to a substantially high level of unmet family planning need in the three most populous areas of the world. They also violate one of

---

[*]Chief Executive Officer, Caribbean Family Planning Affiliation Limited, Saint John's, Antigua.

the basic principles of the United Nations World Population Plan of Action, which affirms that women have the right to complete integration in the development process particularly by means of an equal access to education and equal participation in social, economic, cultural and political life. Evidently, substantial numbers of women are being left out of this integration process through a bondage to pregnancies and childbearing they do not want and, given current technology, appropriate policy instruments and services, can certainly avoid.

A mandate for action

These data do more than validate the family planning agenda of Governments, intergovernmental and non-governmental organizations. They are an eloquent mandate for action. The fact that the majority of women in these countries "want" family planning either to space their births or to limit their family size makes that agenda a binding moral imperative for all concerned. The obligation to meet these unmet family planning needs transcends arguments of social and economic development; it becomes more basic than that. The data are the collective voices of women across three major areas raised to affirm their desire for and entitlement to reproductive rights—rights to plan their families, to space their births and to limit their family size. If Governments need a mandate from the people to act, the voices of these women give them that mandate.

B. ROLE OF INFORMATION, EDUCATION AND COMMUNICATION PROGRAMMES

The intervention most suited for transforming these high levels of need into effective demand is information, education and communication. An important reason that women in many parts of the world do not use family planning is that they do not know about family planning. When they do know, this knowledge is filtered through the prejudgments and attitudes of people that tend to purvey myth, magnify side-effects and skew the balance away from family planning acceptance. The role of IEC is to provide knowledge where ignorance and myth prevail, to empower people with the facts about the principles of family planning, knowledge of methods, their side-effects and the health and economic issues involved in contraceptive use, poor spacing and too large families. The relation between family planning and the economic advantages of small families is often

stressed. IEC programmes should continue to do so. What must be reaffirmed, however, is that family planning is also a basic health issue and therefore a matter for individuals, families and Governments.

Although the role of IEC is to banish ignorance and myth as causes for the non-acceptance of family planning, the philosophy should be based on the premise that family planning is a basic human right involving people's right to know, their right to decide and a socially enabled capability to act on those decisions. To know, people must have knowledge; to decide, people must have options; to act, people must have access to services. Well-planned IEC programmes can give substance to each of these aspects of one's entitlement to family planning. Some of the instruments available are the theatre, the print and electronic media, the extensive use of outreach workers, counselling and other promotional techniques. Depending upon the phase of the programme, the material may focus on creating awareness of the principles and practices of family planning upon motivating change in attitudes and behaviour, upon developing instructional material to improve user compliance or upon popularizing service centres.

C. RESEARCH, MATERIALS DEVELOPMENT AND MANAGEMENT RESEARCH

Effective IEC has three important aspects, two of which are often neglected: (a) research research; (b) the actual development and dissemination of IEC material; and (c) the management and evaluation of the dissemination process. More often than not, in the rush to get IEC materials out, both the research that should precede materials development and the management that should run concurrently with its dissemination are neglected. Because of time constraints, the dictates of donors and the producers' lack of conviction, IEC materials are developed on the basis of feelings rather than on findings.

The Caribbean experience exemplifies this point. In the Caribbean, the IEC thrusts proceeded on the basis that men were opposed to family planning. Conventional wisdom had it that men judged their manhood by the number of children they sired, that men experienced a loss of control when women acquired power over their own reproductive potential and that they opposed family planning for these reasons. This conviction shaped the IEC thrusts of the family planning movement in the region. The bulk of the public education messages —radio and television talks, posters, pamphlets, counselling activities and outreach family planning programmes—were directed to women. The pill, the intra-uterine device (IUD), injectables, tubal ligations and vaginal foams were aggressively promoted among women at risk by every IEC strategy available. Very little was done with men. When research showed that condom use ran a poor third to oral pills and tubal ligations, everyone wondered why.

Recent research indicates that IEC efforts were proceeding on false premises (Heisler and Lewis, 1985). In Barbados, Dominica and Saint Kitts and Nevis, men desired 2.1, 3.1 and 3.1, respectively, which almost coincides with the number of children women desire. These studies also indicate that men are much more supportive of family planning than was generally thought to be true. In these three countries, at least 40 per cent of the males that knew of one family planning method felt that family planning decisions should be made by both partners, and between 67 and 74 per cent of these respondents felt that the "man should be involved in family planning decisions". Data from a series of contraceptive surveys conducted among nationally representative samples of women aged 15-44 provide some corroboration for these views. The majority of the female users of contraceptives had talked to their male partners about family planning and three out of four of them claimed that their partners were in favour of contraceptive use.

In a sense, planners and donors went with their feelings and constructed programmes throughout the Caribbean that fortified prevailing notions of male irresponsibility, marginalized men and missed an opportunity to strengthen the relationships among Caribbean couples with IEC interventions. This experience is not specific to the Caribbean region. It can be found elsewhere. Research was not conducted when it was logical to do so. Research was conducted when it was convenient to do so and it led to inappropriate IEC effort. But an important lesson has been learned. It is necessary to guard against the tendency to do research for the sake of research and to ensure that practical programme implications shall be built into the research design. Similar work is also being done in other parts of the world and they generally reaffirm the need for family planning IEC strategies to be targeted to men in societies where they are prominent in communications networks or household decision-making.

This inattention to context shows up in the nature of the research done in family planning. Both the World Fertility Survey and DHS provide comprehensive data on past, current and projected levels of use on contraceptives and the socio-economic correlates thereof. The importance of these data cannot be denied. Take, for example, the study of fertility preferences of MWRA 0-23 months after their last child (Thapa and others, 1991). The study identifies a large proportion of women not wanting children but not using a contraceptive. This is useful data indeed. They are the basis for powerful advocacy drives with Governments and non-governmental organizations underscoring people's rights and desires to control their fertility.

Relevant questions

Other questions, however, are left unanswered; the critical one is "why". Why are such large proportions of women desired to space their births and limit their family size not doing so. Is it because of supply scarcities? Physical and economic barriers? Social and knowledge constraints? Personality factors? Household power structures, social prescriptions or interpretations thereof? These are the types of questions that research can answer and IEC programmes can build on. These are comments not on the article cited but more on the fact that family planning research has focused substantially on the knowledge, attitudes and practices of women of reproductive age. They have paid little attention to the analysis of the context of such knowledge, attitudes and practice, how those contexts inhibit use or can be made, through innovative IEC, to support and sustain use.

The odd thing about this situation is that the need for more enabling research is constantly acknowledged. It is known that the development of IEC material must take into account the cultural and political sensitivities of society. It is recognized that there is need to identify the most powerful formal and informal publics in society, to find out how they think, to assess how much programme space their attitudes allow and to develop strategies for managing that space. These are prerequisites to developing a work plan for innovative IEC. But these considerations are seldom assigned high priority in IEC programme development. Failure to take into account and to manage the opinions and opposition of these groups either through co-optation, public relations campaigns, message modification and myth-debunking strategies often injure the sensitivities of the publics that shape the behaviour of primary target groups and spoil the approach for future efforts.

IEC programmes, however, need to be more than sensitive. They must also be courageous. The task of developing material that is delicate enough to pass the scrutiny of society's moral custodians yet courageous enough to test the limits of community tolerance for awareness creation, attitude change and behaviour modification is indeed difficult but necessary. Striking the balance between discretion and directness can be very difficult in many societies but IEC workers have a responsibility to the constituency of couples at risk to marshal the creativity and courage needed to convey a clear and convincing message.

Managing IEC programmes

Despite the tendency to think so, the IEC task is not done with the production of material. Experience has shown that the logic and logistics of dissemination are seldom clearly worked out and when they are, strategies and skills for "using" IEC materials are seldom developed.

IEC programmes must be managed. Very often, family staff are trained to show a video to clients but seldom to use those videos in interactive sequences to motivate change. Posters are put in a village but little reinforcing small group activities done with that village to nail down the message they contain. Material is produced and disseminated without a proper analysis of the distribution of people in the society and their demographic flows during the day and sometimes without regard to cultural timing. In some cases, an analysis of the distribution of the population across villages would permit allocation of efforts according to the size of the community; in other cases, during the day, the majority of the adults will flow either into urban areas or to their place of work on farms and plantations. This information can be used to display material or station fieldworkers. In many societies, it is considered *outré* to broadcast certain kinds of messages at specific points of the cultural calendar, e.g., Ramadan, Diwali, Christmas and Lent. Culturally sensitive IEC planning will take these considerations into account. In a word, IEC activities must be treated from the viewpoint of message design and development, the logic and logistics of dissemination, strategies for reinforcing and sustaining the message and for monitoring and evaluating the process. IEC materials are only as good as the management of their use, that is, the quality of the efforts made to manage their design, development, dissemination, use and impact.

Some pivotal questions come to mind. They must be analysed and clarified in the first stage of the IEC development process. Some of these questions concern: (*a*) the infrastructure that exists for IEC work; (*b*) whether the target group is segmented in ways that would make different types of IEC strategies relevant; (*c*) the mix of messages that is needed and the most appropriate media formats for this mix; (*d*) the basic objectives of an IEC intervention—whether it is to create awareness, to change attitudes, to modify behaviour, to popularize service centres or to market those centres. When one thinks of it, these are logical questions to pursue, wonderful opportunities for a meeting of minds between researchers, communications specialists and managers. Their deliberations can lead to decisions as simple as not producing television spots for target groups for whom television is usually not available. It can be as subtle as deciding that even with a given infrastructure, the nature of influence within certain sections of the target community dictates that IEC messages be delivered through primary face-to-face outreach contacts rather than through the mass media. This decision involves making decisions about how target groups are segmented in terms of their capacity to receive formal versus informal, written as opposed to audiovisual messages; and planning the IEC materials accordingly. Lastly, having decided on the objectives of the IEC campaign, one needs also to decide on the mix of media formats most appropriate to accomplish them. For example, posters seem to work quite well in making people aware of family planning. They are less effective in changing attitudes. Radio talks, videos and face-to-face persuasion seem most appropriate for motivating attitude and behaviour change.

D. INFORMATION, EDUCATION AND COMMUNICATION FOR WHOM—PROVIDERS, POLICY MAKERS AND INFORMAL LEADERS?

The logical target groups for family planning IEC interventions are the men and women at risk. But in many parts of the world, large numbers of women that know of family planning and desire to plan their family are not doing so. The observed resistance comes from unexpected origins. Provider competence and attitudes can significantly determine family planning acceptance and continuation rates. A study of physician attitudes towards family planning in Nigeria (Covington and others, 1986) shows that 38.5 per cent of the physicians sampled thought that family planning was foreign to Nigerian culture, while 22.1 per cent felt that it promoted promiscuity. Even more widespread than this is the preference of physicians in many parts of the world to constrain the provision of oral contraceptives to medical personnel. Although no quantitative data are available for the Caribbean, the views expressed by providers in interviews, seminars, workshops and conferences suggest that many have serious reservations about providing contraceptive services to sexually active adolescents. Clinical competence cannot be equated with a social commitment to family planning. IEC programmes must identify the motivational needs of health-care providers and meet those needs.

Acceptance of family planning by individuals is not an end in itself. It is the first step towards institutionalizing the process. Until family planning is institutionalized in the policy and programme frameworks of society, its progress will be subject to the vagaries of extremist movements, economic growth and political expediency. IEC programmes have a fundamental obligation to build a climate of institutional acceptance of family planning through advocacy programmes for family planning as a reproductive right and to have that right enshrined in its policy, programme and basic educational institutions of society.

IEC professionals should be aware that, in some ways, family planning sells itself to policy makers. There are very few instances in society when the decisions made by individuals to achieve personal goals reticulate so nicely with national objectives as is true of family planning. When large numbers of women decide to use family planning, their decision almost immediately redounds to the national benefit—it reduces the pressure on the health system, reduces labour turnover, releases the productive potential of women into the workforce, reduces the budget for maintaining standards and feeds the impetus to development. The argument is there to be made and with appropriate IEC it can and should be.

E. THE IMPACT OF IEC ACTIVITIES

The evaluation of IEC activities is another sorely neglected area. The problem is partially technical. It is very difficult to isolate the effect of an IEC intervention on any of the variables of interest to programme managers, policy makers or donors. It can be done but often requires a level of professional skill and financial resources not available to family planning associations. The problem is partially definitional. Evaluation designs need not be statistically complex to be useful and they need not and should not be only summational. Process evaluation is a key element in the evaluation process because it provides the best chance to learn what elements of the message are relevant, salient, clear and persuasive to the client.

The consequences of not building evaluation as a process into IEC interventions can be costly indeed. In a study on the quality of family planning services in four rural areas in China, Kaufman and others (1992) found a marked difference in providers' perceptions of the information they provided to the clients and clients' apprehension of this information. The authors concluded that "despite the volume of information services organized by the counties and the providers' belief that they inform women about methods and side-effects, many women reported that they were poorly informed about the methods they selected" (Kaufman and others, 1992, p. 77). The result is that when side-effects were experienced, acceptors lacked the preparation to cope with them. But the providers in all probability did discuss the side-effects of IUD use with clients. It is quite possible, however, that it was not in a form that clients were able to hear and remember. Simple methods of process evaluation—getting feedback from clients—to ensure that what was being said was being communicated could have solved the problem.

The value of good IEC is borne out by a number of studies. In a review of studies on the effects of counselling among family planning users, Gallen and others (1987) cite studies in Benin, Brazil, Indonesia, Lebanon and Tunisia attesting to the fact that good counselling leads both to higher family acceptance and to higher continuation rates once family planning is accepted. In a 19-month study in Benin, it was found that multiparous women that received special counselling on the hazards of many births, the benefits of family planning, the availability of family planning methods etc. were more likely to adopt modern methods of contraception than women that just received information on methods alone. In the study at Beirut, Lebanon, 441 women were randomly assigned to two groups, one to receive one-on-one counselling on contraception, the other to receive none. Of the women that returned for the post-partum follow-up, 86 per cent of those that had received one-on-one education chose a family planning method, compared with 52 per cent of the uncounselled group.

The Tunisian study demonstrated the value of face-to-face encounters in the field. According to that study, house-to-house counselling by an outreach worker led to a greater increase in contraceptive use than adding a new service site; and in Indonesia, it was found that 90 per cent of IUD users that received counselling about side-effects before and after insertion were still users, compared with 52 per cent of those receiving counselling after insertion only if they had a complaint. The programme implications of these findings for IEC work are substantial indeed and definitely point to a future programme emphasis on counselling as a strategy for motivating and sustaining family planning acceptance in the developing world. Good IEC is clearly an indispensable element in the provision of quality services to family planning clients in the clinic and in the field.

But IEC is more than counselling. It usually involves the extensive use of the electronic and print media—posters, pamphlets, radio and television spots, drama serials, videos—and the use of fieldworkers working in the community to provide people with information and education, to create awareness and to motivate behaviour change through face-to-face encounters. Each of these strategies is appropriate for different objectives and different target groups. In general, the mass media are considered better suited for creating awareness, while face-to-face encounters are more appropriate for attitude and behaviour modification.

A number of studies carried out in the Caribbean in 1987 and 1988 show the effect of IEC interventions on contraceptive use. Nationally representative samples of women aged 15-44 were asked whether they had attended family planning discussions, discussed family planning with a primary agent, seen a poster, read a pamphlet or heard a family planning broadcast on the radio or television. Respondents were then divided into three groups representing those with low, high and medium levels of exposure to family planning stimuli. Table 14 shows the relation between level of family planning exposure and contraceptive use in selected Caribbean countries.

These data represent a conscious effort to use research to evaluate the effect of IEC programmes in the Caribbean on contraceptive use. The data are simply

TABLE 14. CONTRACEPTIVE USE AMONG WOMEN IN A UNION, AGES 15-44, BY LEVEL OF EXPOSURE TO FAMILY PLANNING STIMULI, SELECTED CARIBBEAN COUNTRIES
(*Percentage using contraception*)

Country	High	Medium	Low
Antigua	53.9	52.8	42.3
Barbados	64.8	55.5	48.1
Saint Vincent and the Grenadines	65.9	58.6	42.3
Saint Lucia	66.1	53.2	35.7
Dominica	50.3	47.1	38.8

Source: Tirbani P. Jagdeo, Caribbean Contraceptive Prevalence Surveys, Nos. 4-8 (New York, International Planned Parenthood Federation, Western Hemisphere Region, 1990).

presented and have proved useful to family planning managers and donors alike. They show a greater tendency for women that were more exposed to family planning IEC interventions to use contraceptives. A further analysis of the adolescent sub-sample of the data for Antigua, Dominica and Saint Lucia show that exposure to family planning stimuli was the most stable predictor of contraceptive use even when employment, education and parity were included in the equation.

Data from Guyana help to test the value of combining face-to-face encounters with mass media interventions in influencing contraceptive use. In Guyana, three variables were used for this purpose: exposure to mass media family planning stimuli, face-to-face contacts and overall exposure. The first variable was created by summing the scores on the variables relating to lectures and mass media interventions and dividing the sum into five exposure categories, zero, low, fair, medium and high. The face-to-face variable was created by counting the number of primary contacts respondents reported and dividing these into categories of zero, 1-2, 3-4, 5-6 and 7-10 contacts. The contacts included family planning workers, parents, sisters, brothers, aunts, uncles, husbands/partners, friends, nurses, teachers and doctors. The overall exposure variable was created by combining the scores on the exposure to family planning stimuli and face to face variables. Table 15 shows the relation between contraceptive use and these exposure variables.

These findings are an impressive endorsement of the value of information and education programmes for shaping attitudes and behaviour in Guyana. They also indicate that although mass media and face-to-face programme interventions are each important in them

TABLE 15. CONTRACEPTIVE USE AMONG WOMEN IN A UNION, AGES 15-44, BY SELECTED INFORMATION, EDUCATION AND COMMUNICATION VARIABLES, GUYANA, 1992
(Percentage)

Exposure to family planning stimuli	User status	
	User	Non-user
None	28.1	71.9
Low	30.4	69.9
Fair	48.1	51.9
Medium	54.4	45.6
High	59.1	40.9
Face-to-face		
None	14.5	85.5
1-2	35.6	64.4
3-4	61.0	39.0
5-6	67.7	32.3
7-10	63.8	36.2
Exposure		
None	13.4	86.6
Low	16.7	83.3
Medium	45.5	54.5
High	52.9	47.1
Very high	68.7	31.3

Source: Tribani P. Jagdeo, "Guyana Contraceptive Prevalence Survey, 1991-92", unpublished; New York, International Planned Parenthood Federation, Western Hemisphere Region, 1992.

selves, their combination produces an overall effect greater than their individual effects.

Looking at these findings in detail, one sees that, in general, contraceptive use increases with people's exposure to mass media stimuli, to face-to-face contacts and to a combination of the two. In fact, contraceptive use doubles as one moves from zero to medium and high mass media exposure levels. Only 28 per cent of those reporting no exposure to mass media interventions were using a method at the time of the survey compared with 54 and 59 per cent of those reporting medium and high levels of exposure. One sees similar patterns in the relation between contraceptive use and face-to-face exposure and overall exposure.

Of even greater interest is the finding that contraceptive use among those reporting no face-to-face discussion on family planning was less than half that of those reporting no mass media exposure. In fact, only 15 per cent of those reporting no face-to-face family planning influence were contraceptors, compared with 28 per cent of those reporting no mass media exposure. It is evident

that although the mass media play a substantial role in shaping contraceptive behaviour in Guyana, face-to-face systems of persuasion seem to effect the critical difference. The data also suggest that a small amount of face-to-face influence makes a greater difference than a small amount of mass media exposure. Contraceptive use jumps from 15 to 36 per cent as one moves from those with zero face-to-face contacts to those with one to two contacts. The corresponding increase in use found in moving from those with no mass media exposure to those with low levels of exposure is negligible, from 28 to 30 per cent.

These data do a number of things. They validate the argument that IEC interventions can and do influence attitudes towards and acceptance of family planning. The data also demonstrate that a substantial unmet need for family planning exists in Africa, Asia, and Latin America and the Caribbean. If the evidence provided on the Caribbean is any indication, then it can be concluded that these unmet needs can be transformed into effective demand by IEC programmes that combine the power of the mass media with the influence of primary encounters in the field. The needs are substantial, as would be the resources—financial, managerial, technical and creative—needed to do the job. A splendid opportunity for international cooperation presents itself, especially for those Governments without the wherewithal to do it alone.

CONCLUSION

This evidence provided in this paper attests to the fact that the Principles and Objectives of the United Nations World Population Plan of Action (14a-14h) are as viable for the 1990s as they were for the 1980s. The evidence also suggests that intensive efforts should be made to bring to the attention of policy makers the DHS findings with regard to the number of exposed women that are not using contraception and would like both to space their births and to limit their family size. It is further suggested that since the data confirm that IEC not only leads to behaviour change but can also sustain that change, family planning programmes should seek the proper balance between "purely" clinical and contraceptive distribution activities and information and education. In other words, policy makers should be a prime target for an international IEC advocacy campaign. An objective of that campaign should be the recognition of family planning both as a means to a

172

better life and as a right in itself; further, all efforts should be made to enshrine those rights in the population policies of Governments and to guarantee that access to the information and services upon which the exercise of those rights depend is provided in an environment that is free, confidential, safe, continuous and reliable. It is further suggested that since the efficient use of scarce IEC resources is linked to the conduct of appropriate research and effective management and evaluation of the IEC process, that Governments, intergovernmental and non-governmental organizations should consciously build these elements into their IEC initiatives. The complete integration of women into the social, economic, cultural and political life of their societies will not happen until women acquire control of their reproductive potential. Effective IEC will empower this process as it will full flowering of the potential of couples as parents and partners within the home and as productive elements in society.

REFERENCES

Covington, Deborah L., and others (1986). Physician attitudes and family planning in Nigeria. *Studies in Family Planning* (New York), vol. 17, No. 4 (July-August), pp. 172-180.

Gallen, Moira, and Cheryl Lettenmaier (1987). *Counseling Makes a Difference*. Population Reports, Series J, No. 35. Baltimore, Maryland: The Johns Hopkins University, Population Information Program.

Heisler, Douglas, and Gary L. Lewis (1985). *The Barbados Male Family Planning Survey Country Report, 1982*. Columbia, Maryland: Westinghouse Public Applied Systems.

_____ (1985). *The Dominica Male Family Planning Survey Country Report, 1982*. Columbia, Maryland: Westinghouse Public Applied Systems.

_____ (1985). *The St. Kitts-Nevis Male Family Planning Survey Country Report, 1982*. Columbia, Maryland: Westinghouse Public Applied Systems.

Jagdeo, Tirbani P. (1990). *Contraceptive Prevalence in Antigua*. Caribbean Contraceptive Prevalence Surveys, No. 5. New York: International Planned Parenthood Federation, Western Hemisphere Region.

_____ (1990). *Contraceptive Prevalence in Barbados*. Caribbean Contraceptive Prevalence Surveys, No. 6. New York: International Planned Parenthood Federation, Western Hemisphere Region.

_____ (1990). *Contraceptive Prevalence in Dominica*. Caribbean Contraceptive Prevalence Surveys, No. 6. New York: International Planned Parenthood Federation, Western Hemisphere Region.

_____ (1990). *Contraceptive Prevalence in St. Lucia*. Caribbean Contraceptive Prevalence Surveys, No. 7. New York: International Planned Parenthood Federation, Western Hemisphere Region.

_____ (1990). *Contraceptive Prevalence in St. Vincent*. Caribbean Contraceptive Prevalence Surveys, No. 4. New York: International Planned Parenthood Federation, Western Hemisphere Region.

_____ (1992). Guyana Contraceptive Prevalence Survey, 1991-92. Unpublished. New York: International Planned Parenthood Federation, Western Hemisphere Region.

Kaufman, Joan, and others (1992). The quality of family planning services in rural China. *Studies in Family Planning* (New York), vol. 23, No. 2 (March/April), pp. 73-84.

Mauldin, Parker W. (1991). Contraceptive use in the year 2000. In *Demographic and Health Surveys World Conference, August 5-7, 1991, Washington, D.C., Proceedings*, vol. II. Columbia, Maryland: IRD/Macro International, Inc.

Thapa, Shyam, and others (1991). Contraceptive use and needs among postpartum women in 25 developing countries: recent patterns and implications. In *Demographic and Health Surveys World Conference, August 5-7, 1991, Washington, D.C., Proceedings*, vol. II. Columbia, Maryland: IRD/Macro International, Inc.

XI. COMMUNITY-BASED DELIVERY SYSTEMS AND SOCIAL MARKETING OF CONTRACEPTIVES

Alfonso López Juárez[*]

A. ROLE OF COMMUNITY-BASED DISTRIBUTION AND SOCIAL MARKETING OF CONTRACEPTIVES

"Man's desire to control his fertility and not to leave child-bearing to chance has been almost universal throughout the ages in widely differing cultures and societies. Some of these attempts have been amazingly rational considering the lack of knowledge concerning human reproductive physiology; other attempts were magical and based on superstitions and taboos." (Suitters, 1967, p. 3)

A certain degree of human control over reproduction and the birth of new human beings can be observed in almost every society (Sauvy, Bergues and Riquet, 1972). The dominant patterns, however, with sparsely populated earth, had until very recently been one of fostering reproduction in order to increase manpower and settle vast and empty areas.

Although in France and other pioneering areas of contraception, the process of adopting contraception as a commonly accepted practice took a long period of time (Sauvy, Bergues and Riquet, 1972), over the past four decades, thanks to the generalization of hormonal methods and intra-uterine devices (IUDs) (IPPF, 1967) and the availability of surgical contraception (Ross, Hong and Huber, 1985), the same process has been accelerated in the majority of countries, in the attempt to promote a rapid decrease in the pace of world population growth.

The most recent available statistics (Population Reference Bureau, 1992) show that the worldwide percentage of women of reproductive age currently married or in union using contraception is 55 per cent; if one considers only "modern methods" (the pill, IUD, sterilization and other chemical and barrier methods), the percentage of contraceptive users is 47 per cent.

From a different perspective, the effort to expand family planning practice has been assessed twice in the past decade, using essentially identical methods (Lapham and Mauldin, 1985; Mauldin and Ross, 1991); and the most impressive finding is the marked upward shift in programme effort scores during the past decade (Mauldin and Ross, 1991). At the beginning of the decade, only 8 countries were assessed as strong in their efforts for family planning, while in 1989 a total of 14 countries were assessed as being strong. The total number of countries with strong or moderately strong programmes increased from 23 to 42, and those with weak and very weak programmes decreased from 65 to 46. In 1982 a total of 40 countries had weak or non-existent effort; but in 1989, only 17 countries were so rated. Interestingly enough, the 14 countries that ranked "strong" in their commitment to family planning in 1989 contain 64 per cent of the population of all developing countries; while the 17 countries with "very weak or no" family planning programmes contain only 4 per cent.

In the component that is relevant for this paper, "service and service-related activities", the average score rose from 25 (weak) to 42 (moderate).

The general conclusion is that acceptance of contraception is rapidly expanding throughout the world; in other words, there was a latent demand for family planning in many countries which has been met by the offer of contraceptives in many ways. Major suppliers of contraceptives are public-health systems and the commercial network, but non-conventional delivery systems, such as community-based distribution (CBD) and social marketing of contraceptives (SMC), have also played a complementary role in the supply of contraceptives.

Role of community-based distribution

Family planning was introduced into the developing world through physicians and clinics: clients were expected to look there for advice and supplies. But health staff and facilities are in short supply in poor countries; and it became clear very soon that in order to increase the number of clients it was necessary to think of alternative delivery systems. One of them, perhaps

---

[*] Director-General, Fundación Mexicana para la Planificación Familiar, Mexico City, Mexico.

the most successful, was introduced in the mid-1960s (Ross and others, 1987); it is based on the involvement of specific individuals or groups within communities. Local residents having such characteristics as willingness to perform a social service, interpersonal skills and sometimes leadership and literacy are usually selected as distributors for contraceptives. They are provided with training and are required to keep some records and in some cases to make periodic home visits.

Over the past two decades, community-based distribution of contraceptives, which has been more specifically described as distribution of contraceptives through non-professional and volunteer staff, has constituted an important way to spread contraceptive practice in developing countries. Already in 1987 more than 70 locations and some 40 countries were reported as CBD sites (Ross and others, 1987).

When the system includes adequate mechanisms to identify, recruit, motivate and train volunteer distributors, to supply and supervise them and adequately to monitor and evaluate the results, it is an effective model, which will certainly continue to be in use during the coming decades.

The role of CBD is to make contraceptives easily available at the village, neighbourhood or even household level, to make them more acceptable by reducing the social distance between provider and consumer and to reduce operation costs. CBD assures effective communication with people in the community, because distributors share the same culture and life perspectives. It also assures reduced distance to outlets and fewer administrative hurdles for clients.

CBD is generally considered effective (Ross and others, 1987) and has been successful mainly in Southern and South-eastern Asia and in Latin America and the Caribbean. Use of CBD increased during the 1980s, as the following scores show:

Region	1982 CBD score	1989 CBD score
Eastern Asia	1.0	1.52
Southern Asia	1.3	1.63
Northern Africa/Western Asia	0.4	0.85
Sub-Saharan Africa	0.3	0.49
Latin America and the Caribbean ..	1.2	1.75
TOTAL	0.73	1.08

Source: The Population Council data bank.
Note: CBD = community-based distribution.

Despite the higher scores in certain regions, some successful programmes are implemented in other regions, and there is no reason to exclude the possibility of implementing the model in many other countries.

The success of CBD seems to depend upon the general effort the country is devoting to family planning activities. It is a good ally for family planning programmes, not a necessary ingredient: several countries with strong or moderate overall programmes manage without a good CBD programme. Ross and others (1987) cite the cases of Cuba, India, Malaysia, Mexico, the Republic of Korea and Taiwan Province of China, among others.

As a matter of fact, CBD is a good substitute for an efficient distribution network in rural areas; therefore, it is superfluous when there is a good retail system, for instance, in rather economically advanced countries, such as Chile, Costa Rica and Singapore.

Among the different services providers, CBD plays a significant role in the countries in which it is used, proportionally larger than the other channels for the provision of services. It is possible that countries which are weak on other aspects of service implementation resort to CBD as a compensation strategy (Ross and others, 1987).

The main idea behind CBD projects—the involvement of the community in family planning programmes —can be used in a wider context and perspective in order to meet the challenges of the future.

Role of social marketing of contraceptives

SMC programmes were created in the late 1960s with the primary aim of supplementing existing public sector distribution systems by making contraceptives available at low cost to low-income groups (Sheon, Schellstede and Derr, 1987).

Unlike CBD, these programmes use existing commercial and retail channels but often take advantage of subsidies or donations in order to compete advantageously with the private sector. In some cases, SMC programmes use private sector resources (Cisek, 1991).

As a matter of fact, CBD and SMC very often overlap in their implementation, because some family planning agencies use both approaches and have very similar

175

mechanisms for supply, monitoring and supervision, as is the case in Colombia (Vernon, Ojeda and Townsend, 1988).

Social marketing programmes have been implemented in more than 30 countries. According to data provided by Mauldin and Ross (1991), compared with those provided by Lapham and Mauldin (1985), a sharp increase in the use of SMC occurred between 1982 and 1989. In 1982, only 17 countries had any score (other than zero) in the social marketing indicator, while in 1989, 37 did. SMC is as widespread as CBD; and in some countries, it has achieved remarkable success. As in the case of CBD, regions of the world in which this type of strategy has been used with most success are Eastern and South-eastern Asia and Latin America and the Caribbean. The strategy has proved successful also in Egypt. A regional comparison of SMC scores is as follows:

Region	1982 SMC score	1989 SMC score
Eastern Asia	0.73	1.02
Southern Asia	0.91	1.33
Northern Africa/Western Asia . . .	0.48	0.71
Sub-Saharan Africa	0.00	0.48
Latin America and the Caribbean	0.87	1.88
TOTAL	0.48	1.01

Source: The Population Council data bank.
NOTE: SMC = social marketing of contraception.

If one looks at the effectiveness or coverage of SMC, in seven countries it represents 5 per cent or more of registered CYPs (DKT International, 1992). In exceptional cases (Egypt and Jamaica), 15 per cent of the market coverage is attributed to social marketing.

As concerns cost effectiveness, it seems that generating sufficient revenue to cover expenses often causes the abandonment of extensive distribution and concentration on a segment of the market that easily can be covered by the private sector. If that is the case, the subsidies that are often inherent to this strategy would be channelled in the wrong direction.

Some spin-off effects related to SMC have been observed, among them the indirect promotion of family planning made through the advertisement and information materials.

An important issue, still unsolved, is whether SMC fills unmet demand or simply siphons off users from other commercial sources (Stover, 1987). Some studies claim, however, that in Latin America significant numbers of first-time users have been attracted to contraception by social marketing (Skidmore and others, 1990).

Possibly the main problem faced by SMC is the conflict between, on the one hand, the profit-oriented mentality, and, on the other hand, the managerial structure and staff prevailing in family planning agencies, which are often welfare-oriented and normally lack commercial experience and decision-making flexibility. It is a conflict between the values governing commercial ventures and those inherent in social services. It is clear that business firms sponsor social marketing of health programmes in which they derive a benefit, as is the case for life insurance companies, which support campaigns encouraging people to jog and to cut down on fats and sugar (Kotler, 1984); but they normally show very little interest in backing social marketing when a small profit is involved. On the other hand, government or non-profit structures are unfit to face the challenge of a commercial venture.

An additional problem, related to the above-mentioned conflict of values, is that the concepts and words used in marketing are very often resented as manipulative and closely linked to the commercial world and thus they constitute a barrier to the acceptance of social marketing by managers and staff of non-profit organizations (McKee, 1988).

The provision of access to low-cost contraceptives in the market-place alongside other routine household goods, the ideal purpose of SMC, has been attempted in a number of countries from the non-profit sector, with mixed results. The ultimate test for SMC (Sheon, Schellstede and Derr, 1987) would be an experiment to meet an unmet demand, a special segment of the market still not covered by other commercial or non-commercial sources.

It seems than even the use of the term "social marketing" is confined to a rather small circle of its practitioners and to a limited number of donor agencies (McKee, 1988). This aspect notwithstanding, a more comprehensive use of the theory and tools of marketing, already suggested in some SMC programmes (Cisek, 1991) can be very useful to meet the challenges of the future.

B. THE TASK STILL TO BE PERFORMED: CHALLENGES FOR CONTRACEPTION IN THE COMING DECADES

Despite the results achieved so far in the spreading of contraceptive practice, the task to be performed in the near future still looks formidable. Large segments of the world population must still begin to practise modern contraception. Variations among different regions of the world are still very wide and are closely correlated with economic, social and modern indicators. Table 16 illustrates this point. If one studies the table—excluding the atypical cases of China and Southern Europe, which would require a separate in-depth analysis—it is fairly obvious that prevalence in the use of modern contraception is correlated to other indicators of "modern" society, with high levels of gross national product per capita, formal health services, urban concentration and good health conditions.

TABLE 16. CONTRACEPTIVE USE PREVALENCE COMPARED WITH OTHER ECONOMIC, SOCIAL AND HEALTH INDICATORS, SELECTED REGIONS

Region, country or area	Prevalence in use of modern contraceptives (percentage)	Gross national product per captia (dollars)	Population living in areas termed urban by that country (percentage)	Adult literacy (percentage)	Infant mortality under age 1 per 1,000 inhabitants	Life expectancy at birth (years)	Access to formal health services (percentage)	Births attemded by health workers (percentage)
China	70	370	26	68	34	70	..	..
Northern America	69	21 580	75	..	8	75	..	99
Northern Europe	69	17 930	83	..	7	75	..	100
Eastern Asia[b]	63	19 888	77	..	7	75	..	92
South America	50	2 180	74	73-95	56	67	63-97	22-98
Caribbean	48	..	58	48-98	54	69	50-99	40-98
South-eastern Asia[c]	45	754	31	79	61	62	78	38
Southern Africa	43	2 390	52	70	57	63	89	77
Central America	42	2 170	64	82	50	68	49	49
Southern Asia[d]	37	297	25	40	96	58	50	29
Southern Europe	34	12 860	68	81-96	12	76	..	86-100
Northern Africa	28	630	43	45-55	72	65	35	40
Western Africa	3	410	23	13-53	111	49	15-50	15-60
Eastern Africa	..	230	19	18-92	110	52	27-100	2-85

Sources: Nafis Sadik, ed., *The State of World Population, 1991: Choice or Chance* (New York, United Nations Population Fund, 1991); Population Reference Bureau, World Population Data Sheet, 1992 (Washington, D.C., 1992).

NOTES: When data were available in both sources, the most recent information was used. Regions of the world and indicators were chosen by the author of this paper for comparison purposes.

[a]Prevalence in the use of modern contraceptives: the percentage of women of reproductive age currently married or in a union using modern contraceptive methods, which include the pill, intra-uterine device, sterilization and other chemical and barrier methods.

[b]Only comparable countries or areas were selected: Hong Kong; Japan; Republic of Korea.

[c]Only comparable countries were selected: Indonesia; Philippines; Thailand.

[d]Only comparable countries were selected: Bangladesh; India; Pakistan.

A very interesting attempt has been made (Mauldin and Ross, 1991) to assess the impact on fertility decline of social setting and programme effort. The main finding is that both factors play major roles in fertility decline.

Another recent study (Cabrera, 1992) suggests that progress in contraceptive practice is improperly presented as the origin of improvement in social conditions; it is, on the contrary, part of the same process and a product of the same social improvement.

In all developing countries, however, one factor—the proportion of the population living in an urban environment—is consistently associated with contraceptive practice.

Table 17 shows the correlation, in selected regions, between the percentage of urban population and the contraceptive use prevalence rate. The task still to be performed for general acceptance of contraception must be centred in traditional societies and mainly in special groups of the population that are difficult to reach with

TABLE 17. CORRELATION BETWEEN PREVALENCE RATES AND
DEGREE OF URBANIZATION

Major area	Preval-ence rate range of variation	Urban population range (percentage)	Correl-ation coeff-icient	Percentage of variation explained by correl-ation
Africa	1-47	5-76	0.50	25
Asia	0-70	8-100	0.52	27
Americas	10-69	21-89	0.55	30
Europe	5-77	30-91	0.23	5

Source: Data from Population Reference Bureau, *World Population Data Sheet, 1992* (Washington, D.C., 1992); calculation by Agustín Porras Macías.

the strategies already in use. The time of promoting the concept of family planning to the general public is over.

In 1989, a review and assessment by the United Nations Population Fund (UNFPA) concluded that the expansion of family planning in the 1990s would require not just additional funding, but different approaches and improved programme planning and operation (Keller and others, 1989).

Among the broad strategies necessary for programme success, mention was made of generating greater demand for family planning services, improving acceptability of services and increasing community participation. Contrary to common belief, demand is not inherent in health and family planning programmes: it has to·be created from the beginning. (Manoff, 1987).

Moreover, lack of demand is not randomly distributed throughout the world. There is almost unanimous consensus in defining some high-priority areas or special challenges for family planning in the next decades.

Countries with low contraceptive use

There is a need to concentrate and to design effective strategies for expanding family planning in countries in which use of contraceptives is low or non-existent. Such countries are located basically in Africa and Western Asia.

Rural areas

Attention should be focused on geographical areas inside the countries in which prevalence is still low.

Those areas are mainly rural or marginally urban; in the latter areas, people, often migrants, live in rural-like settings, in a social and cultural environment similar to that found in rural areas.

As said before, available statistics show that contraceptive use prevalence is strongly correlated with the proportion of truly urban population in every country. Typically, rural areas are outside the mainstream of modern medicine and technical methods of contraception.

It is not easy to find solutions to the complex problems of health and family planning in rural areas. One can find there all the constraints inherent to traditional societies: difficulty of access; dispersion of the population; reluctance of medical personnel to practise in rural areas; low levels of education; traditional supports of high fertility; religious resistance; very limited understanding of the causal relation between family planning and improved infant and maternal mortality; and general lack of resources of all types. Models for service delivery still often rely upon centralized primary health-care strategies, without taking into account local health and economic conditions.

Services for young people

Teenagers have clearly emerged in family planning as one of the underserved groups. There is much documentation about the sexual behaviour of adolescents and the incidence of pregnancy among them (Morris, 1991). There have also been studies about their knowledge of and attitudes regarding sexuality and family planning (Leñero, 1990) but services remain scarce and prejudices of adults prevail in the daily scene.

Currently, most young people do not get information from schools and other programmes; rather, most comes from the media and friends and the information tends to be incomplete and distorted. Almost universally, when reproductive health programmes for youth are launched, they lack the support of national policies and institutions.

Male involvement

The involvement of males in family planning is a widespread concern, but the results are still very limited in the majority of countries. The burden of fertility control by and large remains in the hands of women, as reflected in predominant patterns of contraceptive use.

The most common approach is to convince males about the convenience of supporting their wives in the use of contraceptives. In some cases, efforts have been made, with mixed results, to encourage men to use condoms and to accept vasectomy. A clearer definition of men's role in the further promotion of family planning is still lacking (Keller and others, 1989).

Promotion of women's status

There are several consistent elements in the findings of research on the pattern of forces that conspire to bring down birth rates.

Among the various factors involved that is most closely correlated is improvement in the living conditions of women, in their education, in their acquiring the right to decide when and how many times they should get pregnant and in their status and emancipation. Taking into consideration only one of the many elements involved, the findings of the World Fertility Survey in the 15 most populous developing countries suggest that if women could make their own decisions on the matter, family size would decline by, on average, almost two children and the rate of population growth would fall by up to 30 per cent.

Among the challenges for the decade ahead in the area of women and family planning are: to strengthen the links between population programmes and women's organizations; to use the tools of the gender-analysis framework to ensure that programmes shall be designed appropriately for the gender roles and household decision-making patterns of a given area; to include training in counselling skills for providers of contraceptives; and to ensure that women shall be involved at decision-making levels, not only as clients and distributors of contraceptives (IPPF, 1992). Each of these issues can and should be taken into account in CBD and SMC programmes.

C. COMMUNITY-BASED MARKETING OF CONTRACEPTIVES

In order to use new approaches to meet the challenges of the future, one needs to go beyond the strategies already in use.

Euphemisms and soft words are common with regard to regulation of fertility. Family planning and planned parenthood, for example, are used instead of contraception. Similarly, community-based distribution and social marketing are often used instead of plain descriptions of the activity actually performed—volunteer sales staff or subsidized sales, both concepts which can be given a wider meaning.

The key words, "community" and "marketing" are very rich concepts, which can be used in a comprehensive way to the advantage of the spread of modern contraception to the half of the population which is not yet practising it.

By "community" what is meant here, in a broad sense, is a group of people that may or not live in the same geographical area but share the same subculture: beliefs; traditions; attitudes; knowledge; values; lifestyles; and patterns of behaviour. They can constitute a territorial community or a segment of the population, for instance, young people, males and women of a certain social class in a specific region.

"Marketing" is defined here as the process of planning and executing the conception, promotion and execution of ideas, goods and services in such a way that exchanges are created among marketers and consumers in order to satisfy individual and social objectives (Kotler and Andreasen, 1991).

Community-based marketing seeks the involvement of a representative group of members of the targeted audience in the process of defining the needs or desires which need satisfaction, in designing the type, form and quality of the product and evaluating the acceptance of the product being marketed (Wasek, 1987). Marketing is not simple, nor easy or inexpensive, but it is cost-effective and it provides important information for effective decisions which reduce managerial mistakes and waste of resources.

Depending upon the complexity of the product or the concept, it will require a series of test-refine/retest-refine cycles for most marketing activities, including product or service development and communication strategy, which can be costly and time-consuming. Commercial enterprises assign 10 per cent or more of total revenues to new product development and evaluation. In the population and public health fields, precisely because budgets are limited, one cannot afford the luxury of ignoring marketing principles, because they can help planners avoid costly mistakes and incorrect strategies.

If one uses the concept of community-based marketing of contraception, it opens a wide perspective for future developments. The full meaning of marketing implies an entire set of theoretical and pragmatic tools, which are already tested and very successful in the business world and can serve the cause of family planning.

The purpose of the proposed approach is to use marketing theory and experience in order to help family planning take root in those communities or groups of population that have thus far seemed reluctant to enter or alien to the family planning movement in the world.

To date, family planning programmes have consisted of offering products to a rather passive population: technicians have interpreted people's needs and wishes and have flooded the market with their products. That is the old marketing approach, the product approach. There is need to renovate the methods according to modern marketing practice and to put the strategic emphasis on the consumer, in such a way that family planning programmes become genuinely user-oriented (Cisek, 1991).

Employing the newer aspects of marketing theory is even more useful to spread contraception, because social products are very often more complex and more controversial than commercial products; it is more difficult for the consumer to perceive the satisfaction obtained (Saunders and Smith, 1984).

In the process of marketing contraception to a community or special group, some steps stand out.

Definition of the target population

The regions and countries in the world in which contraceptive use is either low or non-existent are fairly well identified. Within the countries, however, averages and means tend to obscure a very uneven situation: there are vast areas in which traditional culture is still predominant, access to modern health care is poor; and therefore contraceptive practice is very low. It is of utmost importance to identify and precisely define those "high-priority areas" in order to channel efforts and resources in the right direction.

This approach appears to be just common sense, but if one make a detailed analysis of the way in which even major donors focus their attention and channel their resources, it can easily be seen how major decisions are made in aggregate terms, without segmenting the market, and thus fail to address the real target population.

Marketing theory offers a variety of tools by which available information and statistics can be used adequately to target geographical areas in which special attention is needed.

Location of especially needy segments in the contraception market

Groups that constitute a special challenge for family planning—young people and men, for example—are identified in a general way, but marketing theory can help substantially in locating them in a given context, in finding out where they normally meet, how they can be touched by new information and how can they be attracted to contraceptive practices.

In order to promote contraception effectively among especially needy segments of the population, it is necessary to have in-depth knowledge about gender, ages, income levels and lifestyles, and even more about customs, traditions, beliefs and values.

Marketing tools would be of great help, for example, in clarifying:

"whether separate services must be established to win the acceptance of young people or whether adolescents can be reached through the same types of services used for the general public; whether programs can use traditional agents to promote services, or if special promotional networks must be established; and whether unified messages and approaches will be adequate for the adolescent population, or if segmentation will be required to reach both the males and the females, the married and the unmarried, those in school and those out of school, and those who are employed and those who are unemployed." (Keller, 1989, p. 132).

It is also important to find how to change additional attitudes favouring early child-bearing.

Characterization of demand in needy geographical areas and special segments of population

Marketing theory distinguishes several states of demand: what is referred to here are some examples which fit the circumstances often found with regard to family planning:

(*a*) Negative demand, when potential buyers dislike the offered product. In many cases, the demand for vasectomy is negative. In this case, the required action is to make an analysis of why customers dislike the product and how it can be presented in order to be attractive to potential users;

(*b*) Absent demand, when potential users are indifferent to the product. In agricultural societies, in which the value of fertility is predominant, contraceptive practice is often seen with indifference. In this case, the required action is to find the link between the product and the needs and wishes of customers;

(*c*) Latent demand, when there is an intense need or desire, but there is no product to satisfy it. When the variety of supplied contraceptives is poor, it is very often found that couples desire contraception but are not satisfied with the type of methods available. The required action is to assess the market and design a product or service to meet the demand.

Characterization of the demand is a very important step to define the appropriate strategy to market contraception.

Shifting of focus from product to consumer: formative research

The objective should be not to sell supply but to satisfy demand (Manoff, 1987). That is the customer-oriented approach. Innovative techniques have to be used in order to penetrate the hard crust of consumer resistance to reach the rich subsoil of consumer desire and motivation.

Proper marketing emphasizes the consumer's needs, attitudes, constraints and opportunities (Saunders and Smith, 1984). At this point "community-based marketing" begins once the high-priority areas or segments of contraception market have been identified, the action must be based in concrete communities and communication must begin in the community and among the people.

Contraception marketing efforts have to begin communicating with people in order to ascertain their felt needs, desires and perceptions. In other words, the preeminence of "feed-forward" instead of "feedback" has to be established (Manoff, 1987). This approach means that one should listen and learn from people before beginning design of the project, in order to avoid preventable mistakes.

Proper feed-forward involves not only collection of data on community needs, values, tastes and perceptions but also, and primarily, involvement of the community in interpreting the collected data and in the decision about what problems should be tackled and how it should be done.

Sometimes a finding about a local belief determines a complete change of strategy. One study (Nichter and Nichter, 1987) found that the common belief in a region of Sri Lanka was that the peak time for women's fertility was the period of menstruation and that most probably couples were using condoms only during that period. The use of condoms was thus quite ineffective. It seems that this incorrect information is very common in traditional societies.

A central issue that needs clarification in each community is which is the social value met by contraception, because, as Kotler states:

> "Exchange is the central concept underlying marketing. It calls for the offering of value to someone in exchange for value. Through exchanges, various social units—individuals, small groups, organizations, whole nations—attain the inputs they need. By giving up something, they acquire something else in return. This something else is normally more valued than that which is given up, which explains the motivation for the exchange." (1984, p. 5)

In the marketing of contraception, that exchange usually happens between a welfare organization, which offers a concept, a service or a product, and a community. The community, if interested, buys the offer by committing money, time or a change in behaviour (McKee, 1988).

The terms of the exchange have to be clear in every programme. Not every traditional society is capable of monetary exchange and the expectation of economic self-sufficiency is often unrealistic; it implies that contraception brings benefits only to those using contraceptives, while the final benefit of contraception is the improvement of health and levels of living for the entire country; the individual user does not (or should not) necessarily have to pay the full cost of achieving a social benefit (Fox, 1988).

High-quality research is needed using available methods, both quantitative (sample surveys, archival data analysis and closed-end interviews); and qualitative, including ethnographic fieldwork, focus groups discussions and direct observation (McKee, 1988).

In order to obtain meaningful results, promoters of contraception have to stress disciplined observation, guided interviews and informant panels over formal surveys; informed interpretation over statistical analysis; attention to process and intermediate results over "final" outcomes. The objective is to obtain an understanding of the social dynamics of the village life as a necessary basis for every effective innovation.

The process of planning with the community and adapting the organization to the needs identified is sometimes defined as a "learning process" (Korten, 1980); it requires repeated feed-forward and feedback steps.

Once the qualitative research has been conducted in the community or segment of the population, communication strategies and design of messages can be defined. This approach is necessary for penetrating traditional societies or segments of the population in which values, customs and practices are very different from "modern" culture.

It is not implied that this long process is to be undertaken in every single geographical community or group of people. Sample procedures permit obtaining representative findings which can be applied to culturally similar communities or segments of the population.

Design of communications strategy and choice of media and messages

An outstanding study on the application of marketing methodology for a social cause (Solomon, 1981) concludes that face-to-face communication is more important in changing behaviour; however, use of mass media also proved to be very effective. A proper mix of both means, with the available budget in sight, is always recommended.

The classical theory for the diffusion of innovation applies also to contraception: the process flows from knowledge about an innovation, to persuasion, decision, implementation and ultimately, confirmation (Rogers, 1962).

For plain knowledge about contraception and its social legitimization, mass media can be very useful, but in the persuasion and confirmation stages interpersonal communication is paramount.

It must again be emphasized that before trying to begin this process, a lot of dialogue with the people of the community or with the target segment is needed, in order to assess the possibility and circumstances to establish a market in which contraception is seen as valuable and worthy of an exchange in money, time or behaviour.

The choice of the messages requires a careful process based on the interaction with people that adequately represent the target audience. Very often, field messages in family planning are made by staff without testing and results are accordingly very poor. By contrast, a careful selection of proper messages has proved effective in the marketing of contraception (Skidmore and others, 1990).

The choice of media also requires research and dialogue with the community or target group in order to ascertain which media are the most appropriate and cost-effective to reach the target audience.

A typical case in which the adequate message to convey has not yet been found is the issue of male participation in contraceptive programmes:

"Slow progress in involving males may be at least partially explained by a lack of clear understanding of the desired outcome. To date, most efforts have been limited to attempts to win men's support for their spouse's use of contraceptives, by exposing them to information on and arguments about the negative impact of unregulated fertility on the family's health and socio-economic status. Other educational approaches have emphasized the importance of encouraging responsible male behaviour, while still others have promoted vasectomy or condom use. There is only scanty evidence on the efficacy of such efforts—particularly that of gaining male support for female contraception—even in the minority of programmes in which they have been undertaken. Many advocates clearly believe that something beyond mere male acquiescence is required for success. To make real progress will require a more specific definition of the desired outcome and more rigorous testing of the strategies for bringing it about." (Keller and others, 1989, p. 133)

Community-based selection of contraceptive methods

Marketing theory (Carson, 1967), distinguishes four types of consumer goods, according to the way in which they are purchased:

(*a*) *Convenience goods*. These goods are purchased with a minimum of searching; the consumer is familiar with the assortments offered, the goods are readily accessible on shelves or in display racks and there is little to be gained from more extended shopping;

(*b*) *Shopping goods*. These are the goods for which the customer searches; he or she compares the prices, qualities and styles available in a number of stores, perhaps not even knowing specifically what is desired;

(*c*) *Specialty goods*. These goods have special characteristics that encourage customers to make special efforts to find them, and price may be a minor consideration.

(*d*) *Unsought goods*. These are the goods customers do not want, do not know are available or are not seeking for. In modern societies, contraceptives are convenience goods, or in many cases, shopping goods. In traditional societies, contraceptives are unsought goods.

The challenge for family planners is to use marketing theories and tools in such a way that non-clinical contraceptives, such as condoms, spermicides and pills (this last, after the first medical prescription) become shopping goods or better still, convenience goods, on a more widespread basis.

In order to achieve that objective, it is essential to find, with the community's involvement, "user-friendly" methods (Askew, 1992). The modern trend in marketing is to focus the attention on customers' needs, contrary to the traditional approach of focusing on production or service provision and leaving up to customers the task of adapting themselves to the product or service offered to them.

In the field of contraception, the scientific community has mostly used the product-oriented approach; and for many years, there was the dream of an ideal contraceptive that would fit the needs of everyone, everywhere, every time. Currently, all those in the field acknowledge that this magic bullet cannot exist, that the needs of different people have to be met by a broad choice of contraceptives, tailored not only for different people in different situations but also for the same person in different stages or different circumstances of life (Fathalla, 1990).

The lack of contraceptives that fit the customers' needs can be of consequence for the spread and continuity of family planning practice: when people do not get the contraceptives that meet their needs, they may not use contraception, they may discontinue or they may adopt a method that does not match their circumstance and is therefore ineffective.

One particular field in which the lack of a customer-oriented approach is obvious is male participation in family planning. The most recent statistics show that women contraceptive users are three times more numerous than male users. In some countries, this disproportion can be as high as 20 to 1. Some evidence suggests that this imbalance in the men's participation is due more to the lack of a broad contraceptive choice for the male than to the reluctance of men to be more active in family planning.

Feed-forward research is also needed to find out if the contraceptive method, perhaps identified with community involvement, will be accepted in the field. It is far more cost-effective to begin with pilot tests in order to ascertain the acceptance of a particular contraceptive.

Grounding of contraception in the community

Contraception programmes are very often run from outside the targeted communities or groups, by hired staff that may not be part of that subculture. The only means to ensure the permanence of contraception as an accepted and viable practice in a given community or group is to get local people to take an active part and to become the promoters of the new way to look at reproduction.

It should always be remembered that contraception is a very drastic innovation in traditional societies and in special segments. It is an exogenous element which is introduced as alien to that culture. It has to be digested by the community or group and only its own members can help the process.

If the promoters do not belong to the community or group and are not recognized as part of it, the assimilation of new ideas and patterns of behaviour is very difficult. Once the foreigners leave the community or the group, the new practice may more easily be abandoned.

The contraceptive practice will continue only if there is group pressure or approval, that is, if the new custom is grounded in the community or group. That is why it is necessary to overcome the concept of simple distribution of contraceptives and to adopt a wider framework, including cultural change and the community or group adoption of the new pattern of behaviour.

The same structures and institutions present in the daily life of the community must be involved in the new practice. If there is a health agent in the community, person must be involved in the promotion and distribution of contraceptives.

If general practitioners are already acting in the community, most probably one of the best ways to succeed in the marketing of contraception is to recruit them as part of the project. If there are no trained people, the project has to select the most appropriate representatives and provide the necessary training.

The process must end in a formation of a group of local convinced activists, duly supported and trained in their task. Only this endogenous network makes possible the continuation of contraceptive practice after the initial project and the external support ends.

Community or group networks have a special influence on contraceptive knowledge, attitudes and adoption. Experience has shown that adoption is higher when personal networks include more adopters or greater connectedness to the community network. The main community factor identified for providing access to contraceptive knowledge and supplies is the interpersonal dynamics involved. Even pressures or inducements exerted by central Governments or national policies have to be converted into persuasion in face-to-face interaction in order to be effective.

The only way to assure permanence of contraceptive practice in society is to incorporate it into community norms as a pattern of behaviour that is communicated to individuals through the social network. This action is equivalent to enabling the community itself to determine the direction and development of contraceptive practices, to become self-determining in this important aspect of life.

This community self-reliance has to be achieved community by community; it requires intensive work by well-trained community workers but it is the only way effectively to ground contraception in traditional communities (Askew, 1992).

Evaluation of results: summative evaluation

One of the problems of family planning programmes in recent decades has been inadequate evaluation, which can lead to waste of resources and efforts. Paradoxically, social ventures, in which use of scarce resources is critical, allocate little attention and limited resources to the evaluation of results.

Marketing theory can be a great help in providing tools for a careful evaluation of results and cost efficiency of programmes. Methodologies recommended include longitudinal surveys, random sample surveys, control groups, and single interview and multiple interview groups.

Again, as in the case of formative research, it can be conducted taking advantage of random sample procedures, evaluating results in a limited number of conditions and extrapolating results to the whole.

D. CONCLUSIONS

The diffusion of contraception has achieved remarkable results in the past three decades. About half of the couples in the world are currently regulating their fertility.

Community-based distribution of contraceptives has played an important role in making contraceptives available to people living in areas not covered by commercial networks or institutional services.

Social marketing of contraceptives as a means of bringing contraceptives to low-income groups in developing countries, has been tried in a number of countries with mixed results. Its impact on the increase of prevalence in the use of contraceptives and in the demographics of the countries in which it operates is still uncertain, but it undoubtedly constitutes a way to complement the supply of contraceptives.

In order to face the important challenges for family planning in the next decades, there is a need to overcome the partial concepts of CBD and SMC and to use a more comprehensive approach: community-based marketing of contraception.

The proposed community-based marketing of contraception uses the customer-oriented approach, feed-forward research, and emphasizes such important steps as:

(a) Definition of the target population;

(b) Location of especially needy segments of the contraceptive market;

(c) Characterization of the demand in needy geographical areas and special segments of the population;

(d) Shifting of the focus from product to customer;

(e) Design of a communications strategy for appropriate choice of messages and media;

(f) Community-based selection of the contraceptive methods;

(g) Grounding of contraceptive use as accepted practice in the community;

(h) Evaluation of the results.

E. RECOMMENDATIONS

In order effectively to meet the challenges of contraception in the next decades, programmes need to define carefully the target populations, those that are still reluctant to accept the voluntary regulation of fertility.

Proper segmentation of the market not still covered by contraception, such as young people, males and rural or marginal populations, is crucial for the success of family planning programmes.

Family planning programmes should technically characterize the demand they try to cover, in order to use the appropriate marketing tools.

The use of a customer-oriented approach, through feed-forward procedures and formative research in randomly selected communities and groups, will dramatically enhance the chances of succeeding in family planning programmes.

It is strongly recommended to design carefully, with as much community and target group participation as possible, the communication strategy; to choose properly choose the media and messages related to family plan-

ning; and to select the contraceptive products based on the community needs, desires and preferences and test their customer acceptance through pilot projects.

In order to assure permanence of contraceptive practice in the communities and groups, once the introductory programme has ended, it is of the utmost importance to ground contraception practice, relevant information and distribution of methods in the existing networks of social control, information and distribution. For that aspect, real community participation in planning and management of subsequent activities is paramount in order to assure self-reliance.

The summational evaluation, through random surveys and careful analysis of collected data, is of utmost importance and should be implemented for every type of family planning programme in a given social or cultural area, in order to avoid waste of resources and to give priority to successful approaches.

It is suggested that every family planning project should assign at least 10 per cent of the budget to the process of marketing activities, before they can be grounded in the community.

REFERENCES

Askew, Ian (1992). Patterns, determinants and effects of community participation in family planning programmes. Unpublished paper. Dakar, Senegal: The Population Council.

Cabrera, Gustavo (1992). Los límites de la planificación familiar. Paper presented at the International Conference on The Peopling of the Americas, Veracruz, Mexico, 18-23 May. Sponsored by the International Union for the Scientific Study of Population.

Carson, D. (1967). International Marketing: A Comparative Systems Analysis. New York: Free Press.

Cisek, C. (1991). Applying Lessons Learned in Contraceptive Social Marketing to Other Essential Health Products. Washington, D.C.: The Futures Group.

DKT International (1992). Contraceptive Social Marketing Statistics. Washington, D.C.

Fathalla, Mahmoud (1990). Tailoring contraceptives to meet human needs. People (London), vol. 17, No. 3, pp. 3-5.

Fox, Karen F. A. (1988). Social marketing of oral rehydration therapy and contraception in Egypt. Studies in Family Planning (New York), vol. 19, No. 2 (March-April), pp. 95-108.

International Planned Parenthood Federation (1992). Women and family planning: issues for the 1990s. Prepared for the United Nations Expert Group Meeting on Population and Women, Gaborone, Botswana, 22-26 June.

Keller, Alan, and others (1989). Toward family planning in the 1990s: a review and assessment. International Family Planning Perspectives (New York), vol. 15, No. 4 (December), pp. 127-135.

Korten, David (1980). Community organization and rural development: a learning process approach. *Public Administration Review* (Washington, D.C.), vol. 40.

Kotler, Philip (1984). Social marketing of health behaviour. In *Marketing Health Behaviour*, Lee W. Frederiksen, Laura J. Solomon and Kathleen A. Brehony, eds. New York: Plenum Press.

_____ , and Alan R. Andreasen (1991). *Strategic Marketing for Non-profit Organizations*. Englewood Cliffs, New Jersey: Prentice Hall.

Lapham, Robert J., and W. Parker Mauldin (1985). Contraceptive prevalence: the influence of organized family planning programs. *Studies in Family Planning* (New York), vol. 16, No. 3 (May-June), pp. 117-137.

Leñero, L. (1990). *Jóvenes de hoy*. México, D.F.: Pax.

Manoff, R. K. (1987). The selling of health in family planning. In *Family Planning within Primary Health Care*, F. C. Swezy and C. P. Green, eds. Washington, F.C.: National Council for International Health.

Mauldin, W. Parker, and John A. Ross (1991). Family planning programs: efforts and results, 1982-89. *Studies in Family Planning* (New York), vol. 22, No. 6 (November/December), pp. 350-367.

McKee, Neill (1988). Social marketing in international development. Thesis. Miami: The Florida State University, College of Communication.

Morris, Leo (1991). La experiencia sexual y el uso de anticonceptivos entre jóvenes adultos. In *Memoria de la Conferencia Internacional sobre Fecundidad en Adolescentes en América Latina y el Caribe*. New York: The Pathfinder Fund and The Population Council.

Nichter, Mark, and Mimi Nichter (1987). Cultural notions of fertility in South Asia and their impact on Sri Lankan family planning practices. *Human Organization* (Wakefield, Rhode Island), vol. 46, No. 1 (Spring), pp. 18-28.

Potts, Malcolm (1990). Meeting the challenge of a growing population. *People* (London), vol. 17, No. 3, pp. 5-7.

Population Reference Bureau (1992). *World Population Data Sheet, 1992*. Washington, D.C.

Rogers, Everett M. (1962). *Diffusion of Innovations*. New York: Free Press of Glencoe.

Ross, John A., Sawon Hong and Douglas H. Huber (1985). *Voluntary Sterilization: An International Fact Book*. New York: Association for Voluntary Sterilization.

Ross, John A., and others (1987). Community-based distribution. In *Organizing for Effective Family Planning Programs*, Robert J. Lapham and George B. Simmons, eds. Washington D.C.: National Academy Press.

Sadik, Nafis, ed. (1992). *The State of World Population, 1991: Choice or Chance?*. New York.

Saunders, S., and W. A. Smith (1984). *Social Marketing: Two Views, Two Opportunities*. Development Communication Report, No. 47. Washington, D.C.: Clearinghouse.

Sauvy, Alfred, H. Bergues and M. Riquet (1972). *Historia del control de nacimientos*. Barcelona: Ediciones Península.

Sheon, A., W. Schellstede and B. Derr (1987). Contraceptive social marketing. In *Organizing for Effective Family Planning Programs*, Robert J. Lapham and George B. Simmons, eds. Washington, D.C.: National Academy Press.

Skidmore, W., and others (1990). La calidad de atención en el mercadeo comercial y social de los programas de planificación familiar en América Latina y el Caribe. Unpublished paper. Mexico: The Futures Group.

Solomon, Douglas S. (1981). A social marketing perspective on campaigns. In *Public Communication Campaigns*, Ronald E. Rice and William J. Paisley, eds. Beverly Hills, California: Sage Publications, pp. 281-292.

Stover, John (1987). The impact of social marketing programs on contraceptive prevalence: a cross-section time-series analysis. Occasional papers, SOMARC. Washington, D.C.

Sutters, Beryl (1967). *The History of Contraceptives*. Prepared for the International Planned Parenthood Federation. London: The Fanfare Press.

Vernon, Ricardo, Gabriel Ojeda, and Marcia C. Townsend (1988). Contraceptive social marketing and community-based distribution systems in Colombia. *Studies in Family Planning* (New York), vol. 19, No. 6 (November-December), pp. 354-360

Wasek, G. K. (1987). The social marketing approach: concepts and implications for international public health. In *Child Health and Survival: the UNICEF GOBI-FFF Program*, Richard Cash, Gerald T. Keusch and Joel Ramstein, eds. London: Croam-Helm.

XII. FUTURE CONTRACEPTIVE REQUIREMENTS AND LOGISTICS MANAGEMENT NEEDS

United Nations Population Fund

This paper draws substantially on a study undertaken by the United Nations Population Fund (UNFPA) in 1990 and 1991, which estimated contraceptive requirements throughout the developing world (UNFPA, 1991b). In the course of this study, UNFPA worked closely with selected developing countries, especially the most populated; partner agencies and organizations of the United Nations, bilateral agencies and non-governmental organizations. In particular, the Rockefeller Foundation, the Population Council and the Program for Appropriate Technology in Health (PATH) helped in various aspects of the exercise, including development of the methodology used to determine and project contraceptive needs.

During the course of the study, UNFPA convened four expert group meetings at which the objectives, methodology, initial findings and preliminary conclusions of the study were discussed. The overall findings were presented at the Consultative Meeting on Contraceptive Requirements in Developing Countries by the Year 2000, held in February 1991. This meeting, which was attended by 45 participants from over 25 countries, endorsed the major findings of the study and made a number of recommendations. A follow-up consultative meeting, held in May 1991, focused specifically on: more detailed country specific estimates of contraceptive requirements; programme needs for logistics management of contraceptive; options for local production of contraceptives; and future resource needs for contraceptives (UNFPA, 1991a).

The overall results of the exercise formed the basis for the 1991 UNFPA Governing Council paper entitled "Report of the Executive Director on contraceptive requirements and demand for contraceptive commodities in developing countries in the 1990s" (DP/1991/34).

In order to achieve the United Nations medium-variant population projection by the year 2000, contraceptive prevalence in developing countries must rise from 51 per cent in 1990 to 59 per cent in 2000. This means that some 567 million couples must be using some form of contraceptive at the end of the century.

According to this projection, 151 million surgical procedures for female and male sterilization, about 8.8 billion cycles of oral pills, 663 million doses of injectables, 310 million intra-uterine devices (IUDs) and 44 billion condoms will be needed in developing countries by the year 2000.

If the contraceptives required for the period 1991-2000 are purchased in the international market, they will cost about $5 billion. From an annual cost of $399 million in 1990, the bill for contraceptives will rise to $627 million by the year 2000. The cost for specific methods will be $1.9 billion for oral pills, $1.4 billion for sterilization, $888 million for condoms, $594 million for injectables and $278 million for IUDs. Wider use of the contraceptive implant Norplant will make a difference in total contraceptive costs. Norplant will cost about $750 million from 1991 to 2000. By region, the cost of contraceptives required in the 1990s will be about $3.7 billion for Asia and the Pacific, $224 million for Africa, $696 million for Latin America and the Caribbean, and $340 million for the Arab States and Europe.[1]

With regard to the sources of funding, Governments of developing countries paid $242 million for contraceptives in 1990, the private commercial sector provided $69 million and the international donor community contributed $88 million. By the year 2000, Governments of developing countries are projected to pay $320 million, the private sector $109 million and international donors $198 million, a grand total of $627 million for contraceptive requirements. This amount constitutes about one fifteenth of the total required by the year 2000 for supporting population activities, which was set at $9 billion by the Amsterdam Declaration adopted by the International Forum on Population in the Twenty-first Century (UNFPA, 1989). Other components of this $9 billion target include: data collection and analysis; maternal and child health and family planning (MCH/FP) service delivery costs; information, education and communication; population policy formulation and implementation; research; training; and special programmes.

Contraceptives are currently being manufactured locally in at least 23 developing countries and local production is under consideration in at least four others. Subsidiaries of multinational companies are often involved in the local production of oral pills and condoms, while the majority of domestic IUD manufacturing ventures have been undertaken by private companies. In four countries that are major consumers of contraceptives (Brazil, China, India and Indonesia), at least three methods (pills, condoms and IUDs) are produced locally with capacity approaching or exceeding their respective estimated commodity requirements. External assistance agencies have been quite active in supporting the local production of contraceptives.

A. ESTIMATION OF CONTRACEPTIVE REQUIREMENTS

The exercise to project the volume and cost of contraceptives required to reach the fertility goals of the United Nations medium-variant population projection by the year 2000 was carried out in four stages. The first stage involved determining the contraceptive prevalence rates required to achieve the stated goals. The second stage entailed translating these prevalence rates into numbers of contraceptive users by applying the prevalence rates to the number of married women of reproductive age (MWRA). Where estimates of unmarried women using contraception were available from surveys and other sources, they were included in the calculations. The third stage involved calculating the total quantities of different contraceptives required by applying the proportionate unit of the various number of users and new acceptors and the average quantity of each method required annually per user. The last stage produced the total annual cost for each method, by multiplying the quantity required by the unit cost.

Estimates were made for the numbers of contraceptive users for each of 108 developing countries whose combined population makes up almost 100 per cent of that of the developing world. In addition, the number of contraceptive users that would be required to achieve replacement fertility was also estimated. According to the analysis, a contraceptive prevalence rate of 75 per cent of MWRA is necessary to achieve replacement fertility. For the sake of comparison, estimates were also made of contraceptive prevalence and number of users by country to accommodate the United Nations high and low population projections.

Projection of contraceptive use, 1990-2000

United Nations projections suggest that the population of the developing world will reach 5 billion by the year 2000 (see table 18). The 1990 total fertility rate (TFR) in developing countries was approximately 3.8 births per woman and the estimated contraceptive prevalence (the proportion of MWRA practising contraception) was 51 per cent. According to the most recent United Nations medium-variant population projection, TFR will fall to 3.3 births per woman by the year 2000. Reaching this challenging goal will require a substantial increase in both government commitment to and resources for family planning programmes, including programmes in the governmental, commercial and non-governmental sectors.

Two factors account for the large increase in contraceptive users that will be required to reach the United Nations medium population projection. First, there will be a large increase in the number of MWRA during the 1990s; secondly, the proportion of these women using contraception must be increased. During the 1990s, the number of MWRA in the developing countries will increase by about 212 million (28 per cent), from 747 million in 1990 to 959 million in 2000. Thus, even if the level of contraceptive prevalence remains at 51 per cent throughout the decade, implying no decline in the fertility rate, the number of contraceptive users will have to grow by about 108 million.

If TFR in the developing countries is to decline to 3.3 births per woman by the year 2000 and if population growth between 1990 and 2000 is not to exceed 900 million persons, contraceptive prevalence must rise to 59 per cent. This seemingly modest percentage increase, when combined with the large growth in the number of MWRA, requires that the number of contraceptive users increase by 186 million, to reach 567 million in 2000. By far the largest increase in absolute terms will have to take place in Asia and the Pacific (140 million); considerably smaller increases will be required in Latin America and the Caribbean (18 million), sub-Saharan Africa (14 million) and the Arab States and Europe, covering Northern Africa and the Middle East (12 million). Proportionately, however, the greatest increase will have to take place in Africa (158 per cent); large increases will also be required in the Arab States and Europe (84 per cent), Latin America and the Caribbean (45 per cent), and Asia and the Pacific (44 per cent).

TABLE 18. POPULATION OF DEVELOPING COUNTRIES BY SEX, WOMEN AGES 15-49 AND
MARRIED WOMEN OF REPRODUCTIVE AGE, 1990-2000
(Thousands)

| Year | Population | | | | Married women of reproductive age |
	Total	Males	Females	Females aged 15-49	
1990	4 085 640	2 078 530	2 007 100	1 022 308	747 315
1991	4 175 360	2 123 834	2 051 518	1 046 222	768 892
1992	4 265 080	2 169 138	2 095 936	1 070 137	790 469
1993	4 354 800	2 214 442	2 140 354	1 094 051	812 045
1994	4 444 520	2 259 746	2 184 772	1 117 966	833 622
1995	4 534 240	2 305 050	2 229 190	1 141 880	855 199
1996	4 626 736	2 351 640	2 275 096	1 164 628	876 049
1997	4 719 232	2 398 230	2 321 002	1 187 376	896 898
1998	4 811 728	2 444 820	2 366 908	1 210 124	917 748
1999	4 904 224	2 491 410	2 412 814	1 232 872	938 597
2000	4 996 720	2 538 000	2 458 720	1 255 620	959 447

Source: United Nations Population Fund, "Contraceptive requirements and demand for contraceptive commodities in developing countries in the 1990s", report submitted to the UNFPA Consultative Meeting on Contraceptive Requirements in Developing Countries by the Year 2000, 25-26 February 1991 (New York, United Nations Population Fund, 1991).

Meeting the United Nations high population projection (where the fertility rate will decline to 3.7 in the year 2000) requires that contraceptive prevalence increase to 57 per cent by the end of the decade. Under this scenario, the number of contraceptive users must grow by 170 million to reach 551 million. By comparison, reaching the United Nations low-variant population projection (with a TFR of 2.9) will require an increase in contraceptive prevalence to 65 per cent in 2000. The number of users will have to increase by 218 million by the end of the period, or some 32 million more than the medium projection goal of 186 million additional contraceptive users.

Attaining replacement fertility for each country in the world, an objective consistent with TFR decline to 2.1 births per woman in 2000, requires a contraceptive prevalence level of 75 per cent in that year. This rate implies a near doubling in the number of users, from 381 million in 1990 to 720 million in 2000. These two goals will be extremely difficult, if not impossible, to reach, as the data suggest that as much as 80 per cent of the increase will take place in countries where contraceptive prevalence was below 60 per cent in 1990. Reaching replacement fertility levels in countries with contraceptive prevalence of 60 per cent or more in 1990 —including Brazil, China, Colombia, the Republic of Korea, Thailand and Turkey—will require a combined increase of 72 million users.

Projections of users by method

Tables 19 and 20 give numbers and percentages of contraceptive users in 1990 by method and region. The largest number of contraceptive users choosing sterilization are in the Asia and Pacific region—152 million (89 per cent of the developing country total). Among the regions, Asia and the Pacific also has, at 49 per cent, the highest use of sterilization as a proportion of all contraceptive methods. The proportion of use of sterilization is also quite high in Latin America and the Caribbean as a whole, accounting for some 37 per cent of all methods. Asia and Pacific also has the largest number and proportion of IUD users—nearly 83 million, or 27 per cent of all users. This region is followed by the Arab States and Europe, in which more than 20 per cent of all users rely upon IUDs.

The largest number of contraceptive pill users is in Asia and the Pacific, although only 8 per cent of all users there depend upon the pill, a far smaller proportion than in the Arab States and Europe (33 per cent of users), Latin America and the Caribbean (29 per cent) or Africa (26 per cent). Condoms apparently are the choice of only 6 per cent of users in the developing countries, but this estimate is probably too low, given the increasing use of condoms to help prevent the spread of the acquired immunodeficiency syndrome (AIDS).

189

TABLE 19. NUMBER OF CONTRACEPTIVE USERS, BY METHOD AND REGION, 1990
(*Thousands*)

Region	Sterilization			Number of users					
	All	Female	Male	Pill	Inject-ables	Intra-uterine device	Condoms	Other	Total users
Africa	528	523	5	1907	409	481	333	3666	7394
Arab States and Europe	782	766	16	5200	100	3617	1139	4858	15696
Asia and the Pacific	151759	122759	29148	24741	10066	82537	18596	19936	307743
Latin America and the Caribbean	14993	14377	450	11675	806	4526	1630	7314	40778
World	170716	140993	29665˙	45662	12363	92548	22747	36947	380925

Source: United Nations Population Fund, "Contraceptive requirements and demand for contraceptive commodities in developing countries in the 1990s", report submitted to the UNFPA Consultative Meeting on Contraceptive Requirements in Developing Countries by the Year 2000, 25-26 February 1991; New York, 1991.

TABLE 20. PERCENTAGE OF CONTRACEPTIVE USERS, BY METHOD AND REGION, 1990

Region	Sterilization			Percentage					
	All	Female	Male	Pill	Inject-ables	Intra-uterine device	Condoms	Others	Total
Africa	7	7	0	26	6	7	5	50	100
Arab States and Europe	5	5	0	33	1	23	7	31	100
Asia and the Pacific	49	40	9	8	3	27	6	6	100
Latin America and the Caribbean	37	35	2	29	2	11	4	18	100
World	45	37	8	12	3	24	6	10	100

*Source:*United Nations Population Fund, Contraceptive requirements and demand for contraceptive commodities in developing countries in the 1990s", report submitted to the UNFPA Consultative Meeting on Contraceptive Requirements in Developing Countries by the Year 2000, 25-26 February 1991; New York, 1991.

Table 21 shows estimated numbers of users of different contraceptive methods required to meet the United Nations medium-variant population projection goal of reducing TFR to 3.3 births per woman by 2000. Currently, voluntary sterilization is by far the most prevalent method of contraception in the developing countries; IUDs and oral pills are second and third. Among contraceptive users in 1990, 171 million (45 per cent), nearly 141 million of whom (37 per cent of all users) were women, relied upon sterilization. Some 93 million users (24 per cent) relied upon IUDs. Pill users numbered 46 million (12 per cent of the total). Another 23 million users (6 per cent) relied upon condoms and 12 million (3 per cent) upon injectables. Other methods, mostly traditional, were the choice of slightly fewer than 10 per cent of all users.

TABLE 21. NUMBER OF USERS OF CONTRACEPTIVES, BY METHOD, DEVELOPING COUNTRIES, 1990-2000
(*Thousands*)

Year	Sterilization			Pill	Inject-ables	Intra-uterine device	Condoms	Other	Total users
	All	Female	Male						
1990	170 716	140 993	29 665	45 662	12 363	92 548	22 747	36 947	380 925
1991	178 629	147 552	30 976	47 216	12 985	95 000	24 029	41 063	398 820
1992	186 542	154 111	32 287	48 770	13 606	97 452	25,310	45 179	416 715
1993	194 456	160 670	33 599	50 324	14 228	99 904	26 592	49 294	434 611
1994	202 369	167 229	34 910	51 878	14 849	102 356	27 873	53 410	452 506
1995	210 282	173 788	36 221	53 432	15 471	104 808	29 155	57 526	470 401
1996	218 938	180 376	38 324	57 764	16 616	108 853	30 313	57 480	489 725
1997	227 594	186 964	40 427	62 096	17 761	112 897	31 471	57 433	509 049
1998	236 250	193 551	42 530	66 428	18 907	116 942	32 629	57 387	528 374
1999	244 906	200 139	44 633	70 760	20 052	120 986	33 787	57 340	547 698
2000	253 562	206 727	46 736	75 092	21 197	125 031	34 945	57 294	567 022

Source: United Nations Population Fund, "Contraceptive requirements and demand for contraceptive commodities in developing countries in the 1990s, report submitted to the UNFPA Consultative Meeting on Contraceptive Requirements in Developing Countries by the Year 2000, 25-26 February 1991; New York, 1991.

Reliance upon voluntary sterilization has been steadily growing in the developing countries. To reach United Nations medium population projection goals, the number of sterilization users will have to increase from 171 million to 254 million in 2000 (by 49 per cent). The number of IUD users will have to increase from 93 million to 125 million (34 per cent), the number of pill users from 46 million to 75 million (64 per cent), the number of condom users from 23 million to 35 million (54 per cent) and the number of injectable users from 12 million to 21 million (71 per cent).

Arriving at a meaningful estimate of contraceptive acceptors involves a set of assumptions. The first assumption is that since sterilization and IUDs are effective for longer than one year, a substantial proportion of users each year, depending upon the average duration of effective use, are carried over to the following year. Thus, additional acceptors are needed both to make up for those who drop out (e.g., women that pass their child-bearing years), as well as to meet the required overall increase in the number of users. A second assumption, based on empirical studies, is that, on average, an IUD is effectively used for 3.5 years. Thus, the number of annual acceptors is approximately equal to the estimated number of IUD users multiplied by 1/3.5, or 0.2857. Similarly, in terms of statistical categories, sterilization is considered effective from the time of the procedure until the woman passes out of her reproductive years (or no longer cohabits or dies). Thus, the number of new acceptors of sterilization in each time period is estimated to equal 7 per cent of the estimated

number of persons sterilized. A third assumption involves the user continuation rates for oral pills, condoms and injectables, which are known to vary widely. Since such variation in rates markedly influences the calculation of acceptors for oral pills, condoms and injectables, and since the primary interest here is contraceptive commodity requirements, more complex exercises for estimating separately continuing users, discontinuers and new acceptors of these methods are unnecessary.

Increasing the number of contraceptive users opting for sterilization from 171 million to 254 million over the course of the decade will require adding 151 million acceptors. Since sterilization accounts for a very large proportion of contraceptive use, an additional analysis to estimate the number of users and acceptors for the period through 2000 was conducted using a different methodology. The estimates resulting from this analysis were very close to those from the first analysis, 148.7 million acceptors compared with 150.7 million, respectively.

Contraceptive commodity requirements

Table 22 presents estimates of contraceptive commodity requirements in terms of number of sterilization procedures, cycles of oral pills, doses of injectables, IUD insertions and condoms. The estimates are based on the assumption that each user requires 15 cycles of oral pills, four doses of injectables and 150 condoms (125, plus 20 per cent for wastage) per annum. For sterilization, the commodity requirement estimates include mini-

TABLE 22. CONTRACEPTIVE COMMODITY REQUIREMENTS, BY METHOD, DEVELOPING COUNTRIES, 1990-2000
(Thousands, unless otherwise specified)

Year	All	Sterilization Female	Male	Pill cycles (millions)	Inject-ables	Intra-uterine device	Condoms (millions)
1990	11 950	9 870	2 077	685	49 452	26 442	3 412
1991	12 504	10 329	2 168	708	51 938	27 143	3 604
1992	13 058	10 788	2 260	732	54 425	27 843	3 797
1993	13 612	11 247	2 352	755	56 911	28 544	3 989
1994	14 166	11 706	2 444	778	59 398	29 245	4 181
1995	14 720	12 165	2 535	801	61 884	29 945	4 373
1996	15 326	12 626	2 683	866	66 465	31 101	4 547
1997	15 932	13 087	2 830	931	71 046	32 256	4 721
1998	16 538	13 549	2 977	996	75 626	33 412	4 894
1999	17 143	14 010	3 124	1 061	80 207	34 568	5 068
2000	17 749	14 471	3 272	1 126	84 788	35 723	5 242
1991-2000	150 747	123 977	26 645	8 756	662 688	309 780	44 416

Source: United Nations Population Fund, "Contraceptive requirements and demand for contraceptive commodities in developing countries in the 1990s", report submitted to the UNFPA Consultative Meeting on Contraceptive Requirements in Developing Countries by the Year 2000, 25-26 February 1991; New York, 1991).

laparotomy surgical kits, vasectomy kits, Laprocator systems and other supplies. Requirements for IUD insertion and Norplant subdermal implants were also included in the calculations.

Based on the foregoing assumptions, it is estimated that total contraceptive requirements in developing countries between 1990 and the year 2000 are as follows: 151 million surgical procedures for female and male sterilizations; about 8.8 billion cycles of oral pills; 663 million doses of injectable contraceptives; 310 million IUDs; and 44 billion condoms. The numbers appear somewhat less formidable if expressed in terms of annual averages: 15 million sterilization procedures; 876 million cycles of pills; 66 million doses of injectables; 31 million IUDs; and 4.4 billion condoms.

Contraceptive commodity costs

The UNFPA study of contraceptive requirements found that if the projected contraceptives and commodities required by the developing countries are purchased in the international market, the costs will be about $627 million in the year 2000—57 per cent more than the 1990 total of $399 million (see table 23). The total cost will be more than $5 billion. This does not take into account service-delivery costs associated with infrastructure building, payment of service providers or costs for transport, storage and so forth. For specific methods,

total costs over the decade are shown in table 23 below. If contraceptives are not purchased in the international market, costs could vary significantly, depending upon the source of supply, as well as upon the volume and specifications of commodities. In most such circumstances, the costs are likely to be higher.

The highest regional contraceptive costs—$295 million in 1990, rising to $449 million in 2000—will be in Asia and the Pacific. Africa, however, will experience the highest proportional increase—from $11 million to $43 million, or 290 per cent. The commodity cost for Latin America and the Caribbean will increase from $57 million to $82 million, and the cost for the Arab States and Europe region will increase from $22 million to $44 million.

The introduction of Norplant contraceptive implants and their wider use in the coming decade will increase overall contraceptive costs. The UNFPA study of contraceptive requirements assumed that the number of Norplant acceptors would rise from 0.26 per cent of contraceptive users in 1990 to 3.0 per cent in 1995 and that this proportion would cost $750 million for the period 1991-2000. The study also assumed that if Norplant wss not readily available during the period, about two thirds of its potential acceptors will undergo sterilization; the rest would use other methods, primarily traditional ones. If the first assumption proves to be true

TABLE 23. COST[a] OF CONTRACEPTIVE COMMODITIES TO DEVELOPING COUNTRIES IF
IF PURCHASED ON THE INTERNATIONAL MARKET, BY METHOD, 1990-2000
(Millions of dollars)

Year	Sterilization	Pill	Intra-uterine device	Inject-ables	Condoms	Total
1990	113	150	24	44	68	399
1991	118	155	24	47	72	416
1992	124	160	25	49	76	433
1993	129	165	26	51	80	450
1994	134	170	26	53	84	467
1995	139	175	27	56	87	484
1996	145	189	28	60	91	513
1997	151	204	29	64	94	542
1998	157	218	30	68	98	570
1999	162	232	31	72	101	599
2000	168	246	32	76	105	627
1991-2000	1 428	1 913	278	594	888	5,102

Source: "Contraceptive requirements and demand for contraceptive commodities in developing countries in the 1990s", report submitted to the UNFPA Consultative Meeting on Contraceptive Requirements in Developing Countries by the Year 2000, 25-26 February 1991; New York, 1991.

[a]The following unit costs for purchase on the international market were used in estimating overall costs: condoms, $0.0174; oral pills, $0.19; injectables, $0.78; IUDs (CuT 380A), $0.78; sterilization, $8.24; Norplant, $23.00.

and the use of Norplant reaches 3 per cent in 1995, the number of sterilization acceptors will decline by 21 million during the 10-year period and the cost of sterilization will fall by $197 million. Therefore, the net additional costs for introduction of Norplant and expansion of its use between 1991 and 2000 will be about $553 million—a little over 10 per cent of total contraceptive commodity costs over the period.

The overall annual costs per user in 2000 are given below by region (UNFPA, 1991):

(a)   Africa, $1.48;
(b)   Arab States and Europe, $1.57;
(c)   Asia and the Pacific, $1.00;
(d)   Latin America and the Caribbean, $1.38.

The world annual cost of contraceptive commodities per user in 2000 is $1.10. There is some variation by region due to differences in contraceptive method mix. The high rate of use of sterilization and IUD in Asia and the Pacific tends to decrease the average cost per user.

Lastly, the cost estimates presented in this section of the paper were calculated by taking current international public sector prices for contraceptives and adding 15 per cent for shipping. As figure XV shows, public sector

prices for modern contraceptives over the past decade have remained relatively stable in real dollar terms and have thus decreased in constant dollars. This decrease has probably been due to larger bulk purchases and increasing professionalism in procurement. Whether prices will remain low and stable during the 1990s is, however, difficult to predict, especially in view of some recent price increases. If an annual cost increase of 5 per cent is added to the contraceptive requirement estimates of developing countries, costs in the year 2000 would increase from $627 million to over $1.0 billion, and total costs over the period would increase from $5.1 billion to $7.3 billion.

B. PAYING FOR CONTRACEPTIVE COMMODITIES

Costs of contraceptive commodities are paid for by the Governments of developing countries, by the private commercial sector and by donations from international, bilateral and non-governmental organizations. In 1990, the total cost of $399 million was divided so that Governments of developing countries bore $242 million of the cost; the private sector, $69 million; and international donors, $88 million. The estimate for the private sector was derived from a sub-study of some 25 key developing countries where oral contraceptives, condoms,

Figure XIV. Contraceptive prices, 1982-1992

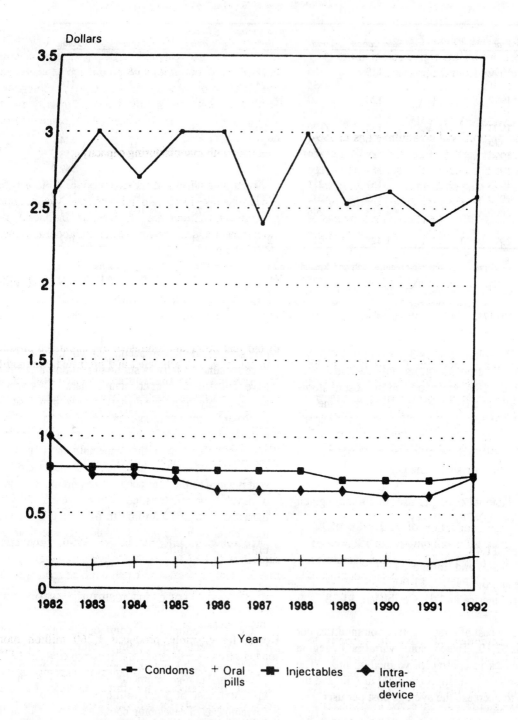

Year

Condoms   + Oral pills   Injectables   Intra-uterine device

Source: United Nations Population Fund, Procurement Unit, 1992.
NOTE: Prices are f.o.b. for a gross (144 pieces) of condoms, one cycle of oral pills, one dose of an injectable and one intra-uterine device.

IUDs and injectables are bought by individuals. This study estimated that in 1990 about one third of oral pills, just over 10 per cent of condoms, 10 per cent of injectables, and 4 per cent of IUDs were obtained from the private sector. This volume represented about one sixth of total costs for contraceptive commodities ($69 million) being derived from the private sector.

Over the course of the 1990s, it is projected that Governments of developing countries will not be able to sustain the same proportional commitment as in 1990 and that the private sector proportion will remain constant. In such a scenario, the donor community would have to raise its support to about one third of total requirements. Thus, by the year 2000, sharing of the total costs of $627 million would have Governments of developing countries providing $320 million; the private sector, $109 million; and the international donor community, $198 million. This would reflect a 9 per cent shift in costs from the Governments to the international donor community, a not unreasonable division given the severity of the economic crises being experienced by most developing countries.

A number of other important factors need to be considered in cost equations for the 1990s. These factors are local production of contraceptives, contraceptive social marketing and public sector cost-recovery schemes, all of which may help reduce or shift the burden of contraceptive commodities costs away from government.

Local production of contraceptives

As of 1990, the production of oral pills, IUDs, condoms and injectables is ongoing or, in a few cases, under serious consideration in 27 developing countries. Affiliates of multinational companies carry out most of the local production; Government-owned and local private companies are responsible for the rest.

Of these 27 countries, 20 have the capacity to produce oral pills, the contraceptive most frequently produced locally. Four other countries are either developing such capacity or considering establishing it. By contrast, only six countries are involved in manufacturing injectables, the method least frequently produced locally. Condoms are second in frequency of production: nine countries produce condoms, most of them in high volume; at least five others are considering new production ventures. Eight countries manufacture IUDs

or have production facilities in advanced stages of preparation; new production ventures are under serious consideration in at least two others.

Multinational companies play a major role in the local production of oral pills (participating in production in 16 of the 20 countries with production capacity) and condoms (five out of nine). Domestic private companies or Governments are involved less frequently in the manufacture of oral pills (8 out of 20 countries) but more often in the production of IUDs (five of the eight countries with manufacturing capacity).

China, Indonesia and Mexico produce all four types of contraceptives locally. In Indonesia and Mexico, non-government ventures are involved; in Indonesia, the Government and the private sector collaborate in local manufacture.

A review of the local production of oral pills, injectables, IUDs and condoms in a core set of 16 developing countries[2] assessed their production capacity in 1990, projected how much the capacity would expand by the year 2000 and contrasted this expanded production capacity with estimated and projected commodity requirements. The 16 countries reviewed account for some 90 per cent of contraceptive requirements in the developing world. The estimates of commodity requirements provided in this section are for all contraceptive users, regardless of whether they obtain their methods from private or public sector sources. Production capacity estimates are based on available data for manufacturers, regardless of whether their products are marketed in the private or the public sector.

According to information for 1990, production capacities in 7 of the 16 countries reviewed are either non-existent or below estimated national requirements for all four methods studied; 6 countries have at most the capacity to produce only one type of contraceptive. Some countries have excess capacity: the Republic of Korea, for example, produced 1,260 million more condoms than its estimated local requirements for 1990. Mexico, in contrast, has production capacity above national requirements for three methods but has inadequate capacity for full-scale condom production; a reported joint venture of Mexico and the Republic of Korea, however, will create what is expected to be the largest condom factory in Latin America. Pakistan has adequate capacity for the production of injectables and Lippes Loop IUDs, although it is dependent upon imports for oral pills, condoms and copper-bearing IUDs.

Furthermore, projected increased requirements for the year 2000 will turn 1990 surpluses into deficits for pill production in China and Indonesia, and for IUDs in China. Shortfalls may occur despite projected expansions in capacity, such as for oral pills in Indonesia, Thailand and Turkey. Among the countries currently with excess production, surplus margins will decline—in Brazil for condoms, Indonesia for IUDs, Mexico for pills and IUDs—primarily because the expansion of capacity will not keep pace with demand.

In some cases, however, excess capacity may be overestimated. Outmoded types of contraceptives—such as high-dosage pills in 21- or 22-day formats, stainless-steel IUDs and certain formulations of injectables—account for a significant portion of excess capacity. In some instances, a large excess capacity—such as in the Republic of Korea for condoms—is used for exportation to developed countries. There appears to be a significant need to expand oral pill production, as a shortfall of oral pills is projected by the year 2000 for 10 of the 13 countries studied that currently produce such contraceptives. Manufacturers in several countries are confident, however, that they can easily expand production to meet rising demand.

Although some countries have an inadequate supply of contraceptives, this is not necessarily due to insufficient production capacity. Rather, it is often the result of the generally poor quality of contraceptive products, inadequate demand and lack of appropriate expertise in the manufacture and distribution of commodities, as illustrated by the cases of Cameroon (orals and condoms) and Colombia (condoms and IUDs).

Estimates of the financial resources required to support local production in these 16 countries up to the year 2000 are extremely difficult to make. However, experience suggests that at least five categories of donor-supported activities are pertinent in estimating the costs of local production: assuring quality control; conducting feasibility studies; upgrading production; expanding existing capacity; and establishing new facilities.

In estimating the costs to the donor community of producing contraceptives locally, variations in local capacity were taken into account. It was found, for example, that in some countries of Asia and Latin America, public or private sector investments might meet most of the costs, although some international donor assistance would be needed to help defray the cost of equipment, technology transfer and training. Most of the countries in Africa, however, would likely require grants to cover 100 per cent of local production. In some countries in the region, concessional loans for initial investments might also play a role.

Ultimately, decisions on local production should hinge on cost considerations—the cost of producing a product locally against the cost of that same product procured on the international market. There may be some flexibility in regard to different components of total cost—for example, the "price" of local costs against the "price" of foreign exchange, but the final product cost should always be a major factor in any such decision.

C. LOGISTICS MANAGEMENT NEEDS

Securing sufficient global funding for contraceptive commodities will not in itself assure access to modern family planning methods for those wishing to use them. An efficient logistics system which maintains a continuous supply line to consumer outlets is essential.

Any logistics management system, be it for the public, non-governmental or private commercial sectors, should be able to accomplish several interrelated functions. First, it must enable managers to determine the volume of contraceptives required for the programme by type, brand and by geographical area. Then the system must ensure that procured contraceptives shall be of the correct quality and standard, and deliver them in the appropriate quantities to the right places in a timely manner to ensure continuity of supply to users. This task will involve the maintenance of a reliable storage and inventory system at all levels in the distribution chain. There must also be a functioning information system which provides necessary and sufficient data to facilitate management decisions. Lastly, the ability to monitor, as required, the quality of stored contraceptives is also important in maintaining consumer confidence.

Forecasting requirements

Forecasting contraceptive requirements can be demographically based or determined by reference to historical data on consumption, modified by an assess-

196

ment of future trends and developments in programme activities and emphasis. In the former case, the estimates of contraceptive consumption will be determined from the number of MWRA in the population and the proportion of these that are, or will be, practising family planning using the different methods available. In the latter case, data on the actual consumption of each product by the end-user is extrapolated to derive future estimates, or, in the absence of accurate and comprehensive service statistics providing actual consumption, information of the quantities distributed from central and/or regional warehouses can act as a surrogate. In both of these consumption-generated exercises, the forecaster will need to be sure that the data relate to a period during which there were adequate supplies at all distribution points to meet demand, because figures of "issued" or "dispensed" contraceptives would understate the real situation had there been rationing or temporary stock depletion. Underestimates lead to stock depletion, inadequate supplies at distribution points and rationing. Overestimates can result in stockpiling (increased expenditures through resources tied up in stocks and extra warehousing), stock deterioration and destruction of stock when expiration dates are passed.

Forecasts also need to be made sufficiently far in advance to facilitate the procurement of supplies in time to maintain availability throughout the system. Contraceptives, especially in the quantities required by national programmes, are not generally available "off the shelf", that is, direct from the manufacturer's stocks. In most instances, the product is manufactured to order and the lead time involved in this production activity, when added to the time required for the completion of tendering procedures, pre-delivery quality testing (as appropriate), shipment from country of origin, clearance through port of arrival and internal transfer to outlets, gives an estimate of the required lead time for procurement activities. It is possible that up to 20 months may be needed from the time of supply planning decisions before the initial distribution of commodities can take place.

Procurement

The quantities of contraceptives to be procured are derived from but are not necessarily equal to the forecasts of contraceptive consumption. The short-term (from one to three years) procurement process must also take into account current stock levels throughout the system, expected deliveries and supplies from other sources, for example, before determining purchase volumes. Failure

to pay attention to these issues may result in the same problems as described above under forecasting.

Contraceptive procurement requires expertise in the areas of product specifications, local and international quality assurance standards and testing procedures, and medical device and pharmaceutical industry practices. Knowledge of the international contraceptive market, the major manufacturers, and public sector pricing policies are also necessary for successful procurement activities. In the absence of donated contraceptives, there are, in general, three procurement options, the selection of which is influenced by the existing organizational structure. These options are: direct competitive procurement; procurement through an intermediate agency; and single-source procurement.

Direct competitive procurement requires expert procurement staff but should result in the lowest price. Procurement through a reputable intermediate agency may be faster (because appropriate business links already exist between the agency and manufacturers which assists in assuring quality) and may be marginally more expensive than competitive procurement (because a handling charge is levied), but should require less in terms of local procurement capability. The third option, single-source procurement, is usually costlier but is useful in circumstances when local staffing and expertise are inadequate to meet the requirements of competitive procurement.

Inventory control

The time-consuming nature of international procurement confirms the vital need for any distribution system to maintain adequate stocks of contraceptives at each level within the system. It is essential to implement stock monitoring and inventory control procedures that ensure that each level shall identify the time at which resupply should be initiated, in order to prevent disruption of supply to the consumer. The credibility of a family planning programme can be compromised by contraceptive shortages or unavailability of stocks, and unreliable supply can contribute to discontinuation of use. The stock level maintained at each distribution point is a function of the consumption at that point and the time that it would take for further supplies to be obtained, the latter being dependent upon such factors as communications, availability of transport and distance from the supply centre to the next level. The implementation of professional inventory procedures is also necessary to ensure that stocks shall be issued in the correct order, thus preventing the ageing of stock and avoiding the necessity to destroy deteriorated stock.

Management information system

The implementation of these interconnecting logistics management activities relies upon the integral components of data collection and record-keeping and the analysis of such information for operational and managerial decisions. Proper maintenance of stock records at each level of the distribution system in conjunction with data on transfers through or out of the system to consumers permits sensible decisions to be reached on requisitioning and resupply. Trends in the use of different types or brands of contraceptives are identified by regular reporting and subsequent monitoring of standard inventory and distribution data. The utilization of appropriate authorizing, issuing and receipt documentation is necessary to secure the integrity of the system and to ensure accountability.

Quality assurance

Following the selection of contraceptive products by relevant authorities, the forecasting process must ensure that appropriate quantities of the types and brands of contraceptives desired by family planning acceptors shall be identified. The procurement process must then ensure that the correct product shall be obtained, first by specifying the exact nature and standards of the contraceptive; and secondly, by assuring quality and compliance with product specifications. This process may require the establishment or utilization of scientific laboratories to verify product acceptability, although in the case of condoms, a number of recognized, independent testing laboratories currently exist to undertake pre-delivery and post-shipment quality assurance testing.

A system in which supplies move regularly and smoothly to the consumer will have less need to monitor quality during the distribution stage. However, and particularly for condoms, testing of quality is appropriate in those circumstances when delays in clearance of shipments or slow movements of stock have caused consignments to remain exposed or stored for long periods of time in unsatisfactory conditions.

Infrastructure and human resources

Product quality and efficacy can deteriorate not only because of prolonged storage (possibly the result of poor inventory control) but also because of unsatisfactory storage conditions. Central, bulk warehousing facilities, especially in tropical climates, need to protect contraceptives from extremes of temperature and humidity, and from exposure to precipitation, sunlight and destructive pests. Proper storage facilities, preferably with controlled environments, along with appropriate handling equipment and trained staff are also essential to the logistics system. It is often the case that there are few staff dedicated to logistics management, and this lack may be due to the relatively low priority given to this activity up to the present.

In order to manage efficiently the resources to be allocated to the provision of contraceptives, as enumerated in the earlier part of this report, commensurate attention must be given to the logistics component of the programme. As demand for family planning increases, so do the complexity and volume of logistics management activities. The strengthening of expanded logistics management systems will thus be a vital factor in assuring that the needs of individual users continue to be met.

D. COUNTRY STUDIES ON CONTRACEPTIVE REQUIREMENTS

In 1991, following on from the global study of contraceptive requirements, UNFPA, in partnership with other interested agencies and organizations, launched an initiative to conduct a series of in-depth studies on contraceptive requirements and logistics management needs in a number of developing countries. In addition to providing the selected countries with a longer term planning instrument to assess their needs in these areas, this exercise will also develop and refine a methodology which would then be available for use by all other countries.

In addition to forecasting contraceptive requirements up to the year 2000, the in-depth studies will focus on the following areas: logistics management needs, including management information systems; options for local production of contraceptives; coordinated procurement of contraceptive commodities; condom requirements for prevention of the human immunodeficiency virus (HIV) and AIDS; and future resource needs.

This initiative has been launched in close partnership with a number of agencies and organizations including the United States Agency for International

198

the World Bank, the World Health Organization Global Programme on AIDS, the Rockefeller Foundation, the International Planned Parenthood Federation, the Population Council and the Swedish International Development Authority. In order to carry out the studies, in-country missions are undertaken with the agreement and full cooperation of the Governments concerned. The global initiative is characterized by a high degree of collaboration and cooperation among its partners, one concrete example of this being the provision by agencies of consultants as mission team members.

To date, three in-depth studies have been completed in India, Pakistan and Zimbabwe. The next in-depth study will be conducted in Nepal, beginning in mid-November 1992; and planning has also been initiated for a further four country studies to be carried out in 1993.

Lastly, an exercise is planned for 1993 to update the global estimates for contraceptive requirements up to the year 2000. This information will be available by the time of the International Conference on Population and Development in 1994.

NOTES

[1]The countries included in the regional divisions used in this chapter do not in all cases conform to those included in the geographical regions established by the Population Division of the Department for Economic and Social Information and Policy Analysis of the United Nations Secretariat.
[2]Bangladesh, Brazil, Cameroon, China, Colombia, Egypt, India, Indonesia, Republic of Korea, Mexico, Pakistan, Philippines, Thailand, Turkey, Viet Nam and Zimbabwe.

REFERENCES

United Nations Population Fund (1989). *Report of the International Forum on Population in the Twenty-first Century, Amsterdam, the Netherlands, 6-9 November 1989.* New York.

_____ (1991a). *Contraceptive Needs and Logistics Management.* New York.

_____ (1991b). Contraceptive requirements and demand for contraceptive commodities in developing countries in the 1990s. Report submitted to the UNFPA Consultative Meeting on Contraceptive Requirements in Developing Countries by the Year 2000, 25-26 February 1991. New York.

Part Six

FAMILY PLANNING AND HEALTH

XIII. SAFE MOTHERHOOD AND CHILD SURVIVAL: THE IMPORTANCE OF FAMILY PLANNING AND THE INTERDEPENDENCE OF SERVICES

*Mahmoud F. Fathalla**

Unwanted high fertility adversely affects the health and welfare of individuals and families, especially among the poor, and seriously impedes social and economic progress in many countries. Women and children are the main victims of unregulated fertility. Too many, too close, too early and too late pregnancies are a major cause of maternal, infant and childhood mortality and morbidity (United Nations, 1984).

Family planning makes a significant contribution to safe motherhood and child survival. The contribution of family planning to health should not, however, be seen as limited to this narrow context. Family planning is an integral component of women's health, apart from its impact on safe motherhood and child survival (Fathalla, 1992).

In the constitution of the World Health Organization (WHO), health is defined as a state of complete physical, mental and social well-being. Although this ideal may not be readily attainable, it serves as a reminder that health is not merely the absence of disease or infirmity. The relation of family planning to health should be viewed in the context of this positive definition of health. The ability to regulate and control fertility is a basic ingredient in the health of women. A woman who is unable to regulate and control her fertility cannot be considered to be in a state of complete physical, mental and social well-being. She cannot have the mental joy of a pregnancy that is wanted, avoid the mental distress of a pregnancy that is unwanted and pursue social health by planning her life, continuing her education and enjoying both a productive and a reproductive career. A woman with an unwanted pregnancy cannot be considered to be in good health, even if the pregnancy is not going to kill her or impair her physical health and even if she delivers the unwanted child alive and with no physical handicap.

While recognizing the basic role of family planning in any strategy for safe motherhood and child survival, one should not lose sight of the basic rationale of family planning for the health of the woman as a woman and not just as a mother.

A. FAMILY PLANNING AND SAFE MOTHERHOOD

"Half a million mothers die each year from causes related to childbirth. Safe motherhood must be promoted in all possible ways. Emphasis must be placed on responsible planning of family size and on child spacing." (United Nations, 1990)

Maternal mortality: the scandal of all times

Data on the magnitude of maternal mortality that became available in the 1980s should have shocked the world. The WHO global estimates indicate that more than half a million women die each year because of complications related to pregnancy and childbirth. All but 4,000 of these deaths take place in developing countries (WHO, 1991). The disparity between maternal death rates in developing and developed countries is greater than for any other health indicator. Moreover, maternal mortality should be looked upon as just the tip of an iceberg of maternal morbidity, suffering and ill health.

Recent information available to WHO suggests that during the past few years pregnancy and childbirth have become somewhat safer for women in most of Asia and parts of Latin America and the Caribbean. In contrast, the situation has changed very little for women in most parts of sub- Saharan Africa (WHO, 1991).

The concern about maternal mortality is not simply because of its magnitude. In fact, it can be argued that

---

*Special Programme of Research, Development and Research Training in Human Reproduction, World Health Organization, Geveva, Switzerland.

maternal mortality, in spite of its magnitude, accounts for only 1.3 per cent of all deaths in developing countries, while infectious and parasitic diseases account for 45 per cent of all deaths (WHO, 1990b). If the concern were simply to reduce mortality in the community, then a smaller investment could save more lives in other areas.

The concern about maternal mortality is mainly because practically all the deaths and sufferings are preventable. The know-how is already available to prevent or effectively to manage all potential life-threatening complications related to pregnancy and childbirth.

The concern about maternal mortality is also because it shows the widest discrepancy between the rich and the poor, when compared with any other health indicator.

Maternal mortality has a particular devastating effect on the family. In a study of the live children born to the mothers that died, it was found that 95 per cent also died within one year (Chen and others, 1974). For every mother that dies, children are left motherless, and their chances of survival, healthy growth and development will be affected. But this statement applies to the death of the mother from any cause and not necessarily from a maternal death. Although in some countries maternal mortality is the commonest cause of death among women of child-bearing age, it generally accounts for from one fourth to one third of all deaths during that period (Royston and Armstrong, 1989).

Maternal mortality is a category by itself. It should not be considered in the general context of disease or in relation to infant, child or adult morbidity and mortality. Pregnancy is not a disease; it is a social function. Although any society would be much better off if people did not develop diseases, no society will survive if women did not get pregnant. Society even imposes on women more pregnancies than they themselves would have wanted. Society has much more of a responsibility for protecting mothers during the pregnancy. Safe motherhood should be discussed on its own or under the role and status of women, as an issue of grave social injustice that should be corrected.

B. FAMILY PLANNING TO SAVE LIVES

Family planning can save the lives of mothers, by preventing the exposure of women to the risks of preg-

nancies which they do not want and by allowing women to plan their pregnancies to take place at times that are more favourable for safe child-bearing.

Prevention of unwanted pregnancy

Prevention of unwanted pregnancy makes a major contribution to decreasing maternal mortality and morbidity, through decreasing unnecessary exposure to the risks of pregnancy and childbirth. The impact of the prevention of unwanted pregnancy on maternal mortality in any community or country largely depends upon two factors: the prevalence of unwanted pregnancy; and the maternal mortality ratio. It is also largely influenced by the availability of safe pregnancy termination services.

Worldwide and particularly in developing countries, prevention of unwanted pregnancy is making a major impact on safe motherhood. The maternal mortality ratio in developing countries is estimated to be, on average, 450 per 100,000 births, that is about 1 maternal death for every 220 births (World Health Organization, 1991). The total fertility rate–the average number of births per woman–in developing countries declined from 6.1 in 1965-1970 to 3.9 in 1985-1990 (Sadik, 1992). This fertility decline is almost completely a result of contraceptive use, the prevalence of which increased over the same period from 9 to 50 per cent. On average, every woman has been able to avoid 2.2 unwanted births. A rough estimate would thus be that in developing countries today 1 out of every 100 women is being saved from an unnecessary maternal death through family planning. It is a rough estimate because women that are using family planning may be at less than average risk of maternal death because of better socio-economic conditions or better access to health services. Nevertheless, the impact must still be great.

Family planning can prevent more maternal deaths than it currently does. There is a large unmet need for contraception in developing countries. A recent study based on data available from the Demographic and Health Surveys provided a conservative estimate of at least 100 million couples or individuals that want contraception but whose needs are not met (Bongaarts, 1991). With an excess unwanted total fertility preventable by family planning of say two children, that is, 200 million births; and given a maternal mortality ratio of 450 per 100,000 births, the number of unnecessary maternal deaths can be roughly estimated at 900,000. It is a rough estimate and probably an underestimate because these women with no access to family planning are likely also to have limited access to maternity services and may be at higher than average risk of maternal death.

Unsafe abortion

All efforts should be made to reduce maternal morbidity and mortality. Governments are urged: "To take appropriate steps to help women avoid abortion, which in no case should be promoted as a method of family planning, and, wherever possible, provide for the humane treatment and counselling of women that have had recourse to abortion" (United Nations, 1984, p. 21).

Figures for induced abortion provide an indication of the level of unmet need for family planning in developing countries. Not all women with an unwanted pregnancy resort to induced abortion, particularly in developing countries where services are either not widely available or not permitted by the legal system. Despite these obstacles, the worldwide estimate is from 36 to 53 million induced abortions performed each year (an annual rate of 32-46 abortions per 1,000 women of reproductive age) (Henshaw, 1990). These figures show the magnitude of the problem of unwanted pregnancy and the unmet need for family planning.

Information on clandestine abortions is too uncertain to give completely reliable estimates. Combining various estimates yields a total of 15 million clandestine abortions. However, since these figures are not fully reliable, the actual number may be as low as 10 million or as high as 22 million (Henshaw, 1990).

It is estimated that of the 500,000 maternal deaths that occur each year throughout the world, from one fourth to one third may be a consequence of complications of unsafe abortion procedures (WHO, 1990a). Contrary to common belief, most women seeking abortion are married or living in a stable union and already have several children. However, in all parts of the world, an increasing proportion of those seeking abortion are unmarried adolescents. In some urban centres in Africa, they represent the majority. WHO estimates that more than half of the deaths caused by induced abortion occur in South-Eastern and Southern Asia, followed by sub-Saharan Africa (WHO, 1990a). It should be stressed that these figures are only estimates; it has not been possible to get true numbers because of the difficulty of distinguishing between deaths from induced abortion and those from spontaneous abortion in countries where induced abortion is illegal.

Unsafe abortion is one of the great neglected problems of health care in developing countries and is a serious concern to women during their reproductive life.

Birth planning

Another potential impact of family planning is enabling a woman to plan her births to take place at optimal times for child-bearing and when any risk to her health will be less. There are medical conditions that can make pregnancy more hazardous and the woman will be well-advised to postpone the pregnancy or to put a limit to child-bearing. For the individual patient, this advice can be very critical. These medical problems are fortunately not very frequent.

It is now an item of general knowledge that maternal mortality is more likely to occur at the extremes of reproductive age and with high-parity births. This would be particularly marked where health care services are inadequate. A number of studies have tried to quantify this potential contribution of family planning. A study in Matlab, Bangladesh, has calculated that maternal deaths per live births could be reduced 14 per cent by eliminating births to women under 20 or over 39, 3.5 per cent by eliminating births at parity 6 or higher and 24.6 per cent by eliminating these two high-risk categories (Trussell and Pebley, 1984). If the births eliminated were redistributed to parities of fewer than 6 and to ages 20-39, maternal deaths per live births would be reduced by 19.3 per cent. The potential impact is in reality much greater, if assessed on the basis of the risk per woman of reproductive age and not per birth. Analysis of the data from the same study shows that eliminating births to women under age 20 or over age 39 and to women with parity of more than 5 would result in a mortality reduction of 55.5 per cent.

Good maternity care does not cover only delivery care and prenatal care. It is not complete without post-partum care and preconceptional care, of which birth planning is a basic component.

Maternal mortality: indicators and measurements

All efforts should be made to reduce maternal morbidity and mortality. Governments are urged: "To reduce maternal mortality by at least 50 per cent by the year 2000, where such mortality is very high (higher than 100 maternal deaths per 100,000 births)" (United Nations, 1984, p. 20).

Current understanding of the important role of family planning in safe motherhood has exposed the inadequacy of the maternal mortality ratio (often incorrectly referred to as a rate) as a useful indicator for progress in safe motherhood (Fortney, 1987). The measurement of maternal mortality, as the number of maternal deaths per 100,000 live births is a ratio of deaths to births, and not a rate. It measures obstetric risk and uses live births as a proxy for the more specific and appropriate denominator, pregnancies, because of the difficulty involved in ascertaining the true number of pregnancies in a population and the relative ease of ascertaining live births.

The maternal mortality rate, on the other hand, is a measure of the number of deaths related to pregnancies per 100,000 women of reproductive age. This rate will measure not only the obstetric risk but also the exposure to risk. A large number of maternal deaths can be prevented by reducing the exposure to unwanted pregnancy. This decline will be adequately reflected in the maternal mortality rate but not in the maternal mortality ratio.

Since the risk of maternal death is a recurrent risk, a more meaningful indicator is the lifetime risk of dying from complications of pregnancy and childbirth. A simple calculation of the lifetime risk is by made by multiplying the maternal mortality rate by 30 (years of reproductive life), but the effective duration of exposure could vary widely (Herz and Measham, 1987). In some parts of rural Africa, this risk can be as high as 1 in 20. In Europe, it is low, at one in several thousand.

Progress towards safe motherhood should be measured as the number of maternal deaths per 100,000 women of child-bearing age (maternal mortality rate) or as the lifetime risk of maternal death. The commonly used maternal mortality ratio of deaths over births is inadequate as it measures only obstetric risk.

Place of family planning in a safe motherhood strategy

No strategy for safe motherhood can be complete without family planning to enable women to avoid unwanted pregnancies and thus not expose themselves to an unnecessary risk, and to enable women to plan their births at optimal times for child-bearing from a health and broad social perspective. It should be noted, however, that even if pregnancies are wanted and planned, they can still carry a risk. Pregnant women must have access to prenatal and delivery care at the primary health care level, for health promotion and for the early detection of high-risk situations. The primary health care level, however, will not be adequate to handle these high-risk situations. Essential obstetric functions should be accessible at the first referral level, and facilities for emergency transport should be available for unpredictable life-threatening complications. Beyond these health measures, advancement of the status of women is essential to enable women, among other things, to take full advantage of these services.

The basic elements (or alphabet) for an integrated strategy for safe motherhood are: advancement of status for all women; birth planning for all women of child-bearing age; community-based prenatal services for all pregnant women; delivery by trained birth attendants for all parturients; essential obstetric functions for women with high risk pregnancies and deliveries; facilities for emergency transport for women with life-threatening complications (Fathalla, 1990).

The basic elements in the strategy for mother's survival are not separate interventions. They are closely interlinked, interdependent and mutually strengthening. Family planning, in particular, strongly interacts with the other elements of safe motherhood strategy.

There is a two-way relation between family planning and advancement of the status of women which is well expressed in the World Population Plan of Action:

"The ability of women to control their own fertility forms an important basis for the enjoyment of other rights; likewise, the assurance of socio-economic opportunities on an equal basis with men and the provision of the necessary services and facilities enable women to take greater responsibility for their reproductive lives." (United Nations, 1984, p. 16)

Family planning interacts with the other elements of maternity care in a number of positive ways. First, prevention of unwanted pregnancies can be expected to ease the load on maternity services. A study in Mexico found that for every peso spent on family planning services, nine pesos were saved in maternal and child health services that were not needed (Nortman, Halvas and Rabago, 1986). Secondly, the planning of births can be expected to decrease the number of high-risk pregnancies which would put less demand on already busy services. Thirdly, where safe abortion services are not readily available, provision of family planning can decrease the load on maternity services imposed by the complications of unsafe abortion. A study in Chile estimated that in 1960, before the introduction of family planning services, 184,000 hospital bed days were used to provide care for abortion cases, for a total expenditure of $1 million (about $10 million today) (Armijo and Monreal, 1965).

The various elements of a safe motherhood strategy are not alternatives to choose from. They are integrated elements in a comprehensive strategy. A country committed to making motherhood safer for its women should pursue all these elements in a mix that is appropriate to the levels of need, demand and resources.

C. FAMILY PLANNING AND CHILD SURVIVAL

"The lives of tens of thousands of boys and girls can be saved every day, because the causes of their death are readily preventable. Child and infant mortality is unacceptably high in many parts of the world, but can be lowered dramatically with means that are already known and easily accessible." (United Nations, 1990)

Significant progress has been made in the past two decades in the area of child survival. In the world as a whole, the infant mortality rate (IMR) declined to 71 per 1,000 live births during the period 1985-1990 (WHO, 1992). Child mortality declined during the same period to 105. Progress, however, has been uneven and the magnitude of the problem remains unacceptable. In the least developed countries almost 200 of every 1,000 children born alive will die before reaching age 5, compared with fewer than 20 in developed countries. The under-five mortality rate for the remaining group of developing countries is about 120 per 1,000 live births.

In all developed countries except South Africa, IMR is fewer than 20 per 1,000 live births, as it is in five of the countries of Eastern Europe (WHO, 1992). On the contrary, IMRs of 100 per 1,000 or higher are still observed in the majority of the least developed countries with only seven of them having IMR below this level and only one with a rate fewer than 50 per 1,000 live births. IMRs for the remainder of the developing

countries are virtually evenly distributed into two groups, those with a rate of 50-99 per 1000 and those with fewer than 50 per 1,000. Indeed, 11 developing countries have already attained IMR of fewer than 20 per 1,000 live births, the level of the developed countries.

Place of family planning in a child survival strategy

It should be a basic right of the child to be born wanted and to be born when conditions are optimal for its survival, healthy growth and development. Family planning, as pointed out by the United Nations Children's Fund (UNICEF), has other health benefits. It can significantly improve the nutritional health of children throughout the developing world. Fewer and more widely spaced births allow mothers more time for breast-feeding and weaning and help prevent the low birth weights which are strongly associated with malnutrition throughout the earliest years of life. Family planning can also improve the quality of life for children. The quality of child care, including play and stimulation as well as health and education, inevitably rises as parents are able to invest more of their time, energy and money in bringing up a smaller number of children (UNICEF, 1992).

The evidence for the potential impact of family planning on child survival is substantive. On the basis of analysis of World Fertility Survey data collected in 41 developing countries, it has been estimated that teenage births carry 24 per cent excess mortality; higher order (7 or more) births, an excess mortality of 21 per cent; and closely spaced births (following a prior birth by less than two years), 52 per cent excess mortality (Hobcraft, 1987).

Birth planning is not enough for child survival. Additional basic elements of a child survival strategy include growth monitoring, oral rehydration, breast-feeding, immunization and food supplementation.

Mothers visiting health services seeking preventive and promotive care for their children should be provided with or have easy access to family planning care.

Place of child survival in a family planning strategy

Does child survival contribute to or is it essential for the success of family planning? This question has received a lot of attention in academic studies and among policy makers. A number of factors can be postulated to link child survival with slowing population growth: the physiological factor (an early infant death will result in the end of breast-feeding and the protection it offers against pregnancy); the replacement factor (the death of a child may prompt the parents to replace the loss with another pregnancy); the insurance factor (parents may insure against anticipated loss by having more children); and the confidence factor (child survival knowledge empowers parents to plan their life and their family). The relation, if any, is difficult to prove in terms of a cause/effect relation. Better child survival can be due to better spacing through family planning; the wider acceptance of family planning can be a result of improved prospects for child survival; or both child survival and family planning may be the result of other underlying factors, such as improved socio-economic conditions and better health services. Moreover, the relation is not consistent (The Lancet, 1990). In Jordan, infant mortality has fallen without a concomitant decline in fertility. In Bangladesh, a country where one fifth of all children die before puberty, the total fertility rate fell from 7.0 to 5.0 between 1975 and 1989.

Although the question of the relation of child survival to family planning can be of academic interest, it is doubtful that it can be appropriate for drawing any policy implications. Whatever the relation may be, both child survival and family planning should be pursued as worthy social goals, without one having to wait for the other. Women should not be denied access to family planning because children die.

At the other extreme is the concern about the demographic implications of child survival. It is sometimes argued that if efforts for child survival are successful, they would ultimately be self-defeating because they would serve only to exacerbate the problem of rapid population growth. The proposition has been put forward that measures for child survival introduced on a public-health scale will only increase the duration of human misery and starvation (King, 1990).

Reduced child mortality, while a desirable social goal in itself, should not be promoted as a necessary and sufficient condition for reduced fertility. Nor should the demographic implications of child survival be accepted as an argument against child survival strategies.

Breast-feeding preferable

Apart from its beneficial effect on child-spacing, scientific evidence has demonstrated the superiority of breast-feeding over other forms of nutrition for the infant.

The prevalence of breast-feeding, especially after three months, is highest in Africa and Asia, and lowest in Europe and the Americas (WHO, 1989a). In industrialized countries, extended breast-feeding is more common among educated, economically advantaged mothers, whereas in developing countries it is greatest among the rural poor, in terms both of prevalence and of duration.

There has been a noticeable improvement in the prevalence and duration of breast-feeding in a number of industrialized countries where a combination of public education, social support and a greater awareness on the part of health workers has made breast-feeding both more attractive and more feasible.

Over the past 30 years, the prevalence of breast-feeding has been falling among the disadvantaged in the developing world, for whom breast-feeding could make a life or death difference. Possible contributing factors are that a large proportion of the population is becoming urbanized, traditional family structures are breaking down and women are entering the labour force in increasing numbers.

If breast-feeding in developing countries continues to decline, the already high rates of infection, retarded growth and development, and mortality and morbidity in infancy and childhood may increase further.

As an example of the interdependence of services, the role of maternity services in protecting, promoting and supporting breast-feeding has recently been highlighted by WHO and UNICEF (WHO, 1989b). It is recommended that every facility providing maternity services and care for newborn infants should:

(a) Have a written breast-feeding policy that is routinely communicated to all health care staff;

(b) Train all health care staff in skills necessary to implement this policy;

(c) Inform all pregnant women about the benefits and management of breast-feeding;

(d) Help mothers initiate breast-feeding within a half-hour of birth;

(e) Show mothers how to breast-feed and how to maintain lactation even if they should be separated from their infants;

(f) Give newborn infants no food or drink other than breast milk, unless medically indicated;

(g) Practice rooming-in and allow mothers and infants to remain together 24 hours a day;

(h) Encourage breast-feeding on demand;

(l) Give no artificial teats or pacifiers (also called "dummies" or "soothers") to breast-feeding infants;

(j) Foster the establishment of breast-feeding support groups and refer mothers to them on discharge from the hospital or clinic.

In developing countries, breast-feeding cannot be excluded from any child health or family planning programme.

Infant mortality: indicators and measurement

WHO and UNICEF have proposed a goal of reduction of 1990 infant mortality rates by one third or to 50 per 1,000 live births, whichever is the greater reduction (United Nations, 1990).

IMR (the number of infant deaths per 1,000 live births) is a good measure of infant and child health care. It is, however, an inadequate measure when the impact of family planning is assessed (Trussell, 1988). Family planning can be expected to decrease teenage births, high-order births and closely spaced births. It will not, however, decrease first births (which are associated with an excess mortality of more than 60 per cent). Because the total number of births will also be reduced through family planning, the relative proportion of first births will increase markedly. The aggregate infant mortality rate may therefore not decrease or may even appear to be increased. This artificial inflation of first births distorts the infant mortality rate, although the actual number of infant deaths decreases. If infant mortality is measured as the number of infant deaths per 1,000 population (rather than live births), the indicator will reflect progress in all components of the child survival strategy.

Infant and child mortality rates inadequately reflect the impact of family planning on infant and child survival. With family planning, the infants and children that are not likely to survive are not born. Using the mortality rate per 1,000 births as the measure, they will be absent not only from the nominator but also from the denominator.

D. REPRODUCTIVE HEALTH: AN INTEGRATED HEALTH-CARE PACKAGE

Traditionally, health aspects of human reproduction have been dealt with through the public health approach of maternal and child health (MCH). Over the past few decades, however, important sociodemo-graphic changes have taken place which have rendered the MCH approach too narrow to meet all the current concerns in this aspect of health. For example, family planning has increasingly become a way of life, with pregnancies fewer and farther between. Women are claiming their right to have their health needs addressed as women and not merely as mothers. Sexually transmitted bacterial and viral infections have assumed epidemic proportions. Adolescents, a rapidly growing population group, have distinctive reproductive health needs which require special attention. Lastly, the reproductive health needs and participation of men also should be considered.

In response to the changed (and changing) situation, the concept of "reproductive health" has emerged, which offers a more comprehensive and integrated approach to the current health needs in human reproduction (Fathalla, 1991).

In the context of the positive definition of health in general, reproductive health in not merely the absence of disease or disorders of the reproductive process. It is a condition in which the reproductive process is accomplished in a state of complete physical, mental and social well-being. This implies that people have the ability to reproduce, that women can go through pregnancy and childbirth safely and that reproduction is carried to a successful outcome, that is, infant and child survival, healthy growth and development. It implies further that people are able to regulate their fertility without risk to their health and that they are able to enjoy mutually fulfilling sexual relations and are safe in having sex.

There is a strong case for integration of the reproductive health care package. The various elements of reproductive health are strongly interrelated, and improvement of one can facilitate the improvement of others (as indeed can the deterioration of one lead to the deterioration of others). Services will be mutually strengthening. They reflect different but closely related needs, concurrent or consecutive, for the same person. Service providers are trained or can be trained to provide several elements of the reproductive health care package. The same infrastructure can support the delivery of several reproductive health services. Fixed costs can be shared resulting in cost efficiency.

Integration versus "bundling" of services

The Concise Oxford Dictionary defines the word "integrate" as "complete (an imperfect thing) by the addition of parts; combine (parts) into a whole". The verb "bundle " (common computer software jargon) is defined as "tie in or make into, a bundle; throw confusedly, esp.".

When services are simply combined or joined together in one way or another, they are not necessarily integrated. In many cases it may be more appropriately labelled as bundling. When services are combined or joined together as a strategy to provide a complete package for services needed, this is integration.

Combining or joining services can operate at three levels: consumers; service providers; and managers. Services may be joined at one level only, at two levels or at the three levels. For the consumers, integration means that they can get the related services they need during the same visit to the health services from the same health provider or a coordinated team of service providers. At the service providers' level, integration means that they have the task of offering not one service but different related services. This definition may or may not coincide with integration from a consumer's perspective. If the same providers are offering the services at different times, this does not respond to the need of the consumers. It only suits the convenience of the providers. At the management level, integration means putting different but related services under the same management. This view may or may not coincide with integration at the service providers' level. Different service providers that are responsible for different services may report to the same management. Alternatively, the same service providers may report to different managements for the different services they offer.

The objective of integration at the consumers level is convenience, better utilization of services and improved quality with continuity and complementarity of the different services offered. The objective of integration at the level of service providers is to exploit the full potential of their capabilities and to leave no excess capacity underutilized. The objective of integration at the management level is to ensure that services shall be mutually strengthening and to achieve cost effectiveness by sharing fixed costs between different services.

Reproductive health care should be provided as an integrated package of services that are mutually strengthening, cost-effective and convenient to the users.

Vertical versus horizontal services

The need for integrated services does not mean that there is no place for vertical services or single-purpose facilities. The department store and the supermarket have not put the specialty shop out of business. Where there is a large demand, a vertical service may prove popular and successful. Also, when special expertise is needed, concentration of the service in one place could result in better quality and could enhance efficiency.

The need for comprehensive health care does not mean an all or none situation. Providing people with some elements of the service is better than providing no services. Services could be built up as resources become available and according to level of need and demand. The best should not be made the enemy of the good.

Family planning for all

The proposition is that the responsible planning of births is one of the most effective and least expensive ways of improving the quality of life on earth - both now and in the future - and that one of the greatest mistakes of these times is the failure to realize this potential (UNICEF, 1992).

The benefits of family planning go far beyond the demographic rationale. It is regrettable that political and religious controversies surrounding the population issue or the abortion issue have sometimes clouded the benefits of family planning for persons, particularly women, desiring to improve their health and the quality of their life. The benefits of family planning should be extended to all. There is enough know-how available to provide quality services that are sensitive to all religious and cultural concerns.

210

It is in this spirit that the WHO has added family planning (the percentage of women of child-bearing age using family planning) as one of the global indicators for monitoring and evaluating progress in the implementation of the health for all strategy (WHO, 1992).

Family planning for all by the year 2000 should be a priority target for all Governments and for the international community. The health of women and children should not be held hostage to any political or ideological debates.

E. SUMMARY

While recognizing the basic role of family planning in any strategy for safe motherhood and child survival, one should not lose sight of the basic rationale of family planning for the health of the woman as a woman and not just as a mother.

Motherhood is a social function and not a disease. Safe motherhood, as an issue, should not be simply discussed under disease morbidity and mortality. It should be discussed on its own or under the role and status of women, as an issue of grave social injustice that should be corrected.

In developing countries, providing family planning services to women that want to avoid unwanted pregnancies is probably saving the life of 1 out of every 100 women. Providing family planning services to women that want to avoid unwanted pregnancies but whose contraceptive needs are not currently met can probably save the lives of no fewer than 900,000 women. Unsafe abortion is one of the great neglected problems of health care in developing countries and is a serious concern to women during their reproductive life Good maternity care does not cover only delivery care and prenatal care. It is not complete without post-partum care and preconceptional care, of which birth planning is a basic component. Progress towards safe motherhood should be measured as the number of maternal deaths per 100,000 women of child-bearing age (maternal mortality rate) or as the lifetime risk of maternal death. The commonly used maternal mortality ratio of deaths over births is inadequate as it measures only obstetric risk.

No safe motherhood strategy can be complete or effective without family planning to help women avoid unwanted pregnancies and to modify the timing of birth to make it more favourable and safer for child-bearing. For pregnancies that are wanted and for unwanted pregnancies that could not be prevented, women must have access to prenatal health care and a trained attendant at delivery. Primary health care must be backed by essential obstetric functions at the first referral level and facilities for emergency transport.

No package for child survival can be adequate without family planning. It will be a grave strategic error to ignore the signals of nature, which has set the planning of births as the basic first-line strategy for child survival. Mothers visiting health services seeking preventive and promotive care for their children should be provided with or have easy access to family planning care. Reduced child mortality, while a desirable social goal in itself, should not be promoted as a necessary and sufficient condition for reduced fertility. Nor should the demographic implications of child survival be accepted as an argument against child survival strategies. In developing countries, breast-feeding cannot be excluded from any child health or family planning programme. Infant and child mortality rates inadequately reflect the impact of family planning on infant and child survival. With family planning, infants and children that are not likely to survive are not born. Using the mortality rate per 1,000 births as the measure, they will be absent not only from the nominator but also from the denominator.

Reproductive health care should be provided as an integrated package of services that are mutually strengthening, cost-effective and convenient to the users.

Family planning for all by the year 2000 should be a priority target for all Governments and for the international community. The health of women and children should not be held hostage to any political or ideological debates.

REFERENCES

Armijo, R., and J. Monreal (1965). The problem of induced abortion in Chile. In "Components of Population Change in Latin America," *The Milbank Memorial Fund Quarterly*, vol. XLIII, No. 4. part 2.

Bongaarts, John (1991). The KAP-gap and the unmet need for contraception. *Population and Development Review* (New York), vol. 17, No. 2 (June), pp. 293-313.

Chen, Lincoln C., and others (1974). Maternal mortality in rural Bangladesh. *Studies in Family Planning* (New York), vol. 5, No. 11 (November), pp. 334-341.

Fathalla, Mahmoud F. (1990). The challenges of safe motherhood. In *Health Care of Women and Children in Developing Countries*, Helen M. Wallace and Kanti Giri, eds. Oakland, California: Third Party Publishing Company.

_____ (1991). Reproductive health: a global overview. *Annals of the New York Academy of Sciences* (New York), vol. 626 (June), pp. 1-10. (1992). Contraception and women's health. *British Medical Bulletin* (London), vol. 49, No. 1 (January), pp. 245-251.

Fortney, Judith A. (1987). The importance of family planning in reducing maternal mortality. *Studies in Family Planning* (New York), vol. 18, No. 2 (March-April), pp. 109-114.

Henshaw, Stanley K. (1990). Induced abortion: a world review, 1990. *Family Planning Perspectives* (New York), vol. 22, No. 2 (March-April), pp. 76-89.

Hertz, Barbara and Anthony R. Measham (1987). *Safe Motherhood Initiative: Proposals for Action*. Washington, D.C.: The World Bank.

Hobcraft, John (1987). Does Family Planning Save Children's Lives? Technical background paper prepared for the International Conference on Better Health for Women and Children through Family Planning, Nairobi, Kenya, 5-9 October, The Population Council.

King, Maurice (1990). Health is a sustainable state. *The Lancet* (London), vol. 336, No. 8716 (15 September), pp. 664-667.

The Lancet (1990). Nothing is unthinkable. *The Lancet* (London), vol. 336, No. 8716 (15 September), pp. 659-660.

Liskin, Laurie (1980). *Complication of Abortion in Developing Countries*. Population Reports, Series F, No. 7. Baltimore, Maryland: The Johns Hopkins University, Population Information Program.

Nortman, Dorothy, Jorge Halvas and Aurora Rabago (1986). A cost-benefit analysis of the Mexican Social Security Administration's family planning program. *Studies in Family Planning* (New York), vol. 17, No. 1 (January-February), pp. 1-6.

Royston, Erica and Sue Armstrong, eds. (1989). *Preventing Maternal Deaths*. Geneva: World Health Organization.

Sadik, Nafis, ed. (1992). *The State of World Population, 1991: Choice or Chance?*. New York: United Nations Population Fund.

Trussell, James (1988). Does family planning reduce infant mortality? An exchange. *Population and Development Review* (New York), vol. 14, No. 1 (March), pp. 171-178.

_____ and Anne R. Pebley (1984). The potential impact of changes in fertility on infant, child and maternal mortality. *Studies in Family Planning* (New York), vol. 15, No. 6 (November-December), pp. 267-280.

United Nations (1984). *Report of the International Conference on Population, 1984. Mexico City, 6-14 August 1984*. Sales No. E.84.XII.8.

_____ (1990). *World Declaration on the Survival, Protection and Development of Children and Plan of Action for Implementing the world Declaration on the Survival, Protection and Development of Children in the 1990s*. Sales No. E.90.XX.USA.1.

United Nations Children's Fund (1992). *The State of the World's Children 1992*. New York: Oxford University Press.

World Health Organization (1989a). The prevalence and duration of breastfeeding. *Weekly Epidemiological Record* (Geneva), vol. 64, No. 42 (October), pp. 321-324.

_____ (1989b). *Protecting, Promoting and Supporting Breastfeeding: The Special Role of Maternity Services*. A joint WHO/UNICEF statement. Geneva.

_____ (1990a). *Abortion: A Tabulation of Available Data on the Frequency and Mortality of Unsafe Abortion*. WHO/MCH/90.14. Geneva.

_____ (1990b). *Global Estimates for Health Situation Assessment and Projections*. WHO/HST/90.2. Geneva.

_____ (1991). New estimates of maternal mortality. *Weekly Epidemiological Record* (Geneva), vol. 66, No. 47, pp. 345-348.

_____ (1992). *Implementation of the Global Strategy for Health for All by the Year 2000, Second Evaluation; Eighth Report on the World Health Situation*. WHO A45/3. Geneva.

XIV. FAMILY PLANNING, SEXUALLY TRANSMITTED DISEASES AND AIDS

Japhet Mati[*]

There are important linkages between family planning, sexually transmitted diseases (STDs) and the acquired immunodeficiency syndrome (AIDS) which suggest that family planning programmes should maintain interest in the control of these diseases. Family planning is practised by sexually active women and men of reproductive age. They are also at risk of coming into contact with STDs as well as heterosexually transmitted human immunodeficiency virus (HIV) infection. Family planning services offer an excellent opportunity to assist in the control of these infections. In most developing countries family planning services are integrated with maternal and child health (MCH), serving women of child-bearing age. Contact can be made with women coming for antenatal care and those bringing their children for immunization and growth monitoring, as well as those coming for family planning services.

Maternal and child health/family planning (MCH/FP) programmes have established an infrastructure which in many countries reaches women living in the rural areas. In addition, counselling is now recognized as an essential part of the family planning information and education. Thus, STD/AIDS information and education can be easily added to the family planning information, education and counselling activities at no additional cost.

Application of the counselling techniques developed for AIDS can also have beneficial effects in the promotion of family planning practice, while the infrastructure created for family planning can be used to avail facilities for early diagnosis and treatment of STDs.

The practice of family planning should play a crucial role in the prevention of vertical transmission of HIV from mother to child, through prevention of pregnancy among women infected with HIV. This is particularly important in sub-Saharan Africa, where according to World Health Organization (WHO) estimates, over 80 per cent of all children with HIV infection acquired during the perinatal period will be born over the next decade (Chin, 1990). Five studies, conducted in Burkina

Faso, Kenya, Rwanda, Zambia and Zaire, reported a similar rate of mother-child transmission of 39 per cent (Prazuck and others, 1990; Datta and others, 1991; Lepage and others, 1991; Hira and others, 1989; Ryder and others, 1988). The high prevalence of infection among women of child-bearing age combined with high fertility rates contribute to the magnitude of perinatally transmitted HIV infection in sub-Saharan Africa.

Another important linkage between family planning and STD/AIDS is that some of the contraceptive methods do have a protective effect against these infections. Use of the condom confers some protection against the transmission of most STDs as well as heterosexually transmitted HIV infection. Certain spermicidal detergents (eg. nonoxynol-9) also have bacterial and virucidal action and may minimize the risk of infection (Louv and others, 1988). Thus, promotion of these family planning methods will assist greatly in the control of STD/HIV infections.

Lastly, fears have been expressed that some of the contraceptive methods (notably, oral contraceptives) may be associated with increased risk of HIV transmission (Plummer and others, 1988; Simonsen and others, 1990). Family planning programmes should be aware of these risks in order to provide appropriate counselling and guidance to the clients. For example, the intra-uterine device (IUD) is known to increase the risk of pelvic inflammatory disease (PID) in those exposed to lower genital tract infections. Hence, women that are at increased risk of contracting STDs (e.g., those having multiple sex partners) need to be advised to use alternative methods for family planning.

A. MAGNITUDE OF THE STD/AIDS PROBLEMS

WHO has recognized the worldwide spread of STDs to be one of the major disappointments in public health in the past two decades (Khanna, Van Look and Griffin, 1992). The "traditional" STDs—gonorrhoea, syphilis

---

*Senior Scientist, Population Sciences, The Rockefeller Foundation, Nairobi, Kenya.

and chancroid–are curable; and in developed countries their incidence has declined. But in the past two decades they have been joined by the "second generation" STDs, which are more difficult to diagnose, treat or control, some having no cure at all at this time. These include chlamydia trachomatis, genital herpes virus, human papilloma virus and HIV. These STDs infections can cause serious complications, which can result in chronic ill health, disability and death. Both the traditional and the second-generation STDs remain prevalent in developing countries. Among some of the reasons that have been advanced for the high prevalence of these infections in developing countries are urbanization, unemployment and poverty, relaxation of the traditional constraints on sexual activity, inadequate facilities for diagnosis and treatment, and emergence of antibiotic-resistant strains. Besides, the age distribution of the population in developing countries is such that there are large numbers of persons in the most sexually active age groups.

The WHO estimates for minimum annual incidence of some STDs worldwide (WHO, 1990) are: gonorrhoea, 25 million; genital chlamydia, 50 million; infectious syphilis, 3.5 million; chancroid, 2 million; trichomoniasis, 120 million; genital herpes, 20 million; genital human papilloma virus, 30 million.

It is estimated that as of early 1992, some 2 million cases of AIDS and from 10 million to12 million HIV infections may have occurred since the beginning of the pandemic in the late 1970s or early 1980s (WHO, 1992). It should be noted that whereas the HIV infection rate appears to be slowing in some industrialized countries, the incidence of new infections is increasing markedly in developing countries, especially in sub-Saharan Africa, but also in Asia, and in Latin America and the Caribbean. It is projected that in the year 2000, a cumulative total from 30 million to 40 million HIV infections and from 12 million to18 million cases of AIDS will have occurred, of which nearly 90 per cent will have occurred in developing countries. By then, 80 per cent of the infections worldwide will be through heterosexual contact. WHO estimates that from 5 million to10 million HIV-infected children will have been born, 80 per cent of them in sub-Saharan Africa (Chin, 1990).

Whereas HIV infection in Europe and Northern America at first affected homosexual men and intravenous drug users, heterosexual transmission is increasingly becoming important. The same pattern is to be seen in some Asian countries, such as Thailand. In sub-Saharan Africa, HIV transmission has been almost entirely heterosexual, although the role of blood transfusion, injections (in medical institutions or by quacks) and skin scarification using contaminated equipment has not been fully evaluated. In Africa, blood transfusion may be the third most important mode of HIV transmission, after heterosexual and perinatal transmission (Jager, Jersild and Emmanuel, 1991). Provision of safe blood transfusion poses great financial and logistic problems to developing countries, and in some of these it will take long before universal screening of all donated blood is possible (Piot and others, 1991; Mhalu and Ryder, 1988). Also, because of the delay in the appearance of the antibody in blood after the infection has taken place, there is a potential risk of passing some infected blood as safe on the ground of a negative antibody test. While these issues need to be addressed, there is need to promote among the medical profession the importance of reducing the need for blood transfusion, through such measures as prevention of anaemia, particularly in children and pregnant women, and improved clinical practices. These concepts will need to be incorporated into the medical and nursing curricula. Means should also be found to make available to developing countries suitable blood substitutes for life-threatening situations.

Because of the potential devastating effects of the AIDS pandemic to human populations, fears have been expressed about the propriety of family planning programmes in those regions hard hit by the pandemic, particularly in Eastern and Middle Africa. However, the demographic rationale apart, it is important to recognize that family planning is also needed for the health and human rights rationale. Family planning services remain important in Africa and other parts of the world, in order to permit couples to plan their family as well as their life, irrespective of the AIDS situation and the level of population growth. To put the impact of AIDS in perspective, WHO has estimated that the upwardly revised projections for AIDS deaths for men, women and children in the decade of the 1990s is equivalent to only about one month's global population growth. Also, the number of women that die each year as a result of unsafe abortion is higher than the number known to have died from AIDS during the 1980s (Khanna, Van Look and Griffin, 1992). Family planning, as mentioned above, should play a crucial role in the prevention of vertical transmission of HIV infection; and while some of the methods (condom and spermicides) remain the only weapon available, other than sexual behavioural change, in the fight against the spread of AIDS.

B. NEED FOR BETTER UNDERSTANDING OF SEXUAL BEHAVIOUR

Research in sexual behaviour has received rather little attention from family planning programmes. By the time the AIDS pandemic appeared, research on sexual behaviour tended to be confined to abstinence practices and adolescent sexuality. A better understanding of sexual behaviour in different sociocultural settings should have important applications in the design and evaluation of educational efforts to encourage self-protective behaviour, a fundamental goal of the campaign against the transmission of STD/AIDS.

Recent research has identified several "high-risk behaviour" groups, (such as prostitutes and their clients, long-distance truck drivers) (Plummer and others, 1991; Mohamed Ali and others, 1990; Nguma, Leshabari and Mpangile, 1990; cited in Caraël, 1991). Common factors in these groups are the number of sex partners, infrequent use of condoms and exposure to other STDs. Available literature suggests that adolescents' behaviour may be described as high risk, since they have been shown to initiate sexual activity early and admit to having had many sex partners. The risk of HIV infection is known to increase with the number of sex partners, and there is evidence that it also linked to certain ulcerative STDs (Plourde and others, 1990). Persons at increased risk of contacting STDs share common sexual behavioural patterns with those at increased risk of HIV infection. This understanding would strengthen the desire for an integrated approach in the control of STDs and AIDS, and the relevance of the involvement of family planning programmes in the common struggle.

There is danger in concentrating STD/AIDS control efforts on these high-risk groups and paying little attention to the "low risk" groups, including the ordinary women attending family planning clinics. Data from Eastern and Middle Africa show that there has been a steady increase in the rates of HIV infection among women attending antenatal clinics and family planning clinics (Ryder and Temmerman, 1991; Mati and others, 1991), thereby rendering the traditional classification of risk categories rather misleading and potentially dangerous. According to Plummer and others (1991), although HIV infection begins by being amplified within the core

groups (high-risk behaviour men and women), it gradually spills over to the lower risk groups, through contact between these in the core group and their regular (low-risk) partners. In a study of women attending family planning clinics in Nairobi (Mati and others, 1991) it was found that, although they did not portray high-risk behaviour (most reported fewer than three lifetime sex partners and the prevalence of STDs was relatively low), the prevalence of HIV infection was, nevertheless, nearly 5 per cent. This means the risk of acquiring HIV infection among such women is determined by the behaviour of their regular sex partners, hence, the need to target men for AIDS control information and counselling.

C. INCLUSION OF STD/AIDS CONTROL MEASURES IN FAMILY PLANNING PROGRAMMES

It has taken a long time for integration of family planning within MCH services to become accepted as the most logical system of extending family planning services to the rural communities in developing countries. In doing so, the cost of setting up a parallel programme for family planning services was avoided, and which has allowed maximization of the utility of physical and human resources. The same argument can be advanced for the inclusion of STD/AIDS control in family planning services in the rural areas.

There were fears that family planning would not receive adequate attention in an integrated system, and similar fears could be expressed with regard to the attention to be given to STD/AIDS control. With good staff training and supervision this obstacle can be overcome. It will be necessary, however, to ensure that the increased work load required by the inclusion of STD/AIDS services shalll not affect the quality of the services being offered, both for family planning and for STD/AIDS control.

It is unfortunate that in some developing countries AIDS control efforts are running parallel to STD control programmes and thereby minimize the impact that limited financial and human resources can have on both AIDS and STDs. Certain STDs (including chancroid, syphilis and gonorrhoea) have been shown to be important risk factors for HIV infection (Laga, Ngila and Goeman, 1991). Hence their control could contribute to the overall prevention of HIV infection. It can be argued from epidemiological principles that because in the general population ("low risk") the prevalence of STDs is not as high as that found among high-risk groups, such as prostitutes, the attributable risk of HIV infection associated with these diseases would be relatively low, so as to make it not cost-effective to invest in STD control as an effort towards control of AIDS. Whereas this may be true in the case of the setting-up of wide-scale screening and treatment facilities for STDs, information, education and counselling about these infections can be provided almost at no additional cost in a joint effort. At the same time, there is need to strengthen STD control programmes for the high-risk groups.

Philosophical differences can be recognized between the family planning and STD/AIDS control approaches to the use of such methods as the condom. Family planning programmes have in the past hesitated to promote the condom not only for contraception but also for protection against STDs, for fear of being seen to be encouraging premarital sex. Thus, for integration of STD/AIDS control into family planning programmes to succeed, it needs to be backed up by re-education of the family planning providers in order to appreciate the wider utility of such methods as the condom and spermicides.

One of the advantages of providing STD/AIDS services at family planning clinics is that in those countries where special centres for STD treatment have been set up, these centres have usually been associated with so much stigma that many persons referred there usually do not go. Therefore, providing services for diagnosis and treatment of STDs at family planning clinics will ensure that treatment is taken. The extent to which STD/AIDS control facilities can be created in such clinics will very much depend upon available resources in the particular country. Emphasis should be on provision of facilities to ensure early diagnosis and treatment (where possible) and appropriate referral. This should involve the setting up of simple laboratories for primary-level diagnosis of such infections as gonorrhoea, trichomoniasis, candidiasis, syphilis and chancroid. These laboratories can be used for provision of Papanicolaou smear screening as well. Cost-effective selective screening should be practised rather than attempts at universal coverage, which few developing countries can afford. It is possible that through the use of a check-list for identification of high-risk behaviour, women at high risk can be identified for screening and some referred to a higher level for more specialized tests. There is need for development of simple quick tests for diagnosis of STDs and HIV at the primary level which can be used in family planning clinics.

The main disadvantage of linking STD/AIDS control to family planning is that these clinics (particularly MCH/FP clinics) are not usually visited by men, and there is little opportunity to reach men with such programmes. In some cultures, men may object to accompanying their spouses to the family planning clinic. Moreover, it is not unusual for a woman to practise family planning without the knowledge of her spouse, in which case she would not be willing to be accompanied to the clinic by her spouse. The compromise will perhaps lie in convincing women of the importance of sharing with their spouses the information and education gained at the clinics, and for the counsellors at these clinics to provide information on those measures that men can take to prevent the spread of STD/AIDS. A WHO document on this issue is an important reference (WHO/MCH/GPA/90.2, 1990). In countries where community-based distribution (CBD) of family planning supplies is practised, it offers additional opportunity to reach men if field activities target men and to provide STD/AIDS information and services (e.g., condom distribution) to men. Social marketing of condoms is another feasible approach.

Linkage of STD/AIDS control with family planning services can be mutually beneficial. The AIDS pandemic has focused attention on the importance of counselling, and several training courses and seminars are available for those involved with AIDS care. Family planning can benefit from the counselling strategies and techniques developed for AIDS. Lastly, as global family planning funding resources diminish, the inclusion of STD/AIDS control in family planning services may provide a new source of funding for certain family planning activities. Bridges are needed between the vertical systems of funding for family planning and STD/AIDS control programmes in developing countries, in order to maximize the effectiveness of the limited financial resources available. In a family planning clinic, facilities already exist for examination of clients for some STDs (e.g., facilities for gynaecological examination and collection of vaginal/cervical specimens, including Pap smears). Considerably fewer additional input items are needed to include STD/AIDS control services in an established family planning clinic than would be needed if these services were confined to other areas in the health system. This situation poses a challenge to the international donor community: the need to broaden their mandates and begin financing family planning and STD/AIDS services in comprehensive programmes.

D. PROMOTION OF CONDOM USE FOR DUAL PROTECTION

Except for those in a few developed countries, such as Japan, family planning programmes have not been able to promote wide utilization of the condom for pregnancy prevention. In the view of the public, condoms have been largely associated with protection against STDs, and are typically used in sexual contacts outside stable unions. This is one of the reasons that although condom use has increased significantly among high-risk groups (especially prostitutes) since the advent of HIV infection control campaigns (Plummer and others, 1991), thet are rarely used by the majority of women attending family planning clinics. In spite of a programme of condom promotion for AIDS control since 1988 at Kenya, a survey carried out in two family planning clinics at Nairobi showed that as late as 1991 only 5 per cent of the clients had ever used a condom and fewer than 2 per cent were currently using this method (Mati and others, 1991).

Family planning services have traditionally recommended the use of condoms when a regular contraceptive method was not practised. There could be considerable difficulties among family planning providers, and among clients as well, with the recommendation that the condom is to be used during sexual intercourse at all times. The other potential difficulty is in appreciating the needs of a woman who is infected with HIV, who not only needs to protect her partner, but who also needs effective contraception. She may need to use a condom as well as another more effective method for pregnancy protection.

Promotion of condom use is one of the few options available in the fight against the spread of STD/HIV. Although abstinence or sex with a mutually faithful uninfected partner is the only totally effective strategy to prevent STD and heterosexually transmitted HIV infections, proper use of a new latex condom with every act of intercourse can reduce, even though it does not eliminate completely, the risk of acquiring HIV. If used properly, condoms provide an effective barrier against sexually transmitted agents. The condom protects the male from infection through contact with secretions of the female genital tract, while for the female the condom protects her from infection transmitted in the semen, urethral discharges or lesions on the penile shaft. The latex condom has been shown to be impermeable to HIV in laboratory tests. Among high-risk groups (e.g. prostitutes) there is significant association between condom use and seronegative status (Mann and others, 1987; Papaevangelou and others, 1988; Krogsgaard and others, 1986; Ngugi and others, 1988). Studies among discordant couples have also shown that condoms could prevent heterosexual transmission of HIV (Feldblum and others, 1990; Kamps and others, 1989).

E. THE FEMALE CONDOM

There is a need for methods that are controlled by the woman, particularly in developing countries where male dominance makes it difficult for women to control the condom use behaviour of male partners. At least three versions of the female condom are in development, two made of latex and a third of plastic. Better refinements of the female condom will improve its acceptability. However, because its cost is likely to be higher than that for the male condom, this may be an important constraint to its widespread availability. It is estimated that, after approval in the United States of America, the plastic female condom will sell at $2 each–from 8 to 20 times the cost of the male condom in developing countries (Network, September 1991).

The plastic female condom, which is expected to be on the market in 1992, consists of a polyurethane plastic tube 17centimeters long, and resembles a large male condom with a ring at both ends. One ring is to be positioned outside the vulva and a second ring inside the vagina, where it settles around the cervix. The insertion of the device is similar to that of the diaphragm. The design of the female condom prevents contact between the vagina and the penis, and separates the vulva from the scrotum and the base of the penis during intercourse.

The plastic condom has undergone extensive testing, and since 1988, more than 1,500 women throughout the world have used it. In the laboratory, the unbroken polyurethane female condom has been shown to be impermeable to organisms smaller than sperm, including HIV, cytomegalo virus (CMV) and hepatitis B virus (Coulter, 1991). Some of the studies have also claimed that the risk of spillage of semen to the vagina is lower with the female condom than with the male. The female condom also compares favourably with male condoms with regard to breakage (Leeper and Conrardy, 1991; Ruminjo, 1991; Monny-Lobe, 1991).

Some of the advantages of the female condom over the male condom include the following:

(*a*) The female condom covers a broader area of the male and female genitalia than the male condom does; it may, therefore, provide better protection against STDs such as Herpes simplex, which can cause lesions in places not covered by the male condom;

(*b*) The female condom may be inserted well in advance of intercourse and thus avoid disruption of the sexual mood;

(*c*) Some men have said they get more pleasure with the female than with the male condom, possibly because the penis moves more freely inside the female condom;

(*d*) The plastic female condom can be use with oil-based lubricants, unlike the latex male condom.

Acceptability studies indicate that the device may be moderately acceptable among a variety of women, ranging from prostitutes to women in long-term monogamous relationships. A study in Kenya conducted by Family Health International suggests that the female condom was somewhat acceptable as a means of family planning (Ruminjo, 1991). In the United States of America, the majority of married or monogamous women participating in an efficacy study rated the female condom more acceptable than other barrier methods, such as the diaphragm or the male condom, and about half said they would continue using the female condom if it were available (Unpublished, quoted by Network, September 1991). In Cameroon, Monny-Lobe (1991) found the female condom to be acceptable among prostitutes, some reporting that they found it easy to use with men that objected to use of the male condom. Thus, the female condom has the potential of being useful in the control of STD/HIV infections.

Some of the disadvantages of the female condom include:

(*a*) Like the male condom, some men and women have complained that it reduces pleasure, and its effectiveness will depend upon the motivation to use it and its being properly used;

(*b*) Some women disliked the shape of the female condom, and some men have reported that they disliked seeing part of the device hanging out of the vagina;

(*c*) Some women have complained that the inner ring caused discomfort;

(*d*) The cost may be prohibitive in developing countries;

(*e*) Because of the high cost of the device, there could be temptation to reuse it; and is the case of prostitutes, this may increase the spread of infections between clients.

Ongoing studies are to establish how long the female condom could be used with repeated washing without increasing the risk of infection transmission. These studies are very important since the female condom can play only a minor role in family planning or STD control in the developing world unless re-use proves feasible and safe (Potts, cited in Network, September 1991a). Accurate data on the efficacy of the female condom in protecting against STD/HIV are also needed.

F. SPERMICIDES AND SPERMICIDAL CONDOM LUBRICANTS

Spermicides constitute a contraceptive option that is entirely under control of the woman. Since they do not require a medical prescription, they are more widely available than most other family planning methods. However, fewer than 3 per cent of family planning users worldwide rely upon spermicides as their primary method. Spermicides usually have been recommended to supplement other methods, such as natural family planning or breast-feeding, or as an adjunct to barrier methods like the condom and diaphragm. Apart from local irritation, reported by a small proportion of users, spermicides are not associated with any notable side-effects. With regard to their efficacy in preventing pregnancy, spermicides have been shown to have a theoretical effectiveness of about 97 per cent, though they have a use effectiveness of only 79 per cent among typical users (Trussel, Hatcher and Cates, 1990). This actual use effectiveness is much lower than that estimated for condoms (88 per cent) and is likely to be as a result of inconsistent use (Network, December 1991). A few minutes are needed to permit the spermicide to dissolve before intercourse commences; otherwise, there is the possibility that sperms reach the cervical canal without contact with the spermicide. It has been shown that nonoxynol-9 (N-9), the active ingredient in most of the spermicides today, cannot penetrate the cervical mucus (Sharman and others, 1986).

Spermicides containing N-9 have been shown *in vitro* to exert protective effects against chlamydia and some viruses, including HIV. As a result of these findings, N-9 has been suggested as one of the agents in the control of HIV transmission. If this proved so clinically, then it would provide a method which is woman-dependent and useful in the prevention of the spread of STD/AIDS. Unfortunately, clinical trials of N-9 spermicides have produced inconsistent results. Data from Kenya, Rwanda and Zambia failed to show any protective effect of N-9 spermicide against HIV infection (Kreis and others, 1989; Kamanga and others, 1991), whereas a study in Cameroon reported a 80 per cent reduction in the rate of HIV infection among consistent users of spermicides (Zekeng and others, 1991).

More recently, Rosenberg and others (1992, cited in *AIDS Weekly*) reported that the contraceptive sponge (impregnated with N-9) and the diaphragm provide more protection against gonorrhoea than the condom does. There was decreased incidence of chlamydia, although this decrease was not statistically significant. In interpreting their findings, the investigators reasoned that it was possible that because women suffer the most severe consequences of STDs–and from contraceptive failure–they are more likely than men to use their method correctly.

There have been a few reports indicating that use of N-9, either for lubrication of condoms or as spermicide, on a repetitive basis (several times a day, as in the case of prostitution), may be associated with microulceration of the vaginal epithelium, which may increase susceptibility to HIV infection (Niruthisard and others, 1991). This irritation seems to be related to the frequency of use and the manner of use, and douching the vagina after every intercourse seemed to protect against the development of colposcopically identifiable lesions (Niruthisard and others, 1991). Vaginal irritation has not featured among women having sexual intercourse less frequently. Thus, when N-9 lubricated condoms and spermicides are used for contraception, they are unlikely to increase the risk of HIV infection.

Other agents that may be useful as spermicides include gossypol and extracts from the neem tree. Gossypol has been shown to have both spermicidal as well as virucidal effect in vitro, and currently a gossypol cream is undergoing clinical trials by the South to South group. The same group is also following on leads suggesting that neem oil has spermicidal and virucidal effects.

G. WHETHER CONTRACEPTIVE PRACTICE CAN INCREASE THE RISK OF HIV INFECTIONS

The question whether contraceptive practice can increase the risk of HIV infection has occupied the minds of researchers as well as those responsible for family planning programmes since a group of investigators at Nairobi first reported an association between the use of oral contraceptive and increased risk of HIV infection in a cohort of prostitutes (Plummer and others, 1988; Simonsen and others, 1990). Fears have been expressed concerning the safety of oral contraceptives and other modern methods of contraception in those countries where transmission of HIV infection is high. Table 24 shows some of the postulated mechanisms for the effect of various contraceptive methods on the risk of HIV infection. Some of these are backed by research while others are purely theoretical. Besides, the distinction between biological effects and behavioural changes that may be associated with the use of an effective method is not easy to make. It can be said immediately that contraceptive methods cannot rank among the important predisposing factors for HIV transmission simply because the prevalence of use of modern contraceptive methods is lowest in the high transmission parts of the world. Some of the biological mechanisms that may play a part in the interaction between hormonal contraceptives and HIV transmission include the following:

(*a*) Increase in the risk of cervical ecotopy which has been associated with use of oral contraceptives (Burns and others, 1975; Goldacre and others, 1978; Oriel and others, 1978; Mati and others, 1991);

(*b*) Increase in leucocytes in vaginal and cervical fluids associated with infections, particularly STDs;

(*c*) Increase in the risk of chlamydia among oral contraceptive users (Hilton and others, 1974; Shafer and others, 1984);

(*d*) Interruption of menstrual patterns and irregular uterine bleeding (leading to a "raw" endometrium) associated with long-acting steroidal methods;

(*e*) Systemic immunological changes associated with steroidal contraceptives (Collins, Campbell and Berber, 1984).

TABLE 24. POSTULATED ASSOCIATIONS BETWEEN CONTRACEPTIVE METHODS AND
TRANSMISSION OF THE HUMAN IMMUNODEFICIENCY VIRUS

Method	Postulated basis for increased risk	Postulated basis for decreased risk
Pill	Cervical ecotopy + STDs (chlamydia) + menstrual spotting, immune suppression	Decreased menstrual bleeding
Injectables and implants	Unsterile equipment Menstrual bleeding	Decreased menstrual bleeding
Intra-uterine devices	STDs + Cervical irritation Uterine inflammation	-
Spermicides	Vaginal/cervical	Antivirucidal action
Condom	Improper use	Mechanical barrier
Voluntary sterilization	Unsterile equipment	-

NOTE: STD = sexually transmitted disease

Data on the association between oral contraceptive use and HIV infection are very limited in quantity and quality.

In sum, present evidence on the relationship between oral contraceptive use and HIV infection remains controversial. A look at those studies with a control group shows that association was apparent among prostitutes but not among women at relatively lower risk of STD/HIV infection. The study by Mati and others (1991) involved a large sample of family planning clients at Nairobi that were at relatively lower risk of STDs compared with the group of women studied by Plummer and others (1988) in the same city. At the moment, it is thought possible that among women exposed to STDs, the added use of oral contraceptives may be associated with increased risk of HIV infection. Consequently, these women these should be advised other methods (not IUD—see above) of contraception. On the other hand, for the general family planning user of oral contraceptives, there seems to be little evidence of increased risk.

The study at Nairobi (Mati and others, 1991) also examined the relation between the use of injectables and IUDs and the risk of HIV infection among the women attending two family planning clinics. None of these methods showed any significant association with in-

creased risk of HIV infection, compared with women that had not used any family planning method at all (injectables, mostly Depo-Provera, odds ratio 1.04, 95 per cent confidence interval, 0.63-1.72; IUD odds ratio 1.20, 95 per cent confidence interval 0.82-1.75). Only 5.2 per cent of the women had ever used a condom, and 1.9 per cent were currently using the condom. This finding could partially explain why condom use was not shown to be associated with significant protection (odds ratio 0.97, 95 per cent confidence interval 0.50-1.90). Other possible explanations include inconsistent and improper use of the condom.

H. BREAST-FEEDING AND HIV INFECTION

Breast milk provides the most balanced and safest food for the infant, and its role in the prevention of gastro-enteritis has been proved. Further, full breast-feeding is associated with prolongation of amenorrhoea, which can provide safe contraception for up to six months post-partum. This means that widespread practice of breast-feeding has the potential of reducing expenditures on contraceptives in developing countries, while at the same time promoting the health of the infant.

Because HIV can pass from blood to breast milk, fears have been expressed that in places where HIV infection is endemic, breast-feeding may be one of the routes for transmission of the virus from infected mothers to their infants. The evidence for transmission of the virus through breast-feeding is limited. In a study in Rwanda (Van de Perre and others, 1991), 219 infants born to 217 at first seronegative mothers were followed up for an average of 16.6 months, during which 16 women seroconverted. Nine of the infants born to these women became HIV-1 positive by polymerase chain reaction, and of these four appeared to have acquired their infection most probably through the mother's breast milk. Similar findings have been reported from the European collaborative study on perinatal transmission. However, a study in Zaire (Ryder and others, 1991) involving 106 children born to largely asymptomatic HIV-1 seropositive women failed to demonstrate a dose-response effect between breast-feeding and HIV-1 transmission, suggesting that the attributable risk is not large for this transmission route.

It is apparent that in developing countries the advantages of breast milk far exceed the possible risk of HIV infection through breast-feeding, and the practice should therefore continue to be promoted. However, it is important for seropositive women to be counselled about the risks involved so that they can make an informed choice.

I. CONCLUSION

Family planning practice is closely linked to sexual behaviour, as is infection with STDs and heterosexually transmitted HIV infection. This important linkage supports the need to broaden the scope of family planning programmes to encompass reproductive health care, including STDs and AIDS control. STD and AIDS control efforts can be enhanced by utilization of the widespread network of family planning clinics, especially in the rural areas of developing countries. These facilities offer unparalleled opportunities to reach women of child-bearing age, when the risk of exposure to STDs and AIDS is greatest. Integration of these services will permit maximization of the limited resources available in developing countries for the control of these infections as well as for family planning. The obvious disadvantage of integration is that services may not reach men directly, and this is an area requiring reorientation of the family planning approach, which has hitherto relied mainly upon contact with women, to permit more interaction with men.

There is need to initiate training activities for the personnel involved in family planning as well as STD/AIDS control services, directed to making them aware of the interrelation between the services they offer, and thereby to promote a closer working relationship. In particular, family planning providers will need to include STD/AIDS information in their information, education and communication material, while the STD/AIDS control workers will need to be able to discuss the contraceptive needs of affected persons. Financial support is urgently needed to assist family planning programmes to add STD/AIDS activities to their existing services. This sevice should, where possible, include selective screening for STDs and AIDS and primary-level treatment facilities for treatable conditions. There is need for the chief players in both the family planning and STD/AIDS programmes to begin coordinating their strategies in developing countries, because this effect can trickle to the grass-roots level. The initiative of integration at the national level can be promoted if the United Nations agencies involved in family planning and those involved in STD and AIDS programmes work closely together. Donor organizations need to broaden their mandates to encompass a broader strategy in their support to programmes in developing countries, and inter-agency coordination at the local level is much needed in order to avoid unnecessary duplication of effort.

Family planning programmes need to recognize the dual advantages associated with condom use –that is, protection against both pregnancy and STD/AIDS–and thus take promotion of its use much more seriously than has been the case so far. Family planning counselling should include discussion on aspects of safer sex, appropriately adapted to suit the needs and behavioural category of the client. Research in sexual behaviour needs to be encouraged in different cultural settings to provide information that can be used in intervention programmes. Already there is evidence that condom use among high risk groups can reduce HIV infection rates. Such efforts need to be applied in national and international programmes. The major constraint in these efforts will remain the cost involved in providing condoms at affordable prices to the consumer.

Lastly, future research in contraceptive technology development should focus on methods that may have additional benefit in the prevention of STD/AIDS, and especially methods that are woman-controlled.

REFERENCES

Burns, D. C., and others (1975). Isolation of chlamydia from women attending clinic for sexually transmitted diseases. *British Journal of Venereal Diseases* (London), (vol. 51, pp. 314-318.

Butlerys, Marc, and others (1990). Risk factors for HIV seropositivity among rural and urban pregnant women in Rwanda. Abstract ThC576. In *VI International Conference on AIDS, San Francisco, 20-24 June 1990; AIDS in the Nineties: From Science to Policy*, vol. 1.

Caraël, Michael, and others (1988). Human immunodeficiency virus transmission among heterosexual couples in Central Africa. *AIDS* (London), vol. 2, No. 3 (June), pp. 201-205.

Chin, James (1990). Current and future dimensions of the HIV/AIDS pandemic in women and children. *The Lancet*, vol. 336, No. 8709 (28 July), pp. 221-224.

Collins, William E., and others (1984). The effect of oral contraceptives in malaria infections in rhesus monkeys. *Bulletin of the World Health Organization* (Geneva), vol. 62, p. 627-637.

Coulter L. (1991). Low particle transmission across polyurethane condoms. Abstract MC3022. In *VII International Conference on AIDS, Florence, June 1991.*

Darrow, William Ward, and others (1988). HIV antibody in 640 US prostitutes with no evidence of introvenous (IV) drug abuse. Abstract 4054. *IV International Conference on AIDS, Stockholm, 12-16 June, 1988,* vol.1. Washington, D.C.: Bio-Data Publishers.

Datta, P., and others (1991). Perinatal HIV-I transmission in Nairobi, Kenya: 5 year follow-up. Abstract MC3. In *VII International Conference on AIDS, Florence, June 1991.*

European Study Group (1989). Risk factors for male to female transmission of HIV. *British Medical Journal* (London), vol. 298, No. 6671, pp. 411-415.

Feldblum, P. J., and others (1990). Anti-HIV efficacy of barrier contraceptives in HIV-discordant couples. Abstract ThC580. In *VI International Conference on AIDS, San Fransisco, 20-24 June 1990; AIDS in the Nineties: From Science to Policy*, vol. 1.

Goldacre, M. J., and others (1978). Epidemiology and clinical significance of cervical erosion in women attending a family planning clinic. *British Medical Journal (London)*, vol. 4, pp. 748-750.

Hilton, A. L., and others (1974). Chlamydia A in the female genital tract. *British Journal of Venereal Diseases* (London), vol. 50, pp. 1-9.

Hira, S. K., and others (1989). Perinatal transmission of HIV-1 infection in Zambia. *British Medical Journal* (London), vol. 299, No. 6710, pp. 1250-1252.

Jager, H., C. Jersild and J. C. Emmanuel (1991). Safe blood transfusion in Africa. *AIDS*, (London) vol. 5, supplement 1), pp. S163-S168.

Kamanga, J. and others (1991). Condom and spermicide use by discordant couples. Paper presented at the Seventh Regular Conference of the African Union Against Veneral Disease and Tieponematoese, Lusaka, Zambia, 17-20 March 1991.

Kamps, B. S., and others (1989). No more seroconversaions among spouses of patients of the Bonn haemophiliac cohort study. Abstract TAP107. In *V International Conference on AIDS, Montreal, 4-9 June 1989; The Scientific and Social Challenge.* Ottawa, Canada: International Development Research Centre.

Khanna, J., P. F. A. Van Look and P. D. Griffin, eds. (1992). *Reproductive Health: A Key to a Brighter Future.* Special Programme of Research, Development and Research Training in Human Reproduction, Biennial Report, 1990-1991. Geneva: World Health Organization.

Kreiss, J., and others (1989). Efficacy of nonoxynol-9 in preventing HIV transmission. Abstract MA036. In *V International Conference on AIDS, Montreal, 4-9 June 1989, The Scientific and Social Challenge.* Ottawa, Canada: International Development Research Centre.

Krogsgaard Kim, and others (1986). Widespread use of condoms and low prevalence of sexually transmitted diseases in Danish non-drug addict prostitutes. *British Medical Journal* (London) vol. 293, No. 6560, pp. 1473-1474.

Laga, M., M. Nzila and J. Goeman (1991). The interrelationship of sexually transmitted diseases and HIV infection: Implications for the control of both epidemics in Africa. *AIDS* (London), vol. 5, supplement 1, pp. S55-S63.

Latif, Ahrmed S., and others (1989). Genital ulcers and transmission of HIV among couples in Zimbabwe. *AIDS* (London), vol. 3, No. 8 (August), pp. 519-523.

Leeper, M. A., and M. Conrardy (1989). Preliminary evaluation of REALITY, a condom for women to wear. *Advances in Contraception* (Dordrect, Netherlands), vol. 5, No. 4, pp. 229-235

Lepage, P., and others (1991). Natural history of HIV-1 infection in children in Rwanda. A prospective cohort study. Abstract WC46. In *VII International Conference on AIDs, Florence, June 1991.*

Louv, William C., and others (1988). A clinical trial of nonoxynol-9 for preventing gonococcal and chlamydial infections. *Journal of Infectious Diseases* (Chicago, Illinois), vol. 158, No. 3 (September), pp. 518-523.

Mann, Jonathan, and others (1987). Condom use and HIV infection among prostitutes in Zaire. *The New England Journal of Medicine* (Boston, Massachusetts), vol. 316, No. 6 (5 February), p. 345.

Mati, J. K. G., and others (1991). Reproductive events, contraceptive use and HIV infection among women users of family planning in Nairobi, Kenya. Abstract WC3095. In *VII International Conference on AIDS, Florence, June.*

Mhalu, F. S., and R. W. Ryder (1988). Blood transfusion and AIDS in the tropics. *Baulliere's Clinical Tropical Medicine and Communicable Diseases* (London), vol. 1, pp. 551-558.

Mohammed Ali, O., and others (1990). Sexual behaviour of long distance truck drivers and their contribution to the spread of STDs and HIV infection in East Africa. Abstract 729. In *VI International Conference on AIDS, San Fransisco 20-24 June 1990; AIDS in the Nineties: From Science to Policy*, vol. 2.

Monny-Lobe (1991). Acceptability of the female condom among a high risk population in Cameroon. Preliminary report submitted to Family Health International.

Musicco, M. for the Italian Partner's Study (1990). Oral contraception, IUD, condom use and man to woman transmission of HIV infection. Abstract ThC 584. In *VI International Conference on AIDS, San Fransisco 20-24 June 1990; AIDS in the Nineties: From Science to Policy*, vol. 1.

Network (1991). *Network: Family Health International* (Durham, North Carolina), vol. 12, No. 2 (September) and No. 3 (December).

Ngugi, E. N., and others (1988). Prevention of transmission of human immunodeficiency virus in Africa: Effectiveness of condom promotion and health education among prostitutes. *The Lancet*, vol. II for 1988, No. 8616 (15 October), pp. 887-890.

Nguma, J. K., M. T. Leshabari and G. S. Mpangile (1991). Implications of the cultural lag in the use of condoms for the prevention of HIV infection among truck drivers in Dar-es-Salaam. Quoted by Michael Caraël and others, *AIDS* (London), vol. 5, supplement 1, pp. S65-S74.

Niruthisard, S., and others (1991). The effects of frequent nonoxynol-o use on vaginal and cervical mucosa. *Journal of Sexually Transmitted Diseases* (Philadelphia, Pennsylvania), vol. 18, No. 3, pp. 176-179.

_____ , and others (1991b). A randomized comparative trial of nonoxynol-9 and placebo for the prevention of gonococcal and chlamydial cervicitics. Abstract C22-028. In *Ninth Meeting of the International Society for STD Research,*

Oriel, J. D., and others (1978). Infection of the uterine cervix with chlamydia trachomatis. *Journal of Infectious Diseases* (Chicago, Illinois), vol. 137, pp. 443-451.

Papaevangelou, G., and others (1988). Education in preventing HIV infection in Greek registered prostitutes. *Journal of Acquired Immune Deficiency Syndromes* (New York), vol. 1, No. 4, pp. 386-389.

Piot, Peter, and others (1991). AIDS in Africa: The first decade and challenges for the 1990s. *AIDS* (London), vol. 5 supplement 1, pp. S1-S5.

Plummer, F., and others (1988). Co-factors in male-female transmission of HIV. Abstract 4554. In *IV International Conference on AIDS, Stockholm 12-16 June*. Washington, D.C.: Bio-Data Publishers.

_____ (1991). The importance of core groups in the epidemiology and control of HIV-1 infection. *AIDS* (London), vol. 5, supplement 1, pp. S169-S176.

Plourde P., and others (1990). Incidence of HIV-1 seroconversion in women with genital ulcers. Abstract ThC571. In *VI International Conference on AIDS, San Fransisco 20-24 June 1990; AIDS in the Nineties: From Science to Policy*, vol. 1.

Prazuck, T., and others (1990). Mother to child transmission of HIV viruses: A cohort study in West Africa (Burkina-Faso). Abstract TH0610. In *VI International Conference on AIDS, San Fransisco 20-24 June 1990; AIDS in the Nineties: From Science to Policy*, vol. 1.

Rosenberg, M., and others (1992). Contraceptive sponge and diaphragm more effective than condom for preventing STDs. *American Journal of Public Health* (Washington, D.C.), vol. 81 (May). ·

Ruminjo, J. (1991). Consumer preference and functionality study of the REALITY condom in a low risk population in Kenya. Final report submitted to Family Health International.

Ryder, Robert W., and M. Temmerman (1991). The effect of HIV-1 infection during pregnancy and the perinatal period on maternal and child health in Africa. *AIDS* (London), vol. 5, supplement 1, pp. S75-S85.

Ryder, Robert W., and others (1988). Perinatal transmission of the human immunodeficiency virus type 1 to infants of seropositive women in Zaire. *The New England Journal Medicine* (Boston, Massachusetts), vol. 320, No. 25 (22 June), pp. 1637-1642.

_____, and others (1991). Evidence from Zaire that breast-feeding by HIV-1 seropositive mothers is not a major route for perinatal HIV-1 transmission but does decrease morbidity. *AIDS* (London), vol. 5, No. 6 (June), pp. 709-714.

Shafer, Mary-Ann, and others (1984). Chlamydia trachomatis: important relationship to race, contraception, lower genital tract infection, and Papanicolaou smear. *Journal of Paediatrics* (St. Louis, Missouri), vol. 104, No. 1 (January), pp. 141-146.

Sharman, Deborah, and others (1986). Comparison of the action of nonoxynol-9 and chlorhexidine on sperm. *Fertility and Sterility*, vol. 45, No. 2 (February), pp. 259-264.

Simonsen, J. Neil, and others (1990). HIV infection among lower socio-economic strata prostitutes in Nairobi. *AIDS* (London), vol. 4, No. 2 (February), pp. 139-144.

Trussel, James, Robert A. Hatcher and Willard Cates, Jr. (1990). Contraceptive failure in the United States: an update. *Studies in Family Planning* (New York), vol. 21, No. 1 (January/February), pp. 51-54.

United States of America, Centers for Disease Control (1992). *AIDS Weekly* (Atlanta, Georgia) (11 May), pp. 7-8.

Van de Perre, Philippe., and others (1991). Postnatal transmission of human immunodeficiency virus type I from mother to infant. *The New England Journal of Medicine*, vol. 325, No. 9 (29 August), pp. 593-599.

World Health Organization (1990). Global estimates for health situation assessment and projections. No. WHO/HST/90.2. Geneva.

_____ (1992). Global strategy for the prevention and control of AIDS 1992 update. Report of the Director-General to the eighty-ninth session of the Executive Board. Geneva.

Zekeng, L., and others (1991). HIV infection and barrier contraception use among high risk women in Cameroon. Abstract C-14-029. In *Ninth Meeting of the International Society for STD Research*.

Part Seven

FAMILY PLANNING AND FAMILY WELL-BEING

XV. FAMILY SIZE, STRUCTURE AND CHILD DEVELOPMENT

Jiang Zhenghua* and Zeng Yi**

The family is the most fundamental unit of society and has long been an important subject of study in social sciences. In common usage, the "family" has at least two clearly distinct meanings, namely, the set of blood relatives and the co-resident domestic group (Brass, 1983). It should be emphasized that the concept of family in this paper refers to "a group of co-residential persons who are related through marriage, blood or adoption".

Filiation has been one of the cornerstones of Chinese society for thousands of years and it is still highly valued in Chinese society. The philosophical ideas of filiation include not only respect for older generations but also the responsibility of children to take care of their parents. Both current marriage law and the current Constitution of China state clearly that children should take care of their parents.

The Chinese family model may be summarized as a "feedback model", which is $F1 \longleftrightarrow F2 \longleftrightarrow F3 \longleftrightarrow Fn$ (F stands for generation). It means that generation $F1$ fosters generation $F2$, generation $F2$ takes care of generation $F1$ when $F1$ is old; the same relation holds between generations $F2$ and $F3$, and so on. In comparison, the Western model may be formulated as a "continued linear model": $F1 \longrightarrow F2 \longrightarrow F3 \longrightarrow Fn$; that is, generation $F1$ fosters generation $F2$ without financial feedback from $F2$ to $F1$, and generation $F2$ fosters generation $F3$, again without financial feedback from $F3$ to $F2$, and so on (Fei, 1983). Consequently, the typical family pattern of Western society is the so-called "nuclear family", consisting of husband, wife and unmarried children. However, the Chinese family structure is not as simple as that, because married children do not necessarily leave the parental home and thus both nuclear and three-generation are important types of family. The Chinese feedback model also implies that the average family size in China is relatively larger than that in Western societies.

Using the most recent data of the 1990 census, this paper tries to investigate the trend of changing family size and structure since the 1950s and their association with population policy.

A. FAMILY SIZE

According to the historical record and some local surveys, the average family size in China in the 1920s, 1930s and 1940s was about 5.3 (statistics of former Ministry of Interior Affairs, cited by Ma, 1984). The average family size in 1953 and 1964 (census years) was 4.3, which is considerably lower than the figures before 1949 (see table 25). This sharp decline was mainly due to the fact that land reform at the beginning of the 1950s broke up some large families, especially those of more than three generations and extended families in which married brothers lived together.

TABLE 25. AVERAGE FAMILY SIZES, CHINA, 1953-1990

Year	Entire country	Rural	Urban
1953	4.30	4.26	4.66
1964	4.29	4.35	4.11
1982	4.43	4.57	3.95
1990	3.97	4.14	3.55

Sources: For 1953, 1964, 1982, Ma Xia, "An analysis on the size of family household and family structure in China", paper prepared for the International Seminar on China's 1982 Population Census, Beijing, 1984, p. 12. For 1990, China, State Statistical Bureau, 1991

The average family size found in the 1982 census was 4.43, which is higher than those in the 1953 and 1964 censuses. The increase in average family size in 1982, compared with 1953 and 1964, cannot be explained by socio-economic development and fertility, declining because the better economic situation and much lower fertility in 1982 would imply a smaller family size under the classic theory. Although there are not enough empirical data to explain this phenomenon

---

*Professor and Director, Population Research Institute, Xi An Jiao Tong University; and Vice Minister, State Family Planning Commission of China, Beijing.
**Professor and Deputy Director, The Institute of Population Research, Peking University.

quantitatively, the authors believe that the serious housing shortage caused by the Cultural Revolution (1966-1976), which stopped most of the social construction during the second half of the 1960s and 1970s, prevented some nuclear units from living away from the larger families.

The average family size decreased to 3.97, as enumerated in the 1990 census. The sharp decrease in family size in 1990 compared with 1982 was mainly caused by the increase in the proportion of small families with one or two children and the improvement of housing supply in the 1980s. At the same time, one should interpret this sharp decline in family size in the 1980s with caution because of possible underenumeration.

As stated in the note "The main figures from the third census of China", published by the State Statistical Bureau, the census enumeration might underestimate the average family size because of an overcount of the number of families. There are two main causes. First, in the so-called "urban-rural" households, some member(s) are state employees, such as local administrative personnel, teachers, doctors or local shop assistants. For those family members that are state employees, commercial food rationing is provided by the State and they have their own separate household register booklets, whereas the other family members (mainly wives and children), that rely upon food provided by local production, have a different type of household register booklet. A family of this type may be registered as two families. Secondly, some urban young couples that are actually living with their parents may have a separate household registration booklet in order to speed up their application for housing and to have some other benefits. The State Statistical Bureau adjusted the 1982 census figure of urban average family size from 3.84 to 3.95 through a post-census sample check. However, the 1990 census figure of urban family size was not adjusted because there was no post-census sample check. Both the 1982 and the 1990 census figures of rural average family size were not adjusted. Obviously, the average family sizes taken from the censuses are somewhat understated. To support this argument, one can compare the average family size from the 1982 One-Per-Thousand Fertility Survey and that from the 1982 census for the provinces of Liaoning, Hebei and Fujian (see table 26). It is generally expected that a well-organized survey, such as China's 1982 One-Per-Thousand Fertility Survey may, in some aspects, pro-

vide more detailed and accurate data than the census. In other aspects, such as total population and its age structure, it may not be the case. The average family size found in the One-Per-Thousand Fertility Survey is consistently higher than that found in the census for all three provinces compared. The present authors believe that the survey figures are more reliable; thus, the average family size in the census is somewhat underestimated. The reason is that the survey interviewers were better trained and were able to follow the instructions correctly; they therefore counted the true membership of each family (Zeng, 1991).

TABLE 26. COMPARISON OF AVERAGE FAMILY SIZE ENUMERATED IN THE 1982 CENSUS AND THE 1982 ONE-PER-THOUSAND FERTILITY SURVEY

Province	Census	Survey
Liaoning	4.1	4.22
Hebei	4.1	4.28
Fujian	4.8	5.02

Sources: For the census, China, State Statistical Bureau, *Important Data From China's Third Population Census*(Beijing, China's Statistical Press, 1982); for the survey, R. Lavely and Li Bohua, "A tentative survey on family structure in Liaoning, Hebei and Fujian provinces, paper presentedat the International Symposium of China's One-Per-Thousand Fertility Survey, Beijing, 1985.

Since there was no adjustment in family size figures in the 1990 census based on a post-census sample check, as was done for the 1982 census figure, the extent of underestimation of family size in the 1990 census figure is more serious than that in 1982.

Whatever the interpretation of the fluctuating figures of average family size enumerated in the four censuses of China from 1953 to 1990 may be, one point is clear: the current average Chinese family is much smaller than before. The remarkable reduction in family size during the 1950s and 1960s, compared with the 1940s and earlier, was obviously due to the far-reaching social structural changes which caused an increase in the proportion of nuclear families, rather than a decline in birth rates, since the fertility level in the 1950s and 1960s did not decrease (the average total fertility rate was 5.44 in the 1940s, 5.88 in the 1950s and 5.68 in the 1960s). The sharp decline in family size in 1990, compared with 1982, 1964 and 1953, is mainly due to the remarkable fertility decline since 1970.

B. FAMILY STRUCTURE

The proportion of nuclear families enumerated in the 1982 census[1] had increased by about 30 percentage points. The families with three or more generations had declined by about 30 percentage points, compared with what was observed in a survey conducted by Li Jing Han in Ding County of Hebei Province in 1930 (quoted by Ma, 1984). Such changes in family structure have a deeply rooted socio-economic background. In old China (before the founding of the People's Republic), parents did not want their children to live separately, because they did not want their land and property to be disintegrated. The poorer families owned very little land and scanty means of production, which were not subdividable. Under the individual ownership system and extremely low productivity levels, it appeared profitable to maintain larger multigeneration families and families in which married brothers lived together. Following the establishment of the People's Republic of China in 1949, feudal landownership was abolished and the land was reallocated. The former large well-to-do families were consequently split up, because they no longer owned large amounts of land, houses and property, which had previously prevented them from disintegrating. The former poorer families received more land, houses and property, as a result of which married brothers were able to live apart and unmarried

brothers were able to get married and leave the large family. Furthermore, as a result of the cooperative movement, members of families no longer worked on the plots of their own land; instead, they worked in a production team under a unified direction, with a collective income distribution. The advantages of maintaining a large family in which married brothers live together, working for private production, was suppressed. Besides, the possible disputes between mothers and daughters-in-law or among sisters-in-law might have encouraged the division of large families (Zeng, 1991).

It is clear that the Chinese family has become a smaller unit and there are fewer extended families, compared with the 1930s. This trend had gone a little bit further in 1990, compared with 1982: the proportion of families with three or more generations declined from 18.8 per cent in 1982 to 18.5 per cent in 1990 (see table 27). However, the three-generation family is still an important family type in China.

For the same reasons that the average family size in the Chinese censuses is likely to be under-estimated, the proportion of families with three or more generations derived from census data may be also somewhat under-estimated. This speculation is supported by the figures given in table 28.

TABLE 27. FAMILY TYPES IN CHINA, 1982 AND 1990

Family type	1982				1990			
	Total	Rural	Town	City	Total	Rural	Town	City
One-person	8.0	7.5	11.3	9.3	6.3	5.9	7.8	7.0
One couple	4.8	4.5	5.7	5.7	6.5	5.8	8.0	8.2
One generation and other relatives and non-relatives	1.2	1.1	1.8	1.7	0.8	0.7	1.2	1.2
Two generations and other relatives and non-relatives	67.3	67.3	67.7	67.2	68.1	68.2	68.5	67.2
Three generations or more	18.7	19.7	13.5	16.1	18.5	19.4	14.4	16.5
TOTAL	100	100	100	100	100	100	100	100

Sources: For 1982, China Population, Statistics Yearbook (Beijing, State Statistical Bureau,1988); for 1987, China, Department of Population Statistics, ed., China 1 per cent Population Sample Survey: National Volume (Beijing, State Statistical Bureau, 1988).

TABLE 28. COMPARISON OF THE PERCENTAGE OF FAMILIES WITH THREE OR MORE GENERATIONS ENUMERATED IN THE 1982 CENSUS AND IN THE 1982 ONE-PER-THOUSAND FERTILITY SURVEY

Province	Census	Survey
Liaoning	14.11	17.45
Hebei	17.07	23.49
Fujian	25.57	29.97

Sources: For the census, China, State Statistical Bureau, *Important Data From China's Third Population Census* (Beijing, China's Statistical Press, 1982); for the survey,
R. Lavely and Li Bohua, "A tentative study on family structure in Liaoning, Hebei and Fujian province", paper presented at the International Symposium on China's One-Per-Thousand Fertility Survey, Beijing, 1985.

The China 1982 census data and other data sources indicate that about 20 per cent of Chinese families are three generations, or other extended families, which is about seven times as large as the percentage in Canada in 1981 (Priest and Pryor, 1984). It should also be pointed out that the majority of the extended families in contemporary China are a three-generation stem family. The joint family with married siblings living together in 1990 only consists of about 1 per cent and the families with four or more generations amount to 0.66 per cent (Zeng, Li and Liang, 1991).

C. RURAL/URBAN DIFFERENCES

In rural areas, the average family size was found to be larger than that in urban areas, except in 1953 (see table 25). The smaller family sizes found in rural areas in 1953 may be explained by the effects of the dramatic change of feudal ownership (land and other property) patterns in the early 1950s. As a result, large families—particularly in the rural areas—were broken up. If one compares rural and urban family sizes in 1982 with those in 1953, onee finds a slight increase in rural family size and a significant decrease in urban family size. This change is due to a more abrupt decline in fertility in urban areas than in rural areas and to the fact that the desirability of having parents live with one married child is more persistent in rural than in urban areas. Urban family size as enumerated in 1982 and 1990 is substantially smaller than rural family size.

Table 27 compares family types in rural areas, towns and cities in 1982 and 1990. In both 1982 and 1990, the proportions of two-generation families in rural areas,

towns and cities were more or less equal. The 1982 proportion of families with three or more generations was much higher in rural areas than in towns and cities, accompanied by a much lower proportion of one-person and one-couple households in rural areas. It is interesting to note that the proportion of families with three or more generation is higher in Chinese cities than in towns. This may have resulted from the fact that the housing shortage is more serious in cities than in towns, preventing some married children from living away from their parents.

D. IMPACT OF POPULATION POLICIES ON FAMILY

As Keyfitz (1984) points out, the political structure of Chinese society is such that policy decisions can be quickly implemented. Hence, population policies exert a major influence on the determinants of family dynamics and population change in China. One might say that demographic determinants, such as current nuptiality and fertility, are to a considerable extent the outcome of population policies. For instance, the "Wan Xi Shao" policies implemented during the 1970s increased the average age at first marriage remarkably, from 20.4 years in 1970 to 22.9 in 1980. When the restriction on age at first marriage of the "Wan Xi Shao" family planning campaign was relaxed by the new marriage law around 1980, the average age at first marriage decreased from 22.8 years in 1980 to 22.2 in 1985 and 22.0 in 1989 (Zeng, 1992).

The current national fertility policy in China is to advocate one child per couple, control of second births and resolute prevention of third births. It does not mean, of course, that all Chinese couples of child-bearing age can have only one child. Since early 1984, revisions of provincial family planning regulations have generally expanded the categories of couples that qualify for approval of a second child. Almost all provinces have begun officially to allow rural couples whose first child was a girl to have a second child. With the approval of the central Government, six provinces and some pioneer areas in the other provinces have even begun to test the policy of universally allowing two children per couple with appropriate spacing.

In the face of the recent increase in birth rates and a large group of young people that are reaching marriageable and child-bearing ages, the Chinese leadership has re-emphasized the importance of controlling population

230

growth and the promotion of one-child families at public occasions. Nevertheless, the Chinese family planning programme is placing emphasis on stabilizing, in the next few years, the existing family planning policies, including continuation of the revisions since 1984 of provincial regulations, which generally expanded the categories of couples that qualify for approval of a second child.

Differential population policies have been implemented in different areas based on the local situation. For instance, control of the second, third and higher order children is stricter in urban areas and for the Han majority than in rural areas and for ethnic minorities. These differential policies are one of the reasons that such large differences in fertility levels and family sizes exist between rural and urban areas and between minorities and the Han majority.

Since the political structure of Chinese society is such that policy decisions can be quickly implemented, population policies have had and will continue to have a major effect on changes in family size and structures in China. The evaluation of the impact of population policies on demographic trends and the investigation of the possible optimal population policies in the future are important tasks for demographers that are interested in population problems in China.

In addition to the impact of population policy on family, socio-economic factors also play important roles in determination of changes in family size and structures. Given the fact that China is a very large country with different socio-economic conditions in various areas, it is a complex undertaking to analyse the relation between the family and social and economic development, which is beyond the scope of this paper. Interested readers may refer to some recent studies on this topic (Guo, 1991; Zeng, Li and Liang, 1992).

E. PROSPECT OF FUTURE CHANGES IN CHINESE FAMILY SIZE AND STRUCTURE

With an efficient family planning network, improved contraceptive services and education, and with people changing attitudes towards a smaller number of desired children, fertility may be expected to continue its gradual fall. One may also expect the mean age at marriage and the divorce level to increase gradually with the process of modernization. Rapid socio-economic development will gradually reduce the desirability of co-residence of parents and married children. Therefore, the Chinese family size will continue to decrease gradually with the expected decrease in fertility and in the desirability of co-residence.

Will desirability of co-residence between parents and married children decrease dramatically? The present authors suspect this is unlikely to occur in the near future. There are two different categories of socio-economic factors which operate in opposite directions.

Among the factors that will reduce the desirability of co-residence are:

(a) Rapid economic development and improvement of education;

(b) Gradual relief of severe housing constraints in the urban areas because of widespread housing construction, which will allow more young people to live away from their parents;

(c) With the relaxation of restrictive policies on migration, the larger scale rural-urban and urban-urban migration;

(d) With the process of urbanization, an increase in the proportion of old people that rely upon pensions or social security, which will reduce the necessity for aged parents to live with one of their married children.

On the other hand, several other factors will be acting in the opposite direction. Under the rural household responsibility system, peasant families became the production unit since the early 1980s. In urban areas, the number of privately owned small shops, restaurants, hotels etc. has grown very rapidly in recent years. Given the very low level of automation in agricultural, private industrial or commercial production, it appears profitable for peasants and privately owned industrial and commercial households in urban areas to maintain larger families for division of labour and mutual care in work and daily life among the family members.

It is unlikely that the pension system will spread rapidly throughout the rural areas in the foreseeable future. A great majority of the peasants will still depend economically upon their children when they are old.

Although there is no officially stated government policy which promotes three-generation families, there is clear evidence that the Chinese Government is in favour of maintaining the three-generation family as a major family type for the sake of upholding a Chinese cultural tradition and because of the savings for the State in old-age care. For instance, both the current Marriage Law and the current Constitution state explicitly that children have full responsibility for caring for their parents in old age.

As discussed earlier, the expected rural-urban or urban-urban migration may result in, on the one hand, the division of some families. On the other hand, it may result in an increase in the number of extended families due to the fact that some young migrants may temporarily live with relatives and because rural-urban migration may aggravate the housing constraints in urban areas.

The ethical tradition of "respect to, and care for the elderly" will continue to play an important role. Psychologically speaking, most old Chinese parents will continue to dislike being alone and prefer to have a warm family environment with a married child and grandchildren living with them. This argument is supported by the persistence of traditional extended families in the industrial-commercial society of Taiwan Province of China.

To summarize, the actual change in Chinese family structure will be the balance of the two above-mentioned categories of factors which act in opposite directions. The authors suspect that the average desirability of co-residence in China is not likely to decrease rapidly; instead, it will decrease slowly in the near future. On the other hand, the tremendous reduced number of births after 1970 will affect the family structure in the coming years. When those children born during the 1970's reach the age of family formation, they will have less chance of leaving the parental home to set up an independent nuclear family, since they have a much smaller number of siblings. Thus, the proportion of nuclear families will decrease in the near future, given that the desirability of co-residence is not likely to decrease dramatically. If fertility continues to drop, when children born under a below-replacement fertility level reach the age of family formation, some elderly parents will not be able to live with any married children even if they wish to do so. At that time, the declining fertility will intensify the effect of the gradually decreasing desirability of co-residence on the increasing proportion of nuclear families. It is, of course, still an open question to what extent and how

quickly the Chinese family structure will change. It certainly deserves further study by both sociologists and demographers.

NOTE

[1] No data on family types were collected in the 1953 and 1964 censuses of China.

REFERENCES

Brass, William (1983). The formal demography of the family: an overview of the proximate determinants. In *The Family*. Occasional paper, No. 31. London: Office of Population Censuses and Surveys.

China, State Statistical Bureau (1982). *Important Data From China's Third Population Census*. Beijing: China's Statistical Press.

_____ (1983). *10 Percent Sampling Tabulation on the 1982 Population Census of the People's Republic of China* (computer tabulation). Beijing: China's Statistical Press. In Chinese.

_____ (1986). Preliminary report on in-depth fertility survey in China, phase 1. Beijing.

_____ (1988a). *China Population Statistics Yearbook, 1988*. Beijing: China's Statistical Press.

_____ (1988b). *Tabulation of China 1% Population Sample Survey: National Volume*. Department of Population Statistics, ed. Beijing: China's Statistical Press.

Fei, Xiaotong (1983). Problem of providing for the senile in the changing family structure. *Journal of Peking University (philosophy and social sciences)* (Beijing), No. 3, pp. 6-15. In Chinese.

Guo, Zhigang (1987). Multivariate statistical analysis of family size in China. *Population and Economics* (Beijing), vol. 8, pp. 40-43.

Jiang, Zhenghua, and others (1984). The preliminary study to the life expectancy at birth for China's population. Paper prepared for the International Seminar on China's 1982 Population Census, Beijing, March.

Keyfitz, Nathan (1984). The population of China. *Scientific American* (New York), vol. 250, No. 2, pp. 22-31.

Lavely, R., and Li Bohua (1985). A tentative survey on family structure in Liaoning, Hebei and Fujian provinces. Paper presented at the International Symposium of China's One-Per-Thousand Fertility Survey, Beijing.

Ma, Xia (1984). An analysis on the size of family household and family structure in China. Paper prepared for the International Seminar on China's 1982 Population Census, Beijing, March.

Priest, G. E., and E. T. Pryor (1984). Household composition: 1982 census of China. Paper prepared for the International Seminar on China's 1982 Population Census, Beijing, March.

Zeng, Yi (1986). Changes in family structure in China: a simulation study. *Population and Development Review* (New York), vol. 12, No. 4 (December), pp. 675-703.

_____, (1992). The methods and application of estimating age at first marriage and the birth intervals using census data. *Population and Economic* (Beijing), vol. 12.

_____ (1991). *Family Dynamics in China: A Life Table Analysis*. Life Course Studies, No. 7. Madison, Wisconsin: The University of Wisconsin Press.

_____, Li Wei and Liang Zhiwu (1992). Current status, regional differentials and dynamic trends of family structure in China. *Journal of Chinese Population Science* (Beijing), vol. 2.

XVI. FERTILITY DECLINE AND FAMILY SUPPORT SYSTEMS

*Napaporn Havanon**

Declines in mortality rates and almost constant high fertility rates have caused rapid population growth in developing countries in Asia, Africa, and Latin America and the Caribbean since the Second World War. Concern over the negative effects of high population growth rates on socio-economic development and the welfare of individuals has led the Governments of a number of developing countries to adopt policies to reduce their rates of population growth. The general strategy followed was to attempt to lower birth rates by encouraging couples to have small families. Lower growth rates brought about by lower fertility were believed to facilitate development at the macro-economic level, while smaller families were thought to benefit both parents and their children directly.

More recently, this conventional argument has been increasingly challenged and currently is the subject of controversy (e.g., National Research Council, 1986). Such debates on population growth and development reflect the complexity of the relation between these two elements and the difficulty of disentangling the causal connections. Nevertheless, efforts to reduce fertility through the promotion of large-scale family programmes are still under way in many countries of the third world. An assessment of whether fertility decline in these developing countries has been beneficial at either the societal or the family level is thus of great importance.

It has been argued that in a situation where family size is a matter of choice, the number of children that a couple has reflects the final outcome of the decision-making process. Confronted with the problems of limited resources, the households will have different strategies to meet their needs. In most cases, the strategy for ensuring household security and welfare involves selecting two or three options rather than making any single, exclusive choice (Grigg, 1980; Morrison, 1980). Long-term planning of family size is one of the mechanisms for adjusting family needs to its available resources. In making a decision about family size, parents seek to maximize both the short- and long-term welfare of the family within a set of resource constraints (Hayami and Kikuchi, 1982; Podhisita, 1985; Havanon, 1992). Short-term concerns are basically related to the immediate consumption and production of a household. These involve parents balancing production and the resources available for the household, on the one hand, and the number of people to support, on the other. Long-term concerns of the family include parents' concerns about the labour requirements of the household, expectations about support from adult children when parents become old and concerns about providing sufficient resources and funds for their children to establish their own lives.

The idea that family size is the final outcome of the decision-making process implies that the relation between family size and family welfare is a product of a deliberate trade-off between the two made at the beginning of child-bearing. In other words, family size and family welfare are simultaneously determined choices. It is thus inappropriate to view the relation between family size and family welfare as if they are causally related. Under this scenario, King (1987) argues that family welfare is the result of decisions by parents and not simply a consequence of family size.

However, one cannot expect that couples can make full calculations about their fertility decisions. How well a couple is able to compare alternative strategies and select the best remains an issue for exploration. The objective of this paper is to explore the linkages between reduced family size and family welfare systems, and to reflect on various aspects of family well-being, including the economic well-being of the family, welfare of the children, wife's employment and parental old-age security.

A. FAMILY SIZE AND ECONOMIC WELL-BEING OF THE HOUSEHOLDS

There has been a considerable debate over whether the number of children is positively or negatively correlated with the economic well-being of the family.

---

*Faculty member, Srinakharinwirot University, Bangkok, Thailand.

Many scholars have argued that within the social settings of less developed countries, children are net economic contributors to parents, at least in the long term (Cain, 1977; Mendosa, 1977; Caldwell, 1977). In these circumstances, couples with many children should eventually be better off than those with only a few. The economic contributions from children may be in the form of providing labour for family farm work or providing income in cash or kind from wage labour in or outside agriculture.

The extent of the contribution that children make to support parents economically will vary with the life cycle stage of both the parents and the children. During the stage when children are still economically dependent, couples with many children may have more financial strains than those with fewer children. However, when some children become young adults or approach the age at which they can make economic contributions to the family, the strains on family finances may be relieved. Thus, in the later stages of the family cycle, couples with more children may be economically better off than those with fewer children. A number of studies in developing countries found that children begin to make contributions to the households at very young ages. For example, in a village in Bangladesh, Cain (1977) found that male children became net producers at age 12 and could compensate for their own cumulative consumption by age 15. Similar results were found in a village in northern Ghana (Mendosa, 1977). Others contend that children are net economic burdens to parents even in peasant societies. A study in a village in rural India found that economic cost outweighed the benefits of sons up to age 16. Even at older ages, local economic opportunities were quite limited, severely restricting sons' abilities to contribute to their parents' income unless urban employment was found (Vlassoff, 1979). Another study that took into account the family cycle stages found that at the aggregate level, the net worth of children in peasant societies was negative. A large family gained economic benefits only in certain stages of the family life cycle (Mueller, 1976).

Studies on the economic utility of children in developing countries have focused on the actual costs and benefits of children and typically estimate from those the net contributions of children to the household economy. Such studies, however, do not provide direct evidence on the relation between the actual number of children and the economic well-being of families. Knowing the net economic contributions of children of different ages to their parents does not inform directly of the cumulative effect of actual family size on economic well-being of the family.

Conceptually, assessments of the economic consequences of family size can be inferred from a comparison of the current socio-economic situations characterizing small and large families while controlling for differences in socio-economic conditions at the beginning of family-building. This model risks not taking into account the simultaneous nature of decisions between family size and choices of levels of economic well-being of the family. However, there are a number of reasons that in many areas of developing countries, family size can be considered a prior determinant of economic well-being. A study purposely designed to assess the impact of family size on wealth accumulation in selected rural villages of Thailand provides a good example of the treatment of family size as largely exogenously determined with respect to levels of accumulated wealth found at the end of a couple's reproductive career. Three main factors are identified (Havanon, Knodel and Sittitrai, 1992).

First, fertility decline in Thailand, as in many other developing countries, has taken place in conjunction with changes in other socio-economic conditions. The emergence of an industrial sector has generated substantial employment and income opportunities outside agriculture, while changes within the agricultural sector have also affected employment opportunities. At the same time, there has been a remarkable change in people's levels of living, accompanied by rising costs of living and of rearing children. Moreover, the causes of social and economic changes tend to be external to ordinary people. It is difficult, if not impossible, for parents to anticipate the future socio-economic situation before their child-bearing begins and accurately to forecast the costs and benefits of having children and other material goods, as well as their resource constraints. For example, some couples may restrict their family size to one or two children due to the lack of job opportunities in the early stage of family-building only to discover later that, when more jobs become available, having fewer children is a disadvantage to family economic well-being.

Secondly, non-economic concerns, such as psychological satisfaction and perceived personal discomfort associated with child-rearing, may play an important role in decision-making about reproductive choices, and economic well-being may not be the primary concern for couples. Some couples may have small families even though the net economic contributions of children are positive, whereas others may have large families even though they anticipate the economic burden of having many children.

Lastly, family size is far from perfectly planned. This is always the case for societies where fertility decline has just begun. Evidence from the Thai study shows that for couples with large families, births were often unplanned and sometimes unwanted. These couples tended to be those that began to have children at a time when modern contraception was only beginning to be known and when thinking about reproductive behaviour as a matter of choice was relatively new. For them, concrete decisions with regard to the number of children to have are likely to have emerged only during the family-building process and within a context of imperfect fertility control.

The measurement of economic well-being is another issue that deserves great attention. The study in rural villages in Thailand used three indicators, including family savings, levels of consumption of modern goods and quality of housing, to reflect the levels of wealth accumulated during the family-building process (Havanon, Knodel and Sittitrai, 1992). The study distinguished economic resources that had been inherited from a couple's parents from wealth that had been accumulated by the couple. The former was treated as part of a couple's economic background, since inherited resources are unlikely to be influenced by the couple's own reproductive behaviour. An assessment of the impact of a reduced number of children on family economic well-being was carried out by comparing couples whose reproductive years corresponded with the decline of fertility in Thailand but who had small and large families. The study found reduced family size to have positive effects on a couple's ability to accumulate wealth. Small-family couples had a better ability to participate in new forms of consumption and thus had more material possessions and better quality houses.

Using consumption patterns as a key measure of family economic well-being runs the risk of selectivity bias. It is possible that differences in consumption patterns between small- and large-family couples may not reflect a greater ability of small-family couples to afford modern goods. It may be that small-family couples are more modern in their tastes than large-family couples. If this is the case, large-family households

should be able to save more than small-family couples because less of their disposable income would be diverted towards consumption. The Thai study found no evidence to suggest that large-family couples are more able to accumulate savings than small-family couples.

An alternative way to assess the impact of family size on economic well-being of the family is to look at the quality of family consumption. Kelley (1981) argues that household saving may not be a good measure of economic well-being in a low-income setting. Formal models assume that larger families save less due to the increasing demands of larger numbers on the household's limited budget. Evidence has shown that within this setting the impact of family size on household spending and saving is relatively small, because low-income families tend to live close to the margin of subsistence. With a larger number of children, these families are likely to adjust the quality of their consumption patterns because these households have relatively little discretion in budget allocations. In a study in a Kenyan urban setting, Kelley (1981) found that the composition of spending for households with larger number of children tends to be in more unproductive forms, away from human capital formation (e.g., schooling, health expenditures) and towards necessities in the form of food and clothing. Kelley concludes that the quality of consumption diminishes with increased family size. For example, the larger family might share more cramped living quarters, consume lower quality items and spend less per capita on food.

B. FAMILY SIZE AND WELFARE OF CHILDREN

Theories of the determinants of fertility presume that the desired number of children is the result of parents balancing the value and cost of children against the resources available for rearing them. The interrelationship of parents and children, therefore, has been studied by sociologists and economists alike in terms of children's costs and benefits for parents. Caldwell (1982), for example, discusses the value and cost of children in terms of the wealth transfer between generations. His theory, known as the "wealth flow theory", is basically concerned with structurally determined relationships between generations. These relationships are believed to determine the nature of the network in which the exchange of goods, services, securities and money takes place. In a pre-transition society, the type of family is an extended one. In this type of family, members of the family share land, budgetary arrangements and/or mutual obligations and guarantees against disaster. In general, different family members enjoy different advantages according to their position in the family structure. The family elder, often the male head of the household, as the dominant decision maker receives higher material advantage, which includes benefits in type and amount of labour activity, in services rendered and in security. In this mode of production, high fertility is advantageous to the elder. Or, as Caldwell notes, the direction of the net wealth flow is from children to parents. A reversal of the flow can occur only when there is a transformation of the familial mode of production to the capitalist mode of production. Mainly, Caldwell proposes that it is the nucleation of the family that leads to the sudden rise in the cost of children and to the subsequent decline in economic returns, particularly in terms of children's labour, to parents. Parents in the capitalist mode of production tend to spend more on their children, particularly for their education, and to demand less from them. The direction of the net wealth flow, then, changes from parents to children.

The model of costs and benefits of children tends to suggest, therefore, that the welfare of their children is not the central issue in parents' motivation to reduce family size. Rather, it is the entire family's welfare that counts in the parents' decision about the number of children they have. The extent to which family size affects children's welfare, independent of other family welfare, has not yet been well documented, either theoretically or empirically. This section explores the linkages between family size and various aspects of children's welfare, including resources provided by parents for children to establish their own lives, children's work roles and their educational opportunities.

In an agricultural society, where land is the most important source of livelihood for people, provision of welfare to their children may be in the form of parents passing their land on to them. Many studies in Thailand, for example, show that parents in rural areas are well aware of the limitations of land resources and are concerned that their land may not be sufficient for subdivision among their children. If they do not limit their family size, their children will be unable to make a living from the land (Knodel, Havanon and Pramualratana, 1984; Podhisita, 1985; Mougne, 1982). However, direct assessment of the impact of family size on the amount of resource transfer, in the form of inheritance, from parents to children is non-existent.

One aspect of children's welfare that has received great attention from a number of studies concerns the linkages between family size and children's work role and educational attainment. There is agreement among many studies that parents send their children to school for both social and economic reasons. The studies in Thailand (Knodel, Havanon and Pramualratana, 1984) and India (Caldwell, Reddy and Caldwell, 1982; Caldwell, Reddy and Caldwell, 1985) show that the motivation for parents to send their children to school arises from the need to find alternative non-agricultural employment. Such employment is seen as a way to improve one's economic situation and to achieve a more comfortable life, and education is considered a prerequisite of those types of jobs. Parents' desire to provide children with a higher degree of education than was typical in the past is interwoven with their aspiration for their children to be socially upwardly mobile so that they will live a more comfortable life when they grow up. Parents believe that better educated children will be in a superior position to obtain more favourable non-farming jobs. Increasing desire for children to be better educated has often been cited as one of the most important factors underlying parents' motivation to limit their family size. According to the new household economics, parents make a trade-off between the number of children they have and the expected investment in education per child. Therefore, larger family size is expected to have a negative impact on children's education.

Extensive empirical assessments of the impact of family size on children's educational attainment in developed countries show the negative link between these two elements (Blake, 1989; Polit, 1982; King, 1987). However, research related to this issue in developing countries is still very scarce due to the limited number of countries that have gone far enough through the process of fertility decline for its consequences to be observed and assessed.

Evidence from Thailand, a developing country that has recently experienced rapid fertility decline, confirms the negative impact of larger family size on children's educational attainment (Knodel and Wongsith, 1991; Knodel, Havanon and Sittitrai, 1990). The explanation for the observed relation relies upon the hypothesis of the dilution model. That is, the larger the number of children, the less the amount of resources (e.g., parental time and attention, material goods, funds) for each child. The study in Thailand provides insights into factors underlying the negative relation between large family size and children's education (Knodel, Havanon and Sittitrai, 1990). In Thai society, the burden of raising children, including paying for their education, falls directly on the parents themselves. Little assistance is provided by other family members and only modest help is given by older siblings to younger siblings among the children themselves. In societies where educational costs are spread among a wider kin network, the trade-off between number of children and resources available may be less significant.

The Thai study also provides useful guidelines for treating the problem of self-selectivity bias when the effects of family size on children's education are estimated. In the survey, couples were asked if they stopped at the number of children they had because they wanted no more or because they were unable to have more. If couples that deliberately have few children are self-selected for characteristics which also lead to educating children at higher levels, the negative relation between family size and educational attainment should exist only for children whose parents deliberately stopped at one or two children, not for children whose parents had small family because they were unable to have more. The results, however, show no difference in the relation between small family size and better educated children for the two types of families.

A general concept in dealing with the relation between schooling and children's work is the incompatibility of roles between these two activities. Time spent in school reduces the child's potential for daily work activities because certain hours are subtracted from the day by school attendance and homework. This hypothesis may not be supported if children do not work for the entire day and if the work they perform does not require a certain schedule. In Bangladesh, Monstead (1977) found that children's work does not seem to decline much for school-going girls, at least under age 16, whereas boys are more frequently relieved from work if they go to school. On the contrary, in Thailand and in southern India, schooling was found to reduce children's help (Knodel, Havanon and Pramualratana, 1984; Caldwell, Reddy and Caldwell, 1985).

Caldwell (1980) notes the effects of the school system on children's welfare not only in terms of changes in activity performed but, more importantly, in terms of changes in children's life experience. School makes children become part of a much larger world. The magnitude of change is so great because it rests not only on what school teaches but on their parents' perceptions. For example, children may cease to perform traditional chores because they feel that such work is at odds with their new learning and status. Parents and other adults may also share some of these feelings and either fail to enforce the performance of traditional work or positively discourage it.

Evidence seems to suggest that the welfare of children, particularly in respect of educational attainment, increases as family size gets smaller. As the opportunity for children to remain in school increases, they are more likely to be relieved from household chores and enter the labour market late, thus enabling them to develop skills and abilities needed for jobs outside home.

C. FAMILY SIZE AND WIFE'S EMPLOYMENT

Although the role of the wife in the family may vary from one society to another, it is well documented that the wife's role is commonly assumed to be confined to the home. In most societies, a wife is expected to be responsible for the domestic caretaking activities regardless of her involvement in economic activities. The husband, in contrast, is normally expected to carry out the role of economic provider. His responsibility for domestic activities, if any, is considered to be only his second priority. Role conflict emerging from the incompatibility between economic and domestic roles, therefore, tends to occur with women rather than with men. One of the most important responsibilities that distracts or deters women from participation in economic activities is the mother's role. Many studies have found that child-bearing and the early stages of child-rearing reduce the amount of time a woman can devote to economic activities.

The linkages between fertility and women's productive role have received significant attention from researchers and public policy makers over the past few decades. Not only would the economic contribution provided by a woman help to increase the economic well-being of the household but, more importantly, participation in economic activities would ensure that the woman is not excluded from developing her potential in the outside work situation as well as having access to and control over economic resources.

Since reproductive and productive activities, in most cases, tend to compete for a woman's limited time, it could be expected that limiting family size would increase women's ability to participate in economic activities. Podhisita and others (1990) propose four situations to describe the potential impact of child-bearing and child-rearing on women's work. First, having a child may prevent a woman from working for the entire period during which she is raising that child. Secondly, the initial demands of caring for a newborn baby may temporarily interrupt a woman's economic activity for only a certain period of time. Once the demands for child care become less intensive, the woman may resume her productive activities. Thirdly, a woman may resume her working activities but child care may interfere with her work by reducing the amount of time that she can devote to it. Lastly, child-bearing and child care may influence a woman's choice of type of work. She may have to switch from jobs that are less compatible to those that are more compatible with rearing children.

A study in two rural areas of Thailand found that reproduction prevents rural Thai women from working for only a very short duration (about three months) following the birth of a child. However, the responsibility of child care interferes with their economic activities, particularly during the breast-feeding period which, on average, takes about 16 months. A nursing mother can fully concentrate on work only when the child is sleeping. Even after the child is weaned, the problem of interference is not completely eliminated. The mother is still periodically distracted from her work by the child's needs. Only when the child has gone to school will the mother be able to participate fully in productive activities (Podhisita and others, 1990). The results from the study in Thailand suggest that, in the short run, reproduction tends to have a significant impact on women's work. The impact of having a child gradually declines as the child approaches school age. Thus, in the long run, the impact of reproduction on women's work may be relatively weak.

It is important to recognize that the linkages between reproduction and women's work found in the study in rural Thailand are relatively straightforward. The fact that almost all rural Thai women work both prior to marriage and during each segment of their child-bearing span, temporarily interrupting from production activities for child-rearing, is not difficult to determine. In some settings, women's participation in work activities is not universal, which leads to the debate about causal direction between women's reproduction and production.

Within this context, women's work may be the determinant of fertility plans. For example, Cramer (1980) found that actual employment reduces actual and expected fertility. Initial employment induces a woman to reduce fertility, which in turn stimulates subsequent employment. In the long run, Cramer (1980) argues that employment is likely to have a substantial effect on fertility. Only in the short run is the causal direction from fertility to employment.

The nature of the linkages between fertility and women's work varies according to a number of factors, including the availability of child care help, substitute labour in the family, availability of jobs, wage levels and cultural norms (King, 1987; Cochrane, Kozel and Alderman, n.d.). In urban areas, where women engage in modern sector employment, role incompatibility between reproduction and production may be stronger than that found in rural areas, where the workplace is often located near the home and work schedules tend to be more flexible. Under the urban scenario, having a baby may deter some women from engaging in economic activities, while, on the other hand, engaging in economic activities may deter other women from child-bearing. In the rural scenario, having a baby may only distract a woman from her work schedule, thus showing only a weak relation between fertility and work.

The availability of child-care help and substitute labour in the family have also been found to be important factors that weaken the negative relation between fertility and women's work (King, 1987). The study in rural Thailand (Podhisita and others, 1990) found a variety of mechanisms that helped minimize the extent to which fertility interrupted or interfered with women's work. Grandparents, close relatives, older children that are not in school, day-care centres and kindergartens can substitute, to some extent, for mothers in taking care of young children, reducing the negative impact of number of children on women's work.

D. FAMILY SIZE AND PARENTAL OLD-AGE SECURITY

Conceptually, parents' concern about the welfare and security of their families and themselves are not restricted to the current consumption of the household, but also include their security and welfare in old age (Caldwell, 1982; Knodel, Havanon and Pramualratana, 1984). In general, in the absence or inadequacy of insurance programmes, families are responsible for taking care of their old members. Many studies in developing countries show that the care of elderly parents by children is an important cultural norm. The expectation of help and support from children is perceived as a fundamental reason for having children. People view children, at least ideally, as a form of security and comfort in old age.

None the less, the adherence to such norms is not perfect or complete. Parents generally do not take their children's support in old age for granted. Social sanctions against those that do not take care of their parents may help maintain the cultural norms to some extent, but parents may prefer to make some arrangements that will ensure their children's support. Nugent (1985) notes that the extent to which children will be loyal to their parents depends upon a number of factors. Parents' capacity to control economic resources and employment opportunities is an important factor. When the household is the unit of production, parents have direct control over employment opportunities of their children; thus, it is not difficult for parents to make arrangements to induce loyal behaviour in their children. Socio-economic changes resulting in a diminishing role of the household as a unit of production may make it more difficult to induce loyalty in children. However, Nugent (1985) argues that even in the presence of outside employment opportunities, the more the economic resources the parents possess, particularly in the form of agricultural land, the more loyal behaviour parents should be able to induce.

Mechanisms traditionally employed by parents in developing countries to induce loyalty in children are largely related to economic resource transfers. White (1976), in his study of rural Java, notes that parents may formally transfer land to children on condition that the children will provide the parents with sufficient rice and cooked food for the remainder of the parents' lifetime. Similarly, in rural Thailand, although parents' lands are supposed to be subdivided and transferred to their children when they establish their own families, parents may arrange to hold some land for themselves. This land may be cultivated jointly by the parents and the children that wish to inherit the land; the produce is usually informally shared between parents and children, even when parents contribute very little to the process of production. In addition, Thai parents tend to keep the family house as their own property during their lifetime. Commonly, the youngest daughter remains in the parental house, assuming the burden of the day-to-day

maintenance of her parents. She inherits the house as part of this arrangement (Moore, 1974).

A qualitative study in rural Thailand also shows that parents do not think that a greater number of children would necessarily bring about an increase in the amount of support received from adult children later in life (Knodel, Havanon and Pramualratana, 1984). Most parents share the opinion that only if their adult children can do well enough economically would they be able to provide economic support for their parents. Providing children either with an adequate education or with economic resources (e.g., cultivated land) is seen as prerequisite to enabling children to gain a better livelihood. With limited resources, having a small number of children would increase the amount of resources available to allow each child to establish their own life more easily.

A direct assessment of the impact of fertility decline on the familial system of support for the elderly has been recently conducted in Thailand (Knodel, Chayovan and Siriboon, 1992). The study shows that fertility decline does not significantly reduce the proportion of the elderly that will co-reside with an adult child. The fact is that even with rapid fertility decline, the proportion of elderly that are likely to be childless or having only one child is still very small. Most elderly parents will have at least two living children and are likely to live with one of them. In this situation, fertility decline may have some impact on the material support provided by children living outside the household since the number of non-co-resident children would decrease substantially. The authors argue, however, that with a small number of children, parents would be able to invest more on the quality of their children's education, which would in turn increase their children's opportunity to achieve economic well-being. All other factors being equal, it could be expected that economically well-off children would be better able to make material contributions to elderly parents than economically worse-off ones.

Results from the studies related to old-age security suggest that in the absence or inadequacy of insurance programmes, as it is the case in most developing countries, children are generally responsible for taking care of their old parents. However, the extent to which the quantity of children would affect parental welfare later in life is unclear. Evidence from some developing countries suggests that the quality of children's resources is an important factor in children's ability to support parents. How parents balance this quality/quantity trade-off in order to maximize the possibility of receiving both material and non-material support from their children is indeed a challenge for further research.

E. DISCUSSION AND IMPLICATIONS

Over the past few decades, a large number of countries in Africa, Asia, Africa, Central America and South America have adopted policies directed tp reducing population growth rates as a means of fostering development and improving family and individual welfare. The objective of this paper is to provide some insights into the impact of fertility decline at the microlevel. It is expected that this understanding will help in assessing the extent to which the rationale behind the policy to reduce fertility and promote family planning is being met.

Family welfare can be broadly defined to include the welfare of the parents, the mother, the individual child and the family as a whole. These various aspects of the welfare of the family and its individual members are actually interrelated. Improvements in one aspect may bring about either a decrease or an increase in other aspects of the welfare system. However, existing studies of the linkages between fertility and family welfare in developing countries tend to focus on each individual aspect of the system, without taking into consideration the mutual relations among those aspects. It is possible that a particular member of the family may improve his/her well-being at the expense of the others. Or some members of the households (such as parents) may try to secure their long-term welfare (that is, old-age security) at the expense of some members' intermediate welfare (e.g., low investment in children's education). Assessments of the interrelations of various aspects of the short-term and long-term welfare of the family and its members deserve special attention for further research on the impact of fertility decline.

Results from the studies purposely designed to assess the impact of fertility decline on family welfare systems in developing countries tend to support the thesis about the negative impact of large family size on the welfare of the family, the parent and the individual child. It is important, however, to recognize that the family welfare system is in itself very broad in scope and that the issues discussed here are limited to only some specific aspects of the welfare system. Some

recommendations for the application of the issues raised in the paper are given below.

One important aspect of the welfare of the family is its economic well-being. There has been considerable research about the economic contribution that children make to the family. The main focus of such studies is to assess the net economic contributions of children of different ages and to determine if the economic costs outweigh the benefits of children. It is assumed that if children are economic contributors to the families, reduced family size would have a negative impact on the economic well-being of the family. Direct assessment of the impact of fertility decline on the actual economic well-being of the family is scarce and limited to only a particular stage of the family life cycle. In addition, most research usually assumes that a household is a cohesive unit in which all family members contribute their separate incomes and resources to the household. It also assumes that each member would subsequently benefit equally from the economic well-being of the household. The extent to which the economic well-being of the whole household is translated into the well-being (that is. the quality of consumption) of its individual members, taking into account differences in sex, age, and/or their relationship to the head of the household, deserves greater attention for future research.

One of the concerns of policies to reduce fertility and promote family planning is children's welfare. Extensive research in developed countries found a negative relation between larger families and several measures of children's welfare, including educational attainment, school achievement, intelligence and physical health (King, 1987). Research in developing countries exploring children's welfare as measured by educational attainment confirms the negative impact of large family size. Other measures have not yet been studied in these countries.

In theory, the welfare of children is affected by a number of factors including: (*a*) household resources; (*b*) household size and composition; (*c*) division of household responsibilities; (*d*) allocation of resources among members; and (*e*) access to resources of family members and relatives residing outside the household (Lloyd and Desai, 1991). The extent to which reduced family size would affect children's welfare, therefore, depends on whether such factors are present or absent in the studied context. Under what circumstances fertility decline would be an advantage or disadvantage for children remains an empirical question for future research.

The cause of fertility decline is another factor that has some implications for children's subsequent well-being. If parents' motivation to have a small family is guided by their aspirations for the quality of their children's well-being, reduced family size would lead to an increase in investment per child. Under this scenario, government policy should also be well prepared to respond to people's needs. For example, if parents' aspiration for their children's education is one of the reasons underlying their fertility decision, long-term plans for making schools available to a large majority of people are of great importance.

The extent to which increased child investment and its relation to the long-term benefit of parents also needs special attention for further research. Past research suggests that sending children to school not only increases the costs of raising children but, in many circumstances, also decreases children's help in domestic and productive activities. However, parents are still willing to send children to school, perhaps, it is argued, for long-term benefits in terms of material support from adult children either while parents can still work or when parents become old. There is a need for more research on the likelihood that children would be willing to support parents and, if so, whether the children are able to provide support for their parents.

Parents may send children to school with the expectation that their children will be able to acquire secure jobs outside agriculture, which, in turn, would increase the children's ability to provide material support for their parents in old age. In a society where children are the main source of old-age security, expansion of the modern sector may be important for economic development policy. Thus, if education does not always guarantee advanced jobs for children, the Government may need to plan for alternative sources of support for its elderly population. Work on the linkages between fertility decline and women's work in countries that have recently experienced fertility decline is extremely is extremely limited. Existing research suggests that childbearing and the early stages of child-rearing interfere with mothers' work. The ways in which families and their individual members, particularly husbands, adjust to mothers' time constraints in different societies and how choices of adjustment in turn affect other aspects of family welfare, such as the household's economic well-being and children's welfare, are important factors for further research.

To the extent that fertility decline has occurred in countries with different levels of socio-economic development, it is important to explore the interweaving of differing levels of socio-economic development, fertility decline and family welfare systems. At what level of socio-economic development would fertility decline become an advantage or disadvantage for parents and their children? To what extent should population policy be accompanied by particular public policies (e.g., expansion of secondary and higher schools, improvements in health-care services and introduction of social security for aging people) so that fertility decline would actually bring about people's well-being?

REFERENCES

Blake, Judith (1989). Number of siblings and educational attainment. *Science* (Washington, D.C.), vol. 245, No. 4913 (7 July), pp. 32-36.
Cain, Mead T. (1977). The economic activities of children in a village in Bangladesh. *Population and Development Review* (New York), vol. 3, No. 3 (September), pp. 201-227.
_____ (1981). Risk and insurance: perspectives on fertility and agrarian change in India and Bangladesh. *Population and Development Review* (New York), vol. 7, No. 3 (September), pp. 435-474.
Caldwell, John C. (1977). The economic rationality of high fertility: an investigation illustrated with Nigerian survey data. *Population Studies* (London), vol. 31, No. 1 (March), pp. 5-27.
_____ (1980). Mass education as a determinant of the timing of fertility decline. *Population and Development Review* (New York), vol. 6, No. 2 (June), pp. 225-255.
_____ (1982). *Theory of Fertility Decline*. New York: Academic Press.
_____ , P. H. Reddy and Pat Caldwell (1982). The causes of demographic change in rural south India: a micro approach. *Population and Development Review* (New York), vol. 8, No. 4 (December), pp. 689-727.
_____ (1985). Educational transition in rural South India. *Population and Development Review* (New York), vol. 11, No. 1 (March), pp. 29-51.
Cochrane, S. H., V. Kozel and H. Alderman (n.d.). Household consequences of high fertility in Pakistan. Unpublished manuscript.
Cramer, James C. (1980). Fertility and female employment: problems of causal direction. *American Sociological Review* (Washington, D.C.), vol. 45, No. 1 (April), pp. 167-190.
Grigg, D. B (1980). *Population Growth and Agrarian Change*. Cambridge, United Kingdom; and New York: Cambridge University Press.
Havanon, Napaporn (1992). Rice, labor and children: an analysis of peasant livelihood strategy in Northeast Thailand. In *Fertility Transitions, Family Structure, and Population Policy*, Calvin Goldscheider, ed. Boulder, Colorado: Westview Press.
_____ , John Knodel and Werasit Sittitrai (1992). The impact of family size on wealth accumulation in rural Thailand. *Population Studies* (London), vol. 46, No. 1 (March), pp. 37-51.

Hayami, Yujiro and Masao Kikuchi (1982). *Asian Village Economy at the Cross Roads: An Economic Approach to Institutional Change*. Tokyo: University of Tokyo Press; and Baltimore, Maryland: The John Hopkins University Press.

Kasarda, John D. (1971). Economic structure and fertility: a comparative analysis. *Demography* (Alexandria, Virginia), vol. 8, No. 3 (August), pp. 307-317.

Kelley, Allen (1981). Demographic impacts on demand patterns in the low-income setting. *Economic Development and Cultural Change* (Chicago, Illinois), vol. 30, No. 1 (October), pp. 1-16.

King, Elizabeth (1987). The effect of family size on family welfare: what do we know? In *Population Growth and Economic Development: Issues and Evidence*, Gale Johnson and Ronald D. Lee, eds. Madison, Wisconsin: The University of Wisconsin Press.

Knodel, John, and Malinee Wongsith (1991). Family size and children's education in Thailand: evidence from a national sample. *Demography* (Alexandria, Virginia), vol. 28, No. 1 (February), pp. 119-131.

Knodel, John, Apichat Chamratrithirong and Nibhon Debavalaya (1987). In *Thailand's Reproductive Revolution: Rapid Fertility Decline in a Third World Setting*. Madison, Wisconsin: The University of Wisconsin Press.

Knodel, John, Napaporn Chayovan and Siriwan Siriboon (1992). The impact of fertility decline on the familial system of support for the elderly: an illustration from Thailand. Research Division Working Paper, No. 36. New York: The Population Council.

Knodel, John, Napaporn Havanon and Anthony Pramualratana (1984). Fertility transition in Thailand: a qualitative analysis. *Population and Development Review* (New York), vol. 10, No. 2 (June), pp. 297-328.

Knodel, John, Napaporn Havanon and Werasit Sittitrai (1990). Family size and the education in the context of rapid fertility decline. *Population and Development Review* (New York), vol. 16, No. 1 (March), pp. 31-62.

Lloyd, Cynthia, and Sonalde Desai (1991). Children living arrangements in comparative perspective. In *Demographic and Health Surveys World Conference, August 5-7, 1991, Washington, DC, Proceedings*, vol. III. Columbia, Maryland: IRD/Macro Systems, Inc.

Mendosa, E. L. (1977). The explanation of high fertility among the Sisala of northern Ghana. In *The Persistence of High Fertility*, vol. 1, *Population Prospects in the Third World*, John C. Caldwell, ed. Canberra: The Australian National University.

Monstead, Mette (1977). The changes division of labor within rural families in Kenya. In *The Persistence of High Fertility*, vol. 1, *Population Prospects in the Third World*, John C. Caldwell ed. Canberra: The Australian National University.

Moore, Frank J. (1974). *Thailand, Its People, Its Society, Its Culture*. New York: HRAF Press.

Morrison, Barrie (1980). Rural household livelihood strategies in Sri Lankan villages. *The Journal of Development Studies* (London), vol. 16 (July), pp. 443-462.

Mougne, Christine (1981). The social and economic correlates of demographic change in a northern Thai community. Unpublished dissertation. University of London, School of Oriental and African Studies.

Mueller, Eva (1976). The economic value of children in peasant agriculture. In *Population and Development*, Ronald Ridker, ed. Baltimore, Maryland: The Johns Hopkins University Press.

National Research Council (1986). *Population Growth and Economic Development: Policy Questions*. Washington D.C.: National Academy Press.

Nugent, Jeffrey B. (1985). The old-age security motive for fertility. *Population and Development Review* (New York), vol. 11, No. 1 (March), pp. 75-97.

Parsons, Donald O. (1984). On the economics of intergenerational control. *Population and Development Review* (New York), vol. 10, No. 1 (March), pp. 41-54.

Podhisita, Chai (1985). Peasant household strategies: a study of production and reproduction in a northeastern Thai village. Doctoral dissertation. Honolulu: University of Hawaii.

_____ , and others (1990). Women's work and family size in rural Thailand. *Asia-Pacific Population Journal* (Bangkok), vol. 5, No. 2 (June), pp. 31-52.

Polit, Denise (1982). Effects of family size: a critical review of literature since 1973. Final report. Washington, D.C.: American Institutes for Research.

Vlassoff, Michael (1979). Labour demand and economic utility of children: a case study in rural India. *Population Studies* (London), vol. 33, No. 3 (November), pp. 415-428.

White, B. (1976). Productivity and reproductivity in a Javanese village. Unpublished doctoral dissertation. New York: Columbia University.

Part Eight

**FUTURE DIRECTION: PEOPLE'S INVOLVEMENT
IN FAMILY PLANNING**

XVII. COMMUNITY PARTICIPATION IN FAMILY PLANNING

*John Cleland**

Public sector provision of family planning services, with attendant education and publicity, originated in Asia in the 1960s. Most of these Asian family planning programmes were centrally organized, had a vertical delivery system that was largely independent of health services, were oriented towards openly quantitative demographic rather than welfare goals, set monthly and annual targets usually expressed in terms of numbers of acceptors and often made use of modest financial incentives to providers and clients. Many programmes achieved spectacular success in reducing fertility but there were also instances of failure, notably the intra-uterine device (IUD) programme in Pakistan in the 1960s and the sterilization campaigns of the Emergency period in India in the 1970s, which may have set back the cause of family planning in that country for half a decade. Moreover, Asian programmes were always vulnerable to criticisms of coercion and of insensitivity to the needs of clients.

The past 15 years have seen an appreciable shift away from endorsement of vertical, target-oriented types of programme among both donors and Governments. In its place has arisen a growing concern that family planning services should be tailored to meet the needs and preferences of their clients. The importance of the "user's perspective" has been emphasized in a number of influential articles (e.g., Zeidenstein, 1980). Accompanying this shift in emphasis has been a strong re-assertion of the need to improve the quality of services (e.g., Bruce, 1990) and a commitment to the concept of community participation.

Parallel changes have occurred in health programmes. The Alma-Ata Declaration of 1978 set an agenda for primary health care, defining the latter as "essential health care made universally accessible to individuals and families in the community by means acceptable to them, through their full participation and at a cost that the community and country can afford". Three years later, the International Conference on Family Planning in the 1980s echoed many of the sentiments of Alma-Ata. The four essential components of an overall strategic approach to family planning in the 1980s were identified in the recommendations of this meeting: user's perspective; community participation; integration of services; and women's status and men's participation. The importance of community participation in family planning was reaffirmed at the International Conference on Population at Mexico City in 1984 and at scores of subsequent smaller meetings. Thus, by the mid-1980s, community participation had become a central theme in the rhetoric of the international family planning movement and similarly in the primary health care movement.

It is not difficult to understand why the idea of community participation proved so attractive to international donors and to Governments. As Stone (1992) points out, it offers the promise of improvements in cost effectiveness. To the extent that communities are willing and able to contribute resources, public sector costs, particularly for outreach services, may be reduced. It also accords with the commonsense view that projects which engage the active participation of clients and potential clients are more likely to succeed than would otherwise be the case. Lastly, the moral appeal of community participation, with its implications of equality and self-reliance, is very strong.

Both for health and even more so for family planning, the community participation concept can draw support from theories of behavioural change (Fincham, 1992). Although mass media can disseminate information quickly and effectively, interpersonal contact is thought to exert much greater influence on behaviour itself. Moreover, local leaders and opinion makers may be far more credible in this regard than outsiders. If the former can be persuaded to support family planning,

*Department of Epidemiology and Population Sciences, London School of Hygiene and Tropical Medicine, London, United Kingdom of Great Britain and Northern Ireland. This paper has benefited from discussion with Henriette Search, Lizzie Smith and Sally Monkman of Marie Stopes International and with Jay Bainbridge and Med Bouzidi of the International Planned Parenthood Federation. Their help is gratefully acknowledged.

legitimation and rapid diffusion of contraceptive practice within communities may occur. Similarly, satisfied users of family planning are known to be effective agents of persuasion. Community participation offers the promise that these benign forces of change can be harnessed and encouraged.

Despite its personal and private nature, family planning, like most other forms of behaviour, is subject to social norms and peer pressure. It requires considerable courage to be the first person in a village to adopt modern contraception and an equal degree of courage to persist with use in the face of disapproval. Once again, community participation offered the possibility of a change in community norms and in the climate of opinion, in such a way that these social obstacles to mass use of contraception could be removed. It is thus no surprise that community participation received such strong endorsement as a cornerstone of family planning in the 1980s.

The purpose of this paper is to assess the substance behind the rhetoric. In the following pages, an attempt is made to answer the following questions. What does community participation mean? What are its strengths and limitations with regard to family planning? What empirical evidence is available to evaluate its contribution? What elements of the community participation idea can and should infuse family planning endeavours of the future; and, conversely, which elements can be rejected as impractical, excessively expensive or even counter-productive?

A. THE MEANING OF COMMUNITY PARTICIPATION

Many attempts have been made to define the somewhat elusive concept of community participation in relation to family planning and health (e.g. Askew, 1989; Rifkin, 1990; WHO, 1991). The common ingredients of most definitions are: (a) community assessment of needs and priorities; (b) community involvement in design, management and implementation of activities; (c) use of community resources; (d) an emphasis on self-reliance and self-help.

It is clear that the common thread linking these ingredients is empowerment: the notion that communities should have a degree of control over the nature of development goals and implementation of activities. It is equally clear that participation is a matter of degree

rather than of absolutes, and it is not difficult to construct a ranking from low level forms of participation—that is, modest empowerment—to high-level forms. Examples of low-level participation might include consultation with the community over the siting of a clinic or choice of local candidates for training as voluntary workers. Intermediate-level participation might take the form of a local consultative committee with a mandate to represent the community in discussions with district health or family planning managers. Higher level participation would include community involvement, not only in project implementation but in planning and design of activities, leading to active control of resources and how they are spent.

These distinctions between low, intermediate and high levels of participation correspond closely to the typology offered by the World Health Organization (WHO) (1991). In this paper, three types of participation are identified. The first type, contributory participation, denotes a situation where communities contribute to preset programmes by means of labour, cash or provision of other resources, such as land. Thus, most systems involving community volunteers fall into this category. The second type is termed "organizational participation", where formal structures exist to facilitate contributions by the community. Village committees and clients' groups fall into this category. The last type of participation is termed "empowerment", where the community exercises control over activities.

Few commentators have specified what they mean by the term "community". The most common assumption appears to be one of the geographical community, a rural village or a low-income urban neighbourhood, for instance. Such communities always contain both sexes and people of all ages. They are also often varied in terms of socio-economic, religious and even cultural groups. As Foster (1982) points out, the view that geographical communities are homogeneous in their needs, priorities and outlooks may often be false, thereby undermining the feasibility and potential of community participation.

It is thus valuable, in any discussion of participation, to broaden the concept of community to embrace naturally occurring groupings of people that come together because of some common characteristic, need or interest. Examples of such social communities include political and religious groups, women's groups, schoolchildren, employees of large companies, adolescent groups and so on. Communities of this type tend to be less disparate in outlook and priorities than geographical communities; hence, participation may be a more realistic proposition.

B. COMMUNITY VIEWS ON PARTICIPATION

As implied in the introduction, resolutions passed at international meetings blithely assume that community members will welcome participation if the opportunity is offered. With regard to primary health care, this assumption has come under repeated recent attack (e.g., Stone, 1992). It has been stressed that the concepts of equality and self-reliance that underlie the idea of participation reflect Western values that have little meaning for many communities. Although all communities want services that meet their requirements and that are accessible and affordable, it does not follow that they feel the need for active involvement in planning or decision-making.

In a rare empirical investigation of the views of communities on participation in family planning activities, Askew, Castro-Perez and Sonthrondhada (1991) undertook a study in four countries: Mexico; Sri Lanka; Thailand; and Zimbabwe. In each country, interviews and focus group discussions were held with several different types of persons: community leaders; community members; community-based distributors; and programme staff. The main conclusion of the study was that there was a marked difference in attitude between those involved in planning and implementing programmes and those in the community that might be expected to participate. Managers and staff vigorously supported the principles of decentralization and community involvement in planning and implementation. They also valued strong leadership and well-defined staff responsibilities, which act against participation.

Community members also favoured participation in the abstract. When concrete issues were explored, however, it became clear that most did not welcome an active role for themselves. Although they were willing to attend local meetings or talk to neighbours about family planning, further involvement was not viewed positively. They felt that participation in planning or decision-making, for instance, should be left to existing community leaders.

These findings forewarn that the community participation ideal may not be as popular with the individuals, that are expected to devote their time, energy and perhaps money, as it is among top government staff and members of international organizations.

C. OPTIMAL CONDITIONS FOR SUCCESSFUL COMMUNITY PARTICIPATION

Flowing from the definition of community participation provided earlier, it is relatively easy to identify the optimal conditions for successful participation:

(a) The proposed activity is seen by the community as high priority;

(b) The activity will benefit most community members;

(c) The activity is not controversial;

(d) Available community resources are appropriate and relevant to the achievement of goals;

(e) The amount of outside technical expertise and resources required is modest;

(f) Management of the activity is relatively straightforward;

(g) The outside sponsor is able and willing to accommodate local variability in design and implementation.

Most of these seven conditions are self-evidently beneficial for successful community participation. Obviously, activities that meet a high-priority expressed need, that will benefit the entire community and that are socially and culturally acceptable are more likely to evoke and mobilize full participation than activities that are of low priority, contentious or will benefit only a few. Similarly, activities that are amenable to local management and are undemanding in external resources and skills are more likely to engender community empowerment than those which are complex to manage and require heavy inputs of skills or financial resources from outside.

How does family planning rate when assessed by these seven conditions? In relation to priority, it fares rather badly. Few communities, whether defined geographically or socially, would attach a top priority to fertility regulation. Employment, education, health, sanitation, irrigation and a myriad of other day-to-day concerns are much more likely than family planning to be perceived as pressing problems and thus as high priorities for community action. It is for this reason, perhaps, that most attempts to promote family planning through community participation are integrated projects. Family planning is typically combined with health, income-generating schemes or informal education in order to broaden the appeal and raise the priority of the project in the eyes of the community.

The second condition concerns the spread of anticipated benefits. Here again, family planning does not rate well, as it brings direct and immediate benefit only to the minority of sexually active persons desiring to delay or avoid pregnancy. This is a severe disadvantage. By comparison, a new road, a processing plant, water-supply, a health centre or a school brings the promise of much wider benefits, thus making it easier to engage the interest and active involvement of the community. Moreover, family planning may lack a ready appeal to community élites, typically older men whose wives have passed beyond the reproductive age span. There may be exceptions. In certain circumstances, the entire community may realize that a continued increase in numbers jeopardizes the welfare of all community members. This sentiment is most likely to arise among isolated communities living in fragile ecosystems. The anthropological literature provides numerous instances of traditional societies, living in such circumstances, that had a very acute sense of the need for population control. The Rendille camel herders of northern Kenya, Eskimo groups and the Tikopian Islanders of the South Pacific are among many examples (Douglas, 1966). The methods of population control, however, employed by these populations were often far removed from contraception. Infanticide was probably the most prevalent mechanism, followed by abortion and severe restrictions on marriage.

Few current family planning programmes attempt to mobilize participation on the basis of a demographic threat to entire community. Indeed, in most circumstances, such an approach would not carry weight because of extensive migration possibilities and because of the existence of modes of production that could, if necessary, support much larger human populations.

The third condition concerns controversiality. Once again, this factor tends to operate against community participation in family planning. The advent of contraception in most societies arouses antagonism as well as support. Opposition may be based on religious belief, conservatism, fears about abuse of new sexual freedoms or health concerns. Doubts about the moral or social acceptability of contraception may act synergistically with health concerns and rumours about side-effects to create a formidable barrier to adoption of family planning. It is for this reason that contraceptive practice may be slow to spread even in societies where many women report that they want no more children. Knowledge of methods and access to services are often insufficient to convert latent demand into correspondingly appropriate behaviour. Legitimation of family planning is also required.

Initial resistance to the idea of family planning and to particular methods represents an obstacle to many forms of community participation. Such activities as health, water and sanitation rarely arouse hostility, though communities may be suspicious of the means (e.g., immunization of children). It is therefore relatively easy to obtain widespread community support. In contrast, family planning may be a divisive factor in communities rather than an activity round which members can come together in common purpose.

Next is the issue of appropriateness and relevance of community resources. Community participation is most likely to succeed when the community already possesses many of the skills and resources to achieve the objective. It is clear that clinic and hospital-based family planning services offer little scope for active community participation. But, of course, mass provision of family planning has moved steadily away from this medical model of service delivery to community-based systems of motivation, distribution and referral. This unshackling of family planning from the strait-jacket of a narrowly clinical approach has vastly increased the potential for true community participation. Communities can hold their own supplies of contraceptives; can nominate community members for training in contraceptive distribution, counselling or referral; and can help in many other ways to ensure that appropriate advice, information and supplies shall be available at the grass-roots level.

There are limits, of course, to the degree of self-reliance that can be achieved. Supplies of contraceptives have to be obtained from outside agencies; and such methods as voluntary surgical sterilization, IUDs and injectables require properly trained medical or paramedical staff. Thus, community participation in family planning has to be a partnership between a sponsor with access to supplies and skills and the community that can perform other functions. The balance of responsibilities can be equitable. Practical aspects of family planning are not formidably complicated. The main contraindications to specific methods, their possible side-effects and their relative advantages and disadvantages are all relatively easy to convey to untrained, lay persons. There is thus no sound reason that the community need be the junior and subordinate partner in any family planning project.

Similarly, the sixth condition, simplicity of management, favours participation in family planning. The need for large capital sums, expensive equipment and managerial rigour all tend to undermine the capacity of communities to develop and implement projects with a high degree of self-reliance. Family planning activities require none of these factors.

The last condition, however, often does act to stifle community participation in family planning. Intrinsic to the concept of participation is the freedom of communities to play a role in determining the nature and range of activities. This freedom implies that the outside sponsor has to tolerate, or even encourage, local variability in procedures, personnel, style of supervision and so on. Government family planning bureaucracies rarely possess this flexibility. Hence high-level community participation involving government agencies is rare. Participatory schemes are more evident in the private sector, because non-governmental organizations tend to be more adaptable and accommodating to community wishes than are government departments.

To conclude this section, family planning has some attributes that favour community participation and others that make participation more difficult. Community participation projects are unlikely to succeed unless their sponsors have a firm and realistic grasp of both the advantages and disadvantages.

D. PARTICIPATION WITH NON-GOVERNMENTAL ORGANIZATIONS: THE IPPF CASE-STUDIES

Rifkin (1990) notes that even though much has been written about community participation, remarkably few studies have attempted to analyse the concept and its implications for programmes. Scrutiny of the main journals on family planning confirms this diagnosis. There are, for instance, very few articles on the subject in either *Studies in Family Planning* or in *International Family Planning Perspectives*. One possible reason for this neglect is that many community participation projects are sponsored by small, local non-governmental organizations, which have few links to larger international organizations and little need or desire to publicize their efforts internationally.

The single most important exception is a series of studies commissioned by the International Planned Parenthood Federation (IPPF). Seven community participation schemes in five Southern Asian countries (Bangladesh, India, Pakistan, Nepal and Sri Lanka) were studied in detail, resulting in the publication of five reports by IPPF. A comparative analysis was also published (Askew, 1988 and 1989), together with a document that summarizes organization and managerial recommendations (Askew and Lenton, 1987). This section of the paper describes and interprets the results of the investigations by Askew and his associates.

Five of the seven projects involved geographically compact areas. The other two (in Pakistan and Sri Lanka) were nationwide schemes in which community participation had been introduced as a key feature. The Sri Lankan scheme involved the training of a team of young female volunteers that acted as a resource for family planning and health. Each team was supervised by a local committee. The Pakistan project comprised a network of family welfare centres which offered health and family planning services. Each centre was managed by a committee of local male leaders.

The emphasis of the case-studies was on organizational features. No formal attempt was made to evaluate impact or cost. Each study was essentially qualitative and involved extensive, unstructured interviewing with community members, local leaders and project staff.

None of the seven projects were concerned with family planning alone. Most (six cases) included maternal and child health; a majority (five cases) had a literacy component; other activities included horticulture (four cases), poultry raising (three cases) and irrigation (three cases). The main reason for integration was the view that family planning alone could not meet the priority needs of the community nor could it, by itself, achieve much in terms of health or welfare. Moreover, it was felt that such activities as poultry-raising offered more potential for true community participation than did family planning. Although these case-studies are drawn from only one region of the world, it seems reasonable to conclude that integration is a common characteristic of community participation projects that involve family planning. This feature immediately raises the issues of the ultimate aims of these projects and their cost effectiveness. If the aim is conceived narrowly in terms of contraceptive prevalence and reduction of unwanted pregnancies or the fertility rate, then it appears unlikely that any project studied was cost-effective. However, family planning is only a means to more general goals of better health and welfare. Thus, it could be argued that project evaluation in narrow demographic terms is inappropriate. Furthermore, community participation can be seen as a desirable goal in its own right. The lesson seems to be that integrated community participation schemes should specify their goals and, from the outset, identify the criteria by which their degree of success can be judged.

All seven projects were sponsored solely or partially by family planning associations. In two cases, the initiative for the project came from local residents, but in the other five cases, the initiative came either from associations or IPPF.

All projects had community committees, often one for management and another for implementation. Selection criteria for membership were usually vague and, in reality, members were typically selected by leaders or élites. As a result, most committee members were elderly men, who were not very knowledgable about family planning. Few committees met regularly; their aims and responsibilities were unclear and, in the judgement of Askew and associates, most were ineffective.

The real powers of planning and decision-making lay in the hands of full-time, salaried project officers, usually employees of the family planning associations. In three cases, a project officer was stationed in the community. In the other cases, the project was run by staff from a district or branch office. Indeed, the main function of the committees appears to have been to endorse and legitimize the decisions of the project officers. Askew and associates speculate on the reasons for this power imbalance. They identify three main reasons: project officers prefer to dominate the planning and management of activities; committee members had little experience of running projects; and sponsoring organizations, which had to provide resources, were not willing to hand over too much power to the communities themselves.

Most projects had two types of workers—full-time, salaried workers and volunteers. The duties of the latter group were usually restricted to educational and motivational activities. Their performance varied greatly. Success in this regard appeared to depend upon the extent of support and status given to them. Thus, regular meetings and provision of training, not surprisingly, enhanced the willingness of the volunteers to work.

Collective action by communities for irrigation, road works and similar labour-intensive activities were common. For family planning, such collective action is not relevant. However, group or communities meetings to discuss family planning were a regular feature.

The amount of resources contributed by the community varied widely, depending, as noted above, upon the success in retaining the active interest and commitment of volunteers. No project, however, was able to raise a significant financial contribution from communities and thus none became self-reliant in this regard.

None of the projects could provide the entire range of family planning services, although in Pakistan, all main methods were available, apart from voluntary surgical contraception. One of the most valuable aspects of most projects was to form links with service organizations, in either the public or the private sector.

In his conclusion, Askew (1989) is careful to stress the many positive features of the seven projects. All of them, for instance, reported higher levels of contraceptive use than found at the national level; and all had achieved a degree of community participation. However, it is clear from the analysis that the participation was at a low level, implying modest empowerment of communities and a very unequal partnership between the community and the sponsor. Two root causes are identified. First, the evidence of the study suggests that it is both difficult and costly to provide sufficient incentives to motivate broad-based and sustained participation in planning and implementing provision of family planning services. Secondly, the family planning associations saw participation primarily as a means to extend outreach information and services. The associations acknowledged the desirability of community empowerment but felt that the achievement of this goal lay beyond their skills and responsibility. In a sobering last sentence, Askew warns that greater care must be taken then in preparing policy and program statements about community participation, because rhetoric implying greater self-reliance could encourage initiatives that are doomed to fail. . ." (1989, p. 202).

E. PARTICIPATION WITH THE PUBLIC SECTOR: THE ASIAN FIVE-COUNTRY STUDY

A second major study of community participation complements the IPPF-sponsored study, because it concentrates on participation within the context of national family planning programmes. Its objectives were to assess the current extent of and future scope for community participation within the national programmes of five mainly Eastern and South-eastern Asian countries (Bangladesh, China, the Philippines, the Republic of Korea and Thailand). The study involved extensive interviewing of policy makers, programme managers, fieldworkers, community leaders and community members in each country. Five reports were issued and an overview of results was published (Askew and Khan, 1990).

All five programmes had elements of decentralization, whereby key decisions about implementation were taken at the district or provincial level. And all had community-based services delivered by full- or part-time outreach workers, often supported by voluntary workers. The latter group thus constitutes one form of active participation. A second form of participation, present in all five countries, was the periodic involvement of local leaders in educational and motivational activities. A fourth mode, organized local committees, was found to be effective only in China. Each village in China has a managerial group, comprising the village head, the local doctor, the local family planning supervisor and representatives from the Women's Federation and the Young Communist League. This group is responsible for translating targets received from above into local plans, organizing motivation, provision of services and collecting information. This arrangement clearly contains elements of community participation and empowerment, because tactics and implementation are decided at the local level. At the same time, the setting of priorities and goals remains firmly in the hands of higher level officials and the real purpose of local committees is to ensure that national policies shall be implemented efficiently at local level. The involvement of village heads in the Indonesian family planning programme may be interpreted in a similar way.

With the partial exception of China, participation by communities in planning and decision-making was found to be almost non-existent. Although village committees, social welfare organizations and women's groups had been used frequently for promotional activities, they remained outside the formal programme structure and did not contribute to decision-making. None of the family planning programmes had developed formal mechanisms by which the views of communities could influence planning or priorities. These functions remained exclusively the domain of professional staff and managers.

Despite this lack of high-level community participation, opinions on the topic were by no means hostile. Most policy makers and managers welcomed the idea of greater community involvement, because they thought that it would increase the acceptability of family planning and utilization of services. Fieldworkers were also generally favourable, although those in the Republic of Korea and Thailand wished to maintain control of planning and targets, because they felt that these matters lay beyond the capabilities of community members. The opinions of community members themselves were also canvassed. Again there was a positive attitude, although most respondents interpreted community participation to mean the involvement of local leaders or midwives only. They also expressed the need for a system of compensation or incentives in support of such active involvement. The conclusions of Askew and Khan (1990) are rather pessimistic with regard to the prospects of higher level community participation in these five national family planning programmes. They doubt that family planning, by itself, is sufficiently compelling to kindle a strong interest in active community participation, unless considerable financial benefits are offered. Furthermore, the tightly controlled organizational structure of the programmes, which are designed to meet national targets, is seen as unconducive to genuine participation.

F. PARTICIPATION IN THE INDONESIAN FAMILY PLANNING PROGRAMME

It is a pity that the study sponsored by the United Nations Population Fund (UNFPA), discussed in the preceding section, did not include Indonesia, because the family planning programme in this county places a particularly explicit emphasis on community participation. As described by Suyono and Shutt (1989), the programme originated in 1970 as a set of clinic-based activities. In 1975, fieldworkers, previously attached to Ministry of Health clinics, were given community-based responsibilities. One of their early duties was to identify, within each village, family planning acceptors who were willing to serve as motivators and contraceptive depot holders on a voluntary basis. A second related initiative was to establish family planning acceptor groups, each containing from 15 to 60 members. The mother's clubs in the Republic of Korea constitute perhaps the closest equivalent found in another country. In 1979, the National Family Planning Coordinating Board (BKKBN) began to provide small loans to the acceptor groups, which in turn established rules of eligibility for granting subloans to members. In 1989, there were 145,780 groups in Indonesia, with 19,410 income-generating schemes. The idea appears similar to the credit arrangements of the Grameen Bank and the Bangladesh Rural Advancement Committee (BRAC), whicj also target women with little access to commercial bank credit and which also use the discipline of a local group to enforce repayment by individuals. In the case of the Grameen Bank and BRAC, however, family planning is a part of an overall aim of improving levels of living, whereas in Indonesia, family planning is a central focus of the credit groups.

Other ways in which community participation. in family planning in Indonesia is being encouraged include the family welfare and youth movements. The goal of the family welfare movement is to expand and enhance the role and status of women, and family planning is one of its 10 main activities. The youth movement is a joint activity of the National Youth Organization and BKKBN; its objective is to accelerate the acceptance of the small, prosperous family norm, particularly among single persons. The long-term goal is to train about 95,000 youth cadres, who will then assist family planning fieldworkers to involve young people from the community in the overall family planning movement.

Several of these moves towards greater integration of family planning with other activities and towards greater community participation were consolidated in the Integrated Family Planning and Health Service programme (Posyandu). This programme was introduced in 1984 and has five components: immunization; prenatal care; management of diarrhoeal diseases;

nutrition; and family planning. Activities are run largely by communities, by means of monthly meetings. By the end of 1988, it was claimed that 85 per cent of children under age 5 were covered by Posyandu services.

The BKKBN planning process also allows for a community contribution. Top-down annual plans and targets are set at annual family planning meetings attended by a range of departments. These are then modified by BKKBN and transmitted to lower levels, in the form of local targets, operational and budget guidelines and programme priorities. There then begins a complementary process of bottom-up planning by which programme proposals flow up from village, subdistrict and regency levels. They are consolidated at the provincial level and forwarded to BKKBN headquarters. Presumably, a stage of reconciliation then takes place when discrepancies between centralized and local plans are resolved.

In the absence of any detailed objective evaluation, it is difficult to assess the degree of success achieved by the various form of community participation in Indonesia. Nevertheless, it is clear from this simple description that the Indonesian programme has gone much further than any other to translate mere rhetoric into substance. The pioneering role of BKKBN in this regard may prove difficult for others to follow. The Indonesian family planning organization is exceptionally confident, strong and imaginative, partially because it can demonstrate its achievements. Moreover, Indonesia has unusually effective structures of local government. No other family planning organization has evolved so rapidly from a single-purpose, vertical programme into a broad social movement that encompasses aspects of health, nutrition, loans, income-generating schemes and women's activities.

G. PARTICIPATION BY SOCIAL GROUPS AND ORGANIZATIONS

Earlier in this paper, it was stressed that high-level community participation in family planning may be more realistic when communities are defined as pre-existing organizations or groupings rather than as geographical clusters. Examples include religious groups, women's organizations, mutual credit societies, youth federations, farmer's cooperatives and a myriad of other institutions that exist in every society. Such groups offer the following advantage for community participation:

(*a*) Members tend to be reasonably homogeneous in terms of interests, outlook and social identification;

(*b*) The ethos of many groups is already one of mutual help and thus groups may be receptive to the idea of participation;

(*c*) Similarly, many groups are already self-reliant in some regard, depending upon members' contributions in cash or kind to support activities;

(*d*) Most groups already possess means of rapid communication among members;

(*e*) To varying degrees, groups already possess some structure and leadership, thereby facilitating contact and subsequent decision-making;

(*f*) Because of this pre-existing structure, an equal partnership with a specialist family planning agency leading to high-level participation is a realistic proposition.

Because of these advantages, community participation in family planning is much more likely to be successful among pre-existing groups or organizations than among geographical communities such as villages or urban neighbourhoods. Social groups constitute valuable entry points for family planning organizations and offer considerable potential for quick and cost-effective dissemination of messages and, to some extent, services.

Sexually active, unmarried persons constitute a target population for family planning advice and supplies where a community participation approach may be particularly rewarding. This is so because conventional service delivery channels, such as specialist family planning clinics, maternal and child clinics or community-based distribution, are often inappropriate. There are many imaginative schemes (though few are properly documented) for reaching the adolescent population through some form of participation. Many use peer leaders: carefully selected young people who receive specialist training and then play a major role in education, counselling and referral among their peers. One of the better known examples is the Community Youth Programme at Monterrey, Mexico (Townsend and others, 1987). Through an operations research design, the cost effectiveness of a peer leader scheme was compared with two other approaches (integrated youth centres and community-based distribution). Under the peer scheme, young volunteers provided sex and family

planning education in schools and other places where young people congregate. Persons interested in learning more or in obtaining contraceptive supplies were referred to professional counsellors. Results of the experiment suggest that the peer scheme was the most cost-effective approach and was particularly successful in reaching young males, hitherto ill-served in terms of family planning access.

Examples of similar schemes come from Kenya and Sierra Leone. The Sierra Leone project was sponsored by the Home Economics Association and funded by Marie Stopes International. Its objective was to promote responsible sexual behaviour among young people by means of a self-sustaining youth-to-youth information programme. At the heart of the project was the training of 200 out-of-school youth leaders, selected from a variety of groups, including social and sports clubs, and religious groups. The project also organized a series of football and volleyball competitive matches and disco sessions, which provided opportunities for extensive publicity. In the Kenya project, the entry point was the National Youth Service, a vocational training scheme for young people. Again, a peer family life education scheme was introduced by training adolescents and providing them with condoms to distribute.

The central principle underlying these youth-oriented projects is that the family planning agency acts as a catalyst for change but relies largely upon group members to act as the agents of change. The agency does not need to create its own infrastructure or a large organization. Rather, it provides specialist training to representatives of the target group.

Despite their apparent success, doubts remain about the sustainability of such schemes that rely upon volunteers. In the context of primary health care, Walt, Perera and Heggenhougen (1989) conclude that large-scale use of volunteers is only successful in the long term under special conditions. Volunteer schemes appear to work best when a strong cultural value is attached to the idea of service; the scheme has a strong, and often authoritarian, underlying structure; and there are large numbers of unemployed young men and women to act as volunteers.

H. CONCLUSION AND FUTURE DIRECTIONS

The main conclusions of this brief review are given below.

Despite more than a decade of international and national statements about the need for community participation in family planning, few family planning organizations, whether in the public or the private sector, have developed effective channels through which the wishes or priorities of their clientele can impinge upon decision-making and resource allocation.

Most large family planning organizations still have structural features of centralized target-setting, hierarchy and standardization that are directly antithetical to community participation. Specifically, these large organizations cannot accommodate the wide local variations in goals and procedures that are an inevitable consequences of community participation.

Much of the rhetoric about community participation has paid little attention to its practical implications. At best, the rhetoric has been superficial. At worst, it has been hypocritical.

The interest of communities to participate actively in family planning services is more modest and conditional than has often been assumed.

As a consequence of the foregoing points, genuine participation by communities in the decision-making, planning and resource allocation processes of family planning programmes is not taking place on a substantial scale.

Most community participation projects with a geographical focus have adopted an integrated approach, whereby family planning is offered alongside health, nutrition, income-generating and other activities. The impact of these integrated projects is difficult to evaluate but their cost effectiveness in terms of fertility regulation alone is probably low. In view of tightening resources for family planning, such integrated projects do not appear to be a sound investment.

The most common form of active community participation is the recruitment and training of local voluntary workers, whose duties typically include counselling, referral and holding supplies of non-clinical contraceptives. Experience, both in the field of primary health care and in family planning, suggests that it is difficult to sustain a large-scale, effective volunteer effort. Schemes of this nature eventually require incentives (financial or otherwise) to retain the interest and commitment of volunteers.

The most promising prospects for community participation concern pre-existing social organizations, such as women's and youth groups, cooperatives and religious organizations. Because such groupings often already possess elements of self-reliance and internal structure, they are potentially powerful vehicles for participation in family planning activities, in equal partnership with specialist family planning agencies.

These rather pessimistic conclusions need not imply gloom and despondency. There are many alternative ways to ensure that family planning programmes shall become more responsive to the needs, preferences and priorities of the people whom they intended to serve. Such responsiveness is surely more fundamental to success than the principle of participation. Greater community consultation may be a more realistic slogan for the 1990s than greater community participation. This implies the training of family planning managers so that they are better able to access the views of their own clientele. Applied research also has a vital role to play: in the initial assessment of needs, in evaluating existing services and in suggesting improvements. Qualitative or interactive methods—focus group discussions, unstructured interviewing and observation —will prove more useful in this regard than structured surveys. The latter have a rather poor record in disclosing dissatisfaction with services and are ill-equipped to suggest improvements.

Another cause for optimism is the often overlooked success of family planning during the past 30 years. Existing programmes have clearly met the need of individuals, perhaps not in an ideal way but certainly in an acceptable manner. The surest way of finding out what people and communities really want is to encourage a diversity of approaches and then to place additional resources behind those that work. The least responsive programmes are those which are most centralized and monolithic in their ideology and structure, because they stifle new approaches. Here again, there are grounds for optimism. Most family planning programmes are now much more pluralistic than they were 10 years ago. For instance, Governments are now more likely to welcome non-governmental organizations as partners rather than as opponents than hitherto. Pluralism is perhaps the best long-term guarantee that family planning programmes will serve rather than impose upon individuals.

REFERENCES

Askew, Ian (1988). *A Comparative Analysis of Community Participation Projects in South Asia with Policy and Programme Recommendation for Family Planning Associations.* London: International Planned Parenthood Federation.

_____ (1989). Organizing community participation in family planning projects in South Asia. *Studies in Family Planning* (New York), vol. 20, No. 4 (July-August), pp. 185-202.

_____ , and Aminur Rohman Khan (1990). Community participation in national family planning programs: some organizational issues. *Studies in Family Planning* (New York), vol. 21, No. 3 (May-June), pp. 127-142.

Askew, Ian, and Cliff Lenton (1987). *Community Participation in Family Planning: Some Suggestions for Organizational Development and Management Change.* London: International Planned Parenthood Federation.

_____ , R. Castro-Perez and A. Soonthrondhada (1991). *To What Extent Should Communities Participate in Family Planning Programmes? A Report of a Study in Four Countries.* Population Studies Centre Occasional Report, No. 12. Exeter, United Kingdom: Exeter University.

Bruce, Judith (1990). Fundamental elements of the quality of care: a simple framework. *Studies in Family Planning* (New York), vol. 21, No. 2 (March/April), pp. 61-91.

Douglas, Mary (1966). Population control in primitive groups. *British Journal of Sociology* (London), vol. XVII, No. 3, pp. 263-273.

Fincham, S. (1992). Community health promotion programs. *Social Science and Medicine* (Tarrytown, New York), vol. 35, No. 3, pp. 239-250.

Foster, George (1982). Community development and primary health care: their conceptual similarities. *Medical Anthropology* (New York), vol. 6, No. 3, pp. 183-195.

Rifkin, Susan B. (1990). *Community Participation in Maternal and Child Health/Family Planning Programmes.* Geneva: World Health Organization.

Stone, L. (1992). Cultural influences in community participation in health. *Social Science and Medicine* (Tarrytown, New York), vol. 35, No. 4, pp. 408-418.

Suyono, Haryono, and M. S. Shutt (1989). *Strategic Planning and Management of Population Programmes: Indonesia Case Study.* Jakarta: National Family Planning Coordinating Board.

Townsend, John, and others (1987). Sex education and family planning services for young adults: alternative urban strategies in Mexico. *Studies in Family Planning* (New York), vol. 18, No. 2 (March-April), pp. 103-108.

Walt, Gill, Myrtle Perera and Kris Heggenhougen (1989). Are large scale volunteer community health worker programmes feasible? The case of Sri Lanka. *Social Science and Medicine* (Tarrytown, New York), vol. 29, No. 5, pp. 599-608.

World Health Organization (1991). *Community Involvement in Health Development: Challenging Health Services.* Technical Report Series, No. 809. Geneva.

Zeidenstein, George (1980). The user perspective: an evolutionary step in contraceptive service programs. *Studies in Family Planning* (New York), vol. 11, No. 1 (January-February), pp. 24-28.

255

XVIII. COST OF CONTRACEPTIVE SUPPLIES AND SERVICES AND COST-SHARING

Maureen A. Lewis[*]

Over the past few decades world population growth has slowed and fertility rates have declined remarkably. Contraceptive use has contributed to that decline and will continue to be a central component of couples' decision-making with regard to family size. The difference now is that despite the rapid decline in mothers' desired number of children, the size of the reproductive age cohort is enormous, reflecting earlier high fertility and implying continued population momentum. Meeting future contraceptive demands will require improved efficiency and targeting of public resources, broader financing from users and greater reliance on private providers.

Historically, contraceptive needs have been perceived as requiring public resources and intervention, and international donors and national treasuries have financed contraceptive services in many countries, particularly in Asia. However, as total demand rises due to demographic factors and shifts in household demand, real international resources—that is, adjusted for inflation—are declining, leaving a gap between estimated demand and available services. This situation is in sharp contrast to earlier periods when funding outstripped the abilities of countries to absorb them effectively.[1] Various options are available to reassess public priorities and activities to maximize returns on investments in family planning and to spread the costs across a broader range of providers and payers. These options are explored in this paper.

Although the divergence appears serious, the degree to which demand can be met is a function of the level of effective demand (number of population at risk that want to contracept), household resources and access of the population to contraceptive services. The role of government resources is particularly relevant to persons that have inadequate or incorrect information about contraception (e.g., adolescents) or those that cannot afford or cannot reach services.[2] Ascertaining how to husband public resources and to target high-risk populations is therefore key to coping with reduced funds and growing demand, as is stimulating individuals and institutions to share the costs of family planning.

This paper first summarizes the projected demand, the costs of reaching potential users and the strengths and weaknesses of existing cost information. The second half considers the financing options for reaching contraceptive goals, including assessment of international resources, demand and current purchasing patterns in developing countries.

A. FUTURE DEMAND FOR CONTRACEPTION

By the year 2000, population in the developing world is expected to increase to 3.8 billion, a 29 per cent increase from 1988 (Janowitz, Bratt and Fried, 1992).[3] The highest rates of growth are in sub-Saharan Africa (42 per cent) and the Middle East (35 per cent), and the slowest rates are in Asia (26 per cent) and Latin America (25 per cent).[4] The rates of growth of married women of reproductive age (MWRA) are expected to exceed overall rates of population growth due to declining fertility and the resultant age distribution biased towards the reproductive ages. As a result, the number of contraceptive users was expected to increase from 192 million in 1980 to 365 million in 1990 and is projected to increase to 514 million by the year 2000 (Cochrane, 1992).

The raw figures tell only part of the story. Although the proportion of women wanting no more children and the proportion wishing to delay their next birth have consistently increased over time, the number of unwanted births has remained high: during the mid-1980s, there were an estimated 11.6 million excess births in an average year (Boulier, 1985). This excess of births is

[*]Economist, Population and Human Resource Division, The World Bank, Washington, D.C., United States of America. The reviews by S. Cochrane, G. Kenney, J. De Beyer and S. Rosenhouse are gratefully acknowledged; and S. Cochrane's assistance to this endeavour is particularly appreciated. Vivian Hon provided able research assistance and Patricia Trapani managed production of the manuscript. The author is, of course, responsible for any errors or omissions.

commonly referred to as the "unmet need for contraception". The highest excess fertility was in Asia and Latin America (more than 20 per cent of all births) and the lowest in sub-Saharan Africa (fewer than 10 per cent) (Boulier, 1985).

The definition and extent of unmet need is difficult to measure but key to projections of family planning demand. Boulier (1985) distinguishes between unmet need for limiting and for spacing births, where limiting refers to "married women wanting no more children who are exposed to the risk of pregnancy and are not using contraception", and spacing to "married women seeking to delay wanted pregnancies who are exposed to the risk of pregnancy and are not using contraception". Upward biases are introduced by underestimates of traditional contraceptive methods (e.g., rhythm and withdrawal) and by the framing of the question concerning intention (rather than the desire) to have another child. Biases in these figures has led to a more refined method for measuring "total potential demand", a composite of "health risk criteria" and "preference criteria".[5]

Total potential demand adjusts "gross" unmet need downward. Comparisons of the somewhat dated Boulier (1985) estimates with updated and adjusted total potential demand figures for three Asian countries shows sharp divergence. Table 29 compares projected unmet total potential demand in 1988 for Thailand, Indonesia and the Philippines (8, 13 and 21.4 per cent, respectively) with Boulier's early 1980s gross unmet need figures and his breakdowns for limiting and spacing (Casterline, 1991; Westoff, 1988; Bongaarts, 1991). The decline can be attributed to measurement differences or expanded services, and the data do not explain the relative importance of either. Since estimates for all countries are not available, these are illustrative examples to demonstrate the importance of using careful measures to avoid inflating unmet need estimates. The extent of demand depends upon a myriad factors and its estimation goes beyond the scope of this paper, but it is important to keep in mind that gross estimates of unmet need are generally upwardly biased and should be tempered accordingly in projecting likely future demand for contraceptives.

TABLE 29. ALTERNATIVE MEASURES OF UNMET NEED, SELECTED COUNTRIES

	Thailand 1981	Indonesia 1976	Philippines 1978
Gross unmet need	20-26	20-31	19-49
Unmet need for limiting	3.5-17.3	10.0-15.3	11.1-29.0
Unmet need for spacing	29-31	10.0-15.3	11.1-29.0

Sources: John Bongaarts, "The KAP-gap and the unmet need for contraception", Population and Development Review (New York), vol. 17, No. 2 (June 1991), pp. 293-313; Bryan Boulier, Evaluating Unmet Need for Contraception: Estimates for Thirty-six Developing Countries, World Bank Staff Working Papers, No. 678, Population and Development Series, No. 3 (Washington, D.C., The World Bank, 1985); Charles Westoff, "The potential demand for family planning: a new measure of unmet need", International Family Planning Perspectives (New York), vol. 14, No. 2 (June 1988), pp. 225-232.

Only couples that want to space or limit births will seek contraception. The financial implications of meeting that estimated unmet need hinge on the costs of family planning services, another complex measurement that is discussed in the next section.

B. COSTS OF FAMILY PLANNING

Estimating costs provides a basis for projecting resource needs for meeting family planning demand and for improving the efficiency and effectiveness of family

planning investments, an element that becomes increasingly important as public resources decline and potential demand rises. Cost data form the basis for: (a) determining the financial requirements of the system; (b) measuring relative efficiency and cost effectiveness of public and private delivery that can guide decisions about how to best achieve objectives; and (c) designing cost containment strategies to husband resources and operate efficiently. At the facility level, cost information is equally important for identifying the savings and managerial modifications needed to improve productivity and to clarify how resources can most appropriately be allocated. Thus, cost data provide the raw material for guiding both policy and programme decision-making and are a necessary ingredient in estimating financial needs of family planning investments over the next decade.

Providing a single "cost" for family planning is complicated by a number of problems: (a) the financing and delivery of services are often different entities encompassing private for-profit institutions, private non-profit groups (e.g., non-governmental organizations), public entities from the national Government or state/provincial government and international donors whose funding is obtained from industrialized Governments; (b) each contraceptive method has different costs associated with production and delivery, and unit costs diverge across methods; (c) delivery is sometimes accomplished in conjunction with other health service deliveries, sometimes vertically and other times as part of private marketing efforts. Shared financing and delivery across providers and financiers (e.g., joint costs) make precise cost estimates difficult, especially when there are joint fixed costs (e.g., building or equipment, staff) or multiple actors in family planning programme implementation (e.g., separate bodies for information, education and communication or social marketing activities).

Finally and most importantly, costs are generally based solely on expenditures, which differ markedly from costs. The first item is purely a budget allocation that is spread across functions (e.g., personnel and equipment); the second represents the resources required to produce a certain output. Hence, the former item can be highly misleading but is the most commonly used measure. The error is compounded by reliance upon financial rather than economic costs. The former costs distort the true value of expenditures by not accounting for: donations (e.g., contraceptives) and volunteers; inefficiencies (e.g., unproductive or absent personnel); depreciation of capital; and the value of external resources (Kenney and Lewis, 1991).[6] Ideally, public programme costs should be measured using a resource cost methodology that calculates the value of actual goods and services received by the patient. This process pinpoints inefficiency and captures the true cost of service provision (Lewis, Sulvetta and La Forgia, 1990). These itemized limitations are important for placing existing cost estimates in perspective and highlighting needed reforms in measuring, calculating and comparing costs.

Estimating costs

Despite the limitations, some general estimates are possible. Aggregate costs offer little information regarding use; and most cost estimates are estimated on a per unit basis, such as per user, per-couple year of protection (CYP) or per birth averted. The most revealing but most complicated method is that of births averted, and cost per CYP is the most commonly used measure.[7] Estimates of cost per user range from about $10 to $20 in 1988 prices. Converting these estimates to cost per birth averted in a sample of 16 countries by estimating fertility in the absence of contraception produced costs ranging from a low of $21 in Colombia (1987 dollars) to $386 in Kenya; 60 per cent of costs in the sampled countries were below $100 (Cochrane, 1992).

Cost per CYP provides a more straightforward and useful basis for estimating and projecting costs because arbitrary assumptions of foregone costs are replaced by measures of contraceptive protection, although it has drawbacks as a measure of output. However, this measure can be adjusted to mitigate some of the difficulties (see Janowitz, Bratt and Fried, 1991), and has the added advantage of producing comparable cost estimates across methods and countries. Table 30 presents public service costs for four methods—female sterilization, oral contraceptives, intra-uterine devices (IUDs) and condoms—relying upon adjusted CYP costs in 1988 dollars. Three types of oral contraceptive distribution—clinic, contraceptive social marketing (CSM) and community-based distribution (CBD)—and CSM condom distribution option are considered.

Costs vary within countries (e.g., in Honduras from $15.10 per CYP for IUDs to $28.70 per CYP for clinically delivered oral contraceptives) and categories (CBD costs range from $8.10 in Peru to $38.5 in Morocco). Relative costs are far from constant, with oral contraceptives in urban Mexico ($23.30) at roughly the same cost as IUDs ($24.9), while in Thailand the costs are $17.10 and $4.20, respectively. Thus, the cost of contraceptive services are far from homogeneous and no single "cost" can be offered even by method. The least costly method also varies, with IUDs cheapest in Honduras, the Philippines and Thailand, female sterilization in Morocco, contraceptive retail sales of oral contraceptives in Bangladesh and Colombia, and oral contraceptives from clinics in rural Mexico. These conclusions, however, are incomplete because the data

TABLE 30. COST OF CONTRACEPTION PER ADJUSTED COUPLE-YEAR OF PROTECTION, BY METHOD, FOR SELECTED COUNTRIES[a]

Region and country	Year	Female sterilization	Oral contraceptives (Constant 1988 dollars)			Intra-uterine device	Condoms CSM
			Clinics	CSM	CBD		
Africa							
Morocco	1987	23.8	--	–	38.5	–	
Zaire	1987	–	–	–	10.0	–	..
Asia							
Bangladesh	1988	11.4	–	7.4	–	–	11.3
Philippines	1984	–	20.2	–	–	8.5	–
Thailand	1988	11.4	17.1	–	–	4.2	–
Indonesia	1989	7.9	–	–	–	–	–
Latin America							
Colombia	1985[b]	6.8	–	6.1	18.1	–	–
Guatemala	1983-84	12.1	–	–	–	–	–
Honduras	1988	17.5	28.7	15.7	24.2	15.1	25.5
Mexico	1988	22.5		–	7.7	..	–
Urban		–	23.3	..	24.9		
Rural		6.6			11.7		
Peru	1986/87	–	–	–	8.1	–	–

Source: Barbara Janowitz, John H. Bratt and Daniel B. Fried, Investing in Future: A Report on the Cost of Family Planning in the Year 2000 (Research Triangle Park, North Carolina, Family Health International, April 1990);

NOTES: CBD = community-based distrilution; CSM/F = contraception social marketing.

[a]Adjusted couple-year of protection accounts for the current value of the stream of costs incurred over the life of the contraceptive and for the age-specific relative risk of pregnancy for each method. Age-specific contraceptive use are from Honduras. See annex I to this paper for description of the data collection, calculation and adjustment for each method.

[b]Data for programmes obtained over the period 1984-1986; 1985 is the average.

are only available for some methods in each country (except Honduras) and only for a handful of countries, but they point to useful orders of magnitude and point up the heterogeneous nature of CYP costs.

Overall costs are greatly affected by service delivery characteristics, which are affected by a number of external programme factors, most notably: (*a*) the extent of user demand; (*b*) population density; (*c*) the mix of contraceptive methods offered; and (*d*) programme characteristics, such as the maturity of the programme, scale of operation and delivery modes.[8] Because these factors vary across communities and time, they account for the wide discrepancies in costs per CYP reported in table 30.

The motivation of potential family planning users will affect the economies of scale of national investment in contraceptive services because outlets are more likely to be frequented and down time minimized with high-volume efforts. Furthermore, outreach efforts that can be very costly are more effective and therefore produce higher returns at lower cost where demand is high. Similarly, population density affects the costs of reaching users. Dispersed populations, such as those in Nepal or the outer islands of Indonesia, are more expensive to reach because they lack the volume and infrastructure upon which to build outlets and consumer volume, both relatively and absolutely. For example, in Indonesia, costs per user in the first group of Outer Islands are twice those in Java and Bali, and five times as great in the more distant islands, which are the least densely populated (Cochrane, 1992).

The range of methods offered is likely to affect contraceptive prevalence and cost per CYP. It is estimated that for every method added to a programme, usage increases by 15 percentage points (Cochrane, 1992). Different methods appeal to different income, age, parity and residence (urban/rural) groups, and maximizing access requires availability of multiple options. For instance, sterilization tends to be favoured by older, higher parity women, and IUDs can meet the needs of women that have difficulty reaching resupply outlets. At the same time, the unique delivery requirements of each method must be added and financed, pushing up costs in the process.

Programme characteristics also affect costs, as does the intensity of effort. For example, some CBD efforts entail house-to-house visits. The costs of such programmes will be higher than static clinic facilities (assuming all staff are paid wages) (Lewis, 1985). Similarly, the maturity of any given programme can influence costs, either because they become more efficient with practice (and unit costs decline) or expand into lower demand or lower density areas (and unit costs rise). Hence, cost estimates of new or expanding programmes must be measured with care and policy or programme guidance tempered with evidence about what will affect costs. A particularly useful but underutilized guide from economics is the relation between average (or unit) cost and marginal cost. The relation indicates that when marginal costs are declining, increases in volume may have very low additional cost; however, if additional (or marginal) costs are high and climbing, then

average costs will understate the cost of additional units. Knowing the direction of marginal costs can then inform policy makers of the expected average and total costs of expanded efforts and thereby guide resource allocation decisions (Kenney and Lewis, 1991).

Cost projections

Forward planning requires reliable demand and cost projections to help Governments intervene appropriately and adequately. Given the sensitivity of the data, their limitations and incomparability just reviewed, projections should be taken with caution. Moreover, the variability in global estimates shown in table 31 suggest the extent of volatility and the sensitivity of estimates to assumptions. Annex table A.5 summarizes the key assumptions underlying the cost estimates and provides additional definitional details. Projections for the year 2000 range from $2,593 million, assuming only public investment and excluding China (Janowitz, Bratt and Fried, 1990), to $10,500 million, including all sources and countries (Population Crisis Committee, 1990). Janowitz, Bratt and Fried (1990) estimate rises to $3,675 million if China is added. This leaves a maximum difference of almost $7,000 million between the minimum and maximum. Excluding the Population

TABLE 31. ESTIMATES OF THE COSTS OF FAMILY PLANNING AND PROJECTS TO 2000
(Millions of 1988 dollars)

Source and country group	1980	1988-1990	2000
Bulatao (1985)			
All countries	..	5 150	8 075
Gillespie and others (1989)			
Excluding China	1 508	2 998	5 226
All countries excluding private sector	..	..	6 256
Janowitz, Bratt and Fried (1990)			
Excluding China	..	..	3 623
Excluding China and private sector	..	1 637	2 593
All countries excluding private sector	..	2 605	3 675
Population Crisis Committee (1990)			
All countries and private sector	1 000	2 795	10 500

Sources: Rodolfo A. Bulatao, *Expenditures on Population Programs in Developing Regions: Current Levels and Future Requirements*, World Bank Staff Working Paper, No. 679 (Washington, D.C., The World Bank, 1985); Duff G. Gillespie and others, "Financing the delivery of contraceptives: the challenge of the next twenty years", in *The Demographic and Programmatic Consequences of Contraceptive Innovation*, Sheldon J. Segal, Amy O. Tsui and Susan M. Rogers, eds. (New Yori, Plenum Publishing, 1989); Barbara Janowitz, John H. Bratt and Daniel B. Fried, *Investing in the Future: A Report on the Cost of Family Plannning in the Year 2000* (Research Triangle Park, North Carolina, Family Health International, 1990); Population Crisis Committee, *1990 Report on Progress Toward Population Stabilization* (Washington, D.C. 1990).

Crisis Committee report (1990), and therefore estimates of private expenditures, the differential is somewhat narrower but still more than twice the second highest estimate of $8,075 million (Bulatao, 1985).[9] Among th estimates, Janowitz, Bratt and Fried are probably the most reliable, given the process of estimation and projections. Moreover, for the purposes of this analysis public sector requirements are the most relevant. Given the above-mentioned upward bias coupled with some of the alternative financing mechanisms discussed below, this probably overstates the total cost, but it is an acceptable "ballpark" estimate for beginning. Moreover, whatever estimate is selected, the magnitude of the cost is staggering.

C. FINANCING FAMILY PLANNING

Public monies have been seen as *sine qua non* of funds for family planning. In some countries, however, contraceptive use is high despite minimal public investment (e.g., Brazil, Colombia and Turkey); in others, consumers have avoided accessible subsidized services in favour of commercial products (e.g., Egypt); and in still others, it appears that public subsidies are "crowding out" private suppliers (e.g., Thailand) (Lewis and Kenney, 1988). Little attention has been given to co-payments (user fees) in public services, and although non-governmental organizations and contraceptive retail sales have played central roles in some countries (e.g., Colombia), the commercial sector has been overlooked as a potential partner and its contributions largely ignored. Given declining donor funds, these types of alternatives are key to ensuring consumer access and targeting of government subsidies to population or geographical groups that are underserved or need special attention. This section summarizes current and expected funding and then explores the financial structure of family planning programmes, users' patterns of consumption and their ability and willingness to pay for services.

Family planning funding sources

International donors have been important sources of funding for some countries but negligible additions in others. For example, donors only contribute 13 per cent of the programme in India, 3 per cent in Malaysia and 20 per cent in the Republic of Korea, with the Government financing the bulk of the costs. Government funding predominates in Indonesia, Mexico, Thailand,

Turkey and Zimbabwe, but in much of the rest of the world international donors and non-governmental organizations, both domestic and international, are the major sources of support (Cochrane and others, 1990). Tracing family planning funding should be straightforward, but it is not. Exact magnitudes are difficult because of poor reporting from some non-governmental organizations and the scattering of funding and expenditure across numerous government bodies.

As demand rises, defining alternative options for financing family planning becomes important. The trends in government expenditures are unclear, although commitment is strong in some countries and public initiatives will be key in the coming decades. However, two issues should be mentioned in this regard. First, how effectively Governments allocate and spend family planning resources is of paramount importance. High expenditures with little impact are simply a misallocation or poorly managed expenditures that could be better spent on other priorities. There is some suggestion that this is the case in countries like Egypt, where returns on heavy public investments are not apparent and commercial providers meet 74 per cent of contraceptive use (Lewis and Kenney, 1988); or India, where high public investment has not met contraceptive use expectations (World Bank, 1992b). Improvements or shifts in which entities deliver family planning and how and where they do so become important during periods of fiscal austerity. Efficiency gained through improving cost effectiveness can lower the cost of delivery, and better incentives and accountability can increase the value of resources (World Bank, 1992a; Kenney and Lewis, 1991).

Secondly, users, employers and health-care providers and insurers can contribute to meeting the costs of family planning. Indeed, in many countries this is already occurring. Government subsidies may even be excessive in some settings. There has been little stimulation of other actors in financing services but there are frequently multiple deliverers of service. Non-governmental organizations are common financiers and deliverers of services, and private providers of both resupply and more permanent methods (IUDs and sterilization) tend to exist in most countries. This subject is discussed below.

Public subsidies for family planning

The degree to which Governments subsidize services varies widely across countries, as does the mix of expenditures across categories. In some countries, especially in Asia, users are given incentive payments to promote family limitation. In others, the Government plays a minimal role, leaving to non-governmental organizations and private providers the task of meeting demand for family planning. Again, accurate and complete data are scarce. Summaries of self-reported data across most countries are a beginning, but different definitions, dispersed funding sources and multiple programmes make consolidation and comparability difficult. Annex II presents data for government expenditures/budgets for family planning for the most recent year available (annex table A.6), and breakdowns for family planning components (table A.7).

The most detailed and complete data available, only for Asian countries, are shown in table 32. They represent a unique effort to define and collect comparable data. Interestingly, the Republic of Korea and Thailand spend the most per MWRA (ages 15-44) at $3.21 and $1.06, respectively. The latter country has had a strong and highly visible programme for many years with heavy support from international donors. The Republic of

Korea has kept a significantly lower profile. Both have contraceptive prevalence rates of about 70 per cent, suggesting an effective, if costly, effort. The Philippines and Viet Nam have the least government effort and some of the lowest contraceptive prevalence rates (table 33).

Table 32 further breaks down expenditures across contraceptives: training; information, education and communication (IEC); and incentives. India and Nepal spend significant proportions (60 and 30 per cent, respectively) on incentives; and Bangladesh, the Republic of Korea and Sri Lanka spend over 5 per cent of their budgets on payments to users (14, 12 and 6 per cent, respectively). Sustaining payments will clearly be costly for these countries, especially the first two; and the relative importance and incentive payments will need to be weighed against other family planning components as per capita resources decline. Some countries in Asia, Bangladesh, China, India, Nepal, the Philippines and Viet Nam, are likely to require greater government efforts to inform and provide services to the low-income population and dispersed rural communities. The private

TABLE 32. PUBLIC SPENDING ON CONTRACEPTIVES, FAMILY PLANNING-RELATED TRAINING, INFORMATION, EDUCATION AND COMMUNICATION ACTIVITIES, AND INCENTIVES, ASIAN COUNTRIES, MOST RECENT YEAR

Country	Expenditure per target population on[a]		Distribution of spending on all four components (percentage)[b]				
	Contraception (dollar)	Four components[c] (percentage per capita GNP)	Contraceptives	Training	IEC	Incentives	Year
Bangladesh	0.57	0.41	74	9	4	14	1990
China[d]	0.11	–	–	–	–	–	1990
India	0.18	0.19	28	5	7	60	1990
Indonesia	0.44	0.16	63	18	20	0	1989
Republic of Korea[e]	3.21	0.09	73	1	14	12	1989
Malaysia	0.49	0.03	88	4	8	0	1990
Nepal	0.22	0.30	49	8	13	30	1990
Philippines	0.09	0.03	65	13	21	1	1986
Sri Lanka	0.25	0.07	82	9	3	6	1990
Thailand	1.06	0.10	82	10	7	0	1989
Viet Nam	0.02	0.06	34	29	37	0	1990

Source: The World Bank, Population Issues in Asia: Context, Policies and Prospects, Report No. 10712/SAS/EAP (Washington, D.C., 1992).
NOTE: IEC = information, education and communication.
[a] The target population refers to married women of reproductive age (15-44).
[b] Row figures may not add up to 100 per cent owing to rounding errors.
[c] The four components of expenditure are: contraceptive commodity; training; IEC activities; and incentives. Incentives refers to payment (in cash and in kind) made to acceptors of family planning (usually sterilization and intra-uterine device (IUD) insertion) and incentives paid to service providers, including doctors, nurses, midwives and other personnel. In Bangladesh and India, the bulk of expenditure on incentives are paid to clients rather than providers, while the opposite is true in the Philippines.
[d] Unlike the other countries, allocations in the programme in China are compulsory, and the pattern of spending may not lend itself easily to cross-country comparisons.
[e] In the Republic of Korea, financial assistance is given to a number of low-income acceptors of sterilization, and free medical services are provided for the preschool child of an acceptor of sterilization if sterilized after one child. These subsidies have been declining steadily since 1986, with the sharpest drop occurring between 1989 and 1990. Subsidies in 1990 were only 34 per cent of what they were in 1989.

TABLE 33. SOURCE OF CONTRACEPTIVE METHODS AMONG MARRIED CURRENT USERS,
SELECTED DEVELOPING COUNTRIES

Major area or region, country and region	Contraceptive prevalence rate (percentage)	Government (percentage	Commercial (percentage)	Non-governmental organizations (percentage)	Other (percentage)
Africa					
Botswana (1988)	33	94.2	4.8	..	1.0
Burundi (1987)	9	86.7	1.8	..	11.5
Ghana (1988)	13	34.7	25.2	17.1	20.0
Kenya (1989)	27	71.0	9.0	18.0	2.0
Liberia (1986)	6	31.1	18.3	48.2	2.3
Senegal (1986)	12	45.0	50.0	-	5.0
Zaire (1984)	64.1[d]	28.7	3.6	3.5	
Zimbabwe (1984)	38	42.8	9.2	46.2	2.0
Asia					
India	40	81.2	18.8[c]	..	-
Indonesia (1987)	48	79.9[d]	12.5	..	7.6
Malaysia (1989)	33	51.7	38.3	3.0	6.9
Nepal (1981)	7	73.9	2.7	20.4	2.9
Pakistan (1985)	12	66.8	26.4	..	5.4
Philippines (1988)					
Rep. of Korea (1985)	70	58.0[e]	42.0	..	-
Sri Lanka (1987)	55	84.4	7.9	2.9	4.8
Thailand (1987)	68	82.0	15.3	1.8	1.1
Viet Nam (1988)					
Latin America and the Caribbean					
Barbados (1985)	37	34.4	33.6	21.6	10.4
Belize (1985)	37	38.0	30.0	..	32.0[f]
Bolivia (1983)	26	7.0	93.0	..	..
Brazil (1986)	65	25.4	60.3	0.5	13.8[g]
Colombia (1986)	65	34.0	42.5	22.1	1.4[g]
Costa Rica (1985)	70	57.8	22.4	..	19.8
Dominican Republic (1986)[h]	50	49.9	49.9	1.0	..
Ecuador (1987)	44	38.0	40.0	15.0	7.0
El Salvador (1987)	46	49.7	38.1	..	12.2
Guatemala (1983)	25	31.8	16.1	30.0	22.4
Haiti (1983)	7[i]	75.0	24.0	..	1.0
Honduras (1984)	35	27.9	36.8	32.9	2.4
Jamaica (1983)	51	66.9	30.2	..	2.9
Mexico (1987)	53[j]	61.9	38.1	..	-
Panama (1979)	61	71.0	19.0	..	10.0[k]
Paraguay (1977)	24	41.0	28.0	8.0	22.0[k]
Peru (1986)	41	56.0	33.0	..	11.0
Northern Africa and Western Asia					
Egypt (1988) ....,....	38	23.1	74.2	..	..
Lebanon (1984)[l]	53	0.9	57.3	41.8	..
Morocco (1987)[m]	36	61.1	21.1	..	17.8
Tunisia (1988)	50	76.7	23.3	..	..

Sources and notes to follow.

TABLE 33 *(continued)*

Sources: Contraceptive Prevalence Surveys and Demographic and Health Surveys for years cited; Donald Bogue and others, *Planificación familiar: necesidades y costos projección, 1985-2000, 15 paises* (Chicago, Illinois, Social Development Center, 1986); United Nations, Economic and Social Commission for Asia and the Pacific, "Emerging issues and regional activities: role of the private sector and non-governmental organizations in population matters", Fifth session, Committee on Population, Bangkok, 17-21 August 1987; Leo Morris and others, *Contraceptive Prevalence Surveys: A New Source of Family Planning Data*, Population Reports, Series M, No. 5 (Baltimore, Maryland, The Johns Hopkins University, Population Information Program, 1981); Fertility and Health Surveys. Some material was updated from Maureen A. Lewis and Genevieve Kenney, *The Private Sector and Family Planning in Developing Countries*, Population and Human Resources Department Working Papers, No. 96 (Washington, D.C., The World Bank, 1988); Susan Cochrane and others, "The economics of family planning", draft, Washington, D.C., The World Bank, 1990; Warren C. Sanderson and Jee-Peng Tan, *Population Issues in Asia*, Asia Technical Department Series, No. 5 (Washington, D.C., The World Bank, 1992).

NOTE: Two dots (..) indicate that data are not available or source not used. Contraceptive source information was given by women that were using contraception at the time of the survey.

[a]Community and home-based distribution are included under the "Government" category unless indicated otherwise.

[b]Including private physicians, hospitals, pharmacies and any other private non-governmental organizations.

[c]Unspecified source; may encompass "non-governmental organizations" when private non-profits are not a category and may include "Commercial" when there is not a separate category.

[d]This figure overstates the government provision of services by including services of non-governmental organizations that are partially funded by Governments. The figures are therefore underestimates for these countries.

[e]Source allocation data are for 1979.

[f]Thirty per cent uncertain as to source of contraceptives.

[g]Including couples using Billings, rhythm or withdrawal methods.

[h]Including women in union as well as married women.

[i]Only 40 per cent of users use modern contraceptive methods.

[j]Prevalence data are for 1982.

[k]Including users of both traditional and modern contraceptive methods.

[l]Source figures for Lebanon pertain only to rural areas.

[m]Including only users of modern methods.

family planning. Similar circumstances are found in Africa, parts of the Middle East and a few Latin American and Caribbean countries (e.g., Haiti and Paraguay). The central role of government is not as clear in countries with a mature programme, high contraceptive prevalence levels and rising female education and incomes.

private sector can contribute, as can users, but income affects the ability to pay, and IEC efforts are needed to inform potential users of the existence and benefits of Who actually pays for contraceptives can be estimated using the Contraceptive Prevalence Surveys (CPS) and Demographic and Health Surveys (DHS). Table 33 summarizes contraceptive prevalence and the source of services for married women currently using contraceptives for a large group of countries. Those obtaining contraceptives from commercial sources obviously pay for them, non-governmental organizations often charge some nominal fee and less frequently government does. Commercial providers supply some proportion of users in virtually every country and play a major role in countries with a strong overall private sector (e.g., Brazil and the Republic of Korea) and those where the Government is either in turmoil (e.g., Lebanon and El Salvador) or disinterested (e.g., Bolivia). Similarly, non-governmental organizations predominate where government programmes are nascent actors and the countries and among the world's poorest (e.g., much of Africa, Nepal and Honduras) or, again, where there is political turmoil (e.g., Lebanon). Colombia is a special case where collaboration between non-governmental organizations (Profamilia) and the Gov-

ernment has extended the non-governmental organization network throughout the country.

These patterns suggest an existing private sector role that in many countries is equal to or exceeds government efforts. Some commercial activity can be attributed to Government/donor-subsidized CSM, but what is important is that the market functioned to relieve the Government of (full) subsidies and of having to deliver services to consumers that are able and willing to pay for contraceptive services. That situation bodes well for possible future efforts to expand reliance upon commercial providers, particularly as urban areas expand and incomes rise.

User contributions for family planning services

What price, if any, is charged in private and public outlets and how these charges relate to income; who purchases contraceptives as opposed to receiving them free or at a negative price (e.g., with incentive payments) and consumer ability and willingness to pay for contraception are the issues that require scrutiny in evolving a fair and effective policy to place greater reliance upon partially subsidized contraceptives and upon more carefully targeted public expenditures.

Pricing of contraceptives

A number of attempts have been made to estimate the prices consumers face for contraceptive services in the public and private sectors (Schearer, 1983; Lewis and Kenney, 1989; Ross and others, 1992; World Bank, 1992b). These data tend to be incomplete, available for only a small number of countries or taken from non-comparable sources (e.g., household surveys, government reports and commercial sector surveys). Each method carries different prices and service arrangements across providers. Table 34 summarizes government policies on charges for the countries that report them; however, as will be seen, policy and practice often diverge. Most public programmes do not impose fees on users. In 20 per cent of programmes, all services carry charges and some services have fees in another 19 per cent.[10]

TABLE 34. POLICES ON CHARGING FOR FAMILY PLANNING SERVICES IN PUBLIC PROGRAMMES, COUNTRIES OR AREAS, 1989

All free		All with charges	Combination
Africa	Asia	Africa	Africa
Burkina Faso	Bangladesh	Benin	Ethiopia
Botswana	China	Congo	Nigeria
Burundi	India	Ghana	Zimbabwe
Cameroon	Nepal	Guinea	
Central African Republic	Philippines	Lesotho	Asia
Chad	Viet Nam	Madagascar	Hong Kong
Kenya[a]		Zaire	Indonesia
Liberia	Latin America		Republic of Korea
Mali	and the Caribbean	Asia	Malaysia
Mauritania	Brazil	Singapore	Pakistan
Mau ritius[c]	Chile	Thailand[b]	Sri Lanka
Mozambique	Costa Rica		Taiwan Province of China
Niger[a]	Ecuador	Latin America	
Rwanda	El Salvador	and the Caribbean	
Sierra Leone	Guyana[d]	Colombia[e]	Latin America
Sudan	Haiti	Guatemala	and the Caribbean
United Republic of Tanzania	Jamaica	Panama	Colombia[c]
Togo	Mexico	Peru	Dominican Republic
Uganda	Nicaragua	Puerto Rico	Venezuela[f]
Zambia	Paraguay		
	Trinidad and Tobago[c]	Western Asia	Western Asia
		Lebanon	Jordan
	Northern Africa and		Syrian Arab Republic
	Western Asia		Turkey
	Algeria		
	Egypt[a]		
	Iran (Islamic Republic of)		
	Morocco		
	Tunisia		

Source: John A. Ross and Stephen L. Issacs, "Cost payments and incentives in family planning programs: a review for developing countries", *Studies in Family Planning* (New York), vol. 19, No. 5 (September-October 1988), pp. 270-283.

[a]1987 data.
[b]All methods are free in rural areas. In urban areas, maximum charges are set for each method.
[c]1984 data.
[d]Guyana Responsible Parenthood Association (GRPA).
[e]Asociacion Pro-Bienestar de la Familia Colombiana (Profamilia).
[f]1988 data.

265

In the private sector, prices cover the cost of services. Table 35 summarizes user payments in public facilities for a sample of Asian countries along with average annual charges per CYP for those clients that pay. Although policies concerning charging for services may vary, the household data summarized in table 35 indicate the existence of fees in the six sample countries. Technically speaking, India and Nepal offer free services, but actual practices clearly deviate from that policy (see table 34).

Also evident is the practice of selectively charging for services. None of the sampled countries charged all users for all methods, and none charged full cost. For example, a larger percentage of Sri Lankan users pay something for oral contraceptives (96 per cent), although the amounts are likely to be modest. Only 15 per cent of users in Indonesia pay anything for oral contraceptives, but in the other four countries, 30-49 per cent make some contribution. The proportion charged also appears to vary, based on evidence from two countries. The importance of payments in relation to income suggests that fees in public facilities are modest. No method, even sterilization, captures close to 1 per cent of per capita gross domestic product. Thus, even for low-income households, current service costs are not excessive, particularly in relation to the lifetime benefits of the expenditure.

TABLE 35. PERCENTAGE OF CLIENTS OF PUBLIC FAMILY PLANNING SERVICES RECEIVING SERVICES WITHOUT CHARGE AND PRICES CHARGED TO PAYING PUBLIC SECTOR CLIENTS, SELECTED ASIAN COUNTRIES

Country	Survey year	Percentage receiving services without charge					Average price charged to paying clients for one year of contraceptive protection[a] (as percentage of per capita gross national product)				
		Pill	Condom	Inject-ables	Intra-uterine device	Sterli-zation	Pill	Condom	Inject-ables	Intra-uterine device	Sterli-zation[b]
India	1986/87	51	30	..	94[c]	..	..	..	..	..	..
Indonesia	1987	85	95	34	86	40	.42	0.37[d]	0.84	0.32	0.64
Malaysia[e]	1988/89	52	52	..	..	..	0.30	0.37	0.33	0.04	0.02
Nepal[f]	1986	69	..	..	..	..	1.22	..	..	..	..
Sri Lanka	1987	4	..	..	..	..	0.16	..	..	..	..
Thailand	1987	59	..	..	..	..	0.26	..	..	..	..
	1984	..	..	..	..	..	0.28	..	0.78	2	0.14

Sources: The World Bank, Population Issues in Asia: Context, Policies and Prospects, Report No. 10712-SAS/EAP (Washington, D.C., 1992); Indonesia, Central Bureau of Statistics and National Family Planning Coordinating Board; and Institute for Resource Development/Westinghouse, National Indonesia Contraceptive Prevalence Survey, 1987 (Jakarta, Indonesia; and Baltimore, Maryland, 1989); Second Malaysia Family Life Survey, 1988/89; Nepal, Ministry of Health; and Westinghouse Health Systems, Nepal Contraceptive Survey Report, 1981 (Kathmandu, Nepal; and Columbia, Maryland, 1983; for Thailand, 1987, Napaporn Chayovan, Peerasit Kamnuansilpa and John Knodel, Thailand Demographic and Health Survey, 1987 (Bangkok, Thailand, Chulalongkorn University, Institute of Population Studies; and Columbia, Maryland, Institute for Resource Development/Westinghouse, 1988); for Thailand, 1984, Teera Ashakul, "Analysis of contraceptive method choice and optimum contraceptive pricing structures", Thailand Development Research Institute Newsletter (Bamgkok), vol. 4, No. 3 (1989), pp. 10-13.

NOTE: Two dots (..) indicate that data are not available.

[a]One year of protection calculated with the following assumptions: 13 pill cycles per year; 100 condoms per year; 2.5 years of use duration for intra-uterine devices; 3 months of protection per injection. For sterilization, length of protection is the difference between age 45 and the average age at sterilization in the population

[b]For female sterilization.

[c]Including 67.2 per cent that received the service with incentive payment and 17.7 per cent that received without charge.

[d]There is some uncertainty on the price of condoms because the survey questionnaire did not specifically solicit information about the number of condoms covered by the reported price. In Indonesia packets have 3 or 12 condoms; the latter number was assumed for this calculation because the other number implies a prohibitively high price for a year of protection, more than 10 times the price of, for example, pills.

[e]Prices differ across two types of public providers, the Ministry of Health and the National Population and Family Development Board, and non-governmental organizations; and the private sector. Data reflect the percentage of women using Ministry of Health or National Board facilities and living in communities where services are provided without charge by these entities. There were too few observations for injectables and intra-uterine devices to compute reliable percentages.

[f]The available survey data do not permit identification of public and private sources, but because most providers fall into the government or non-governmental organization category (which in Nepal is heavily subsidized by the Government), the data provide a rough picture of the extent of free provision.

[g]Data for 1984 are reported in the price per month of protection and were converted to annual prices by simple multiplication.

The findings suggested by these disparate data are that the practice of charging is well established at least in Asia, and that a significant number of countries have a direct policy of charging for family planning. This situation bodes well for introducing fees because there is experience with such practices. Moreover, selectively charging clients is consistent with equity considerations in pricing contraceptives, because this practice allows charging those able to pay and waiving fees for those that cannot.

Subsequent and more sophisticated evidence for Bangladesh (Ciszewski and Harvey, 1991), Indonesia (Molyneaux and Diman, 1991); Jamaica, the Philippines and Thailand (Schwartz and others, 1989); and Thailand (Ashakul, 1989) and produce similar results. The Bangladesh study showed that a 60 per cent rise in price resulted in a 46 per cent drop in condom sales and a 17 per cent decline in oral contraceptive purchases the following year. Users in the lowest income groups were the most severely affected by the price increase. Evidence from Indonesia (Molyneaux and Diman, 1991) bolsters this finding, as higher prices led to decreased contraception among the poor but to switching across methods among the more affluent.

Elasticity of demand for contraceptives

Whether the public sector can charge for services without affecting the demand for and use of contraceptives is at the heart of decisions concerning the imposition of user fees for family planning services. Evidence from health care (Jimenez, 1987; Lewis, 1992) and family planning (Lewis, 1985 and 1986; Sanderson and Tan, 1992) suggests that there is scope for charging users for contraceptives, provided certain criteria are met.

Studies of the elasticity of demand with respect to price measure consumer response to a change (or difference) in contraceptive prices. For every percentage increase in price there is a corresponding percentage change in utilization. If the percentage increase in price is equal to the percentage decline in users "elasticity" will be equal to 1. The lower the "elasticity", the less of the negative effect that can be expected from a price increase.

Evidence from a 1986 survey of 13 studies across eight countries provides some useful conclusions. First, demand is not likely to be much affected by modest changes in fees, as is shown by studies in the Republic of Korea. Secondly, as prices increase, demand becomes more price-sensitive, as indicated by evidence from Taiwan Province of China, showing a negligible effect on demand when free oral contraceptives were priced at $0.13 but a 50 per cent decline when the price rose to $0.21 per cycle. Thirdly, large price changes can have significant effects on demand, as is suggested by a study in the Republic of Korea, where eliminating a $20 fee for sterilization increased acceptors from 10 to 170 per month. Lastly, the poor are more sensitive to price than the rich; in the Brazilian state of Piaui, the introduction of free pills resulted in one half of rural users switching from private providers, but only 2 per cent switched in urban areas (Lewis, 1986).

Table 36 summarizes the elasticity estimates from the above-mentioned studies. Interestingly, only one elasticity is less than 1.0 (Jamaica, condoms) and most are below -0.25, suggesting that modest price increases, in general, do not adversely affect contraceptive use. Further evidence for Thailand analysed by the World Bank (1992b) is depicted in figure XV. The decidedly downward sloping curve is consistent across methods. Some of this finding may be explained by the very low cost of contraceptives (less than 1 per cent of gross national product per capita), but the consistency is no less remarkable. Despite the low levels, however, the balance between the number of users and revenue needs to be kept in perspective. For every price increase, programmes must determine whether the earnings justify the loss of users. Elasticity estimates may assist in that process.

The findings strongly suggest the potential for cost recovery in public facilities, especially for nominal amounts. What is critical to designing, introducing or expanding cost recovery are indications from well-designed studies of potential users' ability and willingness to pay for contraceptives. The studies discussed here provide ample methodological options for undertaking such studies. Because the amount that can be charged varies across countries as well as communities and because the ultimate goal is usually to maximize the number of users, measuring willingness and ability to pay is key to meeting the potentially conflicting objectives of higher revenue and rising contraceptive use.

Cost recovery in public systems and other forms of cost-sharing

Cost recovery in public systems is increasingly contemplated by Governments, and some evidence exists

TABLE 36. PRICE ELASTICITIES AT VARIOUS SAMPLE MEAN PRICES FOR ONE YEAR OF CONTRACEPTIVE PROTECTION, THE PHILIPPINES, JAMAICA, THAILAND AND INDONESIA[a]

| Method | Philippines, 1978[b] | | Jamaica, 1984[b] | | Thailand, 1984[b] | | | | Indonesia, 1987 | | |
| | | | | | Schwartz and others | | Ashakul | | | | |
	Elasticity	Mean price	Elasticity	Mean price	Elasticity	Mean price	Easticity	Mean price	Elasticities own price	Net[c]	Mean price
Condom	-0.15	0.24	-1.09	2.46	-0.56	3.10	-0.25	..	..	..	..
Injection	..	..	-0.79	1.80	-0.16	0.83	-0.29	1.26	-0.49	-0.05	1.06
					-0.25	1.04					
					-0.12	0.52					
Pill	-0.00	0.11	-0.07	0.56	-0.10	0.74	-0.23	1.11	-0.11	-0.02	0.21
					-0.09	0.36					
					-0.04	0.19					
Intra-uterine device	0.01	0.02	..	..	-0.10	0.43	-0.04	0.16	-0.14	-0.03	0.12
					-0.02	0.08					
Sterilization	..	..	..	..	-0.02	0.22	-0.05	0.18	..	..	..
All major methods .					-0.02	0.10					
	..	..	..	..	..	..	..	..	..	-0.12[d]	..

Sources: The World Bank, *Population Issues in Asia: Context, Policies and Prospects*, Report No. 10712-SAS/EAP (Washington, D.C., 1982), based on J. B. Schwartz and others, "The effect of contraceptive prices on the choice of contraceptive method in the Philippines, Jamaica and Thailand", in *Choosing a Contraceptive Method: Choice in Asia and the United States*, Rodolfo A. Bulatao, James A. Palmore and Sandra E. Ward, eds. (Boulder, Colorado, Westview Press, 1989); Teera Ashakul, "Analysis of contraceptive method choice and optimum contraceptive pricing structures", *Thailand Development Research Institute Newsletter* (Bangkok), vol. 4, No. 3 (1989), pp. 10-13; and Jack Molyneaux and Tohir Diman, *Impacts of Contraceptive Prices on Indonesian Contraceptive Choices: Further Analysis for the 1987 Indonesian Demographic and Health Survey*, Andrew Kantner and James Palmer, eds. (Honolulu, Hawaii, East-West Center, forthcoming).

NOTE: Two dots (..) indicate that data are not available.

[a]Mean prices are in units of per capita gross national product, which was $510 for the Philippines in 1978, $1,150 for Jamaica in 1984, $860 for Thailand in 1984 and $450 for Indonesia in 1987.

[b]Elasticities are own price elasticities, reflecting the responsiveness of use probabilities of a given contraceptive to changes in its own price.

[c]Reflects the percentage of change in overall use probability after substitution among contraceptives has been taken into account.

[d]Reflects the percentages change in overall use probability if the prices of all the major contraceptive methods simultaneously rise by 1 per cent.

Figure XV. **Elasticity of demand for contraceptives with respect to their cost, Thailand, 1984**

Elasticity of demand for contraceptives

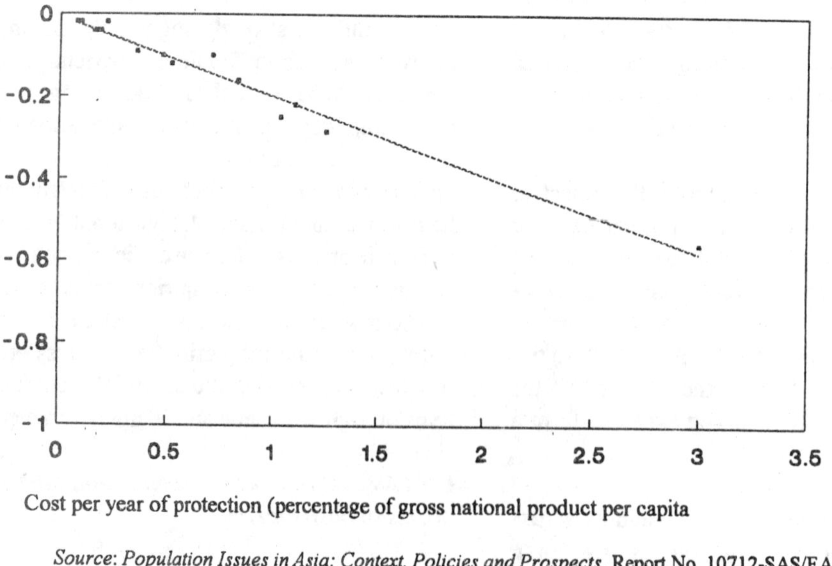

Cost per year of protection (percentage of gross national product per capita

Source: *Population Issues in Asia: Context, Policies and Prospects*, Report No. 10712-SAS/EAP (Washington, D.C., The World Bank (1992).

268

on the possible earnings of such strategies (Lewis, 1987). How much can be recovered will vary according to income and extent of demand. Studies have shown the potential for recovering over 100 per cent of costs in special circumstances with contraceptive social marketing. Otherwise, the proportion tends to fall between 15 and 50 per cent (Lewis, 1987). It is unrealistic, however, to expect that programmes directed to low-income households can or will meet the full cost of services. Moreover, even if users can afford the full cost it is not clear that private sources are less costly and more appropriate, given scarce resources. Hence, public or non-profit programmes directed to these groups will need to price services carefully and to monitor responses to change in order to establish the optimal price where revenues and utilization are maximized.

The importance of targeting cannot be overemphasized. Because of income differences and the implications of low income for contraceptive use, Governments and non-governmental organizations need to reach and target populations that are unaware of contraceptive options, unable to afford contraception or inaccessible to contraceptive messages and services. Whereas middle-income and upper income households have the income and education to make contraceptive decisions, lower income households do not. As public funds become scarcer, a Government must increasingly make trade-offs regarding where to put its marginal dollar. Targeting populations that cannot or will not be reached by commercial providers (e.g., private physicians and nurse out-patient services, pharmacies, private hospitals) and have no alternative sources of supply will use public funds more effectively. Indeed, it is the responsibility of government to serve those populations to enhance social welfare.

At the same time, this course may imply reducing support to programmes for better-off populations. The implications of such reductions may not have serious adverse effects, particularly where high economic growth is coupled with rising contraceptive prevalence rates. For example, there is little reason for women with a secondary education (and therefore of relatively high income) to rely upon subsidized contraceptives. Among women with at least a secondary education, 72, 68, 54 and 50 per cent, respectively, relied upon public sources for supply in Indonesia, Thailand, Mexico and Jamaica from the mid-1980a to the late 1980s (Cross and others, 1991; Lewis and Kenney, 1988). In all four countries, numerous private alternatives are available. This finding suggests either poor targeting or a decision by the Government to underwrite contraception for all women, regardless of whether they were able to afford private services. Targeting would shift resources away from the more affluent to those that must rely upon government programmes.

The other problem with low-cost, accessible contraception for the middle and upper classes is the "crowding out" of private providers because private investors are left with an inadequate market. Zero price is an impossible price to compete against and discourages retailers (e.g., pharmacies) from entering the market. In a similar vein, third-party payers for health care—including insurance companies, company health plans and prepaid group practice (e.g., health maintenance organizations)—have little incentive to pay for contraception if subsidized services are accessible to their enrollees. Sterilizations, in particular, are prime candidates for inclusion in insurance coverage, because they are expensive even for upper income couples. A beginning of this process with support from the United States Agency for International Development, has been made but its full potential and impact need additional experimentation and evaluation (Lewis and Kenney, 1988; Cross and others, 1991). Efforts by government to encourage such coverage and consideration of tax breaks and other incentives to make such decisions attractive are needed. Private insurance is a new policy area for Governments in general, but third-party payers can relieve government not only of costly health care but also of preventive services like family planning that consumers want.

D. CONCLUSIONS AND RECOMMENDATIONS

The evidence compiled in this paper points to some important conclusions. First, the reproductive age cohort is growing rapidly even as overall population growth declines. Simultaneously, donor resources are expected to decline over the next decade, given recent trends and political winds. Secondly, very little is actually known about the extent of unmet need for contraceptives in developing countries because available data are inadequate to the task and therefore measures are flawed. As a result, projected unmet needs must be viewed as orders of magnitude. Thirdly, cost data are also troublesome because of the assumptions underlying them and the inaccuracy built into equating costs and expenditures.

Ways in which to determine financial needs in future are complicated by the data limitations just mentioned. However, under the assumption that resources will be constrained in future, efforts should be made to assess alternative financing arrangements and to improve resource allocation and efficiency of service delivery. Available evidence suggests that among the countries charging for family planning, fees are a small proportion of per capita gross national product. Moreover, studies show that upward adjustments to modest fees have little effect on utilization, indicating possible scope for establishing or raising fees for family planning. These results bolster decision makers' abilities to explore cost-sharing with users. In addition, third-party payers for health care offer another potential financier to share costs with Governments and users.

The recommendations can be summarized as follows:

(*a*) Give more consideration and more careful interpretation to data on costs and unmet needs in order to guide decisions by donors and Governments, and to design effective programmes that promote efficiency and appropriate targeting;

(*b*) Husband resources, by minimizing government subsidies, through raising efficiency (that is, higher output without increasing input) of public programmes, or contracting out to achieve the same thing; targeting resources to those that must rely upon government programmes to ensure access to and affordability of contraceptives; and reducing access of middle-income and upper income users while promoting private alternatives. The decisions entail making trade-offs among programme elements (e.g., incentive payments versus IEC versus contraceptive options) and having available evidence to inform policy makers;

(*c*) Provide better information on price sensitivity of consumers to Governments in order to promote cost-sharing and therefore more and better information on utilization patterns and the effects of price changes on use. Decisions on acceptable trade-offs between revenue and users must be made to guide pricing in this area;

(*d*) Provide incentives to expand or improve private services in order to help ensure a positive climate for increasing private activity in family planning delivery. Removing impediments to private investment in family planning, encouraging its inclusion in health insurance coverage, promoting tax incentives and limiting public "crowding out" by limiting universal free services so that the private sector can flourish are examples of possible initiatives;

(*e*) Give attention and funds to innovations in delivery methods, monitoring of use and other characteristics of family planning, in order to explore new alternatives to place family planning programmes on a firm footing for the next decade. Experimentation and careful evaluation are a priority to guide this process.

NOTES

[1]There appears to be a continuing absorptive capacity problem in a few isolated countries, reflecting poor resource allocation by donors.

[2]For discussions of the economics that define the role of government in family planning delivery and finance, see Lewis (1986) and Lewis and Kenney (1988).

[3]This estimate is based on the United Nations medium-variant population projections.

[4]The countries included in the regional divisions used in this chapter do not in all cases conform to those included in the geographical regions established by the Population Division of the Department for Economic and Social Information and Policy Analysis of the United Nations Secretariat.

[5]The "health risk criteria" identify women with high-risk pregnancies: under age 20 and over 35; of high parity (four or more children); and with closely spaced births (less than 15 months) and not using contraception. "Preference criteria" is equivalent to Boulier's unmet spacing and limiting need.

[6]The limitations of expenditure data in family planning and health are discussed in Kenney and Lewis (1991); Lewis, Solvetta and La Forgia (1990); and in Janowitz, Brett and Fried (1990).

[7]For definition and discussion of these measures, see Cochrane and others (1990).

[8]It should be noted that there are interrelations among these factors. For example, density of demand may be inversely correlated with programme maturity where programmes have reached the population and new demand is therefore low.

[9]The Population Crisis Committee also uses 75 per cent prevalence as its target rather than 55 per cent prevalence as applied in ther other three studies.

[10]The price of services is only one component of client cost. Transportation costs, lost earnings and long waits for services represent other costs for potential contraceptors, and these may exceed any monetary expenditure involved (Lewis, 1985). These costs are even more difficult to measure, but some analytic studies, notably the World Bank's Living Standards Measurement Survey (LSMS), have effectively calculated figures for at least health care.

270

ANNEXES

ANNEX I. SUMMARY OF COST ESTIMATE ASSUMPTIONS

Each cost projection is based on projecting married women of reproductive age (MWRA), rate of contraceptive use among MWRA and cost per user. The assumptions are:

1. *Married women of reproductive age.* Bulatao assumes 734 million MWRA (including China); Gillespie and others; and Janowitz, Bratt and Fried assume 675 million and 654 million (excluding China), respectively (see table A.5);

2. *Contraceptive prevalence rate.* Varies from 50 per cent in 1990 to 58 per cent in 2000 (Bulatao, 1985), from 43 to 52 per cent (Gillespie and others, 1989) and from 39 per cent in 1988 to 48-50 per cent in 2000 (Janowitz, Bratt and Fried).[a]

3. *Cost per user.* Bulatao estimates that cost per user averages $16 for the least developed countries. The United States Agency for International Development (USAID) estimates service cost per user at $18, and commodity costs range from $0.12 per cycle for pills to $16.75 for Norplant.

Bulatao (1985) used expenditure data compiled by Speidel and others to obtain expenditures per capita for countries with data.[b] Expenditure estimates are combined with user estimates to obtain "costs" per user.[c] Projected user costs are in 1980 dollars.

Gillespie and others (1989) made assumptions based on method mix. The service cost per user is estimated at $18 per couple-year of protection, citing Bulatao's expenditure per user data as the source. Gillespie and others (1989) included commodity costs but these costs are only a small portion of total costs (9-12 per cent). Total costs were projected based on the following

assumptions: (*a*) method mix remains constant to 2000; (*b*) there is a slight shift towards Norplant and vaginal rings; (*c*) commodity costs increase from $456 million to $533 million and $602 million in 2000.

Janowitz, Bratt and Fried (1990) differ from the foregoing in these ways:

(*a*) Used costs collected from country visits rather than expenditure data. Previous studies (Bulatao, 1985; Gillespie and others, 1989; and the Population Crisis Committee used government expenditures and donor contributions[d] as a measure of funding available for family planning and contraceptive use to obtain current estimates of per capita funding of family planning. Information that is not available is imputed. Projections on future resource requirements are then made using contraceptive use or fertility targets. Costs were collected from Honduras, Mexico and Thailand from the major providers of contraceptive services. Data for Mexico were obtained through the Social Security Programme; in Honduras, information was collected from the Family Planning Association of Honduras (ASHONPLAFA); and in Thailand, from the Ministry of Health. Costs per method were estimated from direct and indirect costs of service and supplies for each method;

(*b*) Differentiated not only by method but also by delivery system;

(*c*) Used the TARGET model[e] to separate acceptors from users, which enabled them to allocate costs of methods to acceptance and follow-up visits.

TABLE A.5. ASSUMPTIONS UNDERLYING COST PROJECTIONS FOR FAMILY PLANNING TO 2000

Source	Assumed number of married women of reproductive age (millions)	Assumed contraceptive prevalence rate change (percentage)		Assumed cost per user (dollars)
		1980	2000	
Bulatao (1985)	734[a]	50	58	16
Gillespie and others (1989)	675	43	52	18 +
Janowitz, Bratt and Fried (1990)	654[b]	39	48-50	Contraceptive n.a.
Population Crisis Committee (1990)	..	75	16	

Sources: Rodolfo A. Bulatao, *Expenditures on Population Programs in Developing Regions: Current Levels and Future Requirements*, World Bank Staff Working Paper, No. 679 (Washington, D.C., The World Bank, 1985); Duff G. Gillespie and others, "Financing the delivery of contraceptives: the challenge of the next twenty years", in *The Demographic and Programmatic Consequences of Contraceptive Innovation*, Sheldon J. Segal, Amy O. Tsui and Susan M. Rogers, eds. (New York, Plenum Publishing, 1989); Barbara Janowitz, John H. Bratt and Daniel B. Fried, *Investing in the Future: A Report on the Cost of Family Planning in the Year 2000* (Research Triangle Park, North Carolina, Family Health International, 1990); Population Crisis Committee, *1990 Report on Progress Toward Population Stabilization* (Washington, D.C., 1990).

[a]Including China.
[b]Not including China.

The Population Crisis Committee (1990) compiled information on estimated expenditures for family planning in the year 1990: outlays from government budgets; spending on family planning by consumers; and total population assistance received

from bilateral and multilateral sources. Projections were made assuming annual cost of $16 per user and a target contraceptive prevalence rate of 75 per cent.

*Projected prevalence rates assumed were to achieve the United Nations medium-variant population.

[b]Population Crisis Committee (1980) data for 37 countries, Nortman for 22 and Ness for 14. Bulatao's analysis relied mainly upon the Population Crisis Committee, but where data were lacking, they were supplemented with the others. Figures by the Committee are consistently and often substantially higher than the other two.

[c]It is unclear whether these estimates include commodity costs because a large part of the commodities were donated by USAID.

[d]Although information on donor funding is available for many countries, information on national government funding for family planning is often included in health expenditures.

[e]The TARGET model enables one to determine the number of users (and to distinguish between the new acceptors and continuing users) needed to achieve a particular target total fertility rate. In Bulatao (1985) and in Gillespie and others (1989), data were based on current number of current users, regardless of date of initial acceptance of contraceptives.

ANNEX II. CROSS-COUNTRY FAMILY PLANNING BUDGETS AND PROGRAMME EXPENDITURES

TABLE A.6. ANNUAL FAMILY PLANNING AND TOTAL GOVERNMENT BUDGETS, SELECTED COUNTRIES OR AREAS

Major area or region and country or area	Year	Family planning as percentage of		Budget status[a]
		Health budget	Total budget	
Sub-Saharan Africa				
Botswana	1985	0.29	0.01	Expended
Congo	1988	0.02	0.0	Unknown
Ghana	1989	1.02	0.09	Unknown
Kenya	1989	1.19	0.06	Allocated
Mauritius	1989	4.00	0.28	Unknown
Rwanda	1989	9.44	0.42	Expended
Zambia	1989	0.21	0.01	Expended
Zimbabwe	1983/84	27.4	1.49	Unknown
Latin America and the Caribbean				
Dominican Republic	1989	0.8	0.05	Proposed
El Salvador	1989	10.0	1.09	Allocated
Mexico	1984	0.5	0.1	Allocated
Paraguay	1986	0.0	0.0	Unknown
Middle East and Northern Africa				
Islamic Republic of Iran	1989	33.05	2.49	Allocated
Morocco	1989	4.25	--	Proposed
Tunisia	1989	1.83	0.1	Allocated
Turkey	1989	3.24	0.9	Expended
Asia				
Bangladesh	1987	31.69	1.55	Allocated
Hong Kong	1986	0.15	0.01	Unknown
India	1987/88	13.6	0.69	Allocated
Indonesia	1983/84[a]	21.98	0.55	Allocated
Republic of Korea	1989	2.06	0.09	Expended
Malaysia	1986[a]	1.57	0.07	Expended
Nepal	1989/90	18.73	0.50	Allocated
Philippines	1989[b]	..	0.16	Expended
Singapore	1989	1.1	0.04	Unknown
Sri Lanka	1987	1.32	0.05	Allocated
Taiwan Province of China	1989[b]	6.60	0.16	Allocated
Thailand	1987	2.8	0.12	Expended

Source: John A. Ross and others, *Family Planning and Child Survival: Programs as Assessed in 1991* (New York, The Population Council, 1992).

[a]The family planning budget is not included in the Ministry of Budget. Hence, the second percentage column is the ratio of the family planning budget to the separate (health budget).

[b]Not including data for Taipei City.

TABLE A.7. PERCENTAGE DISTRIBUTION OF FAMILY PLANNING PROGRAMME EXPENDITURES,
BY PROGRAMME FUNCTION, SELECTED COUNTRIES OR AREAS

Major area or region and country or area	Year	Total expenditure (thousands of dollars)	Services	Information education and comm- unication	Research	Training	Adminis- tration	Other
Sub-Saharan Africa								
Lesotho	1989	176	39	24	8	17	12	0
Madagascar	1989	258	22	13	1	4	59	1
Mauritius	1989	639	62	6	5	0	13	14
United Rep. of Tanzania	1989	1 600	62	9	3	19	6	0
Togo	1990	1 333	30	5	2	2	20	41
Zaire	1989	356	1	13	1	15	54	17
Zambia	1989	525	80	0	7	13	0	0
Latin America and the Caribbean								
Brazil (BEMFAM)	1989	9 352	35	15	6	1	30	13
Colombia (PROFAMILIA)	1989	9 388	76	1	5	1	17	0
Costa Rica (ADC)	1987	614	23	15	9	7	..	45
El Salvador	1989	7 999	50	15	5	10	15	5
		3 500	26	6	17	6	23	23
Trinidad and Tobago	1989	134	93	7	0	0	0	0
Venezuela	1990	304	71	0	1	0	28	0
Middle East and Northern Africa								
Jordan	1989	1 754	34	1	14	20	31	0
Syria	1989	670	67	15	4	14	0	0
Tunisia	1989	1 085	64	11	11	13	0	0
Turkey	1989	4 000	0	25	19	25	31	0
Asia								
Afghanistan	1989	203	43	5	0	3	17	32
Bangladesh	1989	134 500	22	46	4	4	24	0
Hong Kong	1986	2 257	63	15	1	4	18	0
India 1987/88		31 654	89	4	2	2	4	0
Malaysia	1989	7 531	14	2	3	1	80	0
Pakistan 1989-90		22 300	62	3	4	6	24	1
Philippines	1986	9 862	45	8	4	5	20	18
Republic of Korea	1989	27 332	62	14	2	1	1	21
Singapore	1989	324	46	0	12	11	31	0
Taiwan Province of China	1989	12 846	18	6	1	6	5	64
Thailand	1990	28 240	71	14	1	1	14	0

Source: John A. Ross and others, *Family Planning and Child Survival Programs as Assessed in 1991* (New York, The Population Council, 1992).
NOTE: ADC = Asociación Demográfica Costarricense; BEMFAM = Sociedade Civil Bem-Estar Familiar do Brasil; Profamilia = Asociación Pro-Bienestar de la Familia Colombiana.
*Sometimes based on only one source of funds in the national budget.

REFERENCES

Akin, John S., and J. Brad Schwartz (1988). The effect of economic factors on contraceptive choice in Jamaica and Thailand: a comparison of mixed multinominal logit results. *Economic Development and Cultural Change* (Chicago, Illinois), vol. 36, No. 6 (April), pp. 503-527.

Ashakul, Teera (1989). Analysis of contraceptive method choice and optimum contraceptive pricing structures. *Thailand Development Research Institute Newsletter* (Bangkok), vol. 4, No. 3, pp. 10-13.

Bogue, Donald, and others (1986). *Planificación familiar: necesidades y costos projección, 1985-2000, 15 paises*. Chicago, Illinois: Social Development Center.

Bongaarts, John (1991). The KAP-gap and the unmet need for contraception. *Population and Development Review* (New York), vol. 17, No. 2 (June), pp. 293-313.

Boulier, Bryan (1985). *Evaluating Unmet Need for Contraception: Estimates for Thirty-six Developing Countries*. World Bank Staff Working Papers, No. 678. Population and Development Series, No. 3. Washington, D.C.: The World Bank.

Bulatao, Rodolfo A. (1985). *Expenditures on Population Programs in Developing Regions: Current Levels and Future Requirements*. World Bank Staff Working Papers, No. 679. Washington, D.C.: The World Bank.

Casterline, John (1991). Intergrating health risk consideration and fertility preference in assessing the demand for family planning in the Philippines. Background paper for Philippine sector report.

Chernichovsky, Dov, and others (1991). *The Indonesian Family Planning Program: An Economic Perspective*. Population, Research and External Affairs Working Paper Series, No. 628. Washington, D.C: The World Bank.

Ciszewski, R. L., and P. D. Harvey (1991). The effect of price increases on contraceptive sales in Bangladesh. Washington, D.C.: Population Services International. Mimeographed.

Cochrane, Susan (1992). Internal World Bank memorandum. Mimeographed. Washington, D.C.

_____ , and Frederick Sai (1991). *Excess Fertility*. Health Sector Priorities Review, No. 9. Population, Health and Nutrition Division, Population and Human Resources Department. Washington, D.C.: The World Bank.

Cochrane, Susan, and others (1990). The economics of family planning. Draft. Washington, D.C.: The World Bank.

Cross, Harry E., and others (1991). Contraceptive source and the for-profit private sector in third world family planning. Draft. Washington, D.C.: The Urban Institute.

Gillespie, Duff G., and others (1989). Financing the delivery of contraceptives: the challenge of the next twenty years. In *The Demographic and Programmatic Consequences of Contraceptive Innovation*, Sheldon J. Segal, Amy O. Tsui and Susan M. Rogers, eds. New York: Plenum Publishing.

Janowitz, Barbara, John H. Bratt and Daniel B. Fried (1990). *Investing in the Future: A Report on the Cost of Family Planning in the Year 2000*. Research Triangle Park, North Carolina: Family Health International.

Jimenez, Emmanuel (1987). *Pricing Policy in the Social Sectors: Cost Recovery for Education and Health in Developing Countries*. Baltimore, Maryland: The Johns Hopkins University Press.

Kenney, G. M., and M. Lewis (1991). Cost analysis in family planning: operations research projects and beyond. In *Operations Research: Helping Family Planning Programs Work Better*, Myrna Seidman and Marjorie C. Horn, eds. New York: John Wiley and Sons, Inc.

Lewis, Maureen A. (1985). *Pricing and Cost Recovery Experience in Family Planning Programs*. World Bank Staff Working Papers, No. 684. Washington, D.C.: The World Bank.

_____ (1986). Do contraceptive prices affect demand? *Studies in Family Planning* (New York), vol. 17, No. 3 (May-June), pp. 126-135.

_____ (1987). Cost recovery in family planning. *Economic Development and Cultural Change* (Chicago, Illinois), vol. 36, No. 1 (October), pp. 161-182.

_____ (forthcoming). User fees in public hospitals: comparison of three country case studies. *Economic Development and Cultural Change* (Chicago, Illinois).

_____ , and Genevieve Kenney (1988). *The Private Sector and Family Planning in Developing Countries*. Population and Human Resources Department Working Papers, No. 96. Washington, D.C.: The World Bank.

Lewis, Maureen A., M. Sulvetta and G. La Forgia (1990). *Economic Costs of Hospital Services in the Dominican Republic*. Working Paper No. 3714-06. Washington, D.C.: The Urban Institute.

Merrit, Alice Payne (1992). Family planning goes public. *Integration* (Tokyo), No. 32 (June), pp. 41-43.

Molyneaux, Jack, and Tohir Diman (1991). *Impacts of Contraceptive Prices on Indonesia Contraceptive Choices*, Andrew Kantner and James Palmer, eds. Further Analysis of the 1987 Indonesia Demographic and Health Survey. Honolulu, Hawaii: East-West Center.

Morris, Leo, and others (1981). *Contraceptive Prevalence Surveys: A New Source of Family Planning Data*. Population Reports, Series M. No. 5. Baltimore, Maryland: The Johns Hopkins University Press, Population Information Program.

Population Crisis Committee (1990). *1990 Report on Progress Toward Population Stabilization*. Washington, D.C.

Ross, John A., and Stephen L. Isaacs (1988). Cost, payments and incentives in family planning programs: a review for developing countries. *Studies in Family Planning* (New York), vol. 19, No. 5 (September-October), pp. 270-283.

Ross, John A., and others (1992). *Family Planning and Child Survival Programs as Assessed in 1991*. New York: The Population Council.

Sanderson, Warren C., and Jee Peng Tan (1993). *Population Issues in Asia*. Asia Technical Department Series, No. 5. Washington, D.C.: The World Bank.

Sayila, Alfred (1992). Existing apathy. *Integration* (Tokyo), No. 32 (June), pp. 38-40.

Schearer, S. Bruce (1983). Costs of contraception: detailed review of monetary and health costs. Report for the Panel on Determinants of Fertility in Developing Countries. Washington, D.C.: National Academy of Sciences, National Research Council.

Schwartz, J. B., and others (1989). The effect of contraceptive prices on the choice of contraceptive method in the Philippines, Jamaica and Thailand. In *Choosing a Contraceptive Method: Choice in Asia and the United States*, Rodolfo A. Bulatao, R., James A. Palmore and Sandra Ward, eds. Boulder, Colorado: Westview Press.

United Nations, Economic and Social Commission for Asia and the Pacific (1987). Emerging issues and regional activities: role of the private sector and non-governmental organizations in population matters. Fifth session, Economic and Social Commission for Asia and the Pacific, Committee on Population, Bangkok, 17-21 August 1987.

United Nations Population Fund (1989). *Global Population Assistance Report, 1982-1988*. New York.

Westoff, Charles (1988). The potential demand for family planning: a new measure of unmet need. *International Family Planning Perspectives* (New York), vol. 14, No. 2 (June), pp. 225-232.

World Bank (1991). *New Directions in the Philippines Family Planning Program*. Population and Human Resources Division, Country Department. II, Report No. 9579-PH. Washington, D.C.

_____ (1992a). Effective family planning programs. Population, Health and Nutrition Division, Population and Human Resources Department. Mimeographed.

_____ (1992b). *Population Issues in Asia: Context, Policies and Prospects*. Report No. 10712-SAS/EAP. Washington, D.C.

Yaser, Yasar (1992). Airing method-specific advertisements. *Integration* (Tokyo), No. 32 (June), pp. 16-18.

XIX. CONTRACEPTIVE RESEARCH AND DEVELOPMENT

*Kerstin Hagenfeldt**

The aim of the present paper is to evaluate the most important existing methods of contraception and to review new contraceptive technology in order to develop a background for the 1994 Conference on Population and Development, which will identify issues that will be critical in the future and their policy implications.

The Scientific and Technical Advisory Group of the World Health Organization Special Programme of Research, Development and Research Training in Human Reproduction (WHO/HRP) recommended that the Programme convene a strategic planning group to identify contraceptive research priorities for the future. This group met at Geneva in June 1992 and made recommendations, which are included after each section in this paper.

A. RESEARCH AND DEVELOPMENT OF EXISTING METHODS OF CONTRACEPTION

Voluntary surgical sterilization, intra-uterine devices (IUDs) and oral contraceptive pills are the most widely used methods, accounting for 70 per cent of contraceptive use worldwide. Among users, the proportion of couples using any of these three methods in developing countries is much greater than the corresponding proportion in developed countries, about 81 and 43 per cent, respectively. This finding may reflect to some extent the differing history of contraceptive practice in the two groups of countries but there could also be another reason. Modern methods, particularly clinic-based methods, are very effective but can be associated with side-effects. Thus, where safe pregnancy termination services are widely available and where the health risk of continuing the pregnancy is negligible, a method with a relatively lower efficacy (e.g., condoms) is an accepted trade-off for a more convenient and safer method. The

situation in most developing countries, on the other hand, is such that contraceptive failure can potentially result in a major health hazard—hence the need to use very effective methods (Khanna, Van Look and Griffin, 1992).

Steroidal hormonal contraception

Steroidal hormonal contraception currently used by women includes: (*a*) oral pills; (*b*) injectables; (*c*) implants.

Oral pills

Many millions of women have used oral contraceptives since they became available in the early 1960s. Currently, about 65 million women worldwide are using this highly effective form of contraception. The first pill to be introduced contained high doses of oestrogen and progestagen. There has been a gradual but significant reduction in both components since then. Such reductions have led to a decrease in adverse effects, thus expanding the use of oral contraceptives to a greater range of women. In the late 1960s, progestagen-only contraceptive pills were introduced. These pills made possible the use of oral contraception by women for whom the use of proestrogen was contraindicated or not advisable.

During the time that oral contraceptives have been widely used, they have been studied more thoroughly than any other medication. Much of the data available for evaluation is based on studies of higher dose pills, many of which are no longer in use; and it may be assumed that the pills currently used are even safer than the older ones. The great majority of women that have used oral contraceptives have done so safely, with protection from pregnancy and freedom from major

*Department of Obstetrics and Gynaecology, Karolinska Hospital, Stockholm, Sweden. Background material for this paper has kindly been provided by the following persons: M. Fathalla, Director, Special Programme of Research, Development and Research Training in Human Reproduction, World Health Organization, Geneva, Switzerland; F. P. Haseltine, Director, Center for Population Research, National Institute of Child Health and Human Development, United States Department of Health and Human Services, Bethesda, Maryland; J. M. Spieler, Research Advisor, United States Agency for International Development, Washington, D.C.; C. W. Bardin, Director, Center for Biomedical Research, The Population Council, New York; T. King, Project Director, Family Health International, Durham, North Carolina; H. L. Gabelnick, Director, Contraceptive Research and Development Program, Arlington, Virginia; J. Queenan, The Institute for Reproductive Health, Washington, D.C.

side-effects. The benefits to health and well-being far outweigh the possible side-effects and infrequent complications, which occur in a minority of users. Because oral contraceptives have proved to be so safe and effective, they are available without prescription in many countries.

Recent and ongoing research on oral contraceptives and progestagen-only pills have concentrated on safety aspects; mainly carcinogenesis, the effect on the cardiovascular system, the use of steroid hormonal contraceptives during lactation and the relation between oral contraceptives and infections with a sexually transmitted disease (STD) or the human immunodeficiency virus (HIV).

Carcinogenesis

Research on the relation between steroidal contraceptives and the risk of cancer has been a high priority activity of the WHO/HRP programme since 1979, when the WHO Collaborative Study of Neoplasia and Steroidal Contraceptives was launched. This 13-centre study was initiated because, until then, all data on oral contraceptives and cancer risk came from a few developed countries. The results show that the use of oral contraceptives has a protective effect against cancer of the ovary and endometrium: the woman's risk of developing ovarian cancer is reduced by about 40 per cent and that for endometrial cancer by about 50 per cent. The ovarian effect persists for at least 10 years after stopping the use of oral contraceptives. The endometrial protective effect appears to be maintained for up to 15 years after discontinuation, according to one study. The risk of developing ovarian or endometrial cancer decreases the longer oral contraceptives are used (WHO, 1992b).

The relation between oral contraceptives and breast cancer has been studied extensively in developed countries and more recently in developing countries. Some studies have found a possible link between use for a long duration and increased breast cancer risk among young women. The WHO study indicated that women that had ever used oral contraceptives had an overall and relative risk of 1.15 of developing breast cancer, as compared with women that had never used them. Breast cancer risk was not significantly different in developing, as compared with developed, countries, nor was the risk significantly different among women under age 35, compared with those over that age. Despite continued controversy about the risks in some subgroups of

women, no changes in oral contraceptive use were recommended by a WHO scientific group (WHO, 1992b).

The relation between oral contraceptives and cervical neoplasia is not conclusive. Some of the recent studies provide evidence of a positive relation, particularly for long-term use. Results, however, are difficult to interpret because of a variety of methodological problems of the observational epidemiological studies addressing this relation. Nevertheless, if an increased risk of cancer of the cervix exists, it is small (WHO, 1992b).

Studies on steroid hormones and neoplastic disorders have also been conducted in the United States of America by the Center for Population Research of the National Institute of Child Health and Human Development (CPR/NICHD). A major study has been completed to understand the factors that contribute to the occurrence of cervical cancer. The study focuses on a cervical cancer precursor, cervical dysplasia. The results indicate that sexual activity characteristics probably outweigh oral contraceptive use in cervical dysplasia risk (United States of America, 1991). The question of steroid hormone and breast cancer has also been addressed by CPR/NICHD. New studies will concentrate on other than reproductive and personal demographic risk factors. Further studies of breast cancer in young women should be supported in the future once today's very young oral contraceptive users, in their teens, reach their thirties (CPR, 1991).

Cardiovascular disease

The increases of stroke, myocardial infarction and venous thromboembolism represent important, albeit rare, adverse health effects of oral contraceptives. Most information on this topic comes from developed countries and refers to oral pill preparations that were in common use during the 1960s and 1970s. It is not known, however, whether the observed effects can be extrapolated to developing countries, where risk factors for cardiovascular disease are very different. Also, there is little information about whether the effects are the same for the different patterns of pill use and the different types of low-dose pills, commonly used today or whether changed prescription practices have affected the occurrence of these adverse effects. To address these questions, WHO/HRP is conducting a large multinational case control study of venous thromboembolism, stroke and myocardial infarction in 17 centres in Africa, Asia, Europe and Latin America. The final results of the study should be available in 1994 (WHO, 1992c).

CPR/NICHD is collaborating with WHO in this study. Furthermore, the Center is involved in projects in the United States on the relative risk of acute myocardial infarction and stroke in users of current low-dose oral contraceptives. In addition to establishing relative and attributable risk for cardiovascular disease, a major focus of the projects of CPR is to determine the contribution of oestrogen dose and progestin type and dose to pill-associated risk.

CPR is also involved in studies on the oral contraceptives, cardiovascular risk factors and lifetime prospects for heart disease and diabetes. In this study, the effect of the pill on lipids and lipoprotein metabolism and glucose metabolism is studied.

Lactation

The use of hormonal contraceptives during lactation is practised in both developed and developing countries (WHO, 1981). Hormonal contraceptives may affect the health of the infant, indirectly by modifying the quality and quantity of breast milk or directly as a result of passage of the hormones or their metabolites to the infant through breast milk. Although the studies by WHO/HRP and other groups have shown that oestrogen-containing contraceptives have adverse effects on lactation, the progestogen-only contraceptives appear not to have any consistent effects either on lactation or on infant growth (WHO, 1988). However, the concern has remained that this situation might not be the case for infants that may be ill or whose mothers may be undernourished. In order to address the remaining concerns, WHO/HRP is supporting a multi-centre study on growth and health of infants whose mothers use progestagen-only contraceptives during lactation. The objectives are to assess possible adverse effects of progestogen-only contraceptives on growth, health and development of infants whose mothers have used these contraceptives while breast-feeding the infant. The main study began in 1989 and a final report should be available in 1992 (WHO, 1992c).

In the United States of America. Family Health International (FHI) is also involved in studies on the safety, efficacy and acceptability of progestagen-only pills for lactating women.

Sexually transmitted diseases/HIV and oral contraceptives

Currently, the most important mode of HIV transmission in the world is through heterosexual intercourse. Any factor that may modify the risk of transmission, either upward or downward, is of importance particularly in high-prevalence areas. A study from Nairobi, Kenya, suggests an association between use of oral contraceptives and the risk of acquiring HIV infection (Simonsen and others, 1990). The underlying biological mechanisms for a possible enhancement of HIV transmission by oral contraceptives (or other steroidal contraceptives) are unclear, but they could be related to the presence of cervical ectropion; increased risk of certain STDs, such as chlamydial infection; irregular menstrual bleeding and possibly immunological alterations. Studies on the association of contraceptive use and risk of HIV transmission are difficult because, by necessity, they must be observational and because potential confounding factors complicate their interpretation. A study supported by WHO/HRP on risk factors for HIV acquisition in relation to contraceptive methods used among female sex workers in Bangkok, Thailand, began in October 1990. FHI is also evaluating the relation between various reversible contraceptive methods, particularly oral contraceptives, and HIV infection in women. If logistic problems can be solved, this study will begin as a case-control study screening some 10,000 women attending one or more clinics at Nairobi, Kenya, during a two-year period (FHI, 1992).

CPR/NICHD is undertaking *in vitro* experiments to determine the effects of oral contraceptives on the susceptibility of human lymphocytes to infection with HIV or to the replication of HIV once infected. Although epidemiological studies will best determine any effect of hormonal contraceptives on the acquisition or progression of HIV infection (as described above), *in vitro* studies can provide more timely information than direct clinical studies by offering hypotheses to be tested and can better delineate the mechanism by which these agents may affect the disease process (United States of America, 1991).

Correct use of oral contraceptives

Thirty years after oral contraceptives were introduced, they are still considered one of the most effective reversible methods of birth control. However, recent studies suggest that as many as 15-20 per cent of married users in some developing countries and some 6 per cent of unmarried users in the United States may be getting pregnant, largely because they do not take the pills correctly. FHI is involved in a study of correct use, known as "pill user compliance". Research shows that many women receive confusing instructions, or no instructions at all, on when to begin taking the pill, how many days they should take placebos (or no pills) between cycles and what they should do if they forget to take one or more pills. In many countries, women's failure to use oral contraceptives properly may contribute to increased side-effects, discontinuation and disappointing high pregnancy rates (FHI, 1992). Research and development in this area is therefore of utmost importance. Another area of interest for research and development of oral contraceptive use is removal of service obstacles. Although there is a growing demand for oral contraceptives and other contraceptives in many developing countries, there are often obstacles to obtaining them. Oral contraceptives are suitable methods to be included in community-based services (CBS). Contraindications to their use are few and community workers can be trained in the use of simple check-lists to identify clients that need to be referred to a clinical facility (IPPF, 1992a).

The development of oral contraceptives using new synthetic steroids is in the hands of the pharmaceutical industry. The highest priority for research for WHO/HRP is further epidemiological research, particularly in developing countries. Furthermore, service delivery aspects still need more research and there are still problems involved in acceptability, continuation etc. (WHO, 1992d).

Injectables

Injectable hormonal contraception with long-acting steroidal preparations provides an effective means of fertility regulation and has become an important method of family planning. Current prevalence in less developed regions is 2 per cent of all contraceptives used. Approximately 8 million women throughout the world are using depot-medroxy progesterone acetate (DMPA) as a three-monthly injectable contraceptive (5 million in Indonesia alone and 1 million in Thailand) while more than 1 million women are using the two-monthly injectable norethisterone enanthate (NET-EN). DMPA is now registered as a therapeutic agent in nearly all countries and as a contraceptive agent in at least 83 developed and developing countries. NET-EN is registered as a

contraceptive in at least 57 countries. In some countries, locally produced and non-tested formulations are also available and extensively used. A single injection of an injectable contraceptive can provide highly effective protection against pregnancy for one, two or more months. Delivery is simple, is independent of coitus and ensures periodic contact with medical or other trained health personnel. Ongoing research on injectable contraceptives continues to study the main adverse effect, menstrual irregularities, as well as possible effects on offspring, possible carcinogenesis and metabolic effects.

Menstrual irregularities

One disadvantage of injectables, as perceived by the users, is that they sometimes cause menstrual bleeding to become irregular and unpredictable or occasionally absent altogether. This side-effect, which is not fully understood, is common to all progestagen-only methods, including Norplant (see next subsection). WHO/HRP is studying the mechanisms of endometrial bleeding in order to investigate how it is affected by steroidal hormones and to test various ways of treating these bleeding irregularities. There is no evidence that these menstrual disturbances have adverse health effects. In fact, on average, users of these methods experience less blood loss than with their normal menses and thus are less exposed to the risk of anaemia. However, menstrual irregularities interfere with daily life and for sociocultural reasons are totally unacceptable in some settings.

Effect on offspring

There is evidence from investigations carried out in several countries that DMPA and NET-EN may increase both milk production and the duration of lactation. The question of possible consequences of the transfer of injectable steroids to the breast-fed infant has yet to be solved. It is known that the amounts of steroid transmitted in the milk and absorbed by the infant are small. Although short-term follow-up studies of children breast-fed by mothers using progestagen-only contraceptives have been reassuring, longer term studies are yet to be evaluated.

When discussing possible risks to the infant, inadvertent exposure to DMPA or NET-EN because of injections in women that are already pregnant must be considered. WHO/HRP has funded studies in Israel and Thailand on the possible consequences of exposure of the foetus to contraceptive steroids. The study in Israel was concerned with pubertal development and ended in 1989. The results show no effect on pubertal development from *in utero* exposure to steroidal contraceptives (Jaffe and others, 1988 and 1989). The Thai study used observational historical follow-up methodology and was based on data from interviews of the mothers and from case records of family planning, maternal and child health clinics in hospitals at Chiang-Mai, Thailand (Pardthaisong and Gray, 1991; Gray and Pardthaisong, 1991). The results of the study pertaining to infant survival showed no significantly increased risk of mortality in the first year of life for infants exposed to oral contraceptives *in utero* as compared with infants of control mothers, whereas the infants from DMPA-exposed pregnancies had a somewhat increased risk of dying during the first year of life (relative risk of 1.8, 95 per cent confidence interval, 1.1-3.0). It is therefore necessary to reinforce in all guidelines on use of DMPA or other injectables that the drug should not be administered to pregnant women (Khanna, Van Look and Griffin, 1992).

Carcinogenesis

The WHO Collaborative Study of Neoplasia and Steroidal Contraceptives also includes studies on DMPA. The final analysis of the data collected on DMPA and selected cancer sites is currently being completed. The study, carried out in both developed and developing countries, did not find any significant relation between the use of DMPA and breast cancer in women. Although the study suggests that there may be a small increased risk during the first four years of DMPA use in women under age 35, it did not show any increased risk with duration of use and no extra risk in women that had begun to use DMPA more than five years previously. These results provide reassurance that women that have used DMPA for a long time and initiated use many years previously are not at increased risk for cancer of the breast (WHO, Collaborative Study, 1991a).

Progestagens are supposed to be protective against endometrial cancer and specifically DMPA is used in the treatment of endometrial malignancy. Results from the WHO study show a relative risk of 0.3 for endometrial cancer, which, although not statistically significant, does support the hypothesis that use of DMPA might protect women against this form of cancer (WHO, Collaborative Study, 1991b).

Neither ovarian nor liver cancer has been found with increased frequency among women that have used DMPA (WHO, Collaborative Study, 1991c and 1991d).

The paper on DMPA and cervical cancer has been completed and submitted for publication, and the report on the relation between DMPA use and cancer *in situ* of the cervix is being prepared. Further analysis of adenocarcinoma of the cervix and DMPA use and of breast cancer in relation to reproductive factors, such as lactation, are planned for 1992.

Since the relation between hormonal contraceptives and cancer of the breast and cervix is still not fully resolved, the WHO Scientific Group recommends that further research be undertaken (WHO, 1992b).

Metabolic effects

Despite the intense biochemical research, the only clinical metabolic effect attributed to DMPA is weight gain. No other metabolic effect has associated clinical problems. WHO/HRP has initiated studies on the effects of DMPA and NET-EN on lipid metabolism at Bangkok, Havana and Mexico City. Both DMPA and NET-EN induce changes in lipid metabolism which are unfavourable in terms of arteriosclerotic risk. However, the magnitude of these changes is relatively small and lipid metabolism is only one factor affecting the process of arteriosclerosis. Thus, these results are, on the whole, reassuring (WHO, 1992c).

Currently, DMPA and NET-EN are to be considered safe and effective means of contraception. The most common side-effect, menstrual irregularities, necessitates appropriate counselling for women considering the use of injectable contraception. They should be clearly informed about the advantages and disadvantages, side-effects, costs and alternative contraceptives.

Implants

One of the goals during the past two decades in the development of more effective and acceptable means of steroidal hormonal contraceptives has been to produce an implant releasing the steroid for an extended period of time. This type of device would reduce the risk of patient error, increase compliance and reduce the necessity of repeated contacts with medical personnel while still being a reversible method. The first implant in clinical use is the Norplant system developed by the

Population Council. The Norplant subdermal implant system is a long-acting, reversible, low-dose, progestagen-only contraceptive method which provides protection for five years. The drug, levonorgestrel, is delivered by means of six silastic capsules placed subdermally. Clinical studies began in 1975 in seven countries and further clinical trials have continued in both developed and developing countries. Norplant was first registered for commercial use in 1983 in Finland, the country of manufacture; and since then more than 20 countries, including the United States, have approved the method for distribution. To date, over 55,000 women have participated in studies in 46 countries, and more than 1 million women have used Norplant in countries where it has been approved. Statistically, Norplant has a lower failure rate than the combined pill or most IUDs and its efficacy during the first three years of use can be compared to surgical sterilization. The Postmarketing Surveillance of Norplant is a collaborative project between WHO/HRP, FHI and the Population Council. This is a concurrent cohort study of women accepting Norplant implants for family planning purposes (index subjects) and women choosing IUD or sterilization (control subjects). The index and control subjects are being followed for a five-year period. Clinic visits take place every six months and all health-related complaints and events are recorded as well as shifts to other contraceptive methods. The project is under way in eight participating countries (Bangladesh, Chile, China, Colombia, Egypt, Indonesia, Sri Lanka and Thailand). FHI has also worked with the Program for the Introduction and Adaptation of Contraceptive Technology (PIACT) to coordinate the development of user-oriented education and materials in several countries in order to promote local knowledge and acceptance of Norplant. In addition, programmatic research has been performed to increase the acceptability of Norplant and national information seminars directed to physicians and policy makers have been organized. In collaboration with the Population Council, FHI has developed a worldwide Norplant database (FHI, 1992; Population Council, 1992; WHO, 1992c).

Metabolic studies

Several studies have been undertaken to determine the metabolic and biochemical effects of Norplant. One ongoing WHO study is comparing the effect of Norplant and a non-hormone releasing IUD on lipid metabolism at Bangkok, Jakarta, Mexico City, Singapore and Stockholm. No clinical important changes have been found in the liver, kidney, adrenal or thyroid function. Norplant use has been associated with a slight increase in serum glucose concentration. However, the changes are not of clinical importance, nor are they progressive in magnitude with time (WHO, 1992c).

Service issues

Although Norplant presents obvious advantages for family planning programmes, its introduction poses a number of managerial challenges. First, it is a clinic-based method and requires formal training in insertion and removal. Secondly, it is a progestagen-only method associated with alterations of the menstrual cycle and requiring specific counselling for potential acceptors. The training of medical personnel in the use of the method and of staff responsible for counselling potential acceptors is the most important factor in the successful introduction of the Norplant method (IPPF, 1992b).

Barrier methods and spermicides

Barrier methods of contraception are safe and fairly reliable for couples that are sufficiently motivated to use them consistently. Although they are not as effective as other available contraceptives, barrier methods can play an important role in family planning programmes. Their use often constitutes a first step in contraceptive practice, the user gradually moving towards more reliable methods. The main advantages of barrier contraceptives are that their action is not systemic, they have no known serious short- or long-term side-effects and they do not interfere with lactation. The global spread of STDs, including HIV, has made it more important than ever to create effective contraceptive devices that also provide protection against sexually transmitted diseases.

Male condoms

According to WHO, condom use amounts to 19 per cent of all contraceptive methods in the developed regions but only to 6 per cent in the less developed regions (Khanna, Van Look and Griffin, 1992). Ongoing research has concentrated on efficacy of the condom method and on condom acceptability. Studies have shown that the use of the condom reduces the risk of sexual HIV transmission (Ngugi and others, 1988; Laurian, Peynet and Verroust, 1988). However, the efficacy of the condom in preventing unwanted pregnancies has not been accurately determined. Reported pregnancies vary from fewer than 2 to more than 30 per

100 couple-years (Vessey and others, 1988). In view of this situation, WHO/HRP proposes to undertake a study on the contraceptive use and method effectiveness of the condom among a well-motivated, fertile and sexually active group of people. The project will be conducted in China (Shanghai and Tianjin) and the main phase is expected to commence in 1992 and to involve approximately 3,000 couples to be followed for a 12-month period. Condom acceptability studies were begun in 1989 by WHO/HRP; and in 1991, this male-oriented research was expanded to include a broader set of issues dealing not only with the role of many reproductive decisions within the family but also with behaviour *vis-à-vis* the risk involved in unprotected sexual behaviour. Knowledge of reproductive functions, of methods of contraception and of reproductive risks among men is generally poor. The situation is especially critical among male adolescents. WHO/HRP will continue its efforts to promote research in this area. Ten small-scale studies on how men view the condum, conducted in sub-Saharan African countries, produced interesting findings on who uses condoms, why they are used and why they are not used. The majority of men know about the condom and know that it prevents both pregnancy and disease. There is a large gap, nevertheless, between men's knowledge of the condom and use of the method: far fewer men use the condom than know of it. Policy recommendations from these studies underscore the need for condoms to be promoted as an alternative family planning method and the need to improve the image of the condom as a legitimate and acceptable barrier method for stable couples. These projects also indicate that throughout Africa, more information and education regarding condoms are required. Culture-sensitive information about the condom is often lacking, and the condom should be promoted for safe sex with partners rather than only for high-risk behaviour that men reject or deny. Given the importance of the condom as a contraceptive and disease prevention measure, a substantial effort to educate the public and promote condom sale and use is urgently needed (WHO, 1992c).

New developments

FHI is undertaking a research and development programme to introduce a condom made of synthetic thermoplastic instead of natural latex. This condom is expected to be stronger and better able to withstand the storage conditions in many developing countries, and to be compatible with many kinds of lubricants. The goal is to produce this product at a price that will make it

affordable for widespread use in developing countries. As the quality and reliability of latex condoms provided to family planning and acquired immunodeficiency syndrome (AIDS) prevention programmes in the developing world has become an issue of critical importance, the major donor supplying condoms to these programmes, United States Agency for International Development (USAID), is concerned with assuring product quality and has engaged FHI to undertake a major research effort to evaluate and help improve the latex condom. FHI is also performing acceptability research on small versus standard condoms, on larger condoms and on stronger versus standard condoms. There was no difference in breakage rates of the different condom types. Furthermore, preliminary data show no clear preference for either type of condom. The data suggest that there is great variability in condom breakage rates among individuals regardless of condom type (FHI, 1992). CPR/NICHD is also involved in clinical studies with a new polyurethane condom. These studies will focus on the acceptability of the product when compared with latex condoms (United States of America, 1991).

Female condoms

The female condom, or vaginal sheath, is a barrier method for the prevention of transmission of STDs (including HIV) from men to women and vice versa. The device is under the woman's control and can be inserted some time prior to coitus. In a study conducted by WHO/HRP together with FHI, the female condom was studied among bar- and brothel-based commercial sex workers in Thailand (WHO, 1992c). Together with the Contraceptive Research and Development Program (CONRAD), FHI is also evaluating the female condom and focuses on acceptability and contraceptive efficacy. Studies are being conducted in the United States and Latin America on the female condom Reality (Wisconsin Pharmacal). In January 1992, the studies were reviewed by the advisory panel for medical devices of the United States Food and Drug Administration (FDA). The advisory panel recommended approval of the device pending completion of the clinical study and a final review of the results (FHI, 1992). The main purpose in the development of the female condom is to provide women with the ability to protect themselves against AIDS and other STDs, particularly in situations when men refuse to use condoms. Responding to growing interest in the method, FHI is also supporting acceptability studies in Kenya and Cameroon. WHO/HRP is planning acceptability studies in Zimbabwe that will begin in early 1992 with volunteers from four groups: urban out-patient clinic attenders; urban nurses; rural hospital attenders; and commercial sex workers.

Diaphragm and cervical caps

The most widely used female barrier method is the diaphragm. There is a need for further research to resolve specific issues relevant to diaphragm use, such as whether its contraceptive effect is chiefly due to its role as a barrier to sperm or as a carrier for spermicide. Until more evidence becomes available, the diaphragm should be used together with spermicides in order to ensure maximum contraceptive protection.

The cervical cap may be more suited for some women than the diaphragm; however, it is not widely used and there are few reliable data on its effectiveness. CPR/NICHD is undertaking acceptability and efficacy studies of a new valved cervical cap, which may have the potential of being used either with or without nonoxynol spermicide. Sufficient data may accrue from this study to gain marketing approval from FDA (United States of America, 1991).

FHI is also developing a new barrier method in collaboration with CONRAD. This new method, the Lea's shield, has the potential of being used continuously for 48 hours, preferably without a spermicide. Primary responsibility for the management and monitoring of the project rests with CONRAD. FHI serves as the data manager for this project and will provide statistical analysis of the data once the fieldwork has been completed. FHI is also doing a re-analysis of their contraceptive sponge data, compared with similar studies of the diaphragm and the cervical cap. The results will be available during this year (FHI, 1992).

Spermicides

Spermicidal products (creams, jellies, foams in pressurized containers, foaming tablets or suppositories), when used on their own, are not as effective as other contraceptives, but they do provide additional protection when used in conjunction with a condom or diaphragm. Spermicides can also be useful as backup contraceptive protection for couples relying upon lactational amenorrhoea. Spermicides are well suited for commercial and non-medical distribution as they have no proven systemic side-effects or serious local reactions. Furthermore, evidence suggests that they have a protective effect against certain STDs. There is a need for the development of a variety of improved spermicides both for fertility regulation and for controlling the spread of STDs. In addition to the studies on new condoms, CPR/NICHD has initiated development of spermicide-releasing diaphragms. The two polymers that will be utilized for the matrix of the device are silastic and polyurethane. The spermicide in both products will be nonoxynol-9. Conceptually, such products resemble the Today sponge in that they will be effective over an extended period of time and will not require the addition of a new supply of the spermicide. The effectiveness of these devices may be enhanced by the fact that they represent more of a true barrier than do the sponges. Important issues that can be resolved only through clinical studies are acceptability of such devices and whether they produce significant vaginal irritation. The fact that these diaphragms do not require addition of a spermicide should make them attractive to potential users. The cost effectiveness of such devices can be a problem and will have to be kept in mind during the various developmental phases (United States of America, 1991).

In the spermicide area, CPR/NICHD is supporting research on the development of a long-acting spermicide suppository. The product is designed to release nonoxynol over extended periods of time.

Nonoxynol-9, menfegol and benzalconium chloride have been shown to have *in vitro* bactericidal and virucidal activity in studies conducted in the United States by CPR/NICHD and CONRAD, and there are reports of *in vivo* antichlamydial and gonococcocidal activity. Thus, it would seem obvious that these compounds should be developed as bactericidal and virucidal agents for use in the prevention of STD transmission. The enthusiasm has been halted by reports of vaginal irritation and microulceration in frequent users of nonoxynol-9, which theoretically would put them at greater risk of HIV infection. WHO/HRP has designed studies in female volunteers to evaluate the problem. The study, funded by the WHO Global Programme on AIDS, will be undertaken during 1992 in the WHO collaborating centres at Bangkok, Manila, Chiang Mai, Hat Yai and Khon Kaen. WHO/HRP has also identified a series of compounds originally developed as oral disinfectants that have spermicidal, virucidal and bactericidal properties similar to those of nonoxynol-9. In collaboration with CONRAD, WHO will initiate preliminary toxicological studies in rabbits and rats which would permit phase I studies in humans. CPR/NICHD has developed an animal model using the macaque species. This monkey can be infected with the simian immunodeficiency virus (SIV) through the same routes as in the human. It has been reported that SIV can be transmitted genitally. The amount of virus necessary for 100 per cent infectivity genitally route has been defined and a 50 per cent infectious dose is being defined. This information can then be used to determine the challenge dose for testing the efficacy of spermicides and other compounds in preventing or fostering transmission. Initial studies have demonstrated that contraceptive gel and foam containing nonoxynol-9 provide partial protection against vaginal transmission of SIV to females. Since infected macaques all die of SIV disease, efforts to find a more natural monkey model of disease transmission has led to studies in African green monkey. This monkey develops a persistent long-term infection but does not succumb from the disease. This may be a useful model to evaluate horizontal and vertical transmission of the virus under semi-natural conditions (United States of America, 1991).

There was a consensus in the Strategic Planning Group of WHO/HRP that barrier methods currently represent an important, if not the most important, research area in reproductive health. Therefore, the development and assessment of new methods remains a very high priority for the field. Of equally high priority are the introduction and transfer of technologies. Barrier methods have never been properly introduced; the condom is failing because there is no proper introduction. Introduction is a major interest of, *inter alia*, women groups. Epidemiological research in this field is of high priority, in terms of both contraceptive efficacy and the prevention of STDs, including AIDS. The same high priority should be assigned to social science research, an area in which WHO/HRP appears to be a significant actor (WHO, 1992a).

Intra-uterine devices

The intra-uterine device is one of the most commonly used methods of fertility regulation, especially in developing country programmes. It is estimated that there are more than 80 million IUD users, with some 74 million in China alone (Khanna, Van Look and Griffin, 1992). The new copper- and hormone-releasing IUDs combine high continuation rates with low pregnancy rates. The Population Council has, during the past 20 years,

developed several new models of the copper IUD, the most recent being Copper-T 380A, which now serves as a benchmark for IUD use. The Population Council and WHO/HRP have both conducted large multi-centre studies in both developed and developing countries on the Copper-T 380A, which has shown a failure rate after many years of use of the same level as surgical sterilization. With regard to effectiveness, these modern IUDs have probably reached the maximum level that it is possible to obtain in terms of pregnancy protection.

The main concern with the IUD method during the past 10 years has been the risk of contracting pelvic inflammatory disease (PID). A recent analysis by WHO/HRP, involving data from IUD trials conducted between 1976 and the present, includes information on a large group of IUD users throughout the world. Information collected in these trials include the number of subjects that discontinued IUD use because of PID. Data were analysed from several randomized studies that compared two or more IUDs. A total of 22,908 IUD insertions with 616,790 women-months of experience were included in the analysis. The overall rate of PID was 1.6 cases per 1,000 woman-years of use. PID risk was nearly seven times higher during the 20 days following insertion than during later times, with the risk low and constant for up to eight years of follow-up. Rates varied according to geographical area, with the highest rates in Africa and the lowest in China, and decreased with age. PID rates were lower among women whose IUD was inserted after 1980 than among those whose IUD had been inserted in previous years. These findings indicate that the occurrence of PID among IUD users is strongly related to the insertion process and to the background risk of STDs. They suggest that PID is an infrequent occurrence after the insertion period among appropriately selected women. Because of the increased risk of PID associated with the insertion, IUDs should be left *in situ* up to their maximum life-span and need not be routinely replaced earlier (WHO, 1992c).

CPR/NICHD has pursued studies on the evaluation of the effects of IUDs and other contraceptive methods on the occurrence of infertility. The findings indicate that copper IUDs are safe for certain groups of women, in particular for women with at least one child that are living in a stable and monogamous sexual relationship. Younger women that have no children and may be in an unstable sexual relationship should consider other forms of contraception. The three goals of the project are: *(a)* to measure the reduction in risk and other events requiring IUD removal provided by prophylactic antibiotics; *(b)* to estimate the incidence rate for PID and other events requiring IUD removal; and *(c)* to evaluate the side-effects of the antibiotics used in the study (United States of America, 1991).

One of the side-effects of IUDs identified early in IUD history was the increase in menstrual blood loss following the insertion of the device. Although healthy women do not experience serious health effects of the increased menstrual blood loss, it could be a problem in women with anaemia or bad nutritional status. During the 1970s, one of the research efforts in WHO/HRP was to find solutions to this problem. Several interesting leads were identified while studying the hæmostasis of the uterus and the ætiology of the increased blood loss in IUD users. Due to the change in funding, all basic research in this area was closed down in 1978. The research line has been followed through by other organizations. The Population Council has sponsored the development and clinical testing of IUD which releases 20 mg of levonorgestrel per day. This device has been reported in randomized studies as having a pregnancy rate at five years of 1.1 per 100 woman years (Sivin and others, 1990). Studies on menstrual blood loss have shown a decrease but also a high removal rate for amenorrhoea of nearly 20 per cent. To date there have been more than 70 publications on this device, but very few concern the safety and efficacy of the device in developing countries, where the side-effects of amenorrhoea may not be as acceptable as in some developed countries. WHO/HRP will initiate a randomized, multi-centre, comparative trial of the insertion of the TCU 380A and the 20-mg levonorgestrel-releasing IUD in parous women in 12 centres in 9 countries. It is expected that this study will continue for at least seven years (WHO, 1992c).

Two of the major side-effects of IUDs, namely, pain and cramping, alone or together with bleeding, are thought to be caused by discrepancies between the size of the IUD and the size and shape of the uterine cavity. WHO/HRP is evaluating a new concept in IUDs in which the copper sleeves—which in currently available devices are placed on a plastic frame—are suspended from a nylon suture. The suture is inserted superficially into the uterine muscle at the time IUD is inserted into the uterus, leaving it and the copper sleeves to hang freely from the top of the uterine cavity. This device, Flexi-gard, is currently being compared with the Copper-T 380A in a study involving 28 centres (WHO, 1992c).

Post-placental IUDs

A number of studies have shown that IUD insertion immediately following the removal of the placenta at delivery or at any time from 24 hours to 6 weeks after delivery is associated with a high expulsion rate. This occurrence is probably the result of a combination of the uterus rapidly returning to its usual non-pregnant size and the device being too small, at least in relation to the size of the uterus immediately following delivery. WHO/HRP will begin pilot studies in up to six centres on two novel IUDs that are based on the general concept of the frameless IUD and have been designed specifically for insertion during the early post-partum period.

Due to its positive programmatic implications, post-partum IUD studies are also being taken up by other organizations. In selected developing countries, FHI will assess the safety and efficacy of inserting the Copper-T 380A IUD in the immediate post-placental period.

Basic research in the IUD field

The leads identified in the WHO/HRP research on hæmostasis in the uterus, important aspects when developing IUDs to reduce menstrual blood loss, have been taken up by Chinese scientists. The vast majority of IUD users are in China; thus, most of the innovative research on new IUDs is being conducted in China and IUD research is the first priority of the State Family Planning Commission. The National Institute for Family Planning at Beijing is performing basic research on hæmostatic mechanisms in the uterus and animal studies on hæmostatic drugs to be included in medicated IUDs (China, 1992).

There was general agreement in the Strategic Planning Group of WHO/HRP that further development of the Flexi-gard and post-placental devices is the highest priority in this area. Epidemiological research continues to be a high priority and there is also a place for social science research, especially on issues such as the acceptability of amenorrhoea during the use of a levonorgestrel device (WHO, Collaborative Study, 1991d).

Sterilization

Voluntary surgical sterilization has become an extremely popular and well-established contraceptive procedure, providing the most effective protection against pregnancy for couples desiring no more children. It offers many advantages over other contraceptive methods in that it is a one-time procedure which eliminates the risk of unwanted pregnancy almost completely. It does not entail regular check-ups or the need for expense of continued contraceptive supplies and does not rely upon the sustained motivation of the user for its effectiveness. Also, the risk of complications is small if the procedure is performed according to accepted medical standards. Female and male sterilizations together constitute the most commonly used method for contraception, accounting for over one third of world contraceptive use (Khanna, Van Look and Griffin, 1992). Sterilization is, however, in principle an irreversible method and therefore only of interest to couples that have completed their family size. In most countries where data on contraceptive trends are available, the prevalence of sterilization has increased in recent years. Like other methods, however, sterilization prevalence is unevenly distributed throughout the world. China and India, the two most populous countries, have more than half of the users of this method. In general, female sterilization is far more common than male sterilization and the gap between the two continues to widen. Over the past decade, the development of laparoscopic procedures with the use of rings and clips as well as the refining of the minilaparotomy procedure has decreased complications and side-effects in female sterilization, and the method is now almost always done as an ambulatory procedure.

Sterilization is one of the most popular forms of fertility regulation in the United States, with an estimated 13.6 million women having opted for sterilization or for sterilization of their partner as their contraceptive choice. This fact has prompted CPR/NICHD to investigate the benefits and risks of tubal sterilization. The findings suggest that there are no serious overall health effects of female sterilization. There was no association between any cardiovascular disease, including myocardial infarction and stroke, and sterilization. There was no association between cancer and sterilization. The overall morbidity or mortality of sterilized women was similar to that of women in the population-based comparison group (United States of America, 1991).

Vasectomy

Vasectomy, which is a still simpler surgical procedure, is the contraceptive method that has the lowest incidence of side-effects and the highest effectiveness.

Two main factors limit the acceptability of vasectomy: one is the necessity for a skin incision, which is unacceptable in some cultures; the other is the lack of certain reversibility should the circumstances require this measure. Among many attempts to develop simplified methods to overcome these limitations, research in China, which began in the 1970s, has led to two major technical improvements: the isolation and ligation of the vas through a puncture (non-scalpel) opening in the skin; and the development of a technique for the percutaneous injection into the vas lumen of sclerosing or occluding agents through a hypodermic needle (Zhao, 1990). To study the efficacy and reversibility of silicon vas occlusion, WHO/HRP has initiated a study in baboons at the WHO Collaborating Centre at Nairobi. The study has demonstrated that an injection of silicone directly into the exposed vas deferens achieved total occlusion and azoospermia by one month in 14 of 20 baboons. The plugs are being surgically removed to determine reversibility. The WHO Toxicology Panel has approved the use of silicone in clinical studies to examine the efficacy of vas occlusion (WHO, 1992c).

Two other non-surgical methods, in addition to the percutaneous injection of silicone to form plugs, are used in China for male sterilization: non-scalpel vasectomy; and percutaneous injection of carbolic acid-butyl cyanomethacrylate to block by sclerosing the wall of the vas. A 10-centre study involving 300 men per centre, that were randomly allocated to each method, will study efficacy for two years. The ease and success of reversal of the three methods will be evaluated in subjects requesting a reversal. This study, which is supported by the State Family Planning Commission in China and WHO/HRP, has begun and will be monitored by the National Research Institute for Family Planning at Beijing, where the data will be analysed.

Non-scalpel vasectomy is being studied by FHI in Guatemala, Sri Lanka and Thailand. Studies are ongoing to compare non-scalpel versus standard incision vasectomy in Brazil and Indonesia, and fulguration versus ligation in non-scalpel vasectomy in Mexico (FHI, 1992).

Vasectomy and cancer

Two recent independent studies found a statistical association of vasectomy with prostatic cancer in older men, some of whom had been vasectomized long ago (Rosenberg and others, 1990; Mettlin, Natarajan and

Huben, 1990). Another two studies from the United States and Scotland, found a small increase in risk of testicular cancer after vasectomy (Strader, Weiss and Daling, 1988; Cale and others, 1990). To follow up the reports of increased risk of testicular cancer after vasectomy, WHO/HRP is supporting a historical cohort study based on existing hospital discharge and cancer registers in Denmark. To evaluate research needs and priorities with regard to the relation of vasectomy to cancer of the testis and prostate, WHO/HRP arranged a meeting in 1991; and after reviewing all of the biological and epidemiological evidence available at that time, the expert group concluded that any causal relation between vasectomy and the risk of cancer of the prostate or testis is unlikely. They also concluded that no changes in family planning policies concerning vasectomy are warranted. However, because even a slight increase in risk of prostate cancer would be of concern, the group made recommendations for further research in this area. Such research is also ongoing under the auspices of CPR/NICHD. Both retrospective and prospective data on mortality patterns, 15 years or more following a vasectomy, are being analysed in order to establish the relation between vasectomy and cause of death, including prostate cancer (United States of America, 1991).

Although the work to develop reversible methods for sterilization of the male is in progress, no such step forward has been seen in the female. However, to make sterilization available to larger numbers of women at a lower cost, FHI is working to develop simple, safe and effective non-surgical procedures that could be performed by paramedical personnel. Recent efforts have focused on the development of iodine compounds that may have the ability to occlude the Fallopian tubes. Testing continues to develop formulations that are both safe and effective in preventing unwanted pregnancy (FHI, 1992).

Chinese investigators are studying clinical safety and efficacy of female sterilization by two chemical agents: phenol-mucilage; and phenol-atebrine paste (China, 1992). Studies have also been performed in Chile using the drug quinacrine. All of these methods need repeated instillation of the drugs to reach high effectiveness and are irreversible.

The Strategic Planning Group of WHO/HRP felt that research needs in this area are rather limited, except for some epidemiological issues, for example, long-term consequences of sterilization by quinacrine. There is,

however, still need for the development of a safe chemical method, which can yield, after a single exposure, results comparable to those achieved by minilaparotomy. There is also need for research on the delivery and quality of services and on the social science aspects of female sterilization.

Natural regulation of fertility

Natural family plannin, that is, methods of fertility regulation based on the observation of naturally occurring signs and symptoms of the fertile and infertile phases of the menstrual cycle, is used by a significant number of couples worldwide, at least in some stage of their reproductive life. All of the commonly used methods require periodic abstinence, often quite long, from sexual intercourse. This requirement makes the method unattractive to many potential users, as strong motivation is needed by couples to use it successfully for any length of time. In addition, the successful use of the more effective natural family planning methods requires daily observation and careful record-keeping as well as some understanding of the physiology of both male and female reproduction. Although it is fairly easy to determine the end of the fertile period in women, by detecting a rise in basal body temperature or by detecting predetermined amounts of the ovarian hormone progesterone in the urine, the accurate prediction of impending ovulation, the beginning of the fertile period, is far from straightforward. A great deal of research efforts by diagnostic companies and by agencies, including WHO/HRP, has gone into finding a simple accurate, robust, home-based method for predicting ovulation, as yet with little success. Scientists from Australia have developed a simple instrument that can be used at home to measure the progesterone-increasing levels which mark the end of the fertile period. WHO/HRP has begun a multi-centre study of the home use of this instrument and the daily measurement of the ovarian hormones, compared with the signs and symptoms used in conventional natural family planning methods. If the instrument proves to be accurate and easy to use, further development may be possible to make it suitable for general use. An advantage of this method is that both the beginning and the end of the fertile period are defined using the same method (WHO, 1992c).

The Institute for Reproductive Health (formerly the Institute for International Studies in Natural Family Planning) in the United States, supported by USAID, has continued to implement a broad programme of work which is directed to improving fertility awareness and the acceptability, availability and effectiveness of natural family planning, as well as increasing the acceptability of optimal breast-feeding with focus on its fertility impact. In addition to several training courses for health professionals, the Institute for Reproductive Health has developed simplified and non-competitive assay methods to measure steroid hormones, which can be utilized as a one-step home test. A study on the outcome of pregnancies in users of natural family planning discovered no significant increase in spontaneous abortion rates of women that conceived while using this method compared with other women (Institute for Reproductive Health, 1992).

Lactation

Although breast-feeding has been justly recognized for its nutritional, immunoprotective, antidiarrhoeal and psychological effects on infants, its antifertility effect on the mother has received comparatively little attention. Lactation is not widely promoted as a means of birth-spacing. Increasingly, however, attention is being drawn to this additional benefit of breast-feeding with efforts being made by WHO and other agencies to promote the Bellagio consensus (FHI, 1988; Kennedy, Rivera and McNeilly, 1989), which states that a woman who is fully breast-feeding, is within six months of delivery and is amenorrhoeic has less than a 2 per cent risk of becoming pregnant.

Lactation and its role in the natural suppression of ovulation are thus a major research focus of the WHO Task Force on Methods for the Natural Regulation of Fertility. The aim is to provide health workers and breast-feeding women with advice on the birth-spacing effects of breast-feeding, based on a scientific understanding of biological mechanisms and the behavioural determinants of lactation and infertility. A secondary objective is that novel fertility-regulating methods for women may be developed, as an understanding of the physiology of lactation and infertility increases. A prospective seven-centre study of the relation of breast-feeding practices to the duration of lactational amenorrhoea, in which 3,850 mother-infant pairs will be followed, has been designed to describe at least some of the factors that determine lactation and infertility. Other research includes studies on the effects of maternal supplementary nutrition on the return of ovulation, studies on immunoactivity and bioactivity of pituitary hormones and studies on the interphase between breast-feeding and other methods of contraception (WHO, 1992c).

FHI is also undertaking studies to measure the effectiveness of conscientious breast-feeding in preventing pregnancies in everyday practice. The trials, being conducted in Pakistan and the Philippines, will also provide the insight into various practical aspects of using the method. Under the study protocol, the subjects switch to another method at six months post-partum (or first menstrual bleeding, whichever comes first) and continue to be followed (FHI, 1992). The Population Council is conducting a multi-centre study comparing the progesterone-releasing vaginal ring and the Copper-T 380A in post-partum women (Population Council, 1992).

The Institute for Reproductive Health is continuing the study of lactational amenorrhoea as an important contraceptive method in breast-feeding women in Chile, Ecuador and Honduras.

The WHO/HRP Strategic Planning Group agreed that there is some need for further research on the determinants of lactational amenorrhoea. The introduction and transferral of technologies, particularly of the lactational amenorrhoea method, represents a high priority for the field. There is an important role for social science research and for strengthening of research capacity. With reference to the indices of the fertile period, the group felt that this area is of low priority because of the relatively low scientific feasibility and high development cost (WHO, 1992a).

B. NEW CONTRACEPTIVE TECHNOLOGY

Steroid hormonal methods in women

Vaginal rings

Vaginal rings represent an entirely new approach to contraception. It is the only long-acting method that is under the control of the user. The woman can insert or remove the ring at will without help from a health care-provider. The ring has some other advantages as well. It releases a very small amount of hormones at a constant rate; conversely, the hormone level in the blood falls rapidly when the ring is removed, an advantage in the case of an accidental pregnancy or if the woman wishes to regain her fertility. Vaginal rings are of two types. One delivers a single hormone, a progestogen, and is worn continuously for three months. This ring acts by thickening the cervical mucus, making it impenetrable to sperm; in some women it also inhibits ovulation. WHO/HRP has developed a ring that releases levonorgestrel continuously at a rate of 20 mg. per day. Extensive testing in 19 centres worldwide confirmed its efficacy and acceptability. The main side-effects of the method are irregular menses observed in half of the users, a feature shared by all progestagen-only methods, and a risk of expulsion of the ring, mostly among older women and women of high parity. The efficacy of the ring is also reduced in heavier women. This ring is now produced on industrial scale and will be distributed by Roussel Laboratories, Ltd. once the product licence is granted in the United Kingdom (WHO, 1992c).

The Population Council has developed a ring releasing two hormones, noretindrone acetate and ethinylestradiol, to be used by women that wish to use combined hormonal contraception to block ovulation. Rings releasing various doses of the two hormones are currently under investigation to determine the optimal formulation. The Population Council has also developed a ring releasing the natural hormone progesterone to be used by lactating mothers, and studies are in progress comparing this ring with the Copper-T 380A IUD. More than 600 lactating mothers are using the ring in a multi-centre study, and the efficacy and acceptability of the method should be well documented by the conclusion of the trial (Population Council, 1992).

WHO/HRP is planning to develop rings with zero-order release characteristics to release progesterone at a rate of between 8 and 10 mg. per 24 hours. Approval has been granted by the Toxicology Panel of WHO to commence pharmacokinetic studies. Should adequate release rates be obtained, a phase III clinical trial will begin in 1993. The advantages with the progesterone-releasing rings are that although progesterone is secreted in the milk, it is not readily absorbed orally and has no influence on the child. This method would therefore be suited for breast-feeding women (WHO, 1992c). The Population Council is also developing a ring releasing a new gestagen, ST 1435, which is poorly absorbed by the gastrointestinal tract, to be used by post-partum women (Population Council, 1992).

Transdermal delivery of steroids

The delivery of estradiol through transdermal patches has been very effective in relieving post-menopausal symptoms in women. This route of introducing steroids should have less metabolic side-effects. CPR/NICHD is studying new transdermal patches delivering estradiol and levonorgestrel. The patches are programmed to release the two drugs over a seven-day period, after which a new set of patches is applied. A regimen of the three weeks on and one week off is similar to the administration schedules of the majority of oral contraceptives. If the released drugs inhibit ovulation and the patches do not produce skin irritation, the efficacy of these patches for fertility regulation will be evaluated. Multi-compartment, transdermal drug delivery systems are currently being evaluated in phase I studies (United States of America, 1991).

The Population Council is testing transdermal bracelets designed at the Council with the gestagen ST 1435. The results indicate that the bracelet can deliver a dose of ST 1435 through the skin that inhibits ovulation (Population Council, 1992).

Injectable steroids

To overcome the problems of menstrual irregularity using progestagen-only injectables, WHO/HRP, in collaboration with the pharmaceutical industry, has developed two once-a-month injectables which, like the combined pill, contain two hormones and induce a regular bleeding episode at monthly intervals. Cyclofem (25 mg of DMPA + 5 mg of estradiol cypionate) and Mesigyna (50 mg of NET-EN + 5 mg of estradiol valerate) are both very effective and have the added advantage, compared with the traditional long-acting progestagen-only methods, that fertility returns faster when use is stopped. Both have been extensively tested in multinational clinical trials and are currently being evaluated for introduction into family planning programmes in China, Egypt, Indonesia, Jamaica, Mexico, Thailand and Tunisia. Nearly 6,000 women have been recruited for the introductory trials. Similar trials are planned in Colombia, Costa Rica and Peru. As the use of Cyclofem has become more widespread, the technology for its manufacturing has been developed and transferred by the Concept Foundation to companies in Indonesia and Mexico, and it is hoped that the product will be registered in these countries in 1992. The introduction of Mesigyna has been delayed because of issues relating to the finalizing of agreements and registration. It is anticipated that this product will become available during 1992 (WHO, 1992c).

As with other contraceptive methods, efforts are under way to develop improved injectable formulations with fewer side-effects by lowering the overall steroid dose and by changing the formulation so as to avoid the high peak blood levels that follow the injection. This objective can be achieved with delivery systems, such as microspheres, that slowly release the steroids as they break down. This line of research has been further developed by FHI, which is testing injectable microspheres of noretindrone (NET-90) developed by a pharmaceutical company in the United States (FHI, 1992). WHO/HRP has chosen to develop another line where the size of steroid crystals has been modified so they act as a depot, slowly releasing the drug in the body. Following the multinational synthetic effort of WHO/HRP undertaken in collaboration with CPR/NICHD, which yielded some 230 esters, ester oximes and ethers of norethisterone and levonorgestrel, four compounds have been tested in humans. These studies have been completed and have resulted in the selection of a simple levonorgestrel ester, levonorgestrel butanoate (HRP 002), for further evaluation. The compound has been tested in a phase II comparative clinical trial at Alexandria, Durango, Mexico City and Szeged. Work is continuing to obtain formulations of HRP 002 with different particle size. Three formulations have been tested in monkeys by CPR/NICHD. One was chosen and two-year toxicology studies of this new formulation have begun. A multinational pharmacokinetic study will be undertaken, and HRP 002 will then be studied further in a phase II clinical trial and will be assessed for its metabolic effects (WHO, 1992c).

Implants

The Population Council has proceeded with research on its Norplant system and clinical trials of reformulated Norplant 2 are under way to determine the blood levels of the contraceptive steroid and the equivalency or lack thereof between the reformulated and the old systems. Larger phase III studies have been initiated to measure the efficacy and long-term effects of the reformulated implants. The Population Council has also developed a single implant to release the progestin ST 1435 with an expected duration of effectiveness of at least one year. Prototype devices are undergoing clinical trials at three sites. The initial results are very promising: no pregnancies have occurred in any of the women using the implant. A method for large-scale manufacturing of this implant has been established with a third party and a company interested in marketing the device has been identified (Population Council, 1992). FHI is doing studies on the NET implant (Annulle). This biodegradabable implant developed by a pharmaceutical company in the United States is designed to provide a high level of continuous contraceptive protection for about a year through implantation of NET pellets. A phase II clinical trial comparing the pharmacokinetics of two sets of the pellets is currently ongoing. A review of safety and efficacy data is planned for the next six months (FHI, 1992).

CPR/NICDH has continued its interest in developing biodegradable implants. The concept behind this approach is to develop a drug-releasing device which can be degraded in the body after the drug has been released. The research has resulted in the development of implants made from a biodegradable polymer, caprolactone, which releases approximately 40 mg of levonorgestrel. The initial version of this product, Capronor-I, was evaluated in several countries. The product was intended to provide effective contraception for at least one year. However, careful monitoring of the released drug levels indicated that the release rate decreased at about eight months. These initial studies have shown that the single device was easy to implant and to remove and that women in general were satisfied with it. A newer version of the device, Capronor-II, is now ready for initial clinical evaluation. A phase I study will provide pharmacokinetic results of the system. Further development of the copolymer device, Capronor-III, is essentially a joint venture between NICHD and a pharmaceutical company (United States of America, 1991).

WHO/HRP is no longer undertaking further investigative studies on biodegradabable implants because of the need to rationalize research lines but will work closely with NICHD; and when the newly formulated Capronor device is available, it will undertake its clinical testing. In addition, WHO/HRP provides technical assistance for the clinical testing of a Chinese implant developed by the Shanghai Institute of Rubber Products, which is to be undertaken by the Shanghai Institute of Planned Parenthood Research. This device is a two-rod system designed to release levonorgestrel continuously for a period of five years (WHO, 1992c).

The WHO/HRP Strategic Planning Group considered that, within the next five years, as the number of users of the new once-a-month injectables increases, epidemiological studies should be initiated in the form of post-marketing surveillance, reporting of adverse events and, possibly, cohort studies. Case control studies will be feasible only in a later stage, when the number of users has grown sufficiently large. Apart from epidemiological studies, social science research also represents a high priority as far as the monthly injectable formulations under introduction are concerned. Further development work of high priority is needed on the three-monthly progestagen-only injectable HRP 002, on the progesterone-releasing vaginal ring and on the vaginal delivery system releasing more than 20 mg of levonorgestrel per 24 hours. Basic research should be focused on the mechanism of endometrial bleeding. This basic research and the research on the cultural aspects of acceptability will necessitate the strengthening of research capability, mainly in the form of research training (WHO, 1992d).

Antihormones

Contraception is the first line of defence against unwanted pregnancy. Abortion rates are highest in those countries where information and services of family planning are weakest and where the greatest restraints on the autonomy of women exist. From 35 million to 55 million induced abortions are estimated to take place annually throughout the world; half of them performed by unskilled persons, usually where abortion is legally restricted. In such situations, death may reach or exceed 1,000 per 100,000 abortions. Figures like this provide another indication on the level of unmet need for family planning in developing countries. It is estimated that out of the 500,000 maternal deaths that occur each year throughout the world, as many as from one fourth to one third may be a consequence of complications of unsafe abortion procedures. Unsafe abortion is one of the great neglected problems of health care in developing countries and a serious concern to women during their reproductive lifes. Research on safe methods for the interruption of early pregnancy is therefore an important integral part of research programmes concerned with fertility regulation.

Progesterone is indispensable for normal reproductive function. Because progesterone plays such a key role in the reproductive process, any approach that affects hormone availability to its target cells in the reproductive organs and other tissues would thus have antifertility effects. An effective way of achieving this is through using antiprogestogens (Puri and Van Look, 1991).

Antiprogestogens are compounds that bind with high affinity to the receptor for progesterone. They prevent progesterone from occupying its binding site on the receptor and hence exert an antiprogesterone effect. Although several hundreds of such antiprogestogens have been synthesized to date by various pharmaceutical companies and private investigators, only one of them, Mifepristone (RU486), has been studied intensively in humans. Mifepristone is also the only antiprogestogen currently registered for clinical use—in China and France since September 1988, in the United Kingdom since July 1991 and in Sweden since September 1992. In all four countries, the drug is licensed for use in medical termination of pregnancy with the recommendation that it be administered in conjunction with a uterotonic prostaglandin analogue (WHO, 1992c).

Research to assess the efficacy and side-effects of Mifepristone when used for termination of early pregnancy was begun by WHO/HRP in 1983. For termination of early pregnancy, the regimen currently recommended consists of a single 600-mg dose of Mifepristone followed 36-48 hours later by a suitable prostaglandin preparation. The minimum doses of Mifepristone and of the various prostaglandins that are used in order to ensure a clinically acceptable complete abortion rate have not, however, been established. WHO/HRP continues to support multi-centre trials on different combination regimens of Mifepristone plus prostaglandin with the aim of determining the lowest effective dosage.

Evidence from France, where the combination of Mifepristone plus prostaglandin is the chosen option of some 20-25 per cent of women seeking voluntary interruption of early pregnancy, suggest that this non-surgical approach to inducing abortion fulfils a hitherto unmet need. Small-scale studies conducted mostly in the United Kingdom also confirm that impression. Furthermore, despite greater personal involvement and awareness of the abortion process, the rate of short-term psychiatric morbidity is low and not different from that seen following surgical methods of pregnancy termination. A small acceptability study conducted by WHO/HRP in Hong Kong supports the observations reported from Europe, but further studies are needed to assess in a more systematic and comprehensive manner the acceptability of medical abortion in different populations.

Antiprogesterones are also being tested as contraceptive agents. Ongoing trials on the use of Mifepristone as an emergency post-coital contraceptive are yielding promising results, while research on the effects of the compound when given daily in low doses suggests possible applications of antiprogestagens·as a mini-pill and as a constituent of a sequential contraceptive pill in combination with a progestagen. Other applications of Mifepristone under study include its use in cervical ripening, menses induction and the prevention of implantation.

WHO/HRP has also proceeded with research of other compounds with antiprogestational activity. The preclinical testing is proceeding with HRP 2000 under a collaborative agreement with the patent holder, the Research Triangle Institute in the United States of America. Future research with HRP 2000 will depend upon the interest of a pharmaceutical company to further develop this or a related compound from the same series. WHO/HRP is also supporting work by Mexican investigators on the antiprogestational activity of 5a-dihydro-norethisterone and is funding the synthesis of two new potential anti-progestagens. During the next biennium, WHO/HRP intends to continue its antiprogesterone research along the lines outline above. In the termination of early pregnancy, a multi-centre trial is being planned on the combination of Mifepristone and the orally active PGE1-analogue Misoprostol, in view of the encouraging findings obtained with this combination in two recently reported studies. Other planned clinical investigations include a multi-centre trial on the use of Mifepristone in emergency post-coital contraception and phase I studies on a sequential Mifepristone-medroxyprogesterone acetate regimen for ovulation inhibition and on the potential use of Mifepristone plus Misoprostol as a late luteal once-a-month pill (WHO, 1992c).

The WHO/HRP Strategic Planning Group agreed that further development of a reliable post-coital method and once-a-month pill and studies of various approaches to early pregnancy termination represent the highest priorities for development and assessment in this important area where WHO/HRP is the main, if not the only, actor. An equally high priority is represented by the service needs of medical methods for abortion and of emergency post-coital contraception and the many questions related to acceptability. Some epidemiological studies (surveillance) may also be needed (WHO, 1992a).

Male methods

The first ever multi-centre contraceptive efficacy study of normal men receiving a prototype hormonal regimen, weekly injections of testosterone enanthate, was conducted by WHO/HRP during 1986-1990 and provided convincing evidence that once the laboratory diagnosis of azoospermia has been achieved, normal men were rendered infertile and able to sustain a safe, effective and reversible contraception for at least 12 months (WHO, 1990). It was also found that there were variations in the rate of achievement of azoospermia among men of the same genetic background, and that men in the Chinese centres achieved azoospermia more frequently than those in the Caucasian centres (91 versus 60 per cent). A phase II study to evaluate the likelihood that hormonally induced severe oligozoospermia (≤ 5 million sperm/ml) is associated with an acceptable level of contraceptive efficacy has begun, and 15 centres are currently involved (2 in Australia, 4 in China, 5 in Europe, 2 in South-eastern Asia and 2 in the United States). Progress to date has been good. If this trial demonstrates that the contraceptive efficacy is high even when spermatogenesis is not fully suppressed, the goal of developing a hormonal antifertility agent for men will be greatly simplified. A second hormonal study conducted in five centres in Indonesia was completed by WHO/HRP during the past year. A progestogen used in females, DMPA, was combined with one of two androgens, testosterone enanthate or the longer acting 19-nortestosterone-hexyl-oxy-phenylpropionate. More than 97 per cent of the men achieved azoospermia, which confirmed the earlier reported high efficacy of this treatment in Indonesian men (Pangkahila, 1991).

It is clear that no method based on weekly injections as used in the trials to date would be acceptable. WHO/HRP, in collaboration with CPR/NICHD, has developed a new long-acting testosterone ester, testosterone buciclate (formerly 20 AET-1). Its safety and other properties have been established in animal studies over the past five years. The drug has been tested in hypogonadala patients in a WHO collaborating centre in Germany and has been shown to provide sufficient testosterone to maintain steady blood levels in the normal range over a treatment period of four months. Studies of a single injection of testosterone buciclate in normal men have begun to establish if androgen levels can be raised in a controlled and sustained way to suppress sperm production to the level required for contraceptive efficacy. If this goal is achieved and the new drug continues to be safe, then men may at last have access to a long-acting injectable hormonal method (WHO, 1992c).

The high efficacy achieved in the Indonesian study rekindled interest in long-acting progestogen and androgen combination treatment. WHO/HRP and CPR/NICHD have developed a long-acting levonorgestrel ester (HRP 002), which when simultaneously injected with testosterone buciclate at three-month intervals suppressed sperm production in baboons to azoospermia or severe oligozoospermia. Studies with the objective of establishing the rate of release of levonorgestrel from HRP 002 in normal men are due to begin in 1992. The required androgen supplement will be provided by a single injection of testosterone buciclate. Because of possible ethnic differences, the studies will be conducted in one Caucasian and one Indonesian centre (WHO, 1992c).

Synthesis of gonadotrophin hormone-releasing hormone (GnRH) antagonists continues to be a major focus of the overall synthesis programme of CPR/NICHD. The pivotal role that GnRH plays in regulating the reproductive process suggests that antagonism of this molecule can be utilized as a fertility-regulating agent. Studies by WHO/HRP with an GnRH agonist (Buserelin) induced a completely reversible azoospermia in bonnet monkeys. Studies in monkeys and phase I studies in men have shown that an antagonist is even more potent in the suppression of gonadotropin secretion and sperm production than the agonists. The Nal-Lys GnRH antagonist (called Antide and synthetized by Drs. Folkers and Bowers under contract from the NICHD peptide synthesis programme) is without histamine-releasing side-effects and is the subject of collaborative studies between WHO/HRP and a pharmaceutical company. The study will explore if azoospermia induced by Antide in bonnet monkeys can be maintained by injections of testosterone buciclate. Small studies using GnRH antagonists in men performed by CPR/NICHD suggest that the proportion of treated volunteers reaching azoospermia may be in the range of 90 per cent. However, in order to have a potentially useful product, a compound must have two important properties: *(a)* it must be devoid of local and systemic toxicity; and *(b)* it must be potent enough so that the therapy is cost-effective. Since the decapeptides are expensive to synthetize, a compound that is at least 10 times more potent than the Antide antagonist is needed before one can proceed with extensive male contraceptive studies. Although it is recognized that daily injections of GnRH antagonists can be utilized for limited clinical experimentation, there will be a need to develop more practical routes of administration. Long-

term delivery systems may be the new choice provided that a potent antagonist is available from the synthesis programme (United States of America, 1991).

Another approach to a male contraceptive would be a drug with an action on the normal function of sperm stored in the epididymis. This drug would have to be rapid in onset; and on withdrawal of the drug, normal sperm would return quickly in the ejaculate. The search for drugs with such an action was initiated by WHO/HRP in 1972 and this approach would clearly have some major advantages over hormonal methods. Both WHO/HRP and NICHD have supported basic research in this area. The overall objective is to provide a better understanding of the environment in which sperm is stored prior to ejaculation and to identify mechanisms susceptible to drug intervention. There are always major concerns about any substance that produces histologically demonstrable alterations in the seminiferous epithelium. Primary among these concerns are reversibility and general toxicity. To date all known antispermatogenic drugs have shown sufficient toxic manifestation to render them clinically unacceptable.

Research is, however, proceeding and includes, among others, studies to evaluate plant products. An example is the collaborative study between WHO/HRP and the Chinese National Family Planning Programme on the plant *Tripterygium wilfordii*.

The WHO/HRP Strategic Planning Group agreed that in this area, further development of male methods, epidemiological research (consequences of vasectomy), social science research (acceptability of male methods) and strengthening of research capacity (in andrology) all represent high-priority areas (WHO, 1992a).

Antifertility vaccines

It has been proposed that one method of fertility regulation that would be attractive to both users and providers of family planning services, particularly in developing countries, would be a preparation that is taken once every 12-24 months and is free from side-effects and the use and disposal problems associated with some of the currently available methods. Antifertility vaccines directed against selected reproduction specific molecules—such as those on the spermatozoa, oocytes and the preimplantation embryo—would appear to offer these possibilities, in that prolonged (but not permanent) immune responses generated by such vaccines would inhibit fertilization and the establishment of pregnancy without affecting other body functions. If appropriate molecules are selected, such vaccines would not cause reactions with the endogenous non-target substances, and if designed and developed correctly they would be free of side-effects. Furthermore, they would be easy to administer and comparatively inexpensive. Both WHO/HRP and a number of national and international agencies are funding research on antifertility vaccines (Ada and Griffin, 1991). WHO has concentrated research efforts on the development of vaccines that would work after fertilization has occurred but before pregnancy becomes established. WHO has developed a prototype antifertility vaccine consisting of a conjugate immunogen, formed from a synthetic fragment of the human chorionic gonadotrophin molecule and joined to the diphtheria toxoid as a carrier molecule and an immunostimulant. Phase I trials were performed between 1986 and 1988 in sterilized women. Prior to phase II efficacy studies, it had to be ensured that the vaccine did not produce any abnormalities in the foetus should it fail to prevent pregnancy. Therefore, during 1990 and 1991, teratology studies were conducted in rats and rabbits. Results show that the prototype vaccine had no adverse effects, neither on the pregnant animals nor on the foetuses. WHO/HRP is now in the process of preparing clinicals trials in Sweden to assess the effectiveness of the vaccine, that is, phase II trials.

Although the prototype anti-hCG vaccine appears to be well tolerated and is apparently safe and immunogenic in humans, this version of the vaccine is unlikely to be suited for wide-scale clinical use, because it requires at least two injections at an interval of several weeks to elicit an anti-hCG immune response lasting for from three to six months, depending upon the individual. WHO/HRP is therefore developing an advanced prototype vaccine, which is designed to elicit effective levels of immunity persisting for 12 months or more following a single injection. This new vaccine has the immunogen conjugate and the immunostimulant incorporated into a polymer, designed to release the vaccine slowly over an extended but predetermined period of time. Vaccines of both longer and shorter duration of effect could be produced using the same technology. Dose response and toxicity studies have been carried out in rabbits and baboons to determine the optimal dose of the vaccine and to see that this version of the vaccine is safe for testing in humans. If so, a clinical trial to assess the safety of the advanced prototype anti-hCG vaccine could be initiated. Further modification and improvements

will be needed to make a vaccine suited for large-scale production.

The magnitude and duration of the immunity elicited by vaccines vary from one person to another, largely as a consequence of the genetic diversity of the recipients. Although this variation can be reduced by the use of chemically defined vaccines and selected delivery systems, it will remain an important factor in managing clinical trials of anti-hCG and other antifertility vaccines from phase III stage onwards (WHO, 1992c).

The research that still needs to be done in this area implies that for all practical purposes, this method will not be available to family planning programmes until the end of the twentieth century.

The Population Council has also developed an anti-hCG vaccine consisting of b-hCG conjugated to tetanus toxoid, and phase I clinical trials were completed in 1991. The plans to carry out phase II clinical trials with this vaccine have been delayed (Population Council, 1992). Encouraging data were been obtained during 1990-1991 in the phase II clinical trial of the anti-hCG vaccine developed at the Indian National Institute of Immunology. This vaccine consists of b-hCG combined with ovine a-LH conjugated to either tetanus toxoid, diphtheria toxoid or cholera toxin B-chain. One pregnancy occurred during 928 cycles of exposure in women that had attained the required antibody level (Talwar, 1992).

Another area in the development of an antifertility vaccine is the research on antitrophoblast factors directed to development of vaccines based on non-hormonal antigens of the placenta. The strategy employs a search for tissue-specific antigens expressed on the surface of placental cells. The ultimate objective is to identify, isolate, characterize and evaluate for development those antigens which are restricted to the surface of the trophectoderm of the pre-implantation blastocyst. During 1991, further studies were carried out which show particular promise (WHO, 1992c).

Studies on antigamete vaccines directed against sperm and ovum antigens form a large part of many national and international immunocontraception research programmes. Although an attractive prospect because of their truly contraceptive mechanism of action, antisperm and anti-ovum (*zona pellucida*) vaccines have so far proved disappointing. The basic research is continuing seeking antigens that are involved in and necessary for fertilization and that, in the case of ovum antigens, are expressed only at the periovulatory stage of ovum development. This research is mainly funded by NICHD and USAID but research is ongoing also in other countries, funded by medical research councils and other government agencies (United States of America, 1991; Gabelnick, 1992).

The Population Council is developing a vaccine for men cooperatively with the National Institute of Immunology in India and CPR/NICHD. This vaccine is based on eliciting antibodies that neutralize the biological effects of the GnRH. A second component of this regimen is an androgen that acts synergistically with the vaccine. In the United States, an Investigation of New Drug (IND) application for testing of the vaccine has been approved by FDA. Since this vaccine may have therapeutic effects, the first men to be immunized will be patients with prostate cancer. Clinical trials are in preparation. Additional toxicology tests in rats, rabbits and guinea-pigs, requested by FDA, are ongoing (United States of America, 1991).

The Indian National Institute of Immunology is also developing an anti-GnRH vaccine to be used by women for prolonging post-partum amenorrhoea. Phase I studies are already in progress in India. Concerns have been raised on the unknown effect on the breast-feeding child and the adverse secondary effects, such as those on bone metabolism, which might follow.

An anti-follice stimulating hormone (FSH) vaccine for men is currently undergoing clinical trials in India (Moudgal and others, 1988). This vaccine would have the advantage of not needing testosterone replacement. With both these approaches (anti-GnRH and anti-FSH vaccines), questions still remain about the long-term sequelae of immunity to these target hormones that are continuously present and produced by the hypothalamus and pituitary gland.

Research on contraceptive methods in general and on antifertility vaccines in particular has raised numerous questions, especially of ethical nature, among women's organizations in both developed and developing countries. These concerns were expressed at a meeting arranged by WHO/HRP in Geneva in February 1991 (WHO, 1991) and were addressed at a meeting between scientists involved in antifertility vaccine research and representatives of women from several developed and developing countries held recently at WHO/HRP in Geneva. The meeting concluded that important concerns to be solved before large-scale clinical testing of the most advanced vaccines is undertaken include the lack of user control of the method with the potentiality of abuse, and short- and long-term safety and effectiveness, especially if the vaccine were to be inadvertently given to early pregnant women. It was also stressed that the same rigorous standards for clinical trials that are used in such countries as Australia and Sweden (the countries where phase I and phase II studies of the WHO anti-hCG vaccine are conducted) have to be adopted in any developing country where the method is to be tested.

The Strategic Planning Group of WHO/HRP expressed the view that the future development of the WHO/HRP anti-hCG vaccine should receive the highest priority in the area of antifertility vaccines. There is, however, an important need for social science research on acceptability issues (WHO, 1992a).

C. CONCLUSIONS

The current array of contraceptive methods is far from perfect. Although there has been considerable progress on female methods over the past two decades, the development of new safe and effective male methods remains a high priority. Furthermore, the pandemic proportion of STDs, including HIV, in many areas of the world necessitates a massive effort to improve existing and to develop new barrier methods for both women and men in order to reduce the risk of contracting or spreading STD organisms. Recognizing the importance of breast-feeding, both for the health of children and as a contraceptive method, the scientific community needs to give high priority to the development of methods that do not interfere with lactation, yet give protection against pregnancy. Basic, explorative research is urgently needed to increase the number of contraceptive methods that could be available after the year 2000.

Governments and funding agencies are urged to allocate increased resources for research in human reproduction and fertility regulation, including biomedical research, in order to further improve the safety and efficacy of existing family planning methods, to develop a variety of safe, acceptable and affordable new methods and to address reproductive health problems, including infertility and subfertility, particularly those caused by STDs and environmental pollution. Such research should be sensitive to women's perspectives and to the needs of developing countries. It should include epidemiological research on reproductive health in general and on the balance of health benefits and risks of fertility-regulating agents in particular, as well as social science research on the sociocultural factors influencing the acceptability of various family planning methods in different populations.

REFERENCES

Ada, G. L., and P. D. Griffin, eds. (1991). *Vaccines for Fertility Regulation.* Cambridge, United Kingdom: Cambridge University Press.

Cale, A. R., and others (1990). Does vasectomy accelerate testicular tumour? Importance of testicular examinations before and after vasectomy. *British Medical Journal* (London), vol. 300, No. 6721, p. 370.

China, National Research Institute for Family Planning (1992). *Annual Report, 1991.* Beijing.

Family Health International (1988). Breastfeeding as a family planning method. *The Lancet* (London; and Baltimore, Maryland), vol. 19, No. 2 for 1988, No. 8621 for 29 November, pp. 1204-1205.

_____ (1992). *Contraceptive Technology and Family Planning Research: Semiannual Report, 1 October 1991-March 1992.* Durham, North Carolina.

Gabelnick, H. (1992). Personal communication.

Gray, Ronald, and Tieng Pardthaisong (1991). In utero exposure to steroid contraceptives and survival during infancy. *American Journal of Epidemiology* (Baltimore, Maryland), vol. 134, No. 8 (15 October), pp. 804-811.

Institute for Reproductive Health (1992). *Technical Progress Report, April 1, 1991-December 31, 1991.* Washington D.C.: Georgetown University.

International Planned Parenthood Federation (1992a). *Statement on Community-based Services.* London.

_____ (1992b). *Statement on Norplant Subdermal Contraceptive Implant System.* London.

Jaffe, B., and others (1988). Long term effects of MPA on human progeny: intellectual development. *Contraception* (Stoneham, Massachusetts), vol. 37, No. 6 (June), pp. 607-619.

_____ (1989). Aggression, physical activity levels and sex role identity in teenagers exposed in utero to MPA. *Contraception* (Stoneham, Massachusetts), vol. 40, No. 3 (September), pp. 351-363.

Kennedy, Kathy I., Roberto Rivera and Alan S, McNeilly (1989). Consensus statement on the use of breastfeeding as a family planning method. *Contraception* (Stoneham, Massachusetts), vol. 39, No. 5 (May), pp. 453-459.

Khanna, J., P. F. A. Van Look and P. D. Griffin, eds. (1992). *Reproductive Health: A Key to a Brighter Future.* Special Programme of Research, Development and Research Training in Human Reproduction, Biennial Report, 1990-1991. Geneva.

Laurian, Y., J. Peynet and F. Verroust (1989). HIV infection in sexual partners of HIV-seropositive patients with hemophilia. *The New England Journal of Medicine* (Boston, Massachusetts), vol. 32, No. 3 (19 January), p. 183.

Mettlin, C., Nachiamuth Natarajan and Robert Huben (1990). Vasectomy and prostate cancer risk. *American Journal of Epidemiology* (Baltimore, Maryland), vol. 132, pp. 1056-1061.

Moudgal, N. R., and others (1988). Development of a contraceptive vaccine for the human male: results of a feasibility study carried out in adult male bonnet monkeys (Macaca radiata). In *Contraception Research for Today and the Nineties,* G. P. Talwar, ed. New York: Springer-Verlag, pp. 253

Ngugi, E. N., and others (1988). Prevention of transmission of human immunodeficiency virus in Africa: effectiveness of condom promotion and health education among prostitutes. *The Lancet* (London; and Baltimore, Maryland), vol. II for 1988, No. 8616 (15 October), pp. 887-890.

Pangkahila, W. (1991). Reversible azoospermia induced by an androgen-progestin combination regimen in Indonesian men. *International Journal of Andrology* (Oxford, United Kingdom), vol. 14, pp. 248-256.

Pardthaisong, Tieng, and Ronald H. Gray (1991). In utero exposure to steroid contraceptives and outcome of pregnancy. *American Journal of Epidemiology* (Baltimore, Maryland), vol. 134, No. 8 (15 October), pp. 795-803.

Population Council, Center for Biomedical Research (1992). *Annual Report, 1991.* New York.

Puri, C. P., and P. F. A. Van Look (1991). Newly developed contraceptive progesterone antagonists for fertility control. In *Antihormones in Health and Disease,* M. K. Agarwal, ed. Frontiers of Hormone Research, vol. 19. Basel, Switzerland; and New York: Karger.

Rosenberg, Lynn, and others (1990). Vasectomy and the risk of prostate cancer. *American Journal of Epidemiology* (Baltimore, Maryland), vol. 132, No. 6 (December), pp. 1051-1055.

Simonsen, J. Neil, and others (1990). HIV infection among lower socioeconomic strata prostitutes in Nairobi. *AIDS* (London), vol. 4, No. 2 (February), pp. 139-144.

Sivin, Irving, and others (1990). Long-term contraception with the levonorgestrel 20 mg/day (LNg 20) and the Copper-T 380Ag intrauterine devices: a five-year randomized study. *Contraception* (Stoneham, Massachusetts), vol. 42, No. 4 (October), pp. 361-378.

Strader, Clifton H., Noel S. Weiss and Janet R. Daling (1988). Vasectomy and the incidence of testicular cancer. *American Journal of Epidemiology* (Baltimore, Maryland), vol. 128, No. 1 (July), pp. 56-63.

Talwar, G. P. (1992). Personal communication.

United States of America, National Institute of Child Health and Human Development, Center for Population Research (1991). *1991 Progress Report.* Washington, D.C.: Department of Health and Human Services.

Vessey, Martin P., and others (1988). Factors influencing use-effectiveness of the condom. *The British Journal of Family Planning* (London), vol. 14, pp. 40-43.

World Health Organization (1981). *Contemporary Patterns of Breastfeeding.* Report on the WHO Collaborative Study on Breast-feeding. Geneva.

_____ (1982). Facts about injectable contraceptives; memorandum from a WHO meeting. *Bulletin of the World Health Organization* (Geneva), vol. 60, pp. 199-210.

_____ (1988). Effects of hormonal contraception on breast-milk composition and infant growth. Report of the WHO Task Force on Oral Contraceptives. *Studies in Family Planning* (New York), vol. 19, No. 6 (November-December), pp. 361-370.

_____ (1990). Contraceptive efficacy of testosterone-induced azoospermia in normal men. Report of the Task Force on Methods for the Regulation of Male Fertility. *The Lancet* (London; and Baltimore, Maryland), vol. 336, No. 8721 (20 October), pp. 955-959.

_____ (1991). *Creating Common Ground: Women's Perspectives on the Selection and Introduction of Fertility Regulation Technology.* Geneva.

_____ , Collaborative Study of Neoplasia and Steroid Contraceptives (1991a). Breast cancer and depot-medroxyprogesterone acetate: a multinational study. *The Lancet* (London; and Baltimore, Maryland), vol. 338, No. 8771 (5 October), pp. 833-838.

_____ (1991b). Depot-medroxyprogesterone acetate (DMPA) and risk of endometrial cancer. *International Journal of Cancer* (New York), vol. 49, No. 2 (9 September), pp. 186-190.

_____ (1991c). Depot-medroxyprogesterone acetate (DMPA) and risk of epithelial ovarian cancer. *International Journal of Cancer* (New York), vol. 49, No. 9 (September), pp. 191-195.

_____ (1991d). Depot-medroxyprogesterone acetate (DMPA) and risk of liver cancer. *International Journal of Cancer* (New York), vol. 49, No. 2 (9 September).

_____ (1992a). *Contraceptive Research and Development*. Report of a Strategic Planning Meeting, Geneva, 23-24 June, Special Programme of Research, Development and Research Training in Human Reproduction. Geneva.

_____ (1992b). *Oral Contraceptives and Neoplasia: Report of a WHO Scientific Group*. WHO Technical Report Series, No. 817. Geneva.

_____ (1992c). *Special Programme of Research, Development and Research Training in Human Reproduction*. Annual Technical Report, 1991. Geneva.

Zhao, Sheng-cai (1990). Vas deferens occlusion by percutaneous injection of polyurethane elastomer plugs: clinical experience and reversibility. *Contraception* (Stoneham, Massachusetts), vol. 41, No. 5 (May), pp. 453-459.

XX. RE-EXAMINATION OF THE ROLE OF GOVERNMENTS, NON-GOVERNMENTAL ORGANIZATIONS AND THE PRIVATE SECTOR IN FAMILY PLANNING

*Pramilla Senanayake**

The family planning field has seen many changes over the past two decades, particularly some favourable changes in the attitudes of Governments to enacting population policies, of people and societies to the desirable size of families and of donors to trying to improve levels of living. However, new challenges have emerged for the next 10 years, particularly meeting the growing demand for family planning from those whose needs are not currently being satisfied and from the coming increases in the number of women of reproductive age.

Governments need to continue, and if possible increase, support for family planning programmes over the next decade. They can also remove legal and other barriers to the expansion of services. Governments should also try to adopt a more flexible approach, recognizing the need of adolescents for information and services, copying successful models of service delivery developed by other agencies and giving their backing to moves to improve the position of women in society.

Non-governmental organizations have already taken on the task of creating innovative ways of delivering services. Now their role needs to be reinforced and extended, both to offer a complete range of reproductive and sexual health services, especially to those most in need and those for whom clinic-based services are not relevant, and to incorporate such concepts as quality of care and community involvement. Non-governmental organizations can also lead the way in demonstrating cost effectiveness and in showing the benefits of addressing women's concerns in family planning directly. They should continue their wide-ranging advocacy efforts, including lobbying for reductions in the levels of unsafe abortion and for services for young people.

The private sector needs to continue to cooperate with Governments and non-governmental organizations, pricing contraceptives keenly for distribution through retail outlets in developing countries, as well as making them available for community-based distribution (CBD) and social marketing schemes, where there is plenty of room for expansion over the next few years. Employment-based programmes could also be expanded.

BACKGROUND

A re-examination of the roles of Governments, non-governmental organizations and the private sector in family planning is certainly timely. There have been some considerable, and favourable, changes affecting family planning and population since the World Population Conference held at Bucharest in 1974. First, by 1992, most Governments had enacted population policies and indicated their support for family planning. When the United Nations last reported at the end of the 1980s, 72 per cent of Governments were pursuing policies to support the dissemination of contraceptive information, guidance and supplies, compared with 55 per cent 15 years earlier (United Nations, 1989). Currently, 128 countries give direct support for family planning and only six now limit access. Forty-five countries have a population unit within their planning ministry.

Secondly, there have been remarkable changes in the attitudes of individuals, couples and entire societies about how many children families should have and how to achieve smaller families through spacing of births and stopping child-bearing. The result of these changes has been remarkable declines in fertility levels in some countries. For example, Thailand achieved near-replacement fertility during this period through significant increases in contraceptive prevalence rates and in the use of modern methods. The most recent Demographic and Health Surveys (DHS) suggest that during the past 20 years fertility fell by an average of 40 per cent (Arnold and Blanc, 1990). Even in Kenya, with one of the highest levels of fertility in the world, there is evidence of some substantial decline in recent years (Kenya,

* Assistant Secretary-General, International Planned Parenthood Federation, London, United Kingdom of Great Britain and Northern Ireland.

1989). Contraceptive prevalence has risen steadily, with the use of modern methods increasing since the 1960s from about 10 per cent of couples with the woman of reproductive age to 51 per cent today (UNFPA, 1991).

Another promising development over the Past two decades has been the change in the attitudes of donors. In the 1970s, some funds were given to family planning programmes primarily in order to preserve the political and socio-economic status quo and avert sociopolitical change. Now donors have explicitly declared their concern to alleviate poverty and improve LEVELs of living, and population stabilization and family planning interventions are part of this strategy. Donors have shown much more commitment to family planning and there has been a steady increase in funds allocated to population assistance over the past 20 years. Unfortunately, these increases have failed to keep up with inflation, let alone meet the rising demand for services. Population assistance from donors still represents only 1.3 per cent of their total overseas development assistance–and only 0.004 per cent of their gross national product.

Despite declarations of intent by developed countries and international figures, notably at the International Forum on Population in the Twenty First Century (held in Amsterdam in 1989), funding is still inadequate. The United Nations Population Fund (UNFPA) has estimated that in order to extend family planning services from 381 million couples today (51 per cent of women of reproductive age) to 567 million (59 per cent) by the end of the century–an increase calculated to be necessary in order to keep to the United Nations medium-varient projection for population growth–funding from all sources will need to rise to $9 billion per annum by then; this figure is twice the current level (UNFPA, 1991). Developing countries would have to increase their contribution from $3.5 billion to $4.5 billion, with population assistance from donors needing to go up several-fold.

Meanwhile, demand for services is due to grow even more rapidly from now until the end of the century. According to a recent DHS study of 15 developing countries, 17 per cent of unmarried women had an unmet need for contraception, implying a total for the developing world (excluding China) of 87 million women (Bongaarts, 1991). There can be no doubt that an unmeasured but substantial unmet need also exists among people not married, giving a conservative esti-

mate of at least 100 million couples or individuals whose needs are not being satisfied. Many of those with unmet needs are poor and often living on the margins of society.

Not meeting these needs can only increase the incidence of unsafe abortion, minimum estimates of which reach from 36 million to 53 million a year (Henshaw, 1990). The World Health Organization (WHO) estimates that 150,000-200,000 deaths per annum are the result of unsafe terminations, with many more women suffering permanent ill health. The problem is most acute where abortion is illegal or severely restricted. But even where it is legal, administrative barriers, lack of geographical or financial access to legal services and a scarcity of services or staff to perform them may lead many women to resort to illegal or unsafe abortion.

It is proving difficult, however, for some Governments to continue funding family planning prog-rammes for current users, let alone find additional resources. The collapse of the prices of many products of developing countries, growing external debt, inflation and competing demands on meagre resources are seriously hindering investment in education, health and job creation. These problems are heightened by external debt, which resulted in the 1980s in a cumulative loss of income of close to 40 per cent, compared with growth of gross domestic product in the 1970s. And there is nothing on the horizon which indicates that the economic and financial situation will improve in such countries during the 1990s.

Faced with this situation, many developing countries, especially in Africa and Southern Asia, will decrease allocations to health and family planning. A number of governments have already begun to disengage from family planning programmes in the hope that NGOs and the private sector will fill the vacuum, and this trend is likely to continue.

There have also been signs of a decline in enthusiasm for providing funding or for investing in contraceptive research or development from other quarters, especially in the United States of America: foundations, the National Institutes of Health (NIH), other government agencies and certainly pharmaceutical companies have all been unable to maintain or increase their budgets for family planning, particularly since at the Mexico City Conference in 1984. Additionally, fear of litigation has exacerbated the diminished enthusiasm of drug companies in the United States to market new products. Nevertheless, there is some evidence of a renewal of interest. For example, the United States Food and Drug Administration approved the subdermal implant Norplant in 1991 and in recent months its Fertility and Maternal Health Drugs Advisory Committee has recommended that depot-medroxy progesterone acetate (DMPA) (Depo-Provera) be given approval. NIH has established two new contraceptive research centres and media in the United States are giving the subject much more attention.

The following sections review the roles of Governments, non-governmental organizations and the private sectors in the light of these changes and make some suggestions for expansion of these roles.

A. ROLE OF GOVERNMENTS

As stated earlier, many Governments are currently involved in providing family planning services and usually make the largest financial contribution to national programmes. However, the proportion of programme costs from governments varies remarkably from country to country. China and India, for example, provide about 85 per cent of programme costs, but most Governments contribute much less. Unfortunately, some Governments give low priority to family planning services, which do not receive the necessary support to ensure that they shall be well managed and offer the highest quality services. Financial constraints also often mean that there is a concentration on a small number of methods: for example, sterilization is believed to be cost-effective, although what clients need is a wide range of choices so they can select different methods as their requirements change throughout their child-bearing years.

What often characterizes government services is that they are centrally organized, with a "top down", objective-oriented approach which often leads to a chronic lack of flexibility. Unless workers are well supported, it is difficult for them to sustain their motivation, which can lead to a loss of care for clients. However, Governments may have the resources to offer a wide scope and coverage of services, which in nearly all countries could not be achieved by non-governmental organizations and the private sector. But these Government services are usually less cost-effective than those run by others. For example, they usually require a separate infrastructure, storage, transport and advertising, while non-governmental organizations make use of

existing facilities. And although many Governments have acknowledged that gender equality is a relevant and important issue in the appropriate and effective provision of family planning services, they have yet to move on to concrete action or major support of those taking action.

In some places, there have been concerns about the risk of coercion in Government facilities when the Government has firm demographic targets in mind; there are also suspicions when new methods are introduced. Two of the main deficiencies of government service delivery are that certain areas of need are not being tackled and programmes are not innovative. In addition to being unable to offer quality services where individuals or couples are treated with dignity, most Governments have avoided such issues as adolescent sexuality as it relates to fertility and unsafe abortion. Nor have they attempted to achieve sustainability of services through cost effectiveness, cost-sharing and cost recovery. These omissions are not likely to be rectified for some time.

Removing legal and other restrictions

One step forward would be to design a strategic plan specifying the role of Governments, non-governmental organizations and the private sector. There are some obvious areas where Governments should intervene and could make a major difference by so doing. First, in many places there is still a need to remove legal restrictions or other constraints which hamper the extension of family planning services in some way. For example, in a few countries it is still illegal to disseminate information about contraceptives, and even where the ban has been removed information may not be freely available because of perceived public attitudes or medical profession regulations. In a number of countries, advertising all drugs, including contraceptives, is forbidden, and in most African and Arab countries, social mores do not allow any display of information that relates to sexual matters.

A serious obstacle still exists in many countries where only medical doctors are allowed to provide contraceptives. Since the ratio of medical doctors to population is low and most doctors are in urban areas, the possibility of extending services is limited unless non-doctors are allowed to prescribe oral contraceptives and medical personnel other than doctors are trained to fit intrauterine decices (IUDs) and to perform other family planning procedures. There are also regulations in many developing countries that require drugs, including contraceptives, to be supplied only in pharmacies or medical centres; this requirement often hinders the spread of services in rural areas and prevents community-based distribution.

The majority of contraceptives currently used in many programmes in developing countries are provided free by the United States Agency for International Development (USAID), UNFPA and the International Planned Parenthood Federation (IPPF), and are free of import duties which otherwise would result in high prices for contraceptives and so restrict the expansion of services. In the later 1990s, however, donors may not provide sufficient free contraceptives to meet rising demand, and the import duties problem will have to be faced. These issues are particularly relevant for private sector and social marketing schemes, and where countries embark on the local production of oral contraceptives using imported raw materials.

More freedom for non-governmental organizations

Another area where Governments have a role to play is in allowing more freedom of action to non-governmental organizations and the private sector. For example, family planning associations (FPAs) may need Government approval to charge clients for all or part of services. If FPAs earn revenue from these services, this revenue may be taxed, endangering their status as non-profit organizations. Family planning associations may also need approval to use a Government grant for working with other non-governmental organizations not associated with family planning, in order to encourage them to integrate family planning into some of their other work. Many Governments could also try to emulate non-governmental organizations by decentralizing their programmes.

Empowerment of women

Governments need to adopt more liberal attitudes towards the empowerment of women and towards adolescent sexuality. In some cases this means introducing or changing legislation. For example, only 103 out of 159 States Members of the United Nations have ratified the Convention on the Elimination of All Forms of Discrimination Against Women, in which they agree to eliminate discrimination against women in all civil, political, economic, social and cultural areas, including health care and family planning. Still fewer have really first-class

records on upholding reproductive rights. In a number of countries, there is a need to raise the minimum age of marriage and to ensure that it shall not be overridden. In some countries, abortion and divorce are still illegal; and in others, the consent of a spouse may be required for an abortion, for sterilization or other contraception.

Governments can try to change traditional attitudes and can take a close look at the gender balance in their own agencies, especially those involved in family planning. All institutions involved in family planning should try to collaborate with women's organizations and groups concerned with women's reproductive rights and health, and should incorporate women's perspectives in the design and implementation of programmes. This is especially important as, on the international level, the concern over the environment shifts the emphasis back to the consequences of rapid population growth and away from family planning as a human rights issue.

In sum, Governments should continue to lend support, and if possible increase it, for family planning programmes as an investment for the future and to remove legal barriers to extending services. They should now introduce more controversial programmes tested by non-governmental organizations, including information and services for adolescents, and should support initiatives to remove gender inequalities.

B. ROLE OF NON-GOVERNMENTAL ORGANIZATIONS

The ideal non-governmental organization, on the other hand, is a democratically run body, where responsibility is devolved downward and management is by performance, not objectives. It is generally agreed that non-governmental organizations have certain advantages because of their structure, which allows much greater management flexibility and enables them to adapt easily to changing situations. Non-governmental organizations are also competitive, their workers usually well motivated and good performance can be rewarded, while poor performers usually leave to go elsewhere. Services are cost-effective and make use of the existing infrastructure.

Services

As non-governmental organizations in the family planning field, FPAs have as their starting-point the safeguarding of human rights and the aim that services

300

should be sensitively devised for the communities they serve. But this has not prevented FPAs from taking the lead in introducing programmes that are innovative and that provide ideas and models for Governments and other organizations involved in family planning. For example, FPAs have pioneered new ways of delivering services, such as CBD where trusted members of the community–who could be older married women, leaders of local groups and so on–are trained so they can inform about and distribute contraceptives in their locality. CBD has become one of the success stories of the past two decades and is now accepted throughout the world despite being heavily criticized at first. There are other examples of delivery strategies first introduced by non-governmental organizations, such as the community doctor scheme whereby newly trained physicans are set up in clinics by FPAs in return for their services in the family planning field. Male clinics and youth centres are other innovative ideas coming from the non-governmental organization sector.

FPAs still have an important role to play in identifying neglected sections of the population, such as young people, marginalized groups and environmental refugees and devising suitable approaches to meet their needs. Another way forward is for non-governmental organizations to develop service delivery systems in which such concepts as quality of care, human rights, empowerment of women and community participation are embodied, at an affordable cost. These systems can be promoted to other service providers.

Non-governmental organizations can also show how services can be delivered in a cost-effective way, how part or all of the costs of services can be recovered and how to try to achieve programme sustainability. Some FPAs are already trying to recoup a portion of the costs of services, by charging for all or part of their procedures or by selling contraceptives. One possible new direction may be cross-subsidy, where fees charged at a clinic in a comparatively affluent neighbourhood may be used to subsidize services in a poorer quarter or in a small, remote community where the costs of providing services may be much higher. One FPA that has worked hard at recovering costs is the IPPF affiliate in Colombia, Profamilia, which is about 50 per cent self-sufficient, with 70 per cent of local income coming from fees charged for medical or surgical services.

Non-governmental organizations are well able to adapt business approaches to the social field and new management techniques are being introduced in many FPAs. For example, recent years have seen much more emphasis on quality of care and viewing service delivery from the clients' perspective, which derives in part from the emphasis on quality in the business world. The attention now given to quality assurance in the medical field in the United States of America as a result of concerns over liability lawsuits is in part responsible, but there is recognition that quality services can give a comparative advantage over rival delivery agents and can help minimize scares and rumours. The spread of women's activist organizations, which have raised awareness of health issues, and the gradual increase in the participation of women in family planning have also played a part. Some FPAs have taken up the United States concept of "total quality management", a philosophy that recognizes that customer needs and business goals are inseparable, as an institutional approach to improving service and efficiency in family planning.

As well as continuing to develop in these directions, there are a number of new ways in which the role of non-governmental organizations needs to be redefined and restructured, both in service delivery and in their relationships with Governments, the private sector and the research community.

Empowering communities

The non-governmental organizations must move towards becoming the facilitators of community services, rather than simply the service providers. The role of FPAs needs to be transformed so that their aim will be to empower community networks to deliver locally appropriate services. These networks, which include both the formal and the informal, such as traditional women's networks, women's organizations, unions, youth groups and indigenous community groups, will provide services while FPAs will provide training, programme guidelines, quality control, technical and financial assistance and supplies of contraceptives.

FPAs would need to identify suitable groups and motivate them to become service providers, but this approach would ensure that the expressed needs of community groups should be met with appropriate assistance from FPAs. FPAs would also have the role of "watchdogs", ensuring that services receiving technical assistance should comply with quality assurance standards. Locally applicable measures of performance and community satisfaction would also need to be developed.

Testing innovative approaches

A second emerging function for non-governmental organizations is to extend their role as innovators of new strategies, testing these through operations research. With existing straightforward service delivery handed over to Governments or to local communities, FPAs can concentrate on developing user-centred services. This move would entail building collaborative links with the local research community, becoming a resource centre for local research initiatives and conducting research on sexuality and sexual health needs and attitudes in local communities.

Further experimental work would involve developing alternative approaches to special groups like young people, the handicapped, refugees and other minority groups. Most Governments are still reluctant to tackle such areas as family life and sex education and the integration of related health issues into family planning. Therefore the pioneering role of FPAs needs to continue, especially work on preventing the acquired immunodeficiency syndrome (AIDS) and other sexually transmitted diseases, diagnosis and treatment of reproductive tract infections, sexuality and improving client counselling both in communication style and in content including power relations between men and women that affect the selection and use of contraceptives.

Advocacy

Non-governmental organizations already play a considerable part in advocacy, but again this can take a new direction. Although most Governments now accept the need for family planning, they do not generally recognize all the complex issues relating to sexual and reproductive health. Through their community networking and research, non-governmental organizations can act as intermediaries, voicing to policy makers the real concerns and needs of local communities in respect of sexual and reproductive health.

The points that non-governmental organizations would highlight would include:

(*a*) The unnecessarily high abortion rates, to reinforce the need for family planning services;

(*b*) The rates and consequences of unsafe abortion, and maternal mortality and morbidity as a result of unsafe abortion;

(*c*) Adolescent fertility and the consequences of denying adolescents access to safe services;

(*d*) Age at marriage and the consequences of early marriage, which could be used to campaign for a rise in the age at marriage where child marriages are still permitted;

(*e*) Rates of AIDS and other sexually transmitted diseases, in order to educate Governments and the public on the extent of the problem;

(*f*) Abuses of reproductive rights, including female genital mutilation, enforced sterilization, sexual abuse, etc.;

(*g*) Restrictions on the rights of women to have access to education, employment, control of their own fertility and so on.

Non-governmental organizations need to devise communication programmes that use the media to get across their messages on a wide scale and to produce high-quality materials for clients. There is also a need to rediscover traditional channels of communication, such as folk media.

Other areas where these organizations have begun to act, but where there is much scope to develop their roles, include mobilizing partner organizations. For example, some FPAs already have links with other non-governmental organizations, such as the Red Cross, and with organizations dealing with women's issues, reproductive health and rights, the environment, youth and other organizations, but this work can be done in more countries and with more groups.

Women

Lastly, and most important, non-governmental organizations can be a powerful leading force in dealing with issues related to women in development. For family planning non-governmental organizations this means giving explicit attention to women as clients, service providers and decision makers including applying the tools of the gender-analysis framework to family planning programmes and looking at the gender composition of board members and staff at all levels.

As clients, women need a quality of care approach to services, and where possible the opportunity to have a say about them and how they can be improved. As service providers, women need help in improving their status and self-esteem, whatever this area or level. As decision makers, women need to be present to provide the women's perspective and to help keep women's rights, health, and sexuality at the forefront of programme design and implementation.

The most important tasks for non-governmental organizations are to identify and test new service delivery models and to involve communities in delivering services, as well as to take a leading role in advocacy and promotion of women's perspectives.

C. ROLE OF THE PRIVATE SECTOR

The main characteristic of the private sector is that firms such as pharmaceutical companies take a purely business orientation and are primarily motivated by trying to maximize profits. Nevertheless, the private commercial sector–like some Governments, non-governmental organizations and international organizations–is involved in certain useful activities, such as research, training, product development and manufacture, marketing, provision of services and public relations.

As far as developing new contraceptives is concerned, in recent years pharmaceutical companies have lost their place as the prime agents, as a result of tighter controls on testing and fears of costly lawsuits. Now WHO and a few non-profit organizations have taken the lead. As mentioned above, however, there are some signs that the pharmaceutical companies are beginning to return to this field.

Pharmaceutical companies

There is a particularly high profit margin on contraceptives, in some countries up to 30 per cent, so one way forward would be to try to reduce this margin. Another area where pharmaceutical companies are important is in market research. It is clear that in order to attract current non-users of contraceptives that would like to limit or space their children, efforts need to be made to meet their requirements. Market research is also necessary to determine the demand for particular services and how much, if anything, clients would be prepared to pay for them, as well as where and when they would like them to be available.

Private doctors and pharmacists

The private sector provides contraceptives to more than half the users in many developing countries, through private doctors (e.g., the Republic of Korea) and pharmacists (e.g., Brazil). When pharmacists are well trained, they can do more than just sell products; they can also give information and direct people with special needs to clinics and so provide a useful supplement to clinic services. A recent report suggests that although 15 million couples in developing countries currently obtain their supplies of contraceptives (mostly pills, condoms, injectables and spermicides) through pharmacies the requirements of 85 million couples could be met in this way (Lande, 1989). Family planning associations can help by training pharmacists, and encouraging them to be well stocked and have a range of contraceptives on display. There is also scope to expand the type of outlet stocking contraceptives, in some countries, it is not just pharmacies that market contraceptives, but market traders and others.

Social marketing of contraceptives

There is still much potential for expanding social marketing of contraceptives, since many countries have not yet introduced schemes, and this is obviously a useful direction for the private sector in the future.

Social marketing by non-governmental organizations and the private sector merges commercial and social objectives. Integrating contraceptive distribution into the commercial sector achieves continuity of supply and ease of access because of the multiple distribution or sales points–pharmacies, small shops, supermarkets, bars, hotels and other retail outlets have been used. By subsidizing supplies, the cost to the user is reduced and sales increased. There have been some very successful schemes, notably of pills and condoms in Bangladesh and recently of condoms in a number of African countries, where these supplies have been promoted both for family planning and prevention of human innuno deficiency virus (HIV) infection. Social marketing can also be a useful way of reaching particular groups of people, for example, those with low incomes, or those whose behaviour puts them at higher risk of HIV infection.

Market research to determine product acceptability, the training of vendors, careful pricing and strong promotional campaigns and advertising are essential ingredients, all skills that are the particular province of the commercial sector. Some recent schemes have exhibited built-in sustainability; the contraceptives are not subsidized but bought in bulk at specially negotiated prices, and donor funds are used for heavy initial promotion and advertising, which is scheduled to be phased out after a period of time.

Employment-based programmes

A further area where much more could be done is in employment-based family planning programmes. These programmes have proved particularly useful for promoting male responsibility as well as providing basic health care, including family planning, to workers and their partners. They benefit employees because they are convenient and quick to access; they benefit employers who have a fitter workforce; and they allow other providers to concentrate on reaching those that are unemployed or cannot afford to pay (Rinehart, Blackburn and Moore, 1987).

In general the most effective programmes offer supplies and services as well as information, and offer them directly at the workplace. This is particularly appropriate for such companies as large and medium-sized factories or mining and industrial firms, but there are other schemes whereby employees and their families go to private sector providers who are reimbursed·by employers for the services given. Some recent studies have shown that employment-based schemes can be cost-effective for businesses by preventing sickness and reducing maternity benefits and leave, and child-care costs (Smith, 1990).

Future directions for the private sector should include the adoption of sensitive pricing strategies and extension sales outlets, such as pharmacies. There is scope to develop further both social marketing and employment-based schemes of providing contraception.

D. CONCLUSION

The different sectors involved in family planning already collaborate to a great extent, but there is still much more that still be done. Governments and non-governmental organizations need to get together and build a relationship based on trust. Then, they can move forward by taking a close look at their strengths and weaknesses and trying to learn from each other. There are already several cost-sharing models among

Governments, non-governmental organizations and the private sector. For example, the Government may hand over to such an organization, and then refund one particular activity, such as information, education and communication (e.g. India). The Government may supply a non-governmental organization with free contraceptives, or the Government may provide a service but have FPAs provide training. In Suriname, for example, the association has negotiated with the Government for it to reimburse FPA costs in providing services to low-income clients.

It is clear from surveys that many more women than those currently using contraceptives would like to limit their child-bearing. Also, it can be seen and from the level of abortions that women are still having unwanted pregnancies. It is necessary to attract these non-users with services tailored for their requirements. What is lacking at the moment on all sides–and what should be the ultimate aim–is to put much more emphasis on the clients' point of view and try to improve quality of care. All outlets should be able to offer clients a range of methods, backed by solid counselling and information offered by trained personnel in a suitable manner. Services should be accessible and able to offer continuity of supply; and most importantly, they should be appropriate for local needs.

For many women, especially those who, because they are not completely in control of their own sexuality, have a limited ability to influence their risk of pregnancy or infection with a sexually transmitted disease, family planning services need to be offered as part of a reproductive and sexual health service that will include treatment for reproductive tract infections, infertility and safe abortion services as back up.

REFERENCES

Arnold, Fred, and Ann K. Blanc (1990). *Fertility Levels and Trends.* Demographic and Health Surveys Comparative Studies, No. 2. Columbia, Maryland: Institute for Resource Development/Macro Systems, Inc.

Bongaarts, John (1991). *The KAP-gap and the Unmet Need for Contraception.* Research Division Working Paper, No. 23. New York: The Population Council.

Henshaw, Stanely K. (1990). Induced abortion: a world review, 1990. *Family Planning Perspectives* (New York), vol. 22, No. 2 (March-April), pp. 76-89.

Kenya, Ministry of Home Affairs (1989). *Kenya Demographic and Health Survey, 1989*. Nairobi, Kenya: National Council for Population and Development; and Columbia, Maryland: Institute for Resource Development/Macro Systems Inc.

Lande, Robert E. (1989). Pharmacists and Family Planning. *Population Reports* (Baltimore, Maryland), Series J, No. 37 (November).

Rinehart Ward, Richard Blackburn and Sidney H. Moore (1987). *Employment-based Family Planning Programs*. Population Reports, Series J, No. 34. Baltimore, Maryland: The Johns Hopkins University, Population Information Program.

Smith, Raisa Scriabine (1990). Private sector successes. *People* (London), vol. 17, No. 4, p. 23.

United Nations (1989). *Trends in Population Policy, 1976-1986*. Sales No. E.89.XIII.13.

United Nations Population Fund (1991). *Population Issues Briefing Kit*. New York.

Part Nine

DISCUSSION NOTES

XXI. GENDER PERSPECTIVE IN FAMILY PLANNING PROGRAMMES

United Nations Office at Vienna[*]

The ability of women to control their fertility and choose the number of children they want is widely considered a crucial factor for raising the status of women, as well as improving the health of women and their children along with their economic situation. Equality between men and women in the access to family planning is stressed in article 12 of the Convention on the Elimination of All Forms of Discrimination Against Women:

"States Parties shall take all appropriate measures to eliminate discrimination against women in the field of health care in order to ensure, on a basis of equality of men and women, access to health care services, including those related to family planning." (United Nations, 1988, p. 118)

Although family planning is widely perceived as one of the success stories of development cooperation (Cassen, 1986), and the three past decades have recorded considerable progress in individual family planning (United Nations, 1991b), access to health-care services and family planning is today far from ensured on a basis of equality of men and women, due to cultural factors and the way in which these services are organized.

Although studies have shown that distribution of resources in a society, better access to education and health for both sexes, low infant mortality and measures taken to raise the status of women are factors leading to reduced fertility (Postel, 1992), these issues are not addressed in family planning programmes. Economic development in tandem with distribution of resources and the political will to raise the status of women are important factors for reduced fertility in the long run. Although this point has been recognized in theory, it has only been translated into practice to a limited extent in family planning service delivery. Far too often programmes still operate in a "gender vacuum", to a great extent ignoring the underlying factors that cause women voluntarily or involuntarily to give birth to many children, thus attempting to cure rather than prevent.

Men are also not addressed by family planning programmes to the same extent as women. Therefore, family planning programmes would benefit from taking on a much broader approach, based on gender analysis.

A. GENDER RELATIONS AND FAMILY PLANNING

Whether family planning empowers women or preserves existing gender roles

The attitudes towards family planning have changed radically over the two decades since the World Population Conference was held at Bucharest in 1974. At the time of the Conference, gender or women's issues were not on the agenda to a great extent, and therefore the attitude towards family planning programmes was largely gender-neutral, which is reflected in the World Population Plan of Action (United Nations, 1975). The paragraph in the Nairobi Forward-looking Strategies for the Advancement of Women that mentions family planning was based on the recommendations for the further implementation of the Plan of Action, adopted at the International Conference on Population held at Mexico City in 1984. In accordance with the World Plan of Action, the Strategies stress that all couples and individuals have the basic human right to decide freely and informedly the number and spacing of their children (United Nations, 1989).

However, few women in the world today can exercise their basic human right to decide "freely and informedly" on the number and spacing of their children, or indeed to even influence the size of their families (United Nations, 1991b): men and women are not equal partners in decision-making at either the family level or the national level. Cultural norms, also reflected in national legislation, effectively bar women's participation in, and access to education, paid employment, health care and personal freedom. Processes of lifelong discrimination against women, from birth to death, effectively prevent their full participation in the development process. Modern

---

[*]Division for the Advancement of Women, Vienna, Austria.

medical techniques have opened the road for discrimination against girls even before birth, by enabling selective abortion based on the sex of the foetus (United Nations, 1991b). Young girls are frequently neglected from birth; they receive less food and less medical care, and they are not given access to education and vocational training to the same extent as young boys. As pointed out by the World Bank, women's access to health services is both the outcome of their lower status in society and a determinant of their health and productivity and, so, ultimately their status (World Bank, 1991). According to statistics of the United Nations Education, Scientific and Cultural Organization (UNESCO), the illiteracy rate for women in the developing countries stood at 45 per cent in 1990, and even if illiteracy rates for young women have fallen during the Past two decades, they are still much higher than those for young men (United Nations, 1991B). All this will affect a young woman's chances of supporting herself in the future, and it will help lock her into a dependent position for the rest of her life. Since women are valued mainly as mothers and wives in many cultures, the age at marriage is often very low; and the first pregnancy occurs at an early age, when the woman is neither physically nor psychologically prepared to have children (World Bank, 1991).

Due to their lower status, women often end by being more or less economically dependent upon men all through their lives, whether upon male relatives, husbands or partners. This situation leaves women with reduced bargaining power and little influence on decision-making. In most low-income households, the tasks traditionally "assigned" to women includes most of the reproductive work[1], as well as productive work, often as secondary income-earners. In rural areas, this activity mainly takes the form of agricultural work; and in urban areas, women often work in the informal sector enterprises, located either at home or in the neighbourhood. In addition, women are frequently responsible for community managing[2] work to a great extent, undertaken at a local community settlement level in both urban and rural contexts; inadequate provision of housing and of basic services, such as water and health, forces women to take responsibility for the allocation of limited resources, as an extension of their domestic reproductive role. Since girls are traditionally brought up to carry the main responsibility for most of the reproductive work, they tend to receive less education and thus their chances for wage employment are limited. Studies have shown

that even if a woman works in the informal sector, it does not necessarily mean that she herself controls the income she generates. Therefore, women frequently have limited or no control over their own income or that of their partner or husband income (Faulkner and Lawson, 1991).

A woman's lack of control over her body and sex life often leads to early sexual initiation and greater exposure to sexually transmitted diseases (STDs) and the human immunodeficiency virus/acquired immunodeficiency syndrome (HIV/AIDS), as well as to early and frequent pregnancies (du Guerny and Sjöberg, 1993; and Ford Foundation, 1991). Less educated, poor and physically exhausted mothers are likely to pass on poverty to their children, while better educated mothers are one of the key factors for improving the situation. Studies have shown that women with seven or more years of education tend to marry, on average, four years later and have 2.2 fewer children statistically than women with no schooling (Sadik, 1990). Lack of opportunities early in life will mortgage a woman's potential through all stages of her life. When that happens to a generation, it could mortgage future national development for several decades. Early pregnancies and continued births throughout the productive years, with or without emotional, practical and financial support from the father, leave many women in an economically dependent position, from youth to old age. Family planning programmes tend to overlook not only the gender perspective on family planning but also the age perspective, the different stages of a woman's life which determine her possibilities of making decisions related to fertility. Some of the issues that family planning programmes need to look into are: how to intervene in all stages of a woman's life cycle; how to improve the status of women, in a life-course approach; how to provide sex education for girls (and boys), and how to interfere with the low age at marriage, the lack of education and girls'/women's higher level of economic dependence. These and other questions need to be looked into from a gender perspective.[3]

Until recently, many women's organizations, along with other organizations in the developing countries, were not interested in family planning, claiming that it was a way of blaming poverty on women's fertility (ideas widely shared by feminists and others in the North) (Bondestam and Bergström, 1980). Recently, however, a consensus seems to have been reached that the desire to control the number and spacing of children is almost universal among all women, regardless of economic or social position. The focus has shifted to stressing the importance of increasing women's access to information and services related to family planning. Nevertheless, feminists in the North and the South have raised several critical issues related to family planning programmes and their implementation. Both groups have to a great extent had similar views on family planning recently, but there are also major differences: women of the South have frequently blamed the "northern" feminists for taking on a too individualistic approach to women's fertility, based on their own experience in the highly industrialized countries, which does not necessarily apply to other cultures.

Feminist critics in the North have also raised the question whether development *per se* raises the status of women and what impact reduced fertility has on the status of women. Although studies have shown that the direct links between economic development and raising the status of women are weak, some feminists also stress the negative sides of contraceptive use, pointing at the undesirable side-effects of contraceptives and the fact that contraceptives are almost exclusively designed for women. The feminist network Development Alternatives with Women for a New Era (DAWN) has pointed out, for example, that there is a trend towards making birth control more "woman-centred", thus "letting men off the hook" in terms of their responsibilities for fertility control and placing the burden increasingly on women (Sen, 1985). Since women are the persons giving birth to the children, they are also given the full responsibility for protecting themselves against unwanted pregnancies, a pattern also found in industrialized countries. Other feminists point to the gains in female autonomy and good health, and it has been suggested that any index of the status of women should include access to a free choice of contraception, legal abortion and the right to choose the number of children (Ware, 1992). Therefore, although women on the one side are given the main responsibility for protecting themselves against unwanted pregnancies, many women cannot themselves choose whether to use a contraceptive, due to their gender subordination coupled with poverty, cultural and religious norms, as well as lack of access to and information about contraceptive methods.

Feminists have criticized the lack of understanding among policy makers of the mixed responses to family planning programmes by women in developing countries. While accepting family planning as an instrument for poverty reduction, in combination with other measures, feminists of the North and the South have criticized the methods for carrying out the programmes. Also, while acknowledging the considerable unmet need for family planning today, feminists reject the concept of "control" of their bodies by Governments and international institutions, such as one-baby-per-family quota systems, authoritarian approaches to sterilization and anti-abortion laws. Family planning programmes have been criticized for having too much of a top-down approach towards women, by not involving women enough in the planning and implementation process, as was stressed in the Women's Action Agenda 21:

"We condemn any attempt to deprive women of reproductive freedom or the knowledge to exercise that freedom. We demand women-centred, women-managed comprehensive reproductive health care and family planning, including the right to prenatal care, safe and legal voluntary contraceptives and abortion, sex education and information." (World Women's Congress, 1991, p. 20)

Other issues raised are lack of information and respect, lack of care for user satisfaction and insufficient involvement of users in the design of programmes. Other criticism includes using women as "guinea pigs" for new birth control methods, insufficient contraceptive research, sterilization; and insertion of intra-uterine devices (IUDs) without proper health precaution, information or after-care. It has been pointed out that under third world conditions of sanitation, health care and female nutrition, many of the contraceptive methods being promoted can have serious side-effects and even result in infertility (Sen, 1985). Female sterilization is still the most commonly used method in developing countries (45 per cent compared with 14 per cent in the developed countries), while barrier and natural methods cover only 15 per cent in the developing countries (Sadik, 1990). For female sterilization, when done *en masse* in temporary sterilization camps, is not only hazardous to women's health but is also is frequently carried out without proper information and follow-up. Feminists have also stressed that sterilization is sometimes carried out on poor, young women, without providing them with information about the effects on their future fertility (DAWN, 1988). This action is not compatible with human rights and must be considered a violation of a woman's self-integrity, dignity and body. Access of women to information on contraceptives and, above all, the wide range of available contraceptives, should be improved; and technologies themselves should be better adapted, based on women's and men's experiences. One of the main reasons that women's views are not being taken into account, is because women cannot as easily discuss the family planning service provided, because of their lower status. This situation is something that needs to be acted on in family planning programmes, from a gender as well as from a life-course perspective. Contrary to what situation appears to be the situation right now, women should be empowered to demand better services and Governments should be able to adjust accordingly.

The empowerment of women has not been stressed enough in family planning programmes. Programmes rather tend to be carried out within existing gender roles, rather than attempting to promote equality between the sexes, thus running the risk of being less effective in the long run (United Nations, 1992; and United Nations Office at Vienna, 1992). Women are still perceived to be passively waiting on the sidelines to benefit from policies and programmes, when in reality they are far from passive but are blocked by their lower status and poverty from participating fully in the development process, including deciding on their own fertility. Far to often family planning programmes have tended to take on a welfare approach towards women, seeing them as passive beneficiaries, rather than attempting to involve and empower both women and men to participate actively in the design and implementation of such programmes (United Nations, 1992; and United Nations Office at Vienna, 1992). Caroline Moser (1989) identifies five main policy approaches which highlights how women are perceived in development programmes. Among these, the "welfare approach" or the "efficiency approach" identifies common attitudes: in the first case, women are seen mainly as mothers, as passive receivers; and in the latter, women's economic participation is seen as associated with equity. Neither of these approaches, which are common in development policies and programmes today, recognizes the role of women's full participation in the development process nor that women should also benefit fully from development, on an equal basis with men. Top-down approaches in family planning policies and programmes, based on cost/benefit types of calculations of various risks for women, depending upon the contraceptive method used, are not compatible with a development strategy based on human rights and respect for the individuals concerned.

Shifting from a couple to an individual perspective by bringing men in is currently one of the major feminist ideas. In the Nairobi Forward-looking Strategies for the Advancement of Women, emphasis is put on a greater sharing by men and women of family and health-care responsibilities, and women's access to and control over income to provide adequate nutrition for themselves and their children (United Nations, 1989). Women's Action Agenda 21 also stresses that men should be included as beneficiaries of family planning education and services. The idea is to bring men in to share the economic and practical responsibilities of the family, as well as addressing them to the same extent as women, in family planning programmes.

Family planning programmes currently appear to have an insufficient and rather static view of the family as consisting of a married couple and their children. In reality, however, "family" constellations differ greatly. For example, the number of poor female-headed households is growing; and women are frequently left to raise their children without the support of a partner/husband, for different reasons. Studies in Botswana, Ghana, Kenya, Senegal and Zimbabwe have shown that women actually spend very limited time living with the father of their children, which indicates that the assumption that family members live together in the same household may be appropriate in some settings but very far from reality in others. Labour migration and urbanization, among other factors, are quickly changing and breaking up traditional family networks and structures. Even in the cases when labour migration of men occurs in order to support the family, studies show that the subsequent flow of remittances is typically uncertain, often leaving women to support themselves and their children (Lloyd, 1992). This call for a more realistic view of the family in all its forms, as highlighted by Lloyd, is often stressed by feminists as the right way towards more effective population policies. This point needs to be taken into account in family planning programmes.

How do family planning programmes address men today? Little research and hardly any programmes have centred on men from a gender perspective, largely because of the heavy emphasis on increasing the number of contraceptive users and the variety of contraceptives for women. However, studies have shown that although

312

women often are clear in their understanding of the impact family planning could have on their life, men are frequently more uneasy and suspicious towards family planning and therefore often oppose it (Weekes-Vagliani, 1992). If the influence of men is considered negative and unchangeable, one is implicitly accepting that discrimination against women will always exist (Ford Foundation, 1991). Unless men and women are addressed simultaneously in family planning programmes on the basis of gender analysis, these programmes will continue to operate outside existing gender roles and without attempting to modify them towards equality between the sexes. It is a matter of broadening the goal of family planning, from focusing on population reduction first and foremost within existing gender hierarchies towards also raising the status of women by involving boys and girls, men and women in the process for equality and for a more effective strategy in the long run.

B. STRENGTHENING OF POLICIES AND PROGRAMMES BY INCORPORATING THE GENDER DIMENSION: SOME SUGGESTIONS

In order to be effective in the long run, family planning programmes should focus not only on attempting to reduce fertility within existing gender roles but on changing existing gender roles in order to reduce fertility. Although this point has to some extent been recognized in policy documents, it is less visible in the implementation of family planning programmes. Involving women in the planning and implementation process is prerequisite to improving family planning programmes and the United Nations Population Fund (UNFPA) recommends that women be consulted and involved at every level in the organization of family planning services.

However, shifts in policy approach often occur not only during the formulation stage but also during the implementation process. In other words, planning is one thing; carrying out the plans is something completely different (Buvinic, 1986). By really involving women and men in all stages, this problem could be avoided. This effort will mean involving girls and boys, women and men in all stages of life, using a life-course approach, in order to empower women to gain control over their life and their fertility. Such involvement will entail changing the culturally set gender roles for women and

men into a more balanced sharing of reproductive, productive and community managing and leadership roles, between the sexes (United Nations, 1991a). This objective is not achieved overnight, nor is it impossible. It will require coordination between family planning programmes, Governments and non-governmental organizations, as well as the political will to raise the status of women. In the following discussion, an attempt is made to suggest some ideas for a gender analysis, which could be taken into account in family planning programmes.

As was suggested earlier by the Division for the Advancement of Women, a gender-sensitive approach to family planning could lead to considering integrating several new variables into these programmes. Limiting family planning programmes to the aspects of fertility is not enough; instead, links between the status of women and, for example, education, salaried employment and migration will have to be identified and dealt with. By applying a gender perspective to each of the traditional population variables—that is, fertility, migration and mortality—one could gain new insights and find ways to improve policies and programmes (United Nations, 1992; and United Nations Office at Vienna, 1992).

Setting a new agenda based on gender analysis will mean addressing women and men simultaneously in the gender system that they form in their society. In order to do this, a preliminary analysis of gender relations in the society will have to be performed. Among other measures to be taken, this will mean developing indicators, primarily statistical, and subsequent analysis based on data disaggregated by gender, for a fuller understanding of gender inequality. The research on socio-economic and cultural factors which contribute to high fertility needs to be reinterpreted from a gender perspective. Currently, data are generally available on women as beneficiaries only, and very little attention has been paid to analysis of types of strategies that could be called "transformative and empowering". Research will also have to focus on how to involve boys and men.

The aim of the gender analysis is to identify the current gender roles with which the programme plans to intervene; then, based on this analysis, a framework for the programme can be defined. Such a gender analysis, applied to family planning programmes, could begin by asking some fundamental questions:

(*a*) Which gender roles need to be strengthened or weakened for women and men, respectively, in order to empower women to exercise their basic human right to decide "freely and informedly" on the number and spacing of their children?

(*b*) How can the reproductive and community caring roles of women be redistributed between the sexes? How can men be involved to a greater extent? What other actors could be brought in to organize child care and parental leave, for example?

(*c*) What is the planned outcome of changing these roles, and what may happen if they are not changed: (i) outcome for women; (ii) outcome for men; (iii) outcome for men and women, in the gender system they form; (iv) impact on population growth and on society.

The next step would be to identify how one could intervene on each selected gender role, based on the answers from this analysis, and to organize these interventions into a programme. This step could be done by examining what could be carried out by the family planning programmes and what could be implemented in coordination with other actors. A coherent and collaborative approach is of particular importance in order to include a gender perspective in a multidisciplinary and multiorganizational strategy. The cost of increasing complexity should be examined in the light of the longer term benefits. One institution which needs to be involved is the national machineries for the advancement of women (e.g., ministries for women's rights). These bodies could play an important role in coordinating activities between Governments, non-governmental organizations, academic institutions and other actors.

Ways and means to carry out evaluations of the gender impact of family planning programmes need to be found. Although some development agencies carry out separate evaluations of women in development in their general evaluations, gender impact has not been routinely assessed (Jahan, 1992). As has been demonstrated here, in the case of family planning programmes such evaluation is of crucial importance to the outcome of the programmes. Family planning programmes could be evaluated using the following basic questions:

(*a*) What impact has the programme had on women's health and their socio-economic situation? What are the socio-economic effects of the programme on women,

men, families, individuals, local communities and national societies?

(*b*) What impact has the programme had on the status of women and on gender relations?

(*c*) Should the family planning programme include other demographic variables related to the status of women, such as migration? (United Nations, 1992; and United Nations office at Vienna, 1992).

From these evaluations, important feedback could be gained to improve policies and programmes.

NOTES

[1]"Reproductive work" here means all the unpaid work done (mainly by women, usually considered "women's work") in order to sustain the family: caring for children and sick and old people; cooking; cleaning; shopping (Elson, 1991). Unpaid domestic labour is simply another domestic activity but is seldom seen as such and is not regularly accounted for in production statistics; thus, it remains invisible in the national accounts that provide the statistical counterpart of macroeconomic models (Elson, 1991).
[2]"Community managing work", based on a definition by Moser (1989), means work undertaken at a local community settlement level, mainly by women as an extension of their domestic reproductive role, trying to make up for lack of provision of housing, water and health facilities.
[3]A "gender perspective" means a perspective based on analysis of the socially constructed and culturally variable roles that women and men play in their daily life.

REFERENCES

Bondestam, Lars, and Steffan Bergström, eds. (1980). *Poverty and Population Control*. London and New York: Academic Press.

Buvinic, Mayra M. (1986). Projects for women in the Third World: explaining their misbehaviour. *World Development* (Tarrytown, New York), vol. 14, No. 5 (May), pp. 653-664.

Cassen, Robert, and Associates (1986). *Does Aid Work*? Oxford: Clarendon Press; and New York: Oxford University Press.

de Guerny, Jacques, and Elisabeth Sjöberg (1993). Inter-relationship between gender relations and the HIV/AIDS-epidemic: some possible considerations for policies and programmes. *AIDS* (London), vol. 7, No. 7 (August), pp. 1027-1034.

Development Alternatives With Women for a New Era (1988). *Confronting the Crisis in Latin America: Women Organizing for Change*. Santiago, Chile: Isis International.

Elson, Diane, ed. (1991). *Male Bias in the Development Process*. Manchester, New York: Manchester University Press.

Faulkner, A. H., and V. Lawson (1991). Employment versus empowerment: a case study of the women's work in Equador. *The Journal of Development Studies* (London), vol. 27, No. 4 (July), pp. 16-47.

Figueroa, Blanca (1992). Adding color to life: illustrated health material for women in Peru. In *By and for Women: Involving Women in the Development of Reproductive Health Care Materials*, Valerie J. Hull, ed. Quality/Calidad/Qualité Series, No. 4. New York: The Population Council.

Ford Foundation (1991). *Reproductive Health: A Strategy for the 1990s: A Program Paper*. New York.

Jahan, Rounag (1992). Mainstreaming women in development in different settings: Columbia University/Dhaka University. Paper presented at the Seminar on Mainstreaming Women in Development organized by the Office of Economic Cooperation and Development/Development Assistance Cooperation/Women in Development Expert Group, Paris, 19-20 May.

Lloyd, Cynthia B. (1992). Family and gender issues for population policy. Paper presented at the United Nations Expert Group Meeting on Population and Women, Gaborone, Botswana, 22-26 June 1992.

Moser, Caroline (1989). Gender planning in the third world: meeting practical and strategic gender needs. *World Development* (Tarrytown, New York; and Oxford, United Kingdom), vol. 17, No. 11 (November), pp. 1799-1825.

Postel, Els (1992). The value of women, women's autonomy, population and policy trends. Paper presented at the United Nations Expert Group Meeting on Population and Women, Gaborone, Botswana, 22-26 June 1992.

Sadik, Nafis (1990). *The State of World Population, 1990: Choices for the New Century*. New York: United Nations Population Fund.

Sen, Gita (1985). *Development, Crises and Alternative Visions: Third World Women's Perspective*. Development Alternatives With Women for a New Era Project. New York: Monthly Review Press.

United Nations (1975). *Report of the United Nations World Population Conference, 1974, Bucharest, 19-30 August 1974*. Sales No. E.75.XIII.3.

_____ (1985). *The Mexico City Conference: The Debate on the Review and Appraisal of the World Population Plan of Action*.

_____ (1988). *Human Rights: A Compilation of International Instruments*. Sales No. E.88.XIV.1.

_____ (1989). The Nairobi Forward-looking Strategies for the Advancement of Women. In *Report of the World Conference to Review and Appraise the Achievements of the United Nations Decade for Women: Equality, Development and Peace, Nairobi, 15-26 July 1985*. Sales No. E.85.IV.20.

_____ (1991a). Report of the Seminar on the Integration of Women in Development, Vienna, 9-11 December 1991. Unpublished.

_____ (1991b). *Women: Challenges to the Year 2000*. Sales No. E.91.I.21.

_____ (1992). Priority themes: equality: elimination of de jure and de facto discrimination against women. Report of the Secretary-General to the Commission of the Status of Women E/CN.6/1992/7.

United Nations Office at Vienna (1992). A gender perspective on population issues. Paper presented at the United Nations Expert Group Meeting on Population and Women, Gaborone, Botswana, 22-26 June 1992.

Ware, Helen (1992). Does development lead to greater equality between the sexes? Paper presented at the United Nations Expert Group Meeting on Population and Women, Gaborone, Botswana, 22-26 June 1992.

Weekes-Vagliani, Winifred (1992). *Lessons from the Family Planning Experience for Community-based Environmental Education*. Technical Papers, No. 62. Paris: Office of Economic Cooperation Development Centre.

World Bank (1991). *Gender and Poverty in India*. Washington, D.C.

World Women's Congress for a Healthy Planet (1991). *Official Report of the World Women's Congress for a Healthy Planet, Miami, Florida, 8-12 November*.

XXII. WOMEN: THE ESSENTIAL CONSTITUENCY

Daniel E. Pellegrom[*]

The United Nations declared the decade 1975-1985 the "Decade of Women". Studies and projects were undertaken worldwide to identify critical women's issues and to address those issues through development projects. Although many positive new initiatives resulted during the decade, data gathered from research, during that period and since, suggest that women continue to suffer discrimination in virtually every sphere of their lives.

For example, it is known that being female is life-threatening. A study by the World Health Organization (WHO) shows that wherever food is in short supply, girl children are fed less, breast-fed for a shorter time and taken to doctors less frequently. Females between the ages of one and five years die at much higher rates than males (Bunch, 1992). Data from the World Fertility Survey found that in 23 of the 38 countries surveyed, a preference for male children was the norm (Ladjali and Huston, 1990). When families live in poverty and cannot afford to provide for large numbers of children, girl children are denied and neglected, and the rate of female infanticide rises (Zeidenstein, 1989). One study at Bombay, India documented that 99 per cent of foetuses aborted in that city are female (Bunch, 1992).

Girls that survive past age 5 are often denied education, a principal link to greater economic advancement. Educated women have healthier infants and children, and are more likely to use contraception and space additional births, resulting in fertility declines. As little as three years of maternal education is associated with from 20 to 30 per cent declines in the mortality of children under age 5 (Mosley and Cowley, 1991). The combination of increased female literacy and fertility decline is a powerful deterrent to poverty.

For those women in the developing world that survive infancy and early childhood, the stakes get higher as they approach their reproductive years. In the developing countries, a woman's lifetime risk of death from pregnancy-related causes is between 80 and 600 times greater than her counterpart in the developed countries (Jacobson, 1990). It is estimated that at least 500,000 women worldwide die from pregnancy-related causes each year. Roughly half of those deaths are attributable to unsafe abortion. Women that survive an unsafe abortion often suffer serious complications requiring the use of scarce supplies, such as blood and hospital beds. Hospitals in some developing countries report that as many as 50 per cent of hospital beds at any one time are taken by women suffering from complications of septic abortion.

Women surviving the child-bearing gauntlet often face a life of hardship and poverty. Meanwhile, remaining childless is not a happy option for women in most cultures. Infertility is scorned and when a male partner is infertile, the presumption of infertility falls mercilessly upon the woman. If child-bearing is dangerous, the alternative is social isolation, disapproval and disgrace.

In 1980, women were half the world population, performed two thirds of the work-hours and were recognized for only one third of that work, received 10 per cent of the world income and had 1 per cent of the world property registered in their name (Inter-American Parliamentary Group, 1991). In rich and poor countries alike, female-headed households are on the rise. In many countries of Africa and Latin America, female-headed households account for as much as 50 per cent of all households (Inter-American Parliamentary Group, 1991). In the United States of America, 78 per cent of all Americans living below the poverty level are women or children under age 18. Despite the fact that more than 60 per cent of women in the United States are in the labour force, American women still earn only 64 cents to each dollar earned by a man (Inter-American Parliamentary Group, 1991). Throughout the world, it is harder for women to obtain credit, to arrange for loans or to acquire the skills that would enable them to improve their living situation.

Advances made during the United Nations Decade of Women encouraged those in the field of international family planning. But the seven years since the

---

[*]Pathfinder International, Watertown, Massachusetts, United States of America.

end of that decade have seen an erosion in many areas of maternal and child health. For the first time in many years, maternal and infant mortality rates are beginning to rise and girls' school enrolment is beginning to fall in much of the developing world (Inter-American Parliamentary Group, 1991). Programmes introduced by international financial institutions have not successfully integrated women into economic development. Drastic decreases in funding for education and health programmes have only served to further marginalize women.

Economic development cannot be attained without addressing the issue of the "feminization of poverty". Improving the health and educational status of women contributes to the reduction of poverty and to improved health among the next generation of participants in socio-economic development. Providing access to family planning and universal education to girls and women today will double the human resources tomorrow. Discounting and devaluing the potential contributions of 50 per cent of the world population is not only unfair, it is unproductive.

In planning for the 1994 International Conference on Population and Development, one must avoid repeating the mistakes of the past. If the goal is to achieve universal access to family planning services, it is incumbent upon everyone involved to seek and demand the full participation of women at all levels and in all countries. A feminist vision of development includes an end to all forms of injustice that marginalize and exploit women (Ouellette, 1992).

Those working in international family planning know the realities. Half a million women die each year from causes related to child-bearing. As many as 50 per cent of those deaths result from illegal abortions, many of which occur because women have no access to family planning services. For each death, another 30-40 women suffer impaired reproductive health status (Jacobson, 1990).

Maternal deaths leave hundreds of thousands of children orphaned each year. Since mothers are the primary "producers" of health among children, this tragic loss of maternal life takes a double toll (Mosley and Cowley, 1991). The women that survive the complications of an illegal abortion often find themselves pregnant again within a year. When frequent births occur at short intervals, maternal and child health are

often compromised. Malnutrition and maternal depletion syndrome affect large numbers of women in the developing world (Chen, 1992).

Access to family planning services, including safe abortion services, saves the lives of countless women and children. Failure to communicate these facts effectively and persuasively to broader audiences is the central challenge that must be addressed in looking towards the 1994 International Conference on Population and Development. It is necessary to return to the poignant questions raised at the International Safe Motherhood Conference held at Nairobi in 1987. Why do maternal and infant mortality rates remain so high throughout the developing world? Is it because the majority of these women are poor? (Starrs, 1987).

It must be acknowledged that the causes of maternal mortality and morbidity are:

". . . . deeply rooted in the adverse social, cultural, political, and economic environment of societies, and especially the environments that societies create for women. . . . This discrimination begins at birth and continues through adolescence and adulthood, where women's contributions and roles are ignored and undervalued." (Starrs, 1987, p. 6.2)

If maternal and child health in developing countries is to be improved and the incidence of unwanted pregnancy decreased, comprehensive approaches to reproductive health based on broader human rights issues of justice and equity must be devised (Germain, 1988).

Family planners have compiled the statistics. Those in the field have commissioned the studies, done the research, analysed the data and shared the collective insights from programme experience. They must forcefully reassert to the world at large what they know to be true.

Family planning is a critical health care need. It is sought by women the world over. The separation of abortion from family planning is a denial of health care that causes hundreds of thousands of women to die each year. The United Nations General Assembly declared in 1968 that couples have a basic human right to decide freely and responsibly on the number and spacing of their children. Without the inclusion of abortion as a backup for contraceptive failure, couples cannot freely exercise this right (Jacobson, 1990). Contraceptives reduce the need for abortion, but 7 out of 10 women using a 95 per cent effective contraceptive method would still require at least one abortion in their lifetime to achieve a two-child family (Frejka, 1985).

During the past 12 years, politics in the United States have resulted in policies that reflect an artificial separation of abortion from family planning. These policies, including the Mexico City policy announced at the last International Conference on Population and Development, have compromised the meaning of public health. The tendency for family planners to view their role as programmatic (to be, in effect, apolitical) has, in part, allowed the separation of abortion and family planning to occur. Effective programmes have been undermined and, indeed, threatened by purely political distinctions that distort both goals and accomplishments. Solutions to the reproductive health problems faced by women worldwide are available and cost-effective. To implement these solutions successfully, however, family planners and other health-care providers need to confront the controversial issues head-on and insist upon political commitments that match the problem. It must be recognized that the struggle over abortion is an issue of power, both symbolically and literally. As the politicians in the developed countries debate the issue of "choice", in developing countries, what is at stake is little short of the right to life for women.

REFERENCES

Bunch, Charlotte (1992). Overview of violence against women. In *Violence Against Women: Addressing a Global Problem*. New York: Ford Foundation, Women's Program Forum.

Chen, Lincoln C. (1992). *A New World Health Order: Challenges and Priorities in the 1990's, An Alternative*. Washington, D.C.: Overseas Development Council.

Frejka, Tomas, (1985). Induced abortion and fertility. *International Family Planning Perspectives* (New York), vol. 11, No. 4 (December), pp. 125-129.

Germain, Adrienne (1988). Meeting women's needs. *People* (London), vol. 15, No. 4, p. 23.

Inter-American Parliamentary Group on Population and Development (1991). *The Feminization of Poverty*, vol. 8, No. 6 (July).

Jacobson, Jodi L. (1990). *The Global Politics of Abortion*. Worldwatch Paper, No. 97. Washington, D.C.: Worldwatch Institute.

Ladjali, Malika, and Perdita Huston (1990). Listen to women first. *People* (London), vol. 17, No. 1, pp. 21-23.

Mosley, Henry W., and Peter Cowley (1991). *The Challenge of World Health*. Population Bulletin, vol. 46, No. 4, p. 10. Washington, D.C.: Population Reference Bureau.

Ouellette, Christine (1992). Donor round table. In *Violence Against Women: Addressing a Global Problem*. New York: Ford Foundation, Women's Program Forum.

Starrs, Ann (1987). *Preventing the Tragedy of Maternal Deaths*. A report on the International Safe Motherhood Conference, Nairobi, Kenya, February 1987; cosponsored by the World Bank, World Health Organization and the United Nations Fund for Population Activities. Washington, D.C.: The World Bank.

Zeidenstein, George (1989). Keynote address. In *Proceedings of the International Conference on Adolescent Fertility in Latin America and the Caribbean, Oaxaca, Mexico*.

XXIII. MAKING FAMILY PLANNING WORK: A POLICY MAKER'S CHECK-LIST

Population Crisis Committee[*]

Organized family planning programmes now exist in many developing countries, but their strength and effectiveness vary enormously. Some countries have achieved remarkable success in expanding the use of modern contraception and reducing birth rates; most programmes still have substantial shortcomings.

The organization and management of family planning programmes are critical to their performance. Family planning programmes are often most effective where social and economic conditions generate a strong demand for contraception. But strong programmes can have a powerful impact, even at relatively low levels of social and economic development. Conversely, where programmes have failed to have an impact, it is often because services are weak or inappropriately designed.

Improving existing family planning programmes is often the quickest way to increase levels of contraceptive use. There is no single formula for improving performance. For programmes to be successful, a variety of policy choices affecting the quantity and quality of services must be effectively implemented.

The most important elements of successful family planning programmes are identified below, presented as guidelines for strengthening family planning efforts. Greater attention to these factors by policy makers and programme managers could dramatically improve the effectiveness of established family planning programmes, as well as speed the progress of newly initiated efforts.

A. MAKING FAMILY PLANNING INFORMATION AND SERVICES EASILY AVAILABLE BY LOCATING THEM NEAR POTENTIAL USERS

Availability of family planning information and services is the single most important factor associated with increased use of modern contraception. Studies in numerous countries show that contraceptive use is clearly related to ease of access, particularly knowledge of and distance from a source of services. Scope and density of coverage are therefore critical to programme performance; rural areas, in particular, tend to be underserved.

Expansion of the contraceptive distribution network almost always increases levels of use. In Malaysia, growth in the number of family planning clinics was the most important factor contributing to increased use of contraception. In the Philippines and Pakistan, regional variations in contraceptive use have been largely explained by differences in the density of clinics and personnel. Research in Bangladesh has shown that where family planning outreach workers were at first assigned a very large area, the subsequent addition of staff enabled workers to visit more households on a regular and predictable basis and to spend more time with existing clients, resulting in dramatic increases in levels of contraceptive use.

B. USE OF A VARIETY OF APPROACHES TO PROVIDING FAMILY PLANNING INFORMATION AND SERVICES: CLINICAL, COMMERCIAL AND COMMUNITY-BASED

The specific mix of family planning activities will inevitably differ from country to country. But a combination of complementary approaches is usually necessary to make a full range of contraceptive services widely available and to reach different groups within a society. Multiple channels facilitate access; a study in Thailand, for example, found that areas with four or more different sources of family planning services had significantly higher levels of use than areas where only one source was available.

Multiple delivery systems are necessary because services that rely upon the existing clinical health system alone are usually inadequate to reach the majority of people living in rural areas, as well as the poorest urban areas. Most successful family planning programmes go

---

*Washington, D.C., United States of America.

beyond the public-health system. Private health providers, employer-supported services, commercial sales through pharmacies and retail outlets and community-based distribution (CBD) schemes using a variety of trained lay personnel have helped ensure the widest possible availability of oral contraceptives, condoms and other non-clinical methods.

Specialized services are often needed to reach men and young adults. Different delivery systems are also needed for different contraceptive methods. Clinic-based programmes are still needed for intra-uterine devices (IUDs), implants, sterilization and abortion services, all of which require aseptic techniques and trained health personnel. Clinics are also needed as medical backup for women that initiate contraception through CBD or commercial outlets.

C. PROVISION OF THE BROADEST POSSIBLE CHOICE OF BOTH TEMPORARY AND LONG-ACTING SAFE, EFFECTIVE CONTRACEPTIVE METHODS

Along with ease of access, availability of a range of contraceptive choices may well be the most important factor affecting family planning practice. Providing a variety of methods increases the likelihood that each individual and couple will find a satisfactory method. Different methods are also appropriate at different times in a person's reproductive life. Women that are breast-feeding, for example, need contraceptive methods compatible with lactation.

Introducing a new contraceptive method appears to attract a new clientele and increase overall levels of contraceptive use; a recent study concluded from data for 72 countries that adding one new method increases contraceptive practice by an average of 12 percentage points. A choice of methods is also important to sustained practice of family planning. Discontinuation and method-switching are very common among family planning clients, and programmes need to offer alternatives to clients whose needs may change or who are dissatisfied with their current method.

Very few countries (including some that are highly industrialized) offer the full range of contraceptives available. In many countries, only about two contraceptive methods are widely available. Programmes that include a variety of methods in theory often emphasize a single one in practice, accounting to a large extent for variations in patterns of use among countries. Problems with logistics and supplies, lack of adequate information about certain methods, biases on the part of service providers and restrictive government policies may also limit available choices.

D. MAKING VOLUNTARY CONTRACEPTIVE STERILIZATION FOR BOTH MEN AND WOMEN WIDELY AVAILABLE AT REASONABLE COST AND WITHOUT UNNECESSARY RESTRICTIONS

Most countries with successful family planning programmes offer individuals and couples that want no more children the option of contraceptive sterilization. Worldwide, sterilization is the most popular contraceptive method; high acceptance of female sterilization has contributed to fertility declines in a number of countries. In Brazil (despite tight restrictions), the Dominican Republic, the Republic of Korea, Thailand and the United States of America, more than 20 per cent of couples of reproductive age have chosen sterilization.

Despite its popularity, many couples desiring sterilization cannot obtain it. In some countries, doctors are reluctant to perform sterilization because its legal status is unclear. In many others, trained service providers are not widely available, especially in rural areas. In such countries as Brazil and Honduras, cost is a major obstacle. Unnecessarily restrictive policies, requiring that men or women be a minimum age or have a certain number of children, also serve to discourage couples seeking permanent, effective contraception. Policy makers need to recognize the demand for contraceptive sterilization and remove barriers to access by informed consumers.

E. AVAILABILITY OF SAFE TERMINATION OF PREGNANCIES AS A BACKUP FOR CONTRACEPTIVE FAILURE

Widespread effective contraceptive use can greatly reduce reliance upon abortion. But all contraceptive methods, including sterilization, carry some degree of risk of accidental pregnancy. Thus, even if all couples used modern methods of contraception, some abortions would still be sought in response to contraceptive failure. Given the high mortality rates from abortions performed under unsafe conditions, the most humane approach is to provide ready access to modern contraceptives and safe, legal abortion.

Historically, use of abortion—legal or illegal—has had a significant impact on fertility declines. Liberalization of abortion laws is thought to have played a role in initial birth rate reductions in Japan and in selected countries in Eastern Europe. Abortion has also been widely practised in a number of developing countries or areas where birth rates have fallen significantly, such as Brazil, Cuba, the Republic of Korea, Singapore and Taiwan Province of China. The evidence suggests that some reliance upon abortion for birth control is probably unavoidable, even where levels of contraceptive use are relatively high, given the failure rates associated with current contraceptive technology.

F. WORKING TOWARDS A PARTNERSHIP BETWEEN PUBLIC AND PRIVATE SECTORS TO ENSURE A BROAD ROLE FOR VOLUNTARY AGENCIES, COMMERCIAL OUTLETS AND PRIVATE PRACTITIONERS

In many developing countries, Governments have taken the lead in providing family planning services. Involving a variety of private service providers—commercial distributors, voluntary agencies, private doctors, traditional midwives and pharmacists—not only expands available service outlets but helps reach additional types of clients. Increasing reliance upon such providers can also substantially reduce the costs to Governments. The private sector (which includes commercial and non-governmental groups) can also play an important role in providing family planning information and education to the community.

In some developing countries, the private sector has played a central role in expanding the use of family planning, particularly in urban areas. In most industrialized countries and in some developing countries, such as Brazil and Egypt, the vast majority of family planning services are provided through the commercial sector. Together, the commercial sector and private voluntary agencies are a primary source of non-clinical methods, such as pills and condoms, in many developing countries. Some Governments, however, have tended to overregulate and stifle the development of the private sector. In general, Governments need to seek a more effective partnership with the private sector and to encourage the commercial sector more actively to serve those able to pay for services and supplies.

G. USE OF SENSIBLE COST-RECOVERY MEASURES IN GOVERNMENT-SUBSIDIZED PROGRAMMES WHILE KEEPING SERVICES AFFORDABLE

In virtually all countries, including the United States of America, some people are unable to pay the full cost of private services. In many developing countries, including many in Africa, commercial contraceptive prices are beyond the reach of the majority of people; in Bangladesh, a one-year supply of pills from purely commercial sources costs over $16, compared with an average annual income of $160.

Services for low-income populations need not, however, all be free of charge. Even in the poorest countries, some level of cost recovery is feasible. In many subsidized programmes, minimal charges for contraceptives or clinical services have not proved a major barrier to increased use. The percentage of costs that can be covered by consumers will vary by country and type of programme. In Colombia, where annual income averages about $1,300, social marketing efforts have covered over 100 per cent of costs, while community-based programmes have covered 50 per cent of costs in urban areas and 17 per cent in rural areas.

Evidence from a number of developed and developing countries suggests that abortion services may be the one type of service that can be largely self-sustaining and, in some settings, can even subsidize other family planning and health measures.

Over time, if household income rises, consumers can be expected to assume an increasing share of family planning costs. But the enormous social benefits of family planning are a strong argument for keeping charges modest and for providing services free to those that could not otherwise afford them.

H. LIMITING REGULATORY REQUIREMENTS AND ADMINISTRATIVE RESTRICTIONS ON BOTH PROVIDERS AND CLIENTS TO THOSE PROTECTING THE CLIENT AGAINST HEALTH RISKS OR INVOLUNTARY PROCEDURES

Government policies and regulations can have a powerful impact on family planning practice; policy makers decide which contraceptive methods will be available, under what conditions and who will be authorized to provide them. Policy decisions are too often based on outmoded laws or misperceptions about the health risks of contraceptives. For example, recent studies show that a simplified questionnaire on smoking habits and family history of heart disease, administered by pharmacists or fieldworkers, can effectively screen out most women with contraindications to the pill. As a result, many countries no longer require a prescription for oral contraceptives. In many countries non-physician health personnel have been trained successfully to insert IUDs and perform early pregnancy termination.

Overregulation by Governments can inhibit the commercial importation of contraceptives. Restrictions on advertising can pose a barrier to effective information programmes. Cumbersome procedures for new drug approval and registration can limit access to new contraceptives. Programme restrictions, such as spousal consent or waiting periods, are often inappropriate and create barriers to contraceptive use. Ideally, government policy should provide as wide a range of contraceptives as possible outside medical channels and should minimize other barriers to increased contraceptive practice.

I. EMPHASIZING SYMPATHETIC COUNSELLING AND SYSTEMATIC FOLLOW-UP BY WELL-TRAINED AND COMMITTED WORKERS TO ENSURE EFFECTIVE, LONG-TERM USE OF CONTRACEPTIVES

Many programmes give greater attention to recruiting new clients than to maintaining contraceptive use among existing clients. Yet, continuing and correct use are essential to long-term success for both programmes and their clients. In many developing countries, the use of drugs and devices for birth control is still a new concept. Exaggerated rumours about the side-effects of these new contraceptive methods can lead to high drop-out rates. Negative consumer reactions can undermine programme effectiveness far into the future. Emphasis on high-quality services is critical to building and sustaining family planning use. Accurate information, good counselling and regular follow-up care have been shown to improve consumer satisfaction very significantly.

The way a client is treated by a service provider can be the major factor in determining whether that client becomes and remains a family planning user. Although family planning services need not and should not rely upon physicians, basic technical competence is also very important. This is especially true for clinical methods—if women experience excessive discomfort or medical complications, word of their negative experience will spread quickly in the community. But less tangible factors also matter. Managers play an important role in motivating their staff to provide quality services and in creating an atmosphere conducive to positive interaction between programme staff and clients. Evidence from government and voluntary organization programmes in Bangladesh suggests that conscientious, knowledgeable and caring fieldworkers attract consistently higher numbers of long-term, satisfied clients. When poorly motivated fieldworkers were replaced in one project, levels of contraceptive use rose quickly.

J. MAKING FAMILY PLANNING SERVICES "USER-FRIENDLY": DELIVERING THEM IN A CULTURALLY ACCEPTABLE MANNER AND SETTING

The best services are those adapted to the local cultural setting and sensitive to client needs. In Bangladesh, the Philippines and elsewhere, the gender of service providers has proved important; female outreach workers clearly find it easier to discuss family planning with potential women clients. Differences in language, religion, ethnic origin or social status can also present a problem. In some countries, for example, the social gap between doctors and very poor or illiterate clients is a barrier to effective communication about contraceptive risks and benefits. The attitudes of service providers can also affect performance; studies in several countries show that rude or condescending treatment by clinic staff can be a significant deterrent to potential family planning clients.

The convenience of services is also important. In clinical settings, long waiting times and inconvenient hours can be a major barrier to family planning from the client's perspective—one study in Latin America documented waiting times for first-time clients of up to six hours. On the other hand, when the Matlab project in Bangladesh began to provide injectable contraceptives and IUDs to women in their homes, use of these methods rose significantly.

K. AVOIDING OVERLOADING SERVICE PROVIDERS IN EFFORTS TO INTEGRATE OTHER ACTIVITIES WITH FAMILY PLANNING: NEED TO FOCUS ON SERVICES MOST IN DEMAND AND TO RECOGNIZE CAPACITY LIMITS

There is no factual basis for the perception that family planning programmes must be integrated with health or other activities to succeed. Both free-standing and integrated programmes have been successful—effective implementation, not programme philosophy, has been the key. Ambitious integration schemes have routinely failed when they overtaxed managerial resources or front-line service providers.

A major challenge for multi-purpose programmes is to make sure that family planning is not neglected. Experience suggests that multiple responsibilities can sometimes detract from the delivery of family planning services. When oral rehydration therapy was introduced into the Matlab family planning project in Bangladesh, the percentage of couples using contraception actually declined. In Tunisia, too, integrating family planning with many health measures had a negative impact on family planning. In both cases, workers spent less time on family planning activities and gave them lower priority. In Malaysia, on the other hand, a well-designed integration of health and family planning increased contraceptive use. Integrated activities must be carefully planned and implemented so as to meet clients' felt needs without overextending workers or managerial capacity.

L. USE OF MULTIPLE COMMUNICATION CHANNELS AND MASS MEDIA TO BUILD PUBLIC KNOWLEDGE OF CONTRACEPTION AND SUPPORT FOR RESPONSIBLE PARENTHOOD AND REPRODUCTIVE CHOICE

Reliable, positive information about family planning is crucial. Merely making contraceptives available is not enough. People need to know not just how family planning will benefit them but also where to obtain family planning services and how specific contraceptives actually work, including the specific risks and benefits of each method. Although effective communication between clients and providers is critical to the success of most family planning methods, modern communications networks, especially radio and television, have helped to spread modern technologies for fertility control and smaller family size ideals. Mass communications probably help explain rapid changes in reproductive behaviour in many developing countries, such as Thailand, in recent years.

The strongest programmes include strong public education efforts. Advertising campaigns to raise awareness of specific methods have proved successful in a number of countries. In such countries as China,

India, Indonesia, Mexico and Turkey, media campaigns have played a powerful role. Even where public support for family planning is high, information efforts are needed to counter misinformation about the health risks of contraceptive methods and to provide guides for personal behaviour. Mass media can legitimate open discussion of family planning and help improve women's self-image.

The electronic media now reach millions of people in the developing countries. Yet, many countries do not use mass media to any significant extent to promote the idea of responsible parenthood or to increase contraceptive knowledge and practice. Moreover, many existing public information programmes reach a limited audience, often with patronizing or inappropriate messages. This is an area which deserves much greater attention in coming years.

M. INSTITUTING STRONG MANAGEMENT SYSTEMS TO CREATE ACCOUNTABILITY AND PROVIDE EFFECTIVE ADMINISTRATIVE AND LOGISTICAL SUPPORT

Good management often accounts for the difference between strong and weak family planning programmes. A common problem in both government and private services is that management is often made the responsibility of physicians or other health providers with no interest or training in the managerial process. Management has many different elements, but studies of individual programmes suggest that good supervision and accountability for programme results are the most important to family planning performance.

Frequent and effective supervision is necessary to motivate staff—especially fieldworkers—to carry out their tasks on an ongoing basis. Supervision must be more than just inspection; the Matlab project in Bangladesh has shown that supervisors are most effective where they play a supportive function, providing advice to front-line family planning workers and helping to identify and solve their problems.

Good management requires that senior managers also be able to identify and address problems, as well as to reward good work. For large government programmes, an effective management information system, providing up-to-date information on performance at each level, is needed. Information on continuation rates of new and existing clients, frequency of unwanted pregnancy among contraceptive users and client responses to services offered can all help improve the quality of services. Good information systems are also vital to track the status of contraceptive supplies throughout the distribution system and to prevent sudden shortages.

N. NATIONAL AND LOCAL POLITICAL AND FINANCIAL SUPPORT OF FAMILY PLANNING PROGRAMMES

Political support can play an important role in the success of family planning programmes, even in countries that rely significantly upon private sector activities. Leadership support can help change public attitudes (especially among men), can stimulate demand for services and can remove bureaucratic obstacles limiting access to family planning. Most important, it can determine how seriously government employees take their responsibility to meet programme goals.

Political commitment also affects the resources available to Government-supported family planning services. Only rarely has financial support for family planning been adequate to make good quality affordable services universally available. Although the costs of service programmes will vary, in general, family plan-

ning providers need to allocate $1-2 per capita (of the total population) or $10-20 per acceptor each year.

A comprehensive study of programmes in 93 countries found that existence of a population policy, supportive statements by national leaders and seniority of government managers of family planning programmes were all strongly related to programme performance. In Indonesia, President Suharto has vigorously supported family planning for almost 20 years, including the recent campaign to privatize major programme components. Conversely, in Pakistan and the Philippines, consistent political leadership has been conspicuously lacking and programmes have been much less successful.

To be most effective, national leaders must follow public statements about the importance of family planning with effective community-level action. The success of the Indonesian programme, for example, is largely attributed to its ability to work through existing administrative structures at the village level. Moreover, the level of contraceptive use in Indonesian villages appears related to the level of involvement by local leaders. It is clear that the more supportive the political climate, the more likely the family planning programme is to succeed.

XXIV. FAMILY PLANNING POLICIES AND PROGRAMMES
IN COUNTRIES OF AFRICA

Economic Commission for Africa[*]

At the time of independence in the 1960s, most countries of Africa were preoccupied with accelerating socio-economic development. Population matters and especially family planning programmes were not given much attention. Most of the countries were pronatalist but a few countries showed interest in family planning policies and programmes during the 1960s: Egypt; Ghana; Kenya; Mauritius; and Tunisia. By the end of the 1960s, these countries had adopted family planning policies and programmes to influence demographic trends. The sociocultural values in most African countries encouraged early marriage and child-bearing. At the time of the World Population Conference at Bucharest in 1974, there had not been any significant changes in attitudes among most of the African countries. The belief of Governments in Africa was that socio-economic development would resolve population-related problems.

However, at the African Regional Post-World Population Conference Consultation, held at Lusaka, Zambia, in April 1975, family planning issues were discussed in the context of family formation and reproduction. Consideration was given to the need to prepare young people for marriage and responsible parenthood in order to promote family well-being and happiness. It was pointed out that unwanted pregnancies and abortion needed to be avoided. Population education, both in school and out of school, was seen as a means of preparing the young for responsible parenthood. As research on the interrelations between population variables and socio-economic development became widely disseminated, many Governments began to appreciate the importance and impact of these interrelations.

It was not until 1984 that marked changes in perceptions became very clear with the adoption of the Kilimanjaro Programme of Action on Population by Governments at the Second African Population Conference at Arusha, United Republic of Tanzania. The

recommendations to Governments on fertility and family planning called on African countries to: recognize the usefulness of family planning and child-spacing on the stability and well-being of the family; to integrate family planning services into mother and child health (MCH) services; to incorporate family planning education into training programmes for women, men and youth; to ensure the availability of and accessibility of family planning services to all couples or individuals seeking such services freely or at subsidized prices; to make available a variety of methods to ensure a free and conscious choice by all couples or individuals; to consider setting up family planning outlets which include the utilization of existing health facilities and community-based delivery systems in order to reach those communities, couples and individuals not served by the conventional delivery systems; to educate and motivate the population at the grass-roots level on health and demographic values of family planning; and to improve funding and management for effective implementation of mother and child health/family planning (MCH/FP) programmes.

Since 1984, nearly all countries in Africa have been taking action in varying degrees to reflect these recommendations in their socio-economic development planning. This discussion note briefly describes some of the efforts being made by African countries in implementing the Kilimanjaro recommendations with regard to fertility and family planning, as well as the constraints being met. The impact of family planning programmes on fertility, infant and maternal mortality is highlighted and strategies needed for the future are suggested. It is important to emphasize here that sustainable development cannot be achieved without taking into account family planning policies and programmes as integral parts of overall socio-economic development. The annex to this paper gives information on the efforts that have been or are being made in formulating and implementing family planning and population programmes in some countries of Africa.

---

[*]Population Division, Addis Ababa, Ethiopia.

A. GENERAL PROGRESS SINCE 1984

Countries supporting family planning on health and demographic rationales, include: Algeria; Botswana; Burundi; Cameroon; Central African Republic; Chàd; Côte d'Ivoire; Egypt; Ethiopia; Gambia; Ghana; Guinea; Kenya; Lesotho; Liberia; Madagascar; Mauritius; Morocco; Niger; Nigeria; Rwanda; Senegal; Seychelles; Sierra Leone; Swaziland; Tunisia; Uganda; United Republic of Tanzania; Zambia; and Zimbabwe. However, all countries agree on the need of family planning programmes on the rationale of mother and child health.

Countries that had explicit population and family planning policies and programmes before 1984 include Egypt, Kenya, Ghana, Mauritius and Tunisia. Since 1984, the following countries have formulated and adopted population policies: Guinea (1992); Liberia (1988); Niger (1992); Nigeria (1988); Senegal (1988); and Zambia (1989). Cameroon, the Gambia, Madagascar, Sierra Leone, Togo, the United Republic of Tanzania and Zaire have draft policies awaiting final approval by the Governments.

Since 1984, Ghana and Kenya have taken action to revitalize the implementation of their population and family planning policies by taking various measures, including providing information, education and communication (IEC) programmes intended to convince the population to accept a small family size; increasing the availability of family planning services by involving the private sector to provide services and increasing male involvement in family planning programmes. Some of the countries that have formulated population policies since 1984 have included specific targets for fertility and family planning. The 1988 Senegal population policy includes the introduction of family life education into school curricula and out-of-school youth training programmes. However, the Senegalese population policy has no quantitative targets. Botswana and Zimbabwe, which have no explicit population policies, are implementing very progressive family planning programmes; they are among the African countries with high contraceptive use. These countries are considering the preparation of explicit population policies.

Family planning programmes are implemented in Swaziland to lower fertility and growth even though no population policy exists. In August 1990, the Parliamentary Committee organized a conference on population and national development, which recommended that a national population commission should be created and charged with drafting a population policy. The need to formulate a population policy in the Sudan was voiced at the Third National Population Conference in 1987 and at the two regional population policy workshops held in September and December 1988. Rwanda is among the countries that initiated population and family planning policies to reduce fertility before 1984. MCH/FP programmes are being integrated and contraceptives are available through established clinics and other outlets. In 1986, the Central Committee of the Government's ruling party appealed for a maximum of four children per family and reflected it in the Fourth Development Plan (1987-1991). Recently, the minimum age at marriage was increased to 21 years. Côte d'Ivoire reversed its pronatalist policy in 1989, in favour of family planning.

In its attempts to continue sensitizing African countries on the importance of implementing population and family planning policies and programmes as integral to the overall socio-economic development, the secretariat of the Economic Commission for Africa (ECA) has, since 1984, intensified its research activities on population and development and family planning. For example, in 1991, the secretariat published some guidelines on improving the delivery and evaluation of population and family planning programmes (United Nations, ECA, 1991).

B. CONSTRAINTS

During the 1960s and 1970s, as mentioned earlier, many African countries did not appreciate or accept family planning programmes, even though during that period many donor organizations and Governments were providing money for the programmes. As shown above, during the last half of the 1980s, African countries with family planning programmes were eager to improve their programmes. Many of the countries that did not have a programme eventually accepted such programmes. This momentum has been generated at a time when donor organizations and Governments no longer have the same interest and resources to assist African countries in their population and family planning programmes as they did during the 1960s and 1970s. The impact of the World Bank Structural Adjustment Programmes have hit the health and education programmes which serve as the means of facilitating the implementation of family planning programmes and population policies. Material supplies for family planning services, institutions that provide family planning services and trained personnel are inadequate or lacking.

Other constraints are related to low status of women in terms of education, lack of employment opportunities other than in the traditional agriculture, lack of active involvement of both men and women in family planning programmes, lack of programmes for the youth on reproductive health and family planning, lack of grass-roots involvement and participation at community level, weak political and leadership support to family planning programmes and changed perceptions of population and family planning which have not yet resulted in changed attitudes towards small family size throughout all population segments.

C. IMPACT OF FAMILY PLANNING PROGRAMMES ON FERTILITY, INFANT AND MATERNAL MORTALITY

In Egypt, Morocco and Tunisia, family planning programmes have contributed to increased use of contraception. The increase has been as follows: Egypt, from 24 per cent in 1980 to 38 in 1988; Morocco, from 19 per cent in 1980 to 36 in 1987; and Tunisia, from 31 per cent in 1978 to 50 in 1988. The declines in total fertility among women aged 15-44 in these countries were: Egypt, from 5.2 in 1980 to 4.7 in 1988 (a 10 per cent decline); Morocco, from 5.8 in 1979/80 to 4.6 in 1987 (a 21 per cent decline); and Tunisia, from 5.7 in 1978 to 4.3 in 1988 (a 25 per cent decline). In Botswana, total fertility declined from 7.1 in 1981 to 6.5 in 1984 and to 5.0 in 1988. This decline is associated with contraceptive use of 29 per cent in 1984 and 33 per cent in 1988. In Zimbabwe, there are also indications of fertility decline, from 6.7 in 1969 to 5.5 in 1988. The contraceptive prevalence rate was 38 per cent in 1984 and increased to 43 per cent in 1988. Even in Kenya, where contraceptive use increased from 7 per cent in 1977/78 to 17 in 1984 and 27 in 1989, total fertility declined from 7.7 in 1984 to 6.7 in 1989. In most African countries, contraceptive use is below 10 per cent; and with such low levels, there cannot be any impact on fertility trends.

Where family planning is practised adequately, it helps to space births and contributes to the health of children. Birth intervals of less than two years and births occurring to women before age 20 and above age 35 are all associated with higher infant mortality. Infant mortality could be reduced by 12-22 per cent in Cameroon, Ghana, Kenya, Lesotho and the Sudan if birth intervals were at least two years. Furthermore, infant mortality could be greatly reduced if child-bearing were confined to age range 20-35.

Similarly, use of family planning would reduce maternal mortality among the high-risk groups: women under age 20; women that become pregnant after the fourth child; and women bearing children with less than a two-year birth interval. In developing countries in general, 20-45 per cent of maternal deaths are due to child-bearing. More than 40 per cent of maternal deaths could be avoided in Egypt, Ghana, Kenya, the Sudan and Tunisia if: (a) all married fecund women wanting no more children would use an effective family planning method; and (b) if all women aged 35 years or over would stop having more children.

D. FUTURE STRATEGIES ON FAMILY PLANNING IN AFRICAN COUNTRIES

Future strategies to improve the effectiveness of family planning policies and programmes need to focus on giving adequate attention to: (a) the role of strategic planning; (b) political commitment and strong leadership in support of programmes; (c) the need to change attitudes towards small family size; (d) improvement of the status of women through education, employment and protecting their rights; (e) involvement of males to participate actively and take shared responsibility in family planning programmes; (f) design and implementation of programmes to meet the needs of the youth; (g) involvement of communities, Governments and non-governmental organization in formulating, implementing and financing population and family planning programmes; (h) improvement of socio-economic conditions; (i) setting up of adequate institutional support to programmes; (j) improvement of availability and accessibility to quality family planning services and supplies, with particular emphasis in rural areas; (k) improvement of IEC activities; (l) provision of adequately trained and competent personnel to manage and deliver programmes; (m) provision of adequate material and logistic support to programmes; (n) ensurance of adequate financing of programmes by Governments, communities and non-governmental organizations, and the international community.

In conclusion, it is emphasized that sustainable economic development cannot be achieved without programmes to moderate demographic trends. In this context, strategies on family planning, education and health would be essential in order to moderate demographic trends and improve the health of children and mothers. However, such strategies must complement those which will improve socio-economic conditions in general. The combined efforts of family planning, education and health programmes with socio-economic conditions would have greater impact on improving the well-being of the population.

ANNEX

Country information

A. BOTSWANA

Botswana has had programmes on family planning for some years although it has not yet formally adopted a population policy. In 1984, the Government discussed the need to involve and target males in family planning programmes. The following year, in 1985, government officials stated the need to formulate a population policy for the country. In 1988, the Botswana Family Welfare Association was launched through joint efforts of the Government and non-governmental organizations. Among the objectives of the Association are the provision of family planning services and the fostering of better understanding of responsible parenthood in the interest of the family and the community. In 1989, the Government published general policy guidelines and service standards for family planning (Botswana, 1989). These guidelines provide a comprehensive range of activities to enhance quality services to users of family planning services. They include information, education and communication (IEC), provision of a wide range of contraceptive methods, postnatal care, counselling, follow-up, referral, health screening etc. It is important to observe the progress the country has made in family planning programmes, as reflected in the increase in contraceptive use among married women, from 24 per cent in 1984 to 30 per cent in 1988, of which 29 per cent was for modern methods.

B. BURKINA FASO

In 1985, the Government of Burkina Faso adopted a national plan on family planning. The plan was revised in 1986. Among the objectives of the National Family Planning Plan of Action were to revise regulations of the 1920 law which prohibited abortion and advertisement of contraception; to integrate maternal and child health (MCH) and family planning activities; to educate families on the role of child-spacing; and to facilitate access to contraceptive methods.

C. CAMEROON

In 1985, Cameroon established a National Population Commission, with the responsibility of formulating a national population policy. The Commission drafted a policy in 1988 but it has yet to be approved by the Government. The proposed draft policy

on family planning has the objectives of improving knowledge and use of contraception. It is proposed to increase contraceptive use from 10.5 per cent in 1989 to 50 per cent by the year 2000. It is hoped that the various measures to be taken in the implementation of the proposed national population policy will lead to a reduction in population growth from the current level of 2.9 per cent to 2 per cent by the year 2010.

D. EGYPT

Egypt was the first Arab country to adopt a national population policy in 1963 to lower fertility. Over the years, the Egyptian population policy has undergone several modifications. In 1985, the National Family Planning Council, headed by the country's president, was established and given the responsibility of coordinating all population programmes and policy. The goals for the year 2000 include the attainment of population growth rate of between 1.0 and 1.3 per cent; and total fertility of 3.0. The Egyptian Demographic and Health Survey in 1988 showed a contraceptive prevalence rate of 38 per cent among married women. Major suppliers of contraceptive methods in order of importance are: pharmacies; physicians; government hospitals; government family planning clinics; and government MCH centres. Among the modern methods of contraception in 1988, the main methods used by married women were intra-uterine devices (IUDs) (16 per cent) and the pill (15 per cent).

E. GAMBIA

In the Gambia, the Second Five-Year Plan for Economic and Social Development (1981/82-1985/86) included a statement on population policy to reduce population growth rate. Following the first National Conference on Population Policy, a draft National Population Policy for Social Welfare and Sustained Development was prepared in 1991. Among the main objectives of the draft policy are: reduction of population growth rate and provision of family planning services; and information, education and communication with regard to family planning services and child-spacing. Improving MCH is seen as a means to help reduce population growth rate. Some of the targets are to reduce total fertility to 6.0 in 1996 and to 5.0 by 2000 and to increase contraceptive prevalence to 20 per cent by 1996 and 30 per cent by 2000.

F. GHANA

The Government of Ghana adopted a national population policy in 1969, with reducing fertility and population growth rate as one of the objectives. The last half of the 1980s witnessed strong efforts to revitalize the implementation of the population policy. Some of the activities included programmes to encourage greater male involvement in the family planning programme, establishment of the Population Impact Programme Project at the University of Ghana as an outreach programme, establishment of a social marketing programme for contraceptives and the convening of the National Population Conference in 1989 which made recommendations to strengthen the implementation of the population policy. According to the Ghana Demographic and Health Survey, contraceptive use in 1988 was about 13 per cent among all women but use of modern methods of contraception was low at 5 per cent.

G. GUINEA

Up to 1983, the Government of Guinea was pronatalist, but it reversed this position in 1984 on the conviction that high population growth does not necessarily lead to economic growth. The Government established the Population Planning Unit in the Ministry of Planning in 1984 to formulate, coordinate and evaluate population policies. A national population policy was drafted in 1991 and was approved in 1992. Some of the specific objectives include: integration of demographic variables in socioeconomic development programmes; and reduction of fertility to levels that can be supported by families and society. An increase in use of modern contraceptive methods to 25 per cent by 2010 is one of the specific targets.

H. KENYA

In 1966, a national population policy and family planning programme was announced to reduce fertility and the population growth rate in Kenya. Comprehensive new population policy guidelines were launched in January 1986 to reduce population growth rate. This objective was to be reached by raising the status of women, involving men and local leadership, providing education and motivation, and involving non-governmental organizations in population and family planning programmes. There were concerted efforts during the last half of the 1980s to educate, inform and persuade the population to accept a small family size. Some of the specific activities undertaken included: the President's personal appeal to the population to encourage women to have only four children; provision of family planning at place of work by involving the private sector; inclusion of population education in primary and secondary schools; decentralization of the implementation of population and family planning programmes to the district level; creation of community-based distribution to be implemented by non-governmental organizations. Contraceptive use among all women increased from 15 per cent in 1984 to 23 per cent in 1989. Among married women, the increase for the same period was from 17 to 27 per cent.

K. LESOTHO

The Ministry of Planning of Lesotho, in collaboration with other government ministries as well as non-governmental organizations, convened a workshop on population policy in August 1990. Its objectives were to bring to the attention of

policy makers the interrelations between population issues and socio-economic development and the need to have an explicit population policy. Preparations for the formulation of a population policy including family planning are under way.

L. NIGER

In 1986, a national seminar was convened in the Niger, to discuss population and development and the formulation of a plan of action for a population policy. The results of the seminar were integrated into the 1987-1991 Development Plan. In 1988, the Government issued a decree in support of family planning programmes. Prior to that, family planning had only been tolerated. In the same year, the anticontraception law adopted from the 1920 French law was repealed. In 1992, a national population policy was adopted.

M. NIGERIA

In Nigeria, a national population policy was approved in 1988, to reduce fertility and the population growth rate. Measures to be used include: child-spacing; delayed marriages; provision of family planning and MCH services; greater involvement of males in responsible parenthood; IEC programmes; and enhancement of the status of women. Some targets include the reduction of total fertility from 6.0 to 4.0 by the year 2000.

N. TUNISIA

In Tunisia, acknowledgement of the importance of family planning as an integral part of socio-economic development dates back to 1956. Some of the actions taken since 1984 on family planning are that in 1987, Government announced a family planning policy restricting births to three children per family, although it was not compulsory; and in 1989, family planning allowances were restricted to three children per family. The Office national de la famille et de la population promotes and provides family planning services throughout Tunisia. Although the Government has been the major provider of services, in the 1990s the Government will give a greater role to the private sector in providing family planning services. Family planning is also being integrated into basic health services and other sectors, such as education. In 1988, contraceptive use among married women reached 50 per cent, of which 40 per cent was for modern methods.

O. ZIMBABWE

The Zimbabwe National Family Planning Council Act of 1985 empowered the Council to implement family planning activities throughout the whole country. During the last half of 1990, the Zimbabwe National Family Planning Council undertook a three-month project to promote greater male involvement in family planning activities, using entertainment, radio drama series with family planning messages for six months, motivational and educational talks at mines, farms, factories and villages, and pamphlets on family planning and contraceptive methods directed to men. In order to assess the impact of these efforts, an evaluation survey was conducted at the end of 1989. With a combination of such factors as strong leadership from the president on implementation of the family planning programme to reduce fertility, use of a community-based distribution system to provide family planning services, use of IEC in family planning programmes, good management of the programme, the Zimbabwe family planning programme has so far done well. It is one of the progressive programmes with a contraceptive use of 43 per cent

among married women in 1988, of whom 36 per cent were using modern methods. Those using modern methods were 36 per cent.

REFERENCES

Botswana, Ministry of Health (1989). *Botswana Family Planning: General Policy Guidelines and Service Standards.* Gaborone.
United Nations Economic Commission for Africa (1991). *Guidelines on Improving Delivery of Population and Family Planning Programmes in African Countries.* ECA/POP/TP/91/2, 1.2(ii), Addis Ababa, Ethiopia.

XXV. USE OF DEMOGRAPHIC AND HEALTH SURVEYS DATA FOR FAMILY PLANNING PROGRAMME EVALUATION AND HEALTH ASSESSMENT

*Martin T. Vaessen**

The Demographic and Health Surveys (DHS) programme is a multi-year research project on family planning and maternal and child health funded by the United States Agency for International Development (USAID). Thus far, 55 surveys have been initiated. A final report has been published for 43 of these surveys, and the remaining reports are to be published before August 1993. At the same time, a new series of surveys will be undertaken in 30 countries during the period from October 1992 to September 1997.

DHS generally interviews all women aged 15-49 residing in selected households. In some countries, samples are restricted to ever-married women due to the general absence of fertility and family planning among never-married women.

DHS is representative of the total population of households and of women aged 15-49 in a country and thus provide national estimates for the variables under study. Indeed, sample sizes in many countries have been rather large, to allow for regional estimates in response to requests from programme managers.

Nearly all countries participating in the DHS programme have provided open access to their data. DHS data files are therefore available to responsible researchers and policy makers through the DHS Archive, managed by Macro International, Inc., Columbia, Maryland.

A. CONTENT OF THE DHS

DHS covers a large amount of information; and the data can be extremely useful for studying or evaluating such areas as fertility, infant and child mortality, family planning, immunizations, diarrhoeal disease treatment, breast-feeding, prenatal and postnatal care and the nutritional status of small children and mothers.

It should be noted here that DHS uses two separate questionnaires, one for high (A core) and one for low (B core) contraceptive prevalence countries. The difference between these questionnaires is mainly that the "A" core contains more family planning-related information than the "B core". An abbreviated description of the content of the DHS questionnaires currently in use for the second phase of DHS is given below. Questionnaires for the first phase were somewhat different but cover similar topics.

Household schedule

The household schedule obtains the following information:

(*a*) A listing of all household members and relationship to the head, sex, age, level of education and survivorship of parents;

(*b*) Sources of drinking water and other water and time needed to get it;

(*c*) Type of toilet facility and availability of electricity, radio, television and refrigerator;

(*d*) Number of rooms for sleeping;

(*e*) Material of the floor and ownership of bicycle, motorcycle or motor car.

Individual questionnaire

A schematic overview of the contents of the individual questionnaires, by major topic of study, is given in section B.

---

*Director, Demographic and Health Surveys, Columbia, Maryland, United States of America.

B. Summary of topics of Demographic and Health Surveys II questionnaires

The topics of DHS II questionnaires are summarized below:

Topic	Questions	Respondents
	A. *Respondent's background*	
Mobility	Type of childhood residence	All women
Date of birth and age	Month and year of birth	All women
	Age	All women
Education and literacy	Educational attainment	All women
	Ability to read	All women
Mass media	Weekly newspaper/magazine reading, radio listening and television viewing	All women
		All women
Other	Religion, ethnicity	
	All women	
	B. *Reproduction*	
Lifetime fertility	Total sons and daughters living in household, elsewhere and dead	All women
Birth history[a]	Single or multiple birth status	Women with at least one live birth
	Sex	Women with at least one live birth
	Month and year of birth/age	Women with at least one live birth
	Survivorship status; alive; live with whom dead age at death	Women with at least one live birth
Current and recent pregnancy[a]	Current pregnancy status, months of pregnancy	All women
	Pregnancy wanted then, later or not at all	All women
	Pregnancies not ending in live births since January 1985[b]	All women
Menstruation	Start of last menstrual period	All women
	Knowledge of reproductive cycle in a month	All women
	C. *Contraception*	
Knowledge and use	Knowledge of and ever used each method	All women
	Knowledge of source of each method	All women
First use[a]	First method used[b]	Ever-user
	Source of first method[b]	Ever-user
	Number of living children when first used	Ever-user
Current use[a]	Method	Ever-user
	Duration of use	Current user
	Reason for using[b]	Current user
	Problems in using[b]	Current user
Pill use	Consultation when first used	Pill user
	Brand name, cost	Pill user

332

Topic	Questions	Respondents
Source of current method	Source, travel time, difficulty getting there	Current user of modern method
Use of contraception past five years[a] method	Method Duration of use Reasons for discontinuation	Ever-user Ever-user Ever-user
Use prior to January 1985	Date began use Date stopped use	Ever-user Ever-user
Intention for future use	Reason intending not to use Intend to use in next 12 months, method	Non-user Non-user
Source of preferred method	Source, travel time, difficulty getting there	Non-user, asked for modern method
Media information on family planning	Heard FP message in last month Acceptance of radio and television as media	All women All women

D. Health and breast-feeding

Topic	Questions	Respondents
Fertility planning	Pregnancy wanted then, later or not at all Duration of wait	All births past five years All births past five years
Antenatal care	Consultation, card Months pregnant at first checkup Number of check-ups Tetanus injection (number)	All births past five years All births past five years All births past five years All births past five years
Delivery	Place of delivery Who assisted On time or premature Caesarean section	All births past five years All births past five years All births past five years All births past five years
Health of baby at birth	Birth weight Size of baby	All births past five years All births past five years
Post-partum amenorrhoea and abstinence[a]	Months of amenorrhoea and abstinence	All births past five (+ three) years
Breast-feeding[a]	Ever breast-fed Why never breast-fed Delay before beginning Duration Why stopped Intensity of breast-feeding	All births past five years All births past five years All births past five years All births past five (+ three) years All births past five years Last birth still breast-feeding
Supplemental foods	Foods yesterday/last night Ages at introduction of milk, other liquids and mushy foods Bottle + nipple yesterday/last night	Last birth All births past five years Last birth
Immunizations	Has health card Immunization history Mother's recall: bacillus Calmette-Guérin (BCG), drops by mouth, measles	All births past five years All births with health card All births without health card

Topic	Questions	Respondents
Fever/cough (two weeks)	Fever, cough	All children past five years
	Duration of cough	All children <5 with cough
	Rapid breathing with cough	All children <5 with cough
	Source, treatment	All children <5 with fever/cough
Diarrhoea (24 hours + 2 weeks)	Diarrhoea	All children past five years
	Duration, bloody stools	All children <5 with diarrhoea
	Amount of liquids	All children <5 with diarrhoea
	Source, treatment, oral rehydration therapy (ORT) received	All children <5 with diarrhoea
	Knowledge, attitude, practice questions about ORT	If ORT used

E. *Marriage*

Topic	Questions	Respondents
Marital information and co-residence[a]	Ever married	Ever-married women
	Currently married	Ever-married women
	Husband's residence	Currently in union
	Husband has other wives[c]	Currently in union
	Married once or more than once	Ever-married women
First marriage	Age at first marriage	Ever-married women
	Month and year of first marriage	Ever-married women
Marital history past five years[a]	Months in union[b]	Ever-married women
Sexual activity	Ever had sexual intercourse	Never in union
	Frequency in past four weeks	All women
	Last time had sexual intercourse	All women
	Age at first sexual intercourse	All women

F. *Fertility preferences*

Topic	Questions	Respondents
Reproductive intentions	Want another child	Non-sterilized, currently in union
	Birth-spacing	Non-sterilized, currently in union
Sterilization regret	Reason for regret	Sterilized women/partners
Communication with husband	Woman's and husband's approval of family planning	Currently in union
	Frequency of discussion	Currently in union
Discussion of number of children and husband's preference	Husband's preference same, more or fewer	Currently in union
Post-partum attitudes	Delay after birth	Non-sterilized women/partner
Ideal family size	Ideal number of children	All women

G. *Husband's background and woman's work*

Topic	Questions	Respondents
Husband's education	Educational attainment	Ever-married women

Topic	Questions	Respondents
Husband's work	Type of work (occupation)	Ever-married women
	Agriculture or non-agriculture	Ever-married women
	Work on own/family land or someone else's	Ever-married women
Residential mobility past five years[a]	Type of place of residence past five years and when moved	All women
		All women
Woman's work past five years[a]	Type of work (occupation)	All women
	Employment status	All women
	Earn cash	All women
	Work at home or away from home	All women
	Work prior to January 1985[b]	Not working in January 1985
Child care	Takes youngest child to work (if child born since January 1985)	Currently working women
	Who takes care of child	Currently working women

H. *Weight and length*

Weight, length, and BCG scar	All children born since January 1985
Date of weighing and measuring	All children born since January 1985
Reason for not measuring	All children born since January 1985

[a]Entered in five- to six-year calendar on a month-by-month basis (not for the low-prevalence questionnaire).
[b]Not available in the questionnaire for low-prevalence countries.
[c]Only in questionnaire for low-prevalence countries.

C. SPECIAL MODULES AND QUESTIONS

For some countries, special modules have been added to the individual questionnaire on one or more of the following topics: (*a*) natural family planning; (*b*) social marketing; (*c*) maternal mortality; (*d*) acquired immunodeficiency syndrome (AIDS); (*e*) women's employment; (*f*) causes of death; (*g*) sterilization; (*h*) pill compliance.

In addition, countries have adapted the core questionnaire to their specific circumstances and have introduced questions on topics of particular interest to them.

D. THE SERVICE AVAILABILITY QUESTIONNAIRE

Aside from the individual questionnaire, most Demographic and Health Surveys use a aervice availability questionnaire. This questionnaire collects information about the service environment by visiting the nearest of each type of family planning and health outlets and collects such information as: (*a*) year outlet began functioning; (*b*) number of doctors and nurses; (*c*) methods or services available and year of first availability; (*d*) cost of methods; (*e*) distance and time to outlet.

In addition, there is widely varying further information on the characteristics of services and service providers. In many instances, fieldworkers have actually visited the outlets, while in other instances, particularly in low-prevalence countries, interviews with local residents may have been substituted for the actual facility visit.

E. USES OF DEMOGRAPHIC AND HEALTH SURVEY DATA

The study of most topics discussed at this Expert Meeting would greatly benefit from the use of DHS data. Concrete examples are given below.

Sociocultural milieu, women's status and family planning

DHS data permit the construction of variables relating to sociocultural milieu and women's status from such variables as: household composition; household belongings; educational attainment; religion; region; urban or rural residence; work experience; and fertility. For family planning, data on knowledge, ever-use and current use, method failure or discontinuation, fertility desires and ideal family size are available.

Socio-economic development, importance of social sectors and fertility behaviour.

Variables similar to those listed above can be used to define development and social sector variables, while the birth history permits the calculation of wanted and unwanted fertility rates. Desire for more children and ideal family size can also be incorporated.

Family planning services and unreached population groups

Some information about family planning services is available indirectly from the individual questionnaire through source of contraception questions and knowledge of places where methods can be obtained. More general information is available from the service availability questionnaire. Unreached population groups can be defined using appropriate background variables, such as region, urban or rural, level of education.

Adolescent fertility

Adolescent fertility rates can be calculated by age of the woman and time period before the survey to provide estimates of adolescent fertility and obtain some trend data from the same survey. Also, whether births were wanted or unwanted and the practice of contraception can be related to this topic. Other indicators, such as proportion of women with at least one birth by age x, can readily be constructed.

Community-based distribution and social marketing of contraceptives

Source of supply questions can help define the extent of use of community-based distribution (CBD) and social marketing programmes. In addition, cost data for some methods are available. Furthermore, the reliance of the population upon methods that are not suited for CBD or social marketing programmes can be assessed, for example, the proportions using intra-uterine device (IUD) and female sterilization.

Safe motherhood and child survival: importance of family planning and interdependence of services

DHS data permit the calculation of infant and child mortality rates according to major risk factors such as age of the mother, parity of the birth and length of the birth interval. The effect that family planning can have on these risk factors demonstrates clearly how family planning can be instrumental in increasing safe motherhood and child survival. Data on postnatal and prenatal care and tetanus vaccination are of direct importance to evaluate the safe motherhood environment. Missed opportunities for maternal and child care can be studied.

Family planning, sexually transmitted diseases and AIDS

DHS data generally provide the most up-to-date picture on family planning for most countries where surveys are carried out. In several countries, questions on knowledge about AIDS and its transmission have also been asked.

Family size, structure and child development

Data on family size and structure are available from the household schedule. Data on child development, such as education, nutritional status and vaccination status are available from the individual questionnaire, although mainly for children under age 5.

Fertility decline and family support systems

DHS data can be used to study fertility trends over the past 15 years or so. DHS does not have information on family support systems. Family structure variables, however, are available and might be important for the study of this issue.

Cost of contraceptive supplies and services and cost-sharing

Data on cost of the method currently being used are available from the individual questionnaire for some methods, such as the pill or the condom, mainly to study social marketing issues. The service availability questionnaire can more appropriately serve as the basis for calculating costs of contraceptive methods. This information, however, was not included in all countries.

Re-examination of the role of Government, nongovernmental organizations and the private sector in family planning

Although there are some difficulties in obtaining the exact type of source of supply from contraceptive users, DHS data attempt a distinction between sources which provides a global overview of the "market share" of the different providers as far as current users are concerned. These data, in conjunction with data from service statistics, may be of use in determining problems of drop-outs, method discontinuation etc.

DHS data may be less suited for the study of other topics on this agenda but can be a valuable starting point for understanding the country situation and the issues to be defined or studied further.

F. CONCLUSION

A large body of relevant data is available from the DHS programme to study fertility, family planning and maternal and child issues. The data are generally comparable across countries and can provide a powerful basis for defining policies and programmes. Maximum use of these existing and accessible data should be encouraged.

XXVI. WORLD BANK ASSISTANCE IN POPULATION

The World Bank*

BOX 1. MILESTONES IN WORLD BANK POPULATION WORK

1969	Establishment of Population Projects Department
1970	First World Bank population loan, for $2 million to Jamaica
1976	External advisory panel headed by Bernard Berelson recommends improvements in population work
1979	Lending for health authorized; Population, Health and Nutrition Department established
1979	Annual loan commitments for population exceed $100 million for the first time
1984	*World Development Report* focuses on population
1987	Responsibility for population (and health and nutrition) work devolved to country departments
1987	Women in Development Division established; Safe Motherhood Initiative launched
1991	Loan commitments for population exceed $300 million for the first time, making the Bank the leading funding agency for one year
1992	Population Policy and Advisory Service established

The World Bank made an initial commitment to assisting population and family planning activities in developing countries in 1969. Since then, it has pursued three major avenues to increase interest and action in the population area:

(*a*) Lending in family planning, in population, health and nutrition, and in the related social sectors;

(*b*) Policy dialogue on population, as part of the broad macroeconomic dialogue with Governments and as part of a dialogue on specific sectors;

(*c*) Sector studies for particular countries and regions, as well as more general policy and research work, including, more recently, special grants programmes in population.

World Bank efforts have expanded considerably since the commitment was first made to address population growth as an integral part of development. The nature of the World Bank involvement in population also continues to evolve, as experience and research indicate which approaches succeed and which need modification. A brief review of Bank population activities follows (a summary is given in box 1).

A. HISTORICAL OVERVIEW

The early years

The World Bank began formal involvement in the population sector with the establishment of the Population Projects Department in 1969. During the 1970s, the department funded and supervised 22 projects in 15 countries. Of these, 19 were principally population projects, whereas three combined family planning and nutrition activities. Total lending in this period amounted to $366 million. Assessments of the work accomplished by the department credit it with beginning policy dialogues in many countries, including some where no lending actually took place. Various factors, however, resulted in a relatively low level of lending during this time, including weak country demand, the nascent character of the department and the politically sensitive nature of the issue. Another feature of this period was a concentration on Asia, where 11 of the 19 projects took place.

Health and population

The year 1979 marked a shift in World Bank policy to begin direct lending in the health sector, replacing the

---

*Population and Human Resources Department, Washington, D.C.

Population Projects Department with the Population, Health and Nutrition Department. This change reflected a trend which had already been under way, linking population and health activities more closely, as natural complements sharing many of the same facilities and objectives. Since that time, many World Bank projects have included family planning in larger primary health and nutrition projects.

Between 1979 and 1987, population, health and nutrition activities expanded in all three of the World Bank areas of intervention: lending; policy dialogue; and sector work and research. From fiscal year 1980 to fiscal year 1987, 45 population, health and nutrition projects were approved. Of the $1,209 million committed during these years, approximately $425 million directly financed population activities. The World Bank, together with other donors, played an active role in advising Governments, especially in Africa, on the integration of population issues into development planning. Geographical coverage also expanded, with the advent of lending for health providing the opportunity to support family planning as a part of health provision. This expansion was particularly helpful in Africa and Latin America. A notable example of World Bank research during this period was *World Development Report, 1984* (World Bank, 1984), which focused on population and emphasized its importance to the field of development, and made an important contribution to the International Conference on Population held at Mexico City in 1984.

Reorganization and decentralization

An internal restructuring of the World Bank in 1987 led to the dispersal of population, health and nutrition staff from a single centralized department to the country departments. After an initial downturn in lending following the reorganization, World Bank lending and sector work continued to grow. Figure XVI shows growth in number of new projects, and figure XVII shows annual commitments. Most projects are large and cover multiple years, and the distribution of the funds committed over the years covered by each project (figure XVIII) shows how steady the growth in availability of Bank funds has been.

The World Bank currently has over 50 ongoing projects with substantial population components under supervision, representing a total lending commitment of $963 million for population policy development and

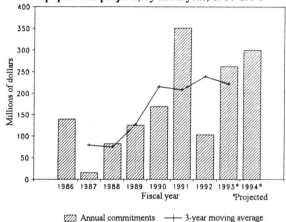

Figure XVI. Annual World Bank commitments for population projects, by fiscal year, 1986-1994

▨ Annual commitments　——+—— 3-year moving average

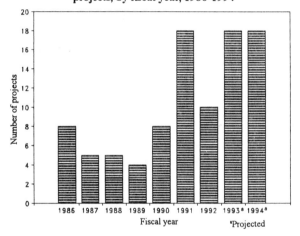

Figure XVII. Number of new World Bank population projects, by fiscal year, 1986-1994

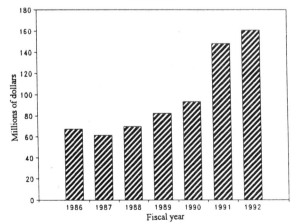

Figure XVIII. World Bank Funds committed for population projects, by approximate year of disbursement, 1986-1992

family planning services. This sum excludes lending for health and nutrition and also excludes social sector lending for such items as female education and infant mortality reduction, which also serve to reduce fertility.

Policy and research work also continue to receive considerable attention, with notable studies conducted on family planning cost effectiveness in Colombia and Indonesia and a major review of family planning programme effectiveness.

Cooperation and collaboration

Over the years, population activities at the World Bank have become more collaborative, as other organizations join in co-financing projects, local communities are integrated into design and implementation activities, and non-governmental organizations are funded to provide service delivery. Indeed, nearly all of the 28 population, health and nutrition operations approved during fiscal year 1991 involve non-governmental organizations, which together with local governments are often included in both project design and implementation. A major focus of many of these collaborative efforts is the establishment of strong institutional frameworks for policy and programme development, at national, local and non-governmental levels.

In addition, population, health and nutrition projects increasingly contain funds for subprojects designed by local governments, community groups and non-governmental organizations. The Nigeria National Population Project, for example, is using its Population Activities Fund to give grants to local organizations for various purposes: to increase family planning use through provision of services; for information, education and communication campaigns; or to strengthen policy makers' commitment to the Nigerian National Population Policy. Inclusion of funds for grants or loans to subprojects fosters grass-roots and community initiatives and involves beneficiaries more directly in project design and implementation.

The World Bank Africa Region provides an illustration of increased coordination with other population-oriented institutions. Together with the United Nations Population Fund (UNFPA), the International Planned Parenthood Federation (IPPF), the World Health Organization (WHO) and the African Development Bank, the Africa Region is funding the Agenda for Action to Improve the Implementation of Population Programs in Sub-Saharan Africa. This initiative, begun and led by African leaders, addresses the dual challenge of high rates of population growth and low rates of economic growth faced by many sub-Saharan African countries.

Under its Special Grants Program, the World Bank joins the United Nations Development Programme (UNDP), UNFPA and WHO in supporting the Special Programme of Research, Development and Research Training in Human Reproduction. The purpose of this organization is to establish new and improved fertility control methods and to strengthen research capacities in developing countries. Another special grants programme funded by the World Bank is the population non-governmental organizations programme, which is designed to encourage collaboration between Governments and those organizations and to strengthen the institutional capacity of the organizations in service delivery. The Safe Motherhood Operational Research fund, executed by WHO, also receives Bank funding, as does the Global Programme on AIDS. The grant programme also supports such population-related initiatives as the Task Force for Child Survival and the Subcommittee on Nutrition of the United Nations Administrative Committee on Coordination.

An intersectoral approach

World Bank experience has shown that the relation between population dynamics and socio-economic development requires a more complex framework for analysis, one that involves many sectors, including health, the social services, women's status, the environment and even economic strategy. Accordingly, the various sectors of the World Bank work together to create the incentives and opportunities for adequate provision of and demand for health care, including family planning services, employment, education and food security. As a result, family planning, health, education and nutrition are often combined in broad social sector projects. Efforts to increase the status and involvement of women in the development process also highlight the synergistic effects of various interventions: literacy and income generation projects can enhance and be enhanced by adequate health and family planning services. The World Bank Safe Motherhood Initiative, for example, combines many interventions to reduce maternal mortality, including the provision of voluntary contraceptive services. The World Bank has also begun to explore the connection between rapid population growth and environmental management, and included a review of the issue in *World Development Report, 1992* (World Bank, 1992).

To benefit from these complementary relations between sectors, 6 of the 18 population, health and nutrition projects conducted in fiscal year 1990 and 10 of the 28 projects in fiscal year 1991 were social development projects, combining population, health or nutrition with education and other sectors. Together, social sector projects account for just under 20 per cent of all World Bank lending. In addition, economic and other sector work, as well as country development strategies, incorporate population considerations, furthering understanding of the linkages between population growth and development and helping operationalize them in future projects.

Research and policy analysis activities in the newly formed Population Policy Advisory Service reflect the widening of the lens used to examine population dynamics. Topics currently on the agenda include various aspects of the macrolevel consequences of population dynamics and the microlevel determinants of household decisions on family size and contraceptive use, including exploratory work on the possible existence and ramifications of market failures in family planning services. More traditional research activities will also continue with the annual development of population projections and other statistical analyses and with further analysis of the effectiveness of family planning programmes.

C. FUTURE OPPORTUNITIES

The development of family planning and population activities at the World Bank has gone from autonomous, strictly population projects to multisectoral efforts coordinated with many other organizations. The trend towards complexity and cooperation will likely continue to develop, as the mechanisms of population dynamics are further illuminated through practical experience and research. The World Bank will attempt to aid that process, through its activities in lending, sector work, policy dialogue and research. Specific areas of focus may include:

(*a*) Action to support countries in supplying and strengthening family planning services, in order to meet the health needs and fertility preferences of their people;

(*b*) Continued collaboration with other donors to build the institutional capacity of Governments for projecting and planning for demographic change;

(*c*) Increased involvement of local communities and non-governmental organizations in projects to promote both family well-being and the development process in general;

(*d*) Concentrated effort to further the integration of population policy into development strategies and economic and sector work, with the overall objective of reducing poverty.

With an eye to these issues, the World Bank will continue to uphold its commitment to aid country Governments in designing and implementing sound population policies and family planning programmes.

REFERENCES

Sai, Fred T., and Lauren A. Chester (1990). *The World Bank's Role in Shaping Third World Population Policy*. Policy Research and External Affairs Working Paper, No. 531. Washington, D.C.: The World Bank.

Simmons, George B., and Rushikesh Maru (1988). *The World Bank's Population Lending and Sector Review*. Policy, Planning, and Research Working Paper, No. 94. Washington, D.C.: The World Bank.

Sinding, Steven W. (1991). *Strengthening the Bank's Population Work in the Nineties*. Policy Research and External Affairs Working Paper, No. 802. Washington, D.C.: The World Bank.

World Bank (1984). *World Development Report, 1984*. New York: Oxford University Press.

_____ (1991). *Population and the World Bank: Implications From Eight Case Studies*. Operations Evaluation Department Report, No. 10021. Washington, D.C.: The World Bank.

_____ (1992). *World Development Report, 1992: Development and the Environment*. New York: Oxford University Press.

XXVII. FAMILY PLANNING PROGRAMMES IN LATIN AMERICA: CURRENT SITUATION AND NEW CHALLENGES

Economic Commission for Latin America and the Caribbean*

The discussion on family planning programmes in Latin America and the Caribbean at first focused on the issue of their legitimacy and their influence on development.[1] However, the progress achieved during the past two decades through these programmes and survey results showing that the new regulating modes of behaviour have become widespread make it necessary to address this matter from a broader perspective. From this point of view, issues concerning the rights of couples to plan their own reproduction—regarded as one of the most significant aspects of human life—should form part of the centre of the debate. Furthermore, the real extent to which family planning programmes can help poor families in their struggle to deal with their circumstances should also be considered.

In this context, and taking into account the role fulfilled by the Centro Latinoamericano de Demografía (CELADE) as part of the Economic Commission for Latin America and the Caribbean, which involves supporting the countries of the major area in matters of technical cooperation for development, this paper is intended to be the institution contribution directed to introducing a set of important issues on this subject. Consequently, this document analyses some relevant facts which turn up in studies, based on surveys, covering women of child-bearing age; at the same time, the study tries to identify the key areas for the future development of the family planning services provided to Latin American and Caribbean couples.

A. THE CONTEXT OF FAMILY PLANNING PROGRAMMES

Institutional support for programmes

The efforts regarding family planning matters in the region, as well as the changes observed in recent years, have been made under diverse institutional contexts. Some countries, such as Costa Rica, the Dominican Republic or Mexico, implemented explicit family planning programmes with official support; other countries, such as Brazil, have had no official policy or direct official support for these programmes; and in others, such as Colombia, private organizations (Profamilia) have played a significant role in spreading knowledge about contraceptive methods and their use. And in still other countries, such as Bolivia, official support has been highly unstable and weak.

Despite this diversity, it is a fact that, with more or less emphasis, the Governments in every Latin American country offer at least some sort of family planning services to women requesting them. At the same time, however, the private sector in the region, including affiliates of the International Planned Parenthood Federation (IPPF) and pharmacies, private physicians and clinics, are a major source of contraceptive services. Indeed, as surveys have shown, in some countries the private sector is more important than the public sector in supplying modern contraceptive methods (Mundigo, 1990).

Mauldin and Ross (1991) recently carried out a study on developing countries in which they analysed the family planning efforts undertaken by countries during the period 1982-1989 and assessed the studies according to four aspects (policies and stage-setting activities, services and service-related activities, record-keeping and evaluation, and availability of contraceptive methods). The authors found "a strong upward shift in effort score ... between 1982 and 1989" (Mauldin and Ross, 1991, p. 199). For the Latin American and the Caribbean area as a whole, the authors found that the total effort indicator had risen by 14 per cent, with increases ranging from 9 to 20 per cent in the different components.

Still, it is worth mentioning that many of the country programmes are considered weak. In this regard, some countries of South America (especially those in the far south of the continent, such as Argentina and Uruguay), have low fertility levels but, according to the parameters evaluated by Mauldin and Ross, their family planning

*Centro Latinoamericano de Demografía (CELADE), Santiago, Chile.

efforts are also limited. The belief that low fertility is a good indicator for the quality of contraceptive services has been questioned through some studies in these countries. For example, it has been shown, at least in Argentina, that women from lower social status had difficulty in practising an effective contraceptive method that was safe for their health and met their personal and family perspectives (Balán and Ramos, 1990).

In general, little is known on the quality of a given service. This element of the family planning programmes in the major area, which do have known effects in increasing coverage and long-term acceptance of specific methods, still seems to have serious deficiencies in most of the countries (Diaz and Halve, 1990; Townsend and Foreit, 1989). Also, not much is known about the degree of deterioration in the quality of the family planning services as a consequence of worsening state attention for the health sector in the 1980s (WHO, 1990).

Fertility change and its proximate determinants

The significant decline in fertility in Latin America and the Caribbean during the past three decades has been prove (Chackiel and Schkolnik, 1990). Fresh data obtained from the Demographic and Health Surveys (DHS) and from other surveys generally show that fertility continues to decrease and that there is a clear-cut relation between total fertility rates and contraceptive prevalence (Arnold and Blanc, 1990). However, an analysis of the change in fertility shows that these changes are not as intense for adolescent fertility (United Nations, 1989a), which shows stable levels and, in certain cases (Brazil and rural areas in Peru), is even rising (Singh and Wulf, 1990). This situation is accounted for by the insignificant change generally observed in the age at first union or at first birth in Latin America in recent years (Singh and Wulf, 1990). From these findings one can infer the sizeable importance of certain cultural patterns as determinants of family formation patterns.

The most important intermediate variable, that is, the variable that influences fertility levels most, is the use of contraceptives; changes in marriage patterns and in the length of breast-feeding have contributed significantly to the decline of fertility (Moreno and Singh, 1990).

An analysis of induced abortion shows that its prevalence in Latin America is very high (Frejka and Atkin, 1990).[2] A more specific study covering three countries (Brazil, Colombia and Peru) concludes that ". . . a high proportion of women in [these countries] are seeking induced abortions; and existing statistics show that many thousands of women are suffering adverse health effects from these procedures" (Singh and Wulf, 1991, p. 13). The same study estimates that in the case of Peru, abortion rates could be increasing. Undoubtedly, one of the reasons that account for this fact in Peru and other countries is related to the non-use of contraception and to method failures, a great proportion of which are probably due to improper use.

B. FAMILY PLANNING SERVICES: CURRENT STATUS OF INFORMATION

There is a lack of basic information on the provision of services in each country; and, therefore, it is very difficult to make a comprehensive diagnosis of the strengths and limitations of family planning programmes in the region. One useful alternative source of information are women's statements in surveys (such as DHS). These are nationally representative surveys conducted among women of reproductive age in 12 countries in Latin America and the Caribbean during the period 1986-1991. Although this information is fragmentary, it nevertheless allows one to describe some important aspects concerning the degree and quality of family planning services.

Knowledge of contraception and the reproductive process

Data from DHS and other national surveys show that women of reproductive age in Latin America and the Caribbean are increasingly acquiring more knowledge on contraceptive methods.[3] In of the 12 countries included in DHS (Brazil, Colombia, the Dominican Republic, Ecuador, El Salvador, Mexico, Paraguay, Peru and Trinidad and Tobago, nearly 90 per cent or more of women currently married or living in consensual union know about some contraceptive method and, more specifically, about a modern one. The exceptions are Bolivia and Guatemala, where one out of four women stated that they had no knowledge of any contraceptive methods.

Similarly, in other countries, where a large number of women claimed to know contraceptive methods, results of DHS and other surveys indicate that when women are asked to provide further information on these methods and their use, large information gaps appear, which account, in part for the high rates of contraceptive failure observed in the so-called "modern and highly efficient" methods.[4] In addition, many women that state that they wish to control their fertility fail to do so for "health-related" or similar reasons, a fact which conceals a certain degree of ignorance about birth control methods that involve no side-effects.

One of the most important elements in this scenario is women's lack of familiarity with reproductive physiology. Significant degrees of misunderstanding about fertile periods have been observed even in countries with high contraceptive prevalence and also among women using contraception. A more radical example of this situation is found in women that resort to periodical abstinence (essentially the calendar method), among which high levels of error in the exact timing of the fertile period have been found. For instance, in the case of users of periodic abstinence in Peru and Bolivia, where this method is used by roughly 40-50 per cent of women, ignorance rates reach 30-40 per cent (Torres, 1992; Loza and Vallenas, 1992). In focus-group sessions conducted in Peru it was found that there are beliefs, rooted in the cultural structure of major population segments, that explain the persistence of this misconception (Fort, 1989).

These findings show that there still are some important contributions to be made by the programmes. There is need to increase knowledge on contraception in countries where ignorance on this issue still affects a significant part of the population and also to foster greater understanding about the methods themselves in countries where knowledge on the proper use of contraceptive methods is apparently high but limited. At the same time, the contribution that family planning programmes can make to women's knowledge of their own reproductive physiology should figure as an important feature of the information, education and communication (IEC) components of the programme. This applies to all women, regardless of the contraceptives they use. Improving women's understanding of reproductive physiology is an important issue in terms of the programmes as such, since it would improve the chances for the proper use of methods and would enable women to choose adequately from available methods.

Contraceptive use

According to DHS, when compared with previous surveys covering the same countries, contraceptive prevalence has risen in proportion to the observed fertility decline. In most of the countries analysed, the percentage of women users of any contraceptive method reached figures ranging from 45 to 65 per cent; in Bolivia and Guatemala, however, this percentage is equal to or lower than 30 per cent. In Guatemala, only one out of five women living in a union was using some contraceptive method at the time of the survey. Among the countries not included in this survey, which have a fertility rate ranging from average to high, are the other Central American countries. In these countries, except in Costa Rica and Panama, fertility is still fairly high and, consequently, the percentage of users is relatively low. Haiti is, perhaps, the extreme case in the region, where prevalence (10 per cent) is the lowest (Cayemites and Chahnazarian, 1989).

The increase of contraceptive prevalence observed in most countries is essentially due to an increase in the use of modern methods. The exceptions are Bolivia, where the increase in traditional methods is equivalent to the rise in modern methods, and Peru, where large numbers of women still use traditional methods (mostly periodic abstinence).

With regard to method mix, results clearly show that sterilization is one of the major methods used by women (Weinberger, 1990; Rutenberg and others, 1991). Except for Bolivia and Peru—where periodic abstinence ranks first—and of Paraguay[5] and Costa Rica—where oral contraceptives are the leading method—sterilization accounts for the largest number of users. In fact, Latin America shows an increasing trend towards the use of sterilization. One of the impressive cases in this respect is the Dominican Republic, where two out of three users of contraceptive methods chose sterilization (Báez, 1992). Among users of sterilization, for one out of three women it was the first and only method they used (Báez, 1992). Oral contraceptives rank second in Brazil, Colombia, the Dominican Republic, Guatemala and Trinidad and Tobago. Conversely, in Ecuador, Mexico and Peru, the intra-uterine device (IUD) occupies second place as the most used method. Only in Trinidad and Tobago (DHS data) and Costa Rica (Oberle and others, 1989) does the condom account for an important part of users (12 and 14 per cent, respectively). In the remaining countries, the prevalence of condoms is less than 2 per cent.[6]

The increasing use of sterilization deserves special attention. The fact that this method is becoming ever more generalized is associated with its use as a way to limit births (rather than spacing them) that prevails in most women using contraception in Latin America (Rutenberg and others, 1991). The question therefore arises whether this "method mix", based exclusively on a single, terminal method, is a desirable model for an entire society. There are some elements of caution in this: if the method is used solely for limiting and not for spacing births then there can be no foreseeable changes in the birth interval, at least as a consequence of contraceptive use. This aspect becomes particularly important whenever the health and survival of the children of female users are employed as the rationale for family planning programmes. Moreover, although most women do claim to be satisfied with sterilization, the appropriateness of resorting to this terminal method in situations of high marital instability and high infant mortality should be evaluated.[7] On the other hand, some hypotheses hold that there is a relation between successive Caesarean sections and sterilization. Perhaps it would be pertinent to determine to what extent this practice is really necessary and whether it encourages an "overmedicalization" of maternal reproductive health, a situation in which women have little to say and therefore have few advantages in matters concerning knowledge on their own reproduction and independence. That is, it is not unreasonable to ask to what extent this phenomenon is contradictory to women's search for greater independence with the goal of achieving broader personal development.[8]

On the other hand, contrary to the questions on knowledge of contraceptives, which did not find any major distinctions according to area of residence and schooling, the use of contraception is prominently related to the fact of belonging to each of the population subgroups defined by the variables under study (Rutenberg and others, 1991). As was to be expected, contraceptive use is lower among less educated women and among those living in rural areas. These results confirm the fertility levels found in these populations.

Another significant element in the study on the degree of contraceptive use is related to the failure rates found in the region. Persistently high failure rates have been found in relation to methods deemed to be highly efficient in some countries (Moreno and Goldman, 1991). Contraceptive failures discourage women from using the methods for spacing births and also, in many cases, may provide the grounds for abortion. Therefore, it is believed that programmes should pay more attention to instructing women on the proper use of all methods, including natural family planning methods. Concerning this subject, further studies should be carried out with specific and controlled populations on the differences in the failure rates among distinct subgroups of the population and on the reasons that account for these failures.

Reproductive preferences and unmet need for family planning

Both the data from the World Fertility Survey and, more recently, those from DHS show that a significant percentage of women wanted no more children than those they had at the time of the interview (Westoff, 1991). This figure is consistent with the number of children that women viewed as ideal, that is, relatively low *vis-à-vis* the fertility rate already observed. Despite the possible deficiencies of the information supplied by women on their reproductive preferences, the survey data show a trend towards an increasingly low number of children in Latin America. The average number of wanted children reported in DHS is close to, or under, four in all countries and close to, or under, three in 7 out of the 10 countries analysed. More importantly, the number of wanted children in most countries does not appear to vary greatly from one social group to another.

This finding shows a trend towards the generalization of small families as a standard accepted by society as a whole, although there are factors that prevent this desired behaviour from becoming effective. In some countries, the decrease in the desired family size is greater than the decline in fertility (Westoff, 1991). According to Westoff, these data may indicate that normative change is leading the decline in fertility.

The above-mentioned study and others evidence the existence of unwanted fertility, either because the pregnancy was unwanted at the time it occurred or because another child was not desired. This unwanted fecundity can be attributed, at least in part, to the existence of an unmet demand, frequently subjacent and not explicit, for contraceptive methods. A way to measure this "unmet need for family planning", developed by Westoff, has made it possible to determine its magnitude in the countries where DHS was carried out.[9] According to the results obtained from the application of this model in these countries, the percentage of women living in a consensual union that can be classified as part of the group with an unmet need for family planning varies from 13 per cent in Brazil to 36 per cent in

Bolivia. These data therefore show that a large number of women are requesting contraceptive methods but are not using them. Therefore, they constitute a group that must be identified in order to ensure the success of the programmes. The significant weight of the demand for spacing births should be underlined. In the Dominican Republic, El Salvador and Guatemala, the demand for spacing births slightly exceeds the demand for limiting births; this fact contrasts with the current use of contraception, which is mainly employed to limit births.

The unmet need for family planning is higher among the most underprivileged and less educated sectors and in rural areas. This situation confirms the need to target programmes in such a way as to meet these needs.[10]. However, one should bear in mind that providing contraceptives will not be enough to transform this unmet need into an effective demand. It has been found, for example, that some of the women in the group of potential users stated that they would not use contraceptive methods in the near future, despite the fact that they were sexually active. In this respect, an area of concern refers to the reasons given by women that do not want to bear (more) children and do not use contraceptives. These reasons include fear of side-effects. Undoubtedly, these fears play a major role and confirm what was previously said about the need to educate the population by providing information on each method, dispelling doubts and mistaken ideas on the proven effects of the use of contraceptive methods on women's health.

C. SOME CHALLENGES FOR FAMILY PLANNING PROGRAMMES: RECOMMENDATIONS FOR THEIR FUTURE COURSE

From the foregoing discussion and taking into account the field experiences in the major area, at this point it may be useful to describe some of the challenges and policy needs regarding family planning programmes.[11].

Expanding and improving the supply of contraceptives

With regard to expanding and improving contraceptive supply, an essential component is to increase the use of reversible/temporary contraceptives that may bring about changes in birth-spacing patterns. The mass use of terminal methods, such as sterilization, cannot be the sole option available to women. Information should be expanded and the use of methods for spacing births should be promoted, including the so-called "natural" methods, which may be effective in controlled circumstances. As Winikoff and Mensch state, "in the long run, the aim should be to increase the options available to women and to ensure flexibility of timing for the use of health services generally and for the adoption of contraception in particular" (1991, p. 306). It has been shown that quality of services can be improved if a wide choice of methods is provided to users (Townsend and Foreit, 1989).

Improvement of information and effective knowledge of the process of reproduction and contraception

The educational and formative aspects of programmes should be strengthened because these are frequently noted for a solely medical approach (Rossetti, 1990). In many countries, there is still a broad margin for reducing fertility by intensifying programmes related to the information/education component. This effort should allow for greater effective knowledge on the proper use of methods, thus contributing to better information on the different contraceptive options available and to the elimination of mistaken concepts about methods and their known side-effects. More emphasis is needed on the positive role that family planning programmes can play in fostering natural breast-feeding, not only because of its contraceptive effect but because of its importance for the child's survival. In addition, awareness should be raised, based on specific studies in each country, on the problems caused by induced abortions and on how to prevent them. For these tasks, the strengthening of information networks among peers seems to be an important way of providing information to women that are not directly reached by the programme. In this endeavour, the importance of information and programmes transmitted through the mass media should be considered.

Targeting of specific populations

The provision of family planning services is one of the tools for eliminating social inequality. Access to information on contraception and the means to implement it cannot be restricted to persons that can afford them. In many countries in Latin America and the Caribbean, women living in rural areas, who are less educated, and lower income women in both urban and rural areas continue to be groups requiring the greatest efforts in contraception. This need is even more urgent when the current framework of structural adjustments carried out by most Latin American countries is taken into account. A greater demand for contraceptive methods could be forthcoming as a result of the wish of prospective parents to postpone births in times of crisis; furthermore, if poverty levels have risen in many countries and, consequently, the real income of the middle class and other wage-earning sectors has been cut back, this change could limit access to contraceptive methods that need to be purchased on the market (oral contraceptives, IUDs etc.).

In this sense, one should bear in mind the significant contribution made by the non-official sector in supplying contraceptive methods and also the possibility of having this sector provide attention to certain priority groups. In addition, programmes involving paid distribution of contraceptive methods to specific groups should not be ruled out.[12]

With regard to the targeting of specific populations, adolescents, as a group requiring particular emphasis, deserve special attention. It has been noted that ". . . one of the central issues underlying adolescent pregnancy is the lack of alternative role options for women other than motherhood, as well as their subordinate role in the society" (Pick de Weiss and others, 1991, p. 80). If this is actually so, one may infer that one of the strategies of family planning programmes should be to deliver more information/education and contraceptive supplies to adolescents. Moreover, these strategies should also help to promote specific programmes, such as education and employment alternatives, because these options can encourage the formulation of attainable life projects.

Inclusion of other health-care services in family planning services

If the area of concern of family planning programmes is extended to the search for a better reproductive health for women and if the difficulties faced by broad segments of women in countries with a deficient health-care system are taken into account, it seems advisable for programmes to expand the services delivered. For example, including the diagnosis and treatment of infections of the female reproductive tract in family planning services would not only have a beneficial effect on the health of mothers and children but could also make an effective contribution to family planning programmes.[13] Moreover, other services, such as Papanicolau (PAP) smears, breast exams, mammogra-

phies and tests for sexually transmitted diseases, including the acquired immunodeficiency syndrome (AIDS), could also be incorporated.

Seeking a more prominent role for men in contraceptive practice and increased male involvement in programmes

It is easy to verify that family planning in Latin America and the Caribbean is based on a medicalized pattern centred around women. This situation is not only the outcome of the will of the persons responsible for the programmes; it also has a cultural basis that prevents men from assuming direct responsibility for contraceptive practice.[14] This matter is an area of study and concern if one considers the effort in which most societies are involved, that is, trying to achieve greater equality between the sexes and trying to encourage equal sharing of the responsibility for the couple's relationship. For example, with respect to adolescent pregnancy, it is believed that "little research has been carried out in Latin America regarding the male's position in this respect and [such research] is urgently needed in order to plan more effective programs that optimize interventions for adolescents in Latin America" (Pick de Weiss and others, 1991, p. 80).

It has been found that even if the concept of men's involvement in family planning programmes has become widely accepted, programme experiences regarding this subject have been scarce (Keller and others, 1989). Apparently, there is a need for more research on the real possibility of male participation in programmes where most of the methods are directed to women.

Improvement of management information systems

Despite the existence of "a nearly universal recognition that improved management is one of the keys to reaching programmatic health and/or demographic objectives" (Keller, 1991, p. 130), the issue of management information systems continues to be a serious problem in most countries. In Latin America and the Caribbean, the outcome of a study in nine countries shows the weakness in the production and use of information geared to programme management, especially in the public sector (Rossetti, 1990). What appears to be needed is to develop a very simple methodology and data-collection procedures that contain actually useful information. The level of the information collected should be directly related to its use.

Taking into account the social and cultural context in family planning programmes

There appears to be agreement in one respect: one of the keys to successful family planning programmes lies in emphasizing the provision of integrated and high-quality family planning services, which should be based on understanding the social and cultural structure where these contraceptive methods will operate (Bongaarts, Mauldin and Phillips, 1990). In this sense, there is a need for community-based programmes, especially in the light of current circumstances in Latin America, where decentralization is viewed as one of the most significant tools to eliminate the concentration of power and achieve productive transformation. An example of the cultural considerations that the programmes should contemplate are the patterns of nuptiality and sexual intercourse between men and women. As a limited example of this, the results of a study on the frequency of sexual intercourse in countries studied by DHS identify important differences among countries. On the basis of these results, Blanc and Rutenberg propose that "... when recommending a method of family planning, service providers should consider whether the use of the particular method is effective for and compatible with the frequency of sexual relations the woman desires" (1991, p. 174). Ignorance concerning such an important aspect could lead to a situation in which contraceptive methods are provided to women that are not exposed to pregnancy.

D. On the rationale of family planning programmes in Latin America and the Caribbean

Nobody denies the demographic impact of family planning programmes, in their role as providers of methods to control fertility and to legitimize a new regulating behaviour that is becoming increasingly widespread. For example, Bongaarts, Mauldin and Phillips (1990) conclude that if unwanted fertility could be eliminated, population growth would be much lower. One of the most conflictive issues in the development of family planning programmes is related to the great significance granted, at least at first, to the need for demographic control as a major rationale. As mentioned previously, recent surveys prove that there is substantial demand for family planning services among women wanting to achieve their desired family size. In addition, several Governments in Latin America and the Caribbean have clearly specified in their official population policies that the fertility ratio should be reduced (United Nations, 1987b, 1989b and 1990). These findings imply that there is no contradiction between government goals and the preferences of individual couples; hence, the rationale of family planning programmes would be focused on human rights and also on matters associated with the elimination of social inequality (CELADE, 1992).

With regard to human rights, human reproduction must be considered a right that couples should be able to exercise freely, based on informed decisions so as to have the number of children that they want. In this sense, the role of the State is to provide the necessary information and methods to enable couples to implement this behaviour. This issue is particularly significant for couples from low-income sectors, that have no easy access to the necessary methods.

Secondly, and related to the foregoing point, it is necessary to underscore the importance of family planning programmes with regard to women's reproductive health and the independence that they can achieve by controlling their own reproduction. Although there is a persisting debate on the role played by family planning as a significant factor that contributes to the decline of infant mortality (Hobcraft, 1992), in several countries these programmes have probably helped to improve maternal health by reducing multiparity in populations that do not control their own fertility. Thus, as Hobcraft states, "... the health rationale for family planning can do no harm, ... [it] can give added impetus to women's pre-existing desires for better control of the timing of births in their own life course..." (1991, p. 1169). On the other hand, as Potter (1988) points out, there are several ways, not always recognized, in which family planning programmes might affect child survival. These are the changes in social composition of births, the reduction of high-risk pregnancies and the more intensive maternity care that comes with increased contraceptive use.

The decline of fertility observed in most Latin American countries has undoubtedly dispelled the great fears of the 1960s and the 1970s concerning the excessive population growth. However, as mentioned previously, there are still many outstanding aspects which need to be solved if the rationale for family planning is centred on the rights of the couple and on the reduction of social inequality with regard to access to methods to control reproduction. It is known that a large part of the actual decline in fertility is due to increased contraceptive use, which is made possible or legitimized through family planning programmes. It is also known that in many countries, these programmes were, and still are, financed in part or to a large extent by international aid. For this reason, international aid is currently as necessary as it formerly was, especially if one considers the economic and social crises that have affected Latin America and the Caribbean.

NOTES

[1] See, for example, Rance's fine summary of this debate with regard to the case of Bolivia (Rance, 1990).

[2] The authors estimate that induced abortions account for one fourth of deliberate fertility control.

[3] For further information on this subject see: DHS data in Rutenberg and others, 1991; World Fertility Survey data in United Nations, 1987b.

[4] For contraceptive failure rates in Latin America, see Moreno and Goldman, 1991.

[5] Data from Paraguay are not included in the report by Rutenberg and others (1991). For information, see Paraguay, 1991.

[6] Figures from more recent surveys do not show major changes in this situation despite the campaigns carried out in recent years in many countries, directed to increasing condom use with a view to preventing AIDS.

[7] For example, one may ask whether a sterilized woman whose union comes to an end and who lives in a setting where a positive meaning is assigned to maternity and paternity, a common situation in many countries, has or does not have a comparative disadvantage in terms of a new union because she has been sterilized.

[8] It could be argued that sterilization increases as a result of women's demand for this procedure because of its safety as opposed to the lack of reliability of reversible methods. Even if this were so, it is necessary to point out that women's attitude in this respect could be modified through the improvement of knowledge on the proper use of non-terminal methods. As suggested below, family planning programmes can make an important contribution in this respect.

[9] Some results of recent surveys have been obtained in the Family Planning Workshop: Current Status and Future Prospects, jointly organized by CELADE and DHS, held at Santiago, Chile, in March 1992.

[10] In the CELADE workshop mentioned in note 9, some detailed studies were carried out which attempt to identify the degree of unmet demand for family planning in various countries in the region. For further details, see Morillo, 1992 (Dominican Republic); Loza and Vallenas, 1992 (Peru); Haussler, 1992 (Guatemala); and Ordoñez, 1992 (Colombia).

[11] For the future course of family planning programmes, the authors follow many of the statements of Keller and hisassociates (1989).

[12] The positive cost/benefit experiences in the mining zones of Peru could provide an adequate example (Foreit and others, 1991).

[13] For example, with regard to female reproductive tract infections, it has been said that the probable consequences of non-diagnosed infections may be blamed on contraceptive methods, which could lead to discontinuation of the method or refusal to use another one.

[14] With regard to the role of men, a study conducted in a poor community at Port-au-Prince found that most men believe that women should be responsible for using contraceptives. Therefore, the extremely low rate of condom use is related to this belief rather than to method availability or to the opinion associated with family planning (Boulos, Boulos and Nichols, 1991).

REFERENCES

Arnold, Fred, and Ann Blanc (1990). *Fertility Levels and Trends*. Demographic and Health Surveys. Comparative Studies, No. 2. Columbia, Maryland: Institute for Resource Development/Macro International, Inc.

Báez, Carlos (1992). República Dominicana: la esterilización como opción única: ¿Una solución? Paper presented at the Family Planning Workshop: Current Needs and Future Prospects, Santiago, Chile, March. Sponsored by Centro Latinoamericano de Demografía and Demographic and Health Surveys.

Balan, Jorge, and Silvina Ramos (1990). Las decisiones anticonceptivas en un contexto restrictivo: el caso de los sectores populares de Buenos Aires. Paper presented at the Seminar on Fertility Transition in Latin America, Buenos Aires, 3-6 April. Sponsored by the International Union for the Scientific Study of Population, Centro Latinoamericano de Demografía and Centro de Estudios de Población.

Blanc, Ann K., and Naomi Rutenberg (1991). Coitus and contraception: the utility of data on sexual intercourse for family planning programs. *Studies in Family Planning* (New York), vol. 22, No. 3 (May/June), pp. 162-176.

Bongaarts, John, W. Parker Mauldin and James Phillips (1990). The demographic impact of family planning programs. *Studies in Family Planning*(New York), vol. 21, No. 6 (November/December), pp. 299-310.

Boulos, Michaelle L., Reginald Boulos and Douglas J. Nichols (1991). Perceptions and practices relating to condom use among urban men in Haiti. *Studies in Family Planning* (New York), vol. 22, No. 5 (September/October), pp. 318-325.

Cayemites, Michel, and Anouch Chahnazarian (1989). *Survie et santé de l'enfant en Haiti: résultats de l'enquête mortalité, morbidité et utilisation des services, 1987*. Port-au-Prince: Ministère du plan, Institut haïtien de l'enfance and the Johns Hopkins University.

Centro Latinoamericano de Demografía (1992). *Políticas de población desde la perspectiva de América Latina y el Caribe*. Series A, No. 262. Santiago, Chile.

Chackiel, J., and Susana Schkolnik (1990). América Latina: transición de la fecundidad en el período 1950-1990. Paper presented at the Seminar on Fertility Transition in Latin America, Buenos Aires, 3-6 April. Sponsored by the International Union for the Scientific Study of Population, Centro Latinoamericano de Demografía and Centro de Estudios de Población.

Diaz, J., and H. Halve (1990). Calidad de la atención en los servicios clínicos de planificación familiar en América Latina. *PROFAMILIA: planificación, población y desarrollo* (Bogotá), vol. 6, No. 16 (June-December), pp. 16-30.

Foreit, Karen, and others (1991). Costs and benefits of implementing family planning services at a private mining company in Perú. *International Family Planning Perspectives* (New York), vol. 17, No. 3 (September), pp. 91-95.

Fort, Alfredo L. (1989). Investigating the social context of fertility and family planning: a qualitative study in Peru. *International Family Planning Perspectives* (New York), vol. 15, No. 3 (September), pp. 88-95.

Frejka, Tomas, and Lucy C. Atkin (1990). The role of induced abortion in the fertility transition of Latin America. Paper presented at the Seminar on Fertility Transition in Latin America, Buenos Aires, 3-6 April. Sponsored by the International Union for the Scientific Study of Population, Centro Latinoamericano de Demografía and Centro de Estudios de Población.

Haussler (1992). Demanda total y necesidad no satisfecha de planificación familiar en Guatemala y su diferenciación étnica. Paper presented at the Family Planning Workshop: Current Needs and Future Prospects, Santiago, Chile, March. Sponsored by Centro Latinoamericano de Demografía and Demographic and Health Surveys.

Hobcraft, John (1991). Child spacing and child mortality. *Demographic and Health Surveys World Conference, August 5-7, 1991, Washington, D.C., Proceedings*, vol. II. Columbia, Maryland: Institute for Resource Development/Macro International, Inc.

_____ (1992). Fertility patterns and child survival: a comparative analysis. *Population Bulletin of the United Nations* (New York), No. 33, pp. 1-31. Sales No. E. 92.XIII.4.

Keller, Alam, and others (1989). Toward family planning in the 1990's: a review and assessment. *International Family Planning Perspectives* (New York), vol. 15, No. 4 (December), pp. 127-135.

Keller, Alam (1991). Management information systems in maternal and child health/family planning programs: a multi-country analysis. *Studies in Family Planning* (New York), vol. 22, No. 1 (January/Febuary), pp. 19-30.

Loza, G., and G. Vallenas (1992). Uso y demanda de métodos anticonceptivos en el Perú. Paper presented at the Family Planning Workshop: Current Needs and Future Prospects. Santiago, Chile, March. Sponsored by Centro Latinoamericano de Demografía and Demographic and Health Surveys.

Mauldin, W. Parker, and John Ross (1991). Family planning programs: efforts and results, 1982-1989. *Studies in Family Planning* (New York), vol. 22, No. 6 (November/December), pp. 350-367.

Moreno, Lorenzo, and Noreen Goldman (1991). Contraceptive failure rates in developing countries: evidence from the Demographic and Health Surveys. *International Family Planning Perspectives* (New York), vol. 17, No. 2 (June), pp. 44-49.

Moreno, Lorenzo, and Susheela Singh (1990). Fertility decline and changes in proximate determinants in the Latin American region. Paper presented at the Seminar on Fertility Transition in Latin America, Buenos Aires, 3-6 April. Sponsored by the International Union for the Scientific Study of Population, Centro Latinoamericano de Demografía and Centro de Estudios de Población.

Morillo, A. (1992). República Dominicana: necesidades insatisfechas y demanda total de métodos de planificación familiar: situación actual y perspectivas futuras. Family Planning Workshop: Current Needs and Future Prospects, Santiago, Chile, March. Sponsored by Centro Latinoamericano de Demografía and Demographic and Health Surveys.

Mundigo, Axel I. (1990). The role of family planning programmes in the fertility transition of Latin America. Document presented at the Seminar on Fertility Transition in Latin America, Buenos Aires, 3-6 April. Sponsored by the International Union for the Scientific Study of Population, Centro Latinoamericano de Demografía and Centro de Estudios de Población.

Oberle, Mark W., and others (1989). Fecundidad y uso de anticonceptivos en Costa Rica, 1987. *Perspectivas Internacionales en Planificación Familiar* (New York), special issue, 1989. New York: The Alan Guttmacher Institute.

Ordoñez, M. (1992). La necesidad insatisfecha y la demanda total de planificación familiar en Colombia, 1990. Paper presented at the Family Planning Workshop: Current Needs and Future Prospects, Santiago, Chile, March. Sponsored by Centro Latinoamericano de Demografía and Demographic and Health Surveys.

Pan American Health Organization (1990). *Las condiciones de salud en las Américas: edición de 1990*, vol. 1. Washington, D.C.

Paraguay, Centro Paraguayo de Estudios de Población; and Institute for Resource Development/Macro Systems, Inc. (1991). *Paraguay, Encuesta Nacional de Demografía y Salud*. Asunción, Paraguay; and Columbia, Maryland.

Pick de Weiss, Susan, and others (1991). Sex, contraception and pregnancy among adolescents in Mexico City. *Studies in Family Planning* (New York), vol. 22, No. 2 (March/April), pp. 74-82.

Potter, Joseph E. (1988). Does family planning reduce infant mortality? An Exchange. *Population and Development Review* (New York), vol. 14, No. 1 (March), pp. 179-187.

Rance, Susana (1990). *Planificación familiar: se abre el debate*. La Paz, Bolivia: Secretaría Técnica del Consejo Nacional de Población.

Rossetti, J. (1990). *Los sistemas de información para la atención materno-infantil y la planificación familiar: la situación en algunos países de América Latina y el Caribe*. CELADE/LC/DEM/R.107. Santiago, Chile: Centro Latinoamericano de Demografía.

Rutenberg, Naomi, and others (1991). *Knowledge and Use of Contraception*. Demographic and Health Surveys Comparative Studies, No. 6. Columbia, Maryland: Institute for Resource Development/Macro International, Inc.

Singh, Susheela, and Deirdre Wulf (1990). *Adolescentes de hoy, padres del mañana: un perfil de las Américas*. New York: The Alan Guttmacher Institute.

_____ (1991). Estimating abortion levels in Brazil, Colombia and Peru using hospital admissions and fertility surveys data. *International Perspectives in Family Planning* (New York), vol. 17, No. 3 (September), pp. 8-13.

Torres Pinto, H. (1992). Hacia el conocimiento ampliado de la planificación familiar en Bolivia según ENDSA, 1989. Paper presented at the Family Planning Workshop: Current Needs and Future Prospects, Santiago, Chile, March. Sponsored by Centro Latinoamericano de Demografía and Demographic and Health Surveys.

Townsend, John W., and James Foreit (1989). Efforts to improve programme performance in Latin America and the Caribbean: lessons learned from operations research. Paper presented at the Seminar on the Role of Family Planning Programmes as a Fertility Determinant, Tunis, June. Sponsored by the International Union for the Scientific Study of Population.

United Nations (1987a). *Fertility Behaviour in the Context of Development: Evidence from the World Fertility Survey*. Population Studies, No. 100. Sales No. E.86.XIII.5.

_____ (1987b). *World Population Policies*, vol. I, *Afghanistan to France*. Population Studies No. 102. Sales No. E.87.XIII.4.

_____ (1989a). *Adolescent Reproductive Behaviour*, vol. II, *Evidence from Developing Countries*. Population Studies, No. 109/Add.1. Sales No. E.89.XIII.10.

_____ (1989b). *World Population Policies*, vol. II, *Gabon to Norway*. Population Studies, No. 102/Add.1. Sales No. E.89.XIII.3.

_____ (1990). *World Population Policies*, vol. III, *Oman to Zimbabwe*. Population Studies, No. 102/Add.2. Sales No. E.90.XIII.2.

Weinberger, Mary Beth (1990). Changes in the mix of contraceptive methods during fertility decline: Latin America and the Caribbean. Paper presented at the Seminar on Fertility Transition in Latin America, Buenos Aires, 3-6 April. Sponsored by the International Union for the Scientific Study of Population, Centro Latinoamericano de Demografía and Centro de Estudios de Población.

Westoff, Charles F. (1991). *Reproductive Preferences: A Comparative View*. Demographic and Health Surveys Comparative Studies, No. 3. Columbia, Maryland: Institute for Resource Development/Macro Systems, Inc.

_____, and Luis H. Ochoa (1991). *Unmet Need and the Demand for Family Planning*. Demographic and Health Surveys Comparative Studies, No. 5. Columbia, Maryland: Institute for Resource Development/Macro Systems, Inc.

Winikoff, Beverly, and Barbara Mensch (1991). Rethinking postpartum family planning. *Studies in Family Planning* (New York), vol. 22, No. 5 (September/October), pp. 294-307.

350

XXVIII. FAMILY PLANNING AND REPRODUCTIVE HEALTH IN SELECTED MEMBER STATES OF THE ECONOMIC COMMISSION FOR EUROPE

*Economic Commission for Europe**

The objectives of this discussion note are: (*a*) to review the current situation with respect to family planning and reproductive health in selected countries of the Economic Commission for Europe (ECE) region; and (*b*) to suggest avenues for future research and policy action in this area for these countries. Geographically,[1] this note focuses on the ECE member States in Eastern Europe and the successor States of the former Union of Soviet Socialist Republics, which are undergoing rapid social, political, and economic change: Albania, Belarus, Bosnia and Herzogovina; Bulgaria; Croatia; Czechoslovakia;[2] Estonia; Hungary; Latvia; Lithuania; Poland; the Republic of Moldova; Romania; the Russian Federation; Slovenia; Ukraine; and Yugoslavia. Compared with other ECE countries, these former centrally planned economies have a great need for research and policy in the domains of family planning and maternal and child health (MCH). These needs are discussed below in sections B and C. Section A briefly addresses some of the commonalities in the economic transition process that currently characterizes these countries.

A. ECONOMIES IN TRANSITION

Although initiated at different times, the transitions from centrally planned to market economies have plagued all of the countries under review with high inflation, collapsing trade, falling output and investment levels and rising unemployment (United Nations, 1991). The severity of these problems, which in some ways resemble those associated with the Great Depression of 1929-1933, and the success of the various stabilization and reform measures designed to resolve them, vary a great deal from country to country; the contrast among problems and reform measures is especially great between Eastern European countries and those in the former Soviet Union. Czechoslovakia, Hungary and Poland are generally considered to be the leading reform countries of Eastern Europe. It is still too early to judge which Soviet successor States are ahead in their development towards an open-market economy.

Increases in the consumer price index of 1991 over 1990 for Eastern Europe (excluding Albania) vary between 35 per cent for Hungary to 344 per cent for Romania (United Nations, 1992b). Comparable inflation figures for the seven successor States to the USSR are unavailable but retail price increases between January 1991 and January 1992 in the four ECE member States of the Commonwealth of Independent States (CIS) are estimated to vary from 487 in Belarus to 873 per cent in the Russian Federation (UNICEF/WHO, 1992). Price increases become even more significant in view of the fact that as of 1989, an estimated 11 per cent of all families in CIS were already living below the poverty line.

Another important aspect of the transition process is the collapse of trade among the members of the former Council for Mutual Economic Assistance, resulting, *inter alia*, in lower production and higher unemployment levels. The domestic output of Eastern Europe in 1991 (excluding Albania), for instance, as measured by the net material product, fell, on average, by about 14 per cent, with considerable differences between individual countries. For the two largest Soviet successor States, the Russian Federation and Ukraine, which together accounted for almost 80 per cent of the aggregate Soviet net material product in 1990, this figure amounts to 11 per cent each.

Rebuilding the productive capacity of the transition economies in Eastern Europe and the former Soviet Union requires a strong recovery of fixed investment. However, gross fixed investment in Eastern Europe (excluding Albania and Yugoslavia) fell, on average, by 23 per cent in 1991, following earlier declines of 2 and 14 per cent, respectively, in 1989 and 1990. Aggregate investment figures for the seven Soviet successor States (members of ECE) are not available. Scattered investment data reported by individual republics register declines roughly in line with their fall in output, for example, 11 per cent in the case of the Russian Federation.

---

*Population Activities Unit, Division for Economic Analysis and Projections, Geneva, Switzerland.

The number of persons registered as unemployed in Eastern Europe more than doubled between December 1990 and December 1991, when it stood at just under 6 million. Unemployment rates in December 1991 were some 10-11 per cent in Bulgaria and Poland, and some 7-8 per cent in Czechoslovakia and Hungary. In the former Yugoslavia,[3] the year-end rate was nearly 20 per cent. Although the accuracy of these figures is uncertain, there seems to be little doubt that joblessness in Eastern Europe has risen dramatically, especially among women and in less developed areas. Open unemployment statistics in the Soviet successor States do not provide a reliable picture of the current extent of unemployment. What does seem clear, however, is that unemployment in these countries is now a serious problem; in the light of experience in Eastern Europe, it is likely to grow rapidly as soon as any real economic restructuring in this part of the ECE region gets under way.

With prices increasing more rapidly than incomes, production declining and unemployment growing, family incomes have fallen dramatically, especially among the poorest families with many children and among pensioners. The erosion of purchasing power for basic commodities and services has meant a growing dependence upon government support for income supplements. Yet, due to mounting difficulties with the balance of payments, these and other public support mechanisms are either being reduced or dismantled. Social safety nets to safeguard the health and nutrition status of the population no longer provide the protection they did under the former Government.

The pervasiveness of health-care systems that reach the most remote areas, high literacy rates, extensive educational systems and extremely high coverage by the mass media offer unparalleled opportunities to harness public action and individual family behaviour to improve the health and nutrition of the most vulnerable groups within the existing constraints. Yet, financial aid and technical assistance from abroad will also be required, in amounts greater than those already provided by the international community.

Women bear a particularly heavy burden during this transition from planned to market economies. More than 80 per cent of women in CIS are employed full-time, mostly in low-paid positions. Food shortages have forced many women to spend time in queues attempting to buy food for their families, in addition to their burden of economic activity and maternal and domestic tasks.

One of the important health issues confronting women in the economies in transition considered here is their heavy dependence upon abortion due to the unavailability of safe, reliable, modern contraceptives.

B. FAMILY PLANNING AND REPRODUCTIVE HEALTH

The political and economic experiences that the countries in Eastern Europe and the former Soviet Union have shared over the past 40-50 years appear to have shaped their current, fairly homogeneous demographic situation. High infant and maternal mortality rates, low fertility and contraceptive prevalence rates and high abortion rates (see table 37) in relation to those in Western Europe are among their common demographic characteristics. The transition to modern family planning, completed for the major part of the rest of Europe, has hardly begun in these countries.

Infant mortality rates (IMRs) in Eastern Europe are approximately 60 per cent higher than those of Western Europe. Albania has the highest IMR, 30.8 per 1,000 births, five times the level in Sweden. Romania and former Yugoslavia follow with 26.9 and 20.2, respectively. Varying between 10.3 infant deaths per 1,000 live births in Lithuania and 19.0 in the Republic of Moldova, IMRs in the four CIS and three Baltic countries do not compare unfavourably with those in Eastern Europe. There are, however, signs of a reversal of the secular trend towards lower levels.

The average maternal mortality ratio in Eastern Europe, excluding Romania, exceeds that of Western Europe by over 50 per cent. Romania has the highest ratio at 170 maternal deaths per 100,000 live births in 1989, which is almost 20 times the ratio in Western Europe. Maternal mortality in Albania is believed to be about 60 deaths per 100,000 live births. Abortion-related maternal mortality for the former USSR as a whole is conservatively estimated at 48 in 1986, varying from 20 to 80 among the individual republics (UNICEF/WHO, 1992).

The average total fertility rate (TFR) for Eastern Europe in 1989 was 2.13, down from 2.69 in 1965. TFR in Western Europe, which in 1965 almost equalled that of Eastern Europe at 2.70, declined to 1.57 in 1989. Albania has consistently had the highest fertility rate in Eastern Europe and recorded TFR of 3.03 in 1990, down from 5.16 in 1970. Studies of the proximate det-

TABLE 37. MOST RECENT AVAILABLE ESTIMATES OF SELECTED DEMOGRAPHIC INDICATORS, ECONOMIES IN TRANSITION

Country	Infant mortality rate (per 1,000) (1)	Maternal mortality ratio (per 100,000) (2)	Total fertility rate (per woman) (3)	Contraceptive prevalence rate (percentage) (4)	Total abortion rate (per 100 live births) (5)
A. Eastern Europe					
	1991	*1989*	*1991*	*1988*	*1990*
Albania	30.8	60	3.03	..	..
Bulgaria	16.9	19	1.74	76	137.5
Czechoslovakia[a]	11.5	10	1.94	95[b]	74.7
Hungary	15.1	15	1.87	73	71.9
Poland	14.7	11	2.06	75	10.6
Romania	26.9	170	1.83	58	315.2
Yugoslavia[c]	20.2	16	1.80	55	96.6
B. Former USSR					
	1990	*1989*	*1988*	*1989*	*1990*
Belarus	11.9	25	2.52	46	101.6
Estonia	12.3	41	2.80	47	74.5
Latvia	13.7	57	2.69	47	75.0
Lithuania	10.3	29	2.70	54	54.3
Republic of Moldova	19.0	34	3.13	28	82.8
Russian Federation	17.4	49	2.70	34	117.5
Ukraine	12.9	33	2.39	46	85.4

Sources: For columns (3) and (4) of panel B, A. A. Avdeyev and I. A. Troitskaya, "Contraception and abortion in the USSR: experience of 1980s", paper presented at the European Demographic Conference, Paris, 21-25 October 1991, tables 3 and 6, respectively; for columns (1), (3) and (5) of panel A, Catherine de Guibert-Lantoine and Alain Monnier, "La conjoncture démographique: l'Europe et les pays développés d'Outre-Mer", *Population* (Paris), vol. 47, No. 4 (juillet-août 1992), pp. 1017-1036, tables 2, 3 and 6a, respectively; for columns (1) and (5) of panel B, United Nations Children's Fund and World Health Organization, "The looming crisis in health and the need for international support", Overview of the reports on the Commonwealth of Independent States and the Baltic Republics prepared by the UNICEF/WHO collaborative missions with the participation of the United Nations Population Fund, the World Food Programme and the United Nations Development Fund, 17 February-2 March 1992, table 1; for column (2) of panel A, *Demographic Yearbook, 1990* (United Nations publication, Sales No. E/F.91.XIII.1), table 17; for column (4) of panel A, *Levels and Trends of Contraceptive Use as Assessed in 1988*, Population Studies, No. 110 (United Nations publication, Sales No. E.89.XIII.4), table 3; for column (2) of panel B, United States Agency for International Development, *USAID Health Profiles* (Arlington, Virginia, Center for International Health Information/International Science and Technology Institute, 1992).

[a]The former State of Czechoslovakia was dissolved on 31 December 1992 and became the independent States of the Czech Republic and Slovakia on 1 January 1993.

[b]Ever-use.

[c]The area of the former State of Yugoslavia currently comprises the independent States of Bosnia and Herzegovina, Croatia, the Federal Republic of Yugoslavia, Slovenia and the former Yugoslav Republic of Macedonia. Data for the period prior to 27 April 1992 refer to the former Socialist Federal Republic of Yugoslavia in terms of its boundaries as they existed prior to that date.

erminants and long-term consequences of these downward fertility trends in many parts of Eastern Europe, as well as in Soviet successor States, would provide a useful basis for further development planning.

It is estimated that fewer than 1 per cent of women in Albania currently use modern contraception. In Romania, only 20,000 women are currently recorded as using modern contraception. The actual rate is probably higher because of unrecorded pill prescriptions by gynaecologists, pills distributed by non-governmental organizations and pills obtained on the black market.

Recently, modern contraceptives have become available to some extent in the former Soviet Union; acceptance rates, however, have been constrained by poor quality, locally made intra-uterine devices that are often rejected or cause side-effects. Low-dose contraceptive pills are unavailable, and condoms are often of inferior quality and their supply is erratic. Estimates by Carl Haub of the Population Reference Bureau of total contraceptive prevalence in the former USSR during 1988 put the number of current users among married women of reproductive age at 31 per cent; of this total, 13 per cent used IUDs, 1 per cent used the pill, 4 per cent used condoms, 1 per cent used spermicides; and 12 per cent opted for more traditional and less reliable methods, such as withdrawal and rhythm.

Family size in countries of Eastern Europe and the former Soviet Union is mostly regulated through abortion, not through modern family planning methods. Abortion rates per 1,000 women aged 15-49 years in 1989 in the seven Soviet successor States vary between 54.3 in Lithuania to 117.5 in the Russian Federation. Romania and Bulgaria have the highest abortion ratios (number of abortions per 100 live births) in Eastern Europe. The number of officially reported abortions in Romania after the legalization of abortion in December 1989 was slightly more than 1 million in 1990, representing almost four abortions to every live birth. In Bulgaria, the problem of abortion is aggravated by a tendency towards early marriages and premarital conceptions. Forty per cent of all first marriages in Bulgaria are to women under age 20, many of whom are already pregnant at the time of marriage. Although from 400,000 to 600,000 abortions are reported in Poland annually, the figures are estimated to be much higher. Polish women have had the right to abortion thus far, but authorities are reluctant to report them, fearing censure from the Catholic Church, which has always played a prominent role in Polish history and culture.

Abortion policies vary within this part of the ECE region. In most countries, abortion is legal; in some, it is illegal except under certain conditions. Policies have changed since the change from a centrally planned economy. For example, in Romania, abortion has been legalized, whereas in Poland, the Catholic Church is pressuring the legislature to make abortions illegal. Religion and tradition are very much a part of the issues surrounding abortion.

Despite the many controversial sides to abortion in the economies in transition, the main problem remains—its prevalence and damaging effects on women's health (Serbanescu, 1990). Many of the problems related to cervical cancer, pelvic inflammation, extra-uterine pregnancy and secondary sterility currently facing millions of women of reproductive age in the economies in transition are abortion-related. Neither contraceptive advice nor a prescription is systematically offered to women after they have had an abortion.

Past government policies in the region generally have not encouraged family planning or modern contraceptive use and have thus contributed to this serious problem. Women in these countries have had to resort to abortion because of lack of knowledge of modern contraceptives and their use, as well as their limited supply and accessibility. Previous Governments in Albania and Bulgaria, for instance, advocated pronatalist policies that encouraged only natural or traditional methods of fertility control, which did not have high success rates.

In conjunction with Governments' shift in attitudes, United Nations Population Fund (UNFPA) programmes in these countries are attempting to remedy these serious problems by promoting family planning and modern contraceptive use. The World Bank is also assisting selected countries in Eastern Europe to restructure their deteriorated health systems. UNFPA assistance to countries in Eastern Europe, totalling $13,188,700 from 1969 to 1991, has been small compared with that in such regions as Africa and Asia, where needs are greatest. With the historical transformations that have recently taken place and the Governments' recognition of the importance of population issues in development planning, one may anticipate an expansion of population activities in the region by UNFPA and/or other international organizations, especially in the areas of family planning and MCH. UNFPA and World Bank needs assessment missions have already been fielded to assist the Governments of Albania, Bulgaria, Poland and Romania in determining their population needs and priorities. A major shift from abortion to modern family planning is needed.

Baseline surveys on knowledge, attitudes and practice of modern family planning must be given high priority. Such survey findings will permit family planning information, education and communication (IEC) programmes to be designed to reach specific groups with specific messages and to produce specific measurable outcomes. Family planning information should be disseminated widely among couples in the region to reverse their suspicions about modern contraceptive methods.

Population and family planning policies are lacking in the economies in transition and current efforts to educate the public regarding modern contraception are insufficient. Demographic surveys concentrating on aspects of fertility, family planning and reproductive health are therefore urgently needed in all these countries to obtain better quantitative and qualitative data on the supply and demand of family planning services. The results of these surveys will be instrumental in preparing national contraception policies, implementation strategies including comprehensive IEC campaigns and training packages for health workers at all levels.

Policies that promote birth-spacing through family planning can play a critical role not only in reducing infant mortality but also in increasing the predictability of the family-building process and in improving the health status of women by decreasing their need for abortion.

C. SUGGESTIONS FOR FUTURE RESEARCH AND POLICY ACTION

On the basis of the preceding review of current family planning and MCH needs in selected ECE countries, the following recommendations are made:

1. ECE member States in Eastern Europe and the former Soviet Union should be assisted to the fullest extent possible by the international community at large to conduct national reproductive health surveys for the proper assessment of family planning knowledge, attitudes and practice among couples. These national surveys may be conducted as part of the UNFPA-supported project on fertility and family surveys in countries of the ECE region. The ECE Population Activities Unit in Geneva is currently implementing this survey;

2. Efforts towards improving IEC on reproductive health should begin immediately, particularly in the lower socio-economic groups. Special efforts to educate the public about family planning should begin through every possible means, from mass media to individual counselling. There is an urgent need to disseminate family planning information to the public to enhance women's knowledge and to reverse their suspicions about modern contraception;

3. Training programmes should be organized for medical and health-care professionals in the region to enhance their trust in modern contraceptive methods and to help overcome institutional barriers obstructing the transition from abortion to modern family planning. These training programmes should be organized throughout the region for medical and health-care professionals at all levels to improve their knowledge of, and trust in, modern contraceptive methods. This effort will help reorient health-care systems throughout the economies in transition from the delivery of abortion-centred services to the provision of contraception-based services;

4. Well organized national family planning programmes that use both public and private resources are needed to assure every access for all interested persons to modern, safe services through family planning centres throughout the region. Increased availability through importation and/or local production, as well as affordability of modern contraceptives, are problems that need to be resolved in order to improve the usage of these methods among all couples in the region and help decrease problems associated with unintended pregnancy. Extra funds will be needed to address these problems.

NOTES

[1]The countries included in the regional divisions used in this chapter do not in all cases conform to those included in the geographical regions established by the Population Division of the Department for Economic and Social Information and Policy Analysis of the United Nations Secretariat.

[2]The former State of Czechoslovakia was dissolved on 31 December 1992 and became the independent States of the Czech Republic and Slovakia on 1 January 1993.

[3]The area of the former State of Yugoslavia currently comprises the independent States of Bosnia and Herzegovina, Croatia, Slovenia, the former Yugoslav Republic of Macedonia and the Federal Republic of Yugoslavia.

REFERENCES

Avdeyev, A. A., and I. A. Troitskaya (1991). Contraception and abortion in the USSR: experience of 1980s. Paper presented at the European Demographic Conference, Paris, 21-25 October.

de Guibert-Lantoine, Catherine, and Alain Monnier (1992). La conjoncture démographique: l'Europe et les pays développés d'Outre-Mer. *Population* (Paris), vol. 47, No. 4 (juillet-août), pp. 1017-1036.

Serbanescu, M. (1990). A brighter future for three million Romanian women? *Entre nous: The European Family Planning Magazine* (Copenhagen), No. 14/15 (June).

United Nations (1989). *Levels and Trends of Contraceptive Use as Assessed in 1988*. Population Studies, No. 110. Sales No. E.89.XIII.4.

_____ (1991). *Economic Bulletin for Europe*, vol. 43. Sales No. E.91.II.E.39.

_____ (1992a). *1990 Demographic Yearbook*. Sales No. E/F.91.XIII.1.

_____ (1992b). *Economic Survey of Europe in 1991-1992*. Sales No. E.92.II.E.1.

United Nations Children's Fund and World Health Organization (1992). The looming crisis in health and the need for international support. Overview of the reports on the Commonwealth of Independent States and the Baltic Republics prepared by the UNICEF/WHO collaborative missions with the participation of the United Nations Population Fund, the World Food Programme and the United Nations Development Programme, 17 February-2 March 1992.

United States Agency for International Development (1992). *USAID Health Profiles*. Arlington, Virginia: Center for International Health Information/International Science and Technology Institute.

XXIX. FAMILY PLANNING POLICIES AND PROGRAMMES: LESSONS LEARNED

Economic and Social Commission for Western Asia[*]

In the Amman Declaration on Population in the Arab World, 25-29 March 1984, the Governments were invited to the adoption of the principle of comprehensive planning based on a clear conception of population policy.

Out of the components of population policy was the reproduction component, which includes:

(*a*) Creation of a favourable socio-economic environment for the achievement of birth rates consistent with the desired population growth rates;

(*b*) The formulation, by Arab Governments wishing to reduce fertility rates, of population guidelines for their development plans with a view to encouraging couples to have a small number of children by expanding education, enhancing the status of women, increasing the participation of women in organized economic activity, reducing infant mortality rates, providing social security and making family planning services accessible to couples that want them.

A. GOVERNMENTS' PERCEPTIONS RELATED TO POPULATION POLICY FACTORS

Population policies are too often confused with family planning. Family planning should be regarded as a service within an overall population policy, taking into consideration such factors as demographic patterns, fertility levels, social and economic conditions and religious and cultural heritage (Salas, 1979).

In fact, Governments could provide family planning services through information and facilities. General health services in many cases provide the best framework for family planning. Moreover, this service could be provided by means of non-governmental and private channels (Salas, 1979).

Hence, a discussion of family planning is part of a review of population policy of the area under study.

This section reviews the Governments' perceptions of population policy factors for member countries of the Economic and Social Commission for Western Asia (ESCWA) during the period 1976-1989.

Population growth

Table 38 shows three groups in relation to Governments' perceptions of population growth.

Group I: rates satisfactory with no intervention

Group I consists of five countries: Bahrain; Jordan; Lebanon; the Syrian Arab Republic; and Yemen. During the follow-up period 1976 to 1989, the Governments' perceptions, with one exception, were that the rates were satisfactory with no intervention to change them. The exception wsa Jordan, which at the last point changed its view to consider the growth rate too high but still did not undertake positive intervention.

Group II: rates too low

Three countries viewed their rates as too low and intervened to raise them during the entire period 1976-1989: Oman; Qatar; and Saudi Arabia.

Kuwait considered the ratio too low from 1976 to 1987, but in 1989 it saw the rates as satisfactory and began to intervene to maintain that rate of growth.

Group III: rates too high with intervention to lower

Group III has only one country, Egypt, as it is the only Government in the ESCWA region which established its own population policy in the 1960s.

Fertility

As is shown in table 39, the ESCWA countries can be classified into the three following main groups with respect to Governments' perceptions and policies concerning national fertility and access to effective fertility regulation.

---

[*]Amman, Jordan.

TABLE 38. GOVERNMENTS' OVERALL APPRAISAL OF RATES OF POPULATION GROWTH AND INTERVENTION TO INFLUENCE RATES, ESCWA REGION, 1976, 1980, 1986 AND 1989

	Rates too low		Rates satisfactory				Rates too high	
	No direct intervention reported (1)	Intervention to raise rates (2)	Intervention to raise rates (3)	Intervention to maintain rates (4)	No direct intervention reported (5)	Intervention to lower rates (6)	Intervention to lower rates (7)	No direct intervention reported (8)
Bahrain								
1976	–	–	–	–	X	–	–	–
1980	–	–	–	–	X	–	–	–
1987	–	–	–	–	X	–	–	–
1989	–	–	–	–	X	–	–	–
Democratic Yemen								
1976	–	–	–	–	–	–	–	X
1980	–	–	–	–	–	–	–	X
1986	–	–	–	–	X	–	–	–
1989	–	–	–	–	X	–	–	–
Egypt								
1976	–	–	–	–	–	–	X	–
1980	–	–	–	–	–	–	X	–
1986	–	–	–	–	–	–	X	–
1989	–	–	–	–	–	–	X	–
Iraq								
1976	–	–	–	–	X	–	–	–
1980	–	–	–	–	X	–	–	–
1986	–	X	–	–	–	–	–	–
1986	–	X	–	–	–	–	–	–
Jordan								
1976	–	–	–	–	X	–	–	–
1980	–	–	–	–	X	–	–	–
1986	–	–	–	–	X	–	–	–
1989	–	–	–	–	–	–	–	X
Kuwait								
1976	X	–	–	–	–	–	–	–
1980	X	–	–	–	–	–	–	–
1986	–	X	–	–	–	–	–	–
1989	–	–	–	X	–	–	–	–
Lebanon								
1976	–	–	–	–	X	–	–	–
1980	–	–	–	–	X	–	–	–
1986	–	–	–	–	X	–	–	–
1989	–	–	–	–	X	–	–	–
Oman								
1976	–	X	–	–	–	–	–	–
1980	–	X	–	–	–	–	–	–
1986	–	X	–	–	–	–	–	–
1989	–	X	–	–	–	–	–	–

357

TABLE 38 (continued)

	Rates too low		Rates satisfactory				Rates too high	
	No direct intervention reported (1)	Intervention to raise rates (2)	Intervention to raise rates (3)	Intervention to maintain rates (4)	No direct intervention reported (5)	Intervention to lower rates (6)	Intervention to lower rates (7)	No direct intervention reported (8)
Qatar								
1976	–	X						
1980	–	X	–	–	–	–	–	–
1986	–	X	–	–	–	–	–	–
1989	–	X	–	–	–	–	–	–
Saudi Arabia								
1976	–	X	–					
1980	–	X	–	–	–	–	–	–
1986	–	X	–	–	–	–	–	–
1989	–	X	–	–	–	–	–	–
Syrian Arab Republic								
1976	–	–	–	–	X	–	–	–
1980	–	–	–	–	X	–	–	–
1986	–	–	–	–	X	–	–	–
1989	–	–	–	–	X	–	–	–
United Arab Estimates								
1976	–	X	–	–	–	–	–	–
1980	–	X	–	–	–	–	–	–
1986	–	–	X	–	–	–	–	–
1989	–	–	–	–	–	–	–	X
Yemen[a]								
1976	–	–	–	–	X	–	–	–
1980	–	–	–	–	X	–	–	–
1986	–	–	–	–	X	–	–	–
1989	–	–	–	–	X	–	–	–
ESCWA region								
1976	1	4	–	–	6	–	1	1
1980	1	4	–	–	6	–	1	1
1986	–	5	1	–	6	–	1	–
1989	–	5	–	1	4	–	1	2

Sources: For 1976, *World Population Trends and Policies: 1979 Monitoring Report*, vol. II, *Population Policies*, Population Studies, No. 70 (United Nations publication, Sales No. E.78.XIII.4); for 1980, *World Population Trends and Policies, 1981 Monitoring Report*, vol. II, *Population Policies*, Population Studies, No. 79 (United Nations publication, Sales No. E.82.XIII.3); for 1986, Global Population Policy Data Base, 1987, Population Policy Paper, No. 9 (United Nations publication, ST/ESA/SER.R/71); for 1989, *Global Population Policy Data Base, 1989*, Population Policy Paper, No. 28 (United Nations publication, ST/ESA/SER.R/99).

[a]On May 22 1990, Democratic Yemen and Yemen merged to form a single State. Since that date they have been represented as one Member of the United Nations with the name "Yemen". For some statistical data which predate the merger, it has been necessary to refer occasionally to the former States of Yemen and Democratic Yemen.

TABLE 39. GOVERNMENTS' PERCEPTIONS AND POLICIES REGARDING NATIONAL FERTILITY AND ACCESS TO EFFECTIVE FERTILITY REGULATION, ESCWA REGION, 1976, 1980, 1986 AND 1989

Country and inquiry year	Government perceptions of the acceptability of current fertility and of the desirability of intervention to change it					
	Rates not satisfactory too low; higher rates desirable	Rates satisfactory				Rates not satisfactory too high; lower rates desirable
	Intervention to raise rates, appropriate incentives and disincentives implemented to raise rates	Intervention to change rates not appropriate				Intervention to lower rates, appropriate, incentives and disincentives implemented to lower rates
		No incentives or disincentives implemented	Incentives and disincentives implemented to maintain rates	No incentives or disincentives implemented		
	(1)	(2)	(3)	(4)	(5)	(6)
Bahrain						
1976	–	–	–	–	X[a]	–
1980	–	–	–	–	X[a]	–
1986	–	–	–	–	X[b]	–
1989	–	–	–	–	X[b]	–
Democratic Yemen[b,c]						
1976	–	–	–	X	–	–
1980	–	–	–	X	–	–
1986	–	–	–	–	–	X
1989	–	–	–	–	–	X
Egypt[b]						
1976	–	–	–	–	–	X
1980	–	–	–	–	–	X
1986	–	–	–	–	–	X
1989	–	–	–	–	–	X
Iraq						
1976	–	–	X[b]	–	–	–
1980	X[d]	–	–	–	–	–
1986	–	–	–	–	X[d]	–
1989	–	–	–	–	X[d]	–
Jordan						
1976	–	–	–	–	X[b]	–
1980	–	–	–	–	X[b]	–
1986	–	–	–	X[a]	–	–
1989	–	–	–	–	X[b]	–
Kuwait[d]						
1976	–	–	X	–	–	–
1980	–	–	X	–	–	–
1986	–	–	–	–	–	X
1989	–	–	–	–	–	X
Lebanon						
1976	–	–	–	X[a]	–	–
1980	–	–	–	X[a]	–	–
1986	–	–	–	X[a]	–	–
1989	–	–	–	X[b]	–	–

TABLE 39 (*continued*)

Country and inquiry year	Rates not satisfactory too low; higher rates desirable	Rates sastisfactory			Rates not satisfactory too high; lower rates desirable
	Intervention to raise rates, appropriate incentives and disincentives implemented to raise rates (1)	Intervention to change rates not appropriate			Intervention to lower rates, appropriate, incentives and disincentives implemented to lower rates (6)
		No incentives or disincentives implemented (2)	Incentives and disincentives implemented to maintain rates (3)	No incentives or disincentives implemented (4) (5)	

Government perceptions of the acceptability of current fertility and of the desirability of intervention to change it

Country and inquiry year	(1)	(2)	(3)	(4)	(5)	(6)	
Oman[d]							
1976	–	–	X	–	–	–	
1980	–	–	X	–	–	–	
1986	–	–	X	–	–	–	
1989	–	–	X	–	–	–	
Qatar[d]							
1976	–	–	X	–	–	–	
1980	–	–	X	–	–	–	
1986	–	–	X	–	–	–	
1989	–	–	X	–	–	–	
Saudi Arabia[e]							
1976	–	–	X	–	–	–	
1980	–	–	X	–	–	–	
1986	–	–	X	–	–	–	
1989	–	–	X	–	–	–	
Syrian Arab Republic[b]							
1976	–	–	–	X	–	–	
1980	–	–	–	X	–	–	
1986	–	–	–	X	–	–	
1989	–	–	–	X	–	–	
United Arab Emirates[e]							
1976	–	–	X	–	–	–	
1980	–	–	X	–	–	–	
1986	X	–	X	–	–	–	
1989	–	–	X	–	–	–	
Yemen[b,c]							
1976	–	–	–	X	–	–	
1980	–	–	–	X	–	–	
1986	–	–	–	–	–	X	
1989	–	–	–	–	–	X	
ESCWA region							
1976	–	–	6	4	2	1	13
1980	1	–	5	4	2	1	13
1986	1	–	3	3	2	4	13
1989	–	–	4	2	3	4	13

Sources and notes to follow.

TABLE 39 (*continued*)

Sources: For 1976, *World Population Trends and Policies: 1979 Monitoring Report*, vol. II, *Population Policies*, Population Studies, No. 70 (United Nations publication, Sales No. E.78.XIII.4); for 1980, World Population Trends and Policies: 1981 Monitoring Report, vol. II, *Population Policies*, Population Studies, No. 79 (United Nations publication, Sales No. E.82.XIII.3); for 1986, Global Population Policy Data base, 1987, Population Policy Paper, No. 9 (United Nations publication, ST/ESA/SER.R/71); 1989, Global Population Policy data base 1989. Population Policy Paper No. 28 (ST/ESA/SER.R/99).

ᵃAccess not limited and indirect support provided.

ᵇAccess not limited and direct support provided.

ᶜOn 22 May 1990, Democratic Yemen and Yemen merged to form a single State. Since that date they have been represented as one Member of the United Nations with the name "Yemen". For some statistical data which predate the merger, it has been necessary to refer occasionally to the former States of Yemen and Democratic Yemen.

ᵈAccess not limited and no support provided.

ᵉAccess limited and no support provided.

Group I: fertility rates satisfactory

Group I is divided into two subgroups:

(a) Incentives and disincentives implemented to maintain rates. Oman, Qatar, Saudi Arabia and United Arab Emirates considered fertility rates to be satisfactory and implemented measures to maintain those rates. In addition, Iraq is in this group at the first point, 1976, and Kuwait is during the period 1976-1980.

(b) As in (a) but with no intervention. This subgroup includes Lebanon and the Syrian Arab Republic; and Democratic Yemen and Yemen were included during 1976-1980.

Group II: Rates not satisfactory; too high, lower rates desirable

Group II is subdivided as follows:

(a) With no intervention. This group includes Bahrain and Jordan, as well as Iraq during the last three years, 1987-1989.

(b) With intervention to lower rates by implementing incentives and disincentives. In this subgroup are Egypt throughout the period 1976-1989; and Democratic Yemen, Kuwait and Yemen during the last three years, 1987-1989.

As concerns contraceptive use in Saudi Arabia, there was limited access to contraceptives and no support was provided.

In the countries in the Persian Gulf area, except Bahrain and Saudi Arabia, there was no limited access to contraceptive use, but no support was provided. The countries in which there was access to contraceptive use and direct support was provided included Democratic Yemen, Egypt, Jordan, the Syrian Arab Republic and Yemen.

B. JORDAN: POPULATION AND FAMILY PLANNING POLICIES AND PROGRAMMES

The Jordan Family Planning and Protection Association (JFPPA) introduced its voluntary family planning information and contraceptive services in 1972 (UNFPA, 1985), with branches and clinics providing family planning education and services in the major cities.

In 1979, the Government of Jordan became involved in family planning activities with the inception of United Nations Population Fund (UNFPA) family planning project. It was felt that the health benefits of family planning for mothers and children were not recognized. The project, which integrates family planning with mother and child health (MCH) services, educates mothers about breast-feeding, child-spacing and health, in classes conducted at MCH clinics. Contraceptives are provided for the mothers on request.

The Jordan Fertility and Family Health Survey of 1983 showed that 26 per cent of married women were using contraceptives at the time of interview. The most popular methods were the intra-uterine device (IUD) and pills. Main sources of contraceptive methods were private physicians and pharmacies (57.5 per cent), public hospitals (9.9 per cent), JFPPA (2.1 per cent), and MCH and health centres (1.6 per cent).

The Survey also indicated that 28 per cent of married women were in need of family planning services, that is, did not wish to become pregnant. The survey suggests that there is a large pool of potential contraceptive users, that may become users as attitudes towards contraception change.

The Jordan Population and Family Health Survey of 1990 indicated that 35 per cent of currently married women were using any method of contraception. This proportion is much higher than those in 1983 and 1976, which were 26 and 24 per cent. It was observed that the increase in contraceptive use is accompanied by a decline in the total fertility rate (TFR) from 7.7 children per woman in 1976 to 6.6 in 1983 and to 5.6 in 1990 (Zou'bi, Poedjastoeti and Ayad, 1991).

C. POPULATION POLICY IN THE SYRIAN ARAB REPUBLIC

The Syrian Arab Republic has no formal population policy; however, the Government is very much concerned about the overall well-being and general health of the population. In order to provide the necessary health care, an elaborate infrastructure has been developed during the past two decades. In 1982, the country had nearly 230 health centres (hospitals), 12 of which were specially designed to provide MCH services. On average, each centre serves a population of 70,000 in urban areas and 27,000 in rural areas. Family planning services are available for needy mothers in these centres, more particularly in the MCH units (Syrian Arab Republic, 1982).

D. YEMEN POPULATION AND FAMILY PLANNING POLICY

On 21 August 1991, the presidential decree No. 356/1991 introduced the first national population strategy of Yemen (unified Yemen).[1] This strategy includes the following targets:

(a) To reduce the crude death rate by about 50 per cent during the next 10 years, that is, to increase expectation of life at birth ($e°_o$) from 46 years in 1990 to reach 60 years in the year 2000;

(b) To reduce TFR to reach 6.0 live births per woman in the targeted year 2000, compared with 8.3 in 1990;

(c) To reduce infant mortality rates from the current level of 130 per 1,000 live births in 1991 to be 60 per 1,000 in the year 2000, and to reduce the maternal deaths by 50 per cent during the period 1991-2000;

(d) Consistent with the targets mentioned above, to reach an annual growth rate of 2 per cent by the year 2000, compared with 3.1 per cent in 1991.

E. FAMILY PLANNING IN EGYPT

Family planning policy

Women living in Mediterranean countries used in ancient times and are still using pieces of sea sponge dipped in vinegar or salted water into the vagina as a contraceptive (Fahmy, 1981).

In Egypt, oral pills were used in 1962 and were locally manufactured in 1965. The Population Council reported that Egypt was the first developing country to use the pills on a large popular scale (Fahmy, 1981).

In fact, the various stages of family planning policies in Egypt can be characterized by some distinguished activities.

1937: Al Azher fatwa[2] that birth control not in conflict with rule of Islam

Egypt was among the first group of developing countries to recognize the importance of population in relation to development. In 1937 the Happy Family Society, a group of university professors, obtained on official fatwa (interpretation of a legal point in Islam) to the effect that birth control, under certain conditions, does not conflict with the rule of Islam (Egypt, 1977). In the meantime, the Egyptian Medical Association discussed the issues of the population crisis, and the Society called for family planning. The call was supported by the press and Egyptian physicians began to test the contraceptives (Fahmy, 1981).

1945: inclusion of family planning services in Child Society

The Child Society of Ma'adi Association included family planning services in its health activities in 1945. The Society took the initiative and tested the contraceptives together with a remedy for sterility. It is noteworthy that the services offered by this Society were the first family planning services to be provided by a private association in Egypt. However, these efforts were later abandoned because of strong opposition (Egypt, 1977).

1953-1955: establishment of National Population Commission

The beginning of government interest in the population question dates back to 1953, when the Egyptian Council of Ministers approved of the establishment of the National Population Commission, under the chairmanship of the Minister of Social Affairs. Three committees were organized within the Commission to study the demographic, economic and medical implications of population changes. The medical committee was authorized to experiment with family planning services under certain conditions. In 1955, eight family planning clinics were organized for this purpose under the authority of the Ministry of Public Health (Rizk and others, 1980). One of those clinics were under the supervision of the Muslim Women's Association, which implies that Islam does not oppose the exercise of family planning. These centres required—to offer services—the approval of the husband, the existence of a number of children and proof that contraception was necessary for economic or medical reasons. On the other hand, publishing the location of these centres was not permitted (Fahmy, 1981).

1955-1961: public opinion against family planning

Even though the Egyptian Government created the Nation Population Commission in 1953, its opinion was clearly inclined towards the support of social and economic development to raise the level of living of the people. The population element as a factor affecting developmental goals remained unrecognized. The progress of the few family planning clinics slowed and public opinion was generally against adoption of population policy.

1962: recognition of population problem in the national charter

The year 1962 could be considered the beginning of a new stage in that a government document issued in this year (the National Charter) included the first announcement about the Government's stand towards family planning. The National Charter stated that the problem of population increase was the most serious obstacle that confronted Egypt in its attempts to raise the level of production in the country through effective means (Egypt, 1962).

1964: beginning of non-governmental family planning activities

The few clinics that had been providing family planning services under government auspices since 1955 encouraged several non-governmental voluntary organizations to establish their own family planning clinics. Family planning associations were created at Cairo and Alexandria in 1964 and became active in conducting field surveys and research projects related to knowledge, attitude and practice (KAP) of family planning, in addition to provision of contraceptives.

1965: establishment of Supreme Council for Family Planning

The establishment of the Supreme Council for Family Planning by presidential Decree in 1965 marks the beginning of adoption of a population policy. The Council Chairman was the Prime Minister and its membership included the Ministers of Health, Higher Education, National Guidance, Wakfs,[3] Planning, Local Administration and Agriculture; the Deputy Minister of Social Affairs and the Director of Central Agency for Public Mobilisation and Statistics (CAPMAS). The Council appointed an executive committee for family planning activities.

The objectives of the Supreme Council were: *(a)* to set a comprehensive plan for family planning in the country; *(b)* to study, encourage and coordinate activities related to population questions and their relation to social, economic and medical settings; *(d)* to develop cooperation between the different administrations participating in the programme (Rizk and others, 1980).

The first national population policy (fertility reduction) was declared in 1965 (Egypt, 1980). This policy centred on one aspect of population problem, growth, and was directed to fertility reduction. In February 1966, a family planning programme was developed on the national level as the instrument of this policy. It adopted a medical orientation, conforming with family planning programmes in existence at that time.

Subsequently, the national population policy went through two successive stages of development.

1973: the socio-economic approach to fertility reduction

The second phase of the policy, which was fully developed in 1973, can be called the "socio-economic approach" to fertility reduction. Although fertility reduction was still the primary concern, the policy recognized the role of socio-economic variables in relation to fertility and identified nine factors as critical fertility influences which have to be manipulated simultaneously (Egypt, 1980). These influences are:

(a) The socio-economic standard of the family;

(b) Education;

(c) The status of women (stressing participation of women in the wage-earning labour force outside the agricultural and domestic fields;

(d) Mechanization of agriculture;

(e) Industrialization (with emphasis on agro-industries);

(f) Infant mortality (with improvement of nutrition and sanitation as basic elements);

(g) Social security;

(h) Information and communication; and

(I) Family planning delivery services.

1975: the development approach to population problem

The third phase, which began in 1975, may be called the "development approach" to the population problem. It was an elaboration of the previous phase and was developed on the basis of greater realization of the magnitude and implications of population growth, the limits within which it can be reduced and a better understanding of both population and the socio-economic environment. This last phase differs from previous policy phases in defining the population problem in its entirety, in terms of growth, distribution and characteristics.

The policy relates population activities to the three hierarchical levels of administration—the central, governorate and community levels. The policy takes the community as its platform for action, and programmes are designed to transfer the responsibility for implementing population and family planning policy to the local administration and community. In this respect, efforts capitalize on a law decentralizing the Government's responsibilities (Egypt, 1980).

1986-1991: objectives of the national population policy

The objectives of the national population policy exceeded quantitative expectations for the past five year (1986-1991). The contraceptive prevalence rates achieved were 34 per cent of currently married women of child-bearing age in 1986/87, 41 per cent in 1988/89 and 54 in 1990/91. When the rates are compared by geographical area, the urban governorate shows a 64 per

cent contraceptive prevalence rate in 1986/87, reaching 87 in 1990/91, while the upper Egypt governorate shows the lowest rates, 21 per cent in 1986/87 and 33 in 1990/91 (table 40). In 1991, protected women totalled 4,193,792 woman/years (table 41). Those women-years of protection were distributed among different contraceptive devices, as given in table 41. IUDs protected 68 per cent of the total protected women, oral pills were next at 25 per cent, then condoms at 6 per cent and all the other devices at only 2 per cent (Egypt, 1991).

The above-mentioned achievement of the objectives of the national population policy (Egypt, 1992) was due to the collaborated efforts of the ministerial, national and executive bodies. This policy has been thoroughly studied, resulting in some amendments in the quantitative objectives. In addition, it devoted more attention to some new fields, such as youth and environment.

First, with regard to quantitative objectives, some examples of the goals of the new population strategy, in various fields, are given below:

(a) Family planning. The objective of the new strategy is to increase the contraceptive prevalence rate from 47.6 per cent in 1991 to 55 in 1997 and then to 59 in 2002, to reach 65 per cent in 2007. The strategy is also intended to reduce the birth rate from 32.2 per cent in 1991 to 27 in 1997 and 26 in 2002, to reach 25 per cent in 2007;

(b) Maternal and child care. The goal of the strategy is to reduce the number of dead infants from 43.5 per cent in 1991 to 37 in 1997 and 30 in 2002, to reach 23 per cent in 2007. It is hoped to reduce child mortality under age 5 from 6.1 per cent in 1991 to 5 in 1997 and 4 in 2002, to reach 3 per cent in 2007. As concerns maternal care, the objective is to reduce the rate of maternal deaths due to pregnancy and labour, from 260 to 120 per 100,000 live births in 1997 to 80 in 2002, until it reaches only 50 per 100,000 live births;

(c) Woman and development. As concerns women and development, the goal is to reduce the percentage of illiteracy among females from 57 in 1991 to 45 in 1997 and 33 per cent in 2002, until it declines to 22 per cent in 2007;

(d) Mass communication and population communication. The strategy is directed to promoting the efficiency of personal communication, particularly at the

level of rural areas, and working to vary the content of information materials so as to suit the different environmental conditions of various categories of targeted people;

(e) Work and labour. The strategy is intended to reduce the relatively increasing rate of unemployment for those aged 15 or over. This rate goes from 14.6 per cent in 1991 to 16.6 in 1997 and to 18.6, until it reaches 20.6 per cent in 2007;

(f) Youth encouragement. The strategy is also directed to encouraging youth to settle in new cities where it has been noted that the proportion of youths, as compared with the total population was 25 per cent in 1991. The objective is to increase this percentage from 30.5 in 1997 to 32.5 in 2002, and to reach 34.5 in 2007. The strategy also attempts to remedy the negativism phenomenon among youth, in particular, drug abuse and extremism;

(g) Environment. The strategy is directed to reducing the population density in overcrowded areas, as well as providing all the means of attraction to inhabit the new cities. For instance, the strategy works at reducing the population density in the inhabited areas;

(h) Education and eradication of illiteracy. The strategy is intended to reduce the percentage of drop-outs in primary education from 1.7 per cent in 1991 to 1.0 in 1997. This phenomenon is expected to come to an end by 2007. As for illiteracy, the goal is to reduce the percentage of illiteracy from 46 per cent in 1991 to 37 in 1997 and 28 per cent in 2002, to reach 19 per cent in 2007;

(i) Land utilization. The strategy is intended to control urban expansion at the expense of agricultural lands. About 20,000 feddans are lost annually because of urban expansion.

Secondly, to achieve the goals of population programme, more effective methods were considered in the policy (Egypt, 1992), such as:

(a) Reducing the fertility rate. The policy concentrated on local industrialization for the means of family planning and coping with modern development by introducing the most suitable methods. Special attention was given to providing deprived areas with family planning services, in rural areas;

(b) Maternal and child care. The new policy concentrates on promoting the performance level in the field of maternal and child care, benefiting from the projects, which lead to increasing the number of those benefiting from the provided services as well as setting and implementing integrated plans of social and health care for mothers and children;

(c) Family protection. The goal of the policy is to study and revise legislation in the coming period; this policy influences upbringing values, and implements and issues legislation while supporting the tendency to have a small family. This policy is also intended to broaden coverage of social insurance, pensions and social security, as well as to support the programmes of old-age care which secure stability;

(d) Promoting the status of woman. The goal is to be achieved by encouraging women to participate in public life, establishing suitable kindergartens for children, supporting the activities dealing with the projects of productive families and assuring the importance of education and training as well as eliminating illiteracy, especially of rural women;

(e) Preparing and promoting youth.[4] This policy was intended to utilize youth as pioneers in the field of population and family planning; especially in the local societies, in addition to the dissemination and strengthening of the concept of small family;

(f) Education and eradication of illiteracy. The policy is very concerned with the issue of school dropouts, especially among females. It also draws attention to the support of personal efforts and to the contribution of society to overcome this phenomenon;

(g) Personal communication. The policy concentrates on the importance of personal communication as a way of persuasion that is more effective, especially in rural societies and public zones. This is achieved through benefiting from the efforts of local leaders. The policy also emphasizes the role of houses of worship, as they are considered religious, social, health and cultural centres.

(h) Development of rural societies. The policy views the importance of the role of each of the local educational organizations in promoting rural societies through coordination among the programmes of these institutions;

TABLE 40. ESTIMATED NUMBERS OF CURRENTLY MARRIED WOMEN OF CHILD-BEARING AGE, 15-49 YEARS, NUMBER OF PROTECTED WOMEN AND CONTRACEPTIVE PREVALENCE RATE, EGYPT

Geographical area	1986/87	1988/89	1990/91
Urban Governorate			
Currently married women aged 15-49	1 481 101	1 547 102	1 598 671
PW	903 135	1 083 311	1 386 104
CPR (percentage)	61	70	87
Lower Egypt			
CMCB	3 098 268	3 270 252	3 414 968
PW	1 026 436	1 392 219	1 913 104
CPR (percentage)	33	43	56
Upper Egypt			
CMCB	2 660 652	2 800 132	2 942 892
PW	458 086	643 647	979 465
CPR (percentage)	21	23	33
Frontier Governorate			
CMCB	83 981	113 504	97 156
PW	13 656	20 953	37 827
CPR (percentage)	16	18	39
Total Egypt			
CMCM	7 324 001	7 730 990	8 053 686
PW	2 491 312	3 140 129	4 316 441
CPR (percentage)	34	41	54

Source: Calculated from Egypt, National Population Council, *Annual Analytical Statistical Report, 1991* Cairo, 1991), p. 72.

NOTE: CMCB = currently married women of child-bearing age (15-49);

$$PW = \text{women/years protected} = \frac{\text{Number of oral pills}}{13} + \frac{\text{Number of IUD}}{2.5} +$$

$$\frac{\text{Number of condoms}}{100} + \frac{\text{Number of diaphragm}}{1} + \frac{\text{Number of jellies and creams}}{100} \times 18$$

$$+ \frac{\text{Number of foam tablets}}{100} + \frac{\text{Number of injections}}{4}$$

$$CPR = \text{contraceptive prevalence rates} = \frac{\text{Number of women/years protected} \times 100}{\text{Mid-year estimated women of child-bearing age}}$$

TABLE 41. ESTIMATED NUMBER OF PROTECTED WOMEN,
WOMAN/YEARS OF PROTECTION, BY CONTRACEPTIVE METHOD,
EGYPT, 1991

Contraceptive method	Women-years of protection	Percentage distribution
Oral pills	1 012 029	24.9
Intra-uterine devices	2 849 832	68.0
Condoms	263 744	6.3
Cups	2 423	0.1
Jelly and creams	609	0.01
Foam tablets	25 018	0.6
Injections	40 137	1.0
TOTAL	4 193 792	100.0

Source: Egypt, National Population Council, *Annual Analytical Statistical Report, 1991* (Cairo, 1991), p. 10.

(i) Population distribution. This policy is concerned with the costs, the social and the economic revenue of the settlement policy together with setting up detailed integrated and scheduled programmes.

(j) Environmental protection. This is considered a new field which raises environmental awareness through education and environmental communication. This field is also involved setting legislation and regulations. The goal is to protect both humans and the environment, as well as to provide some balance between them;

(k) Research and population information. The current policy attends to the setting of integrated systems of data and population information at the national level, emphasizing the local level and utilizing it in planning and implementing this policy;

(l) Management of population programmes. The policy is concerned about setting up an integrated organizational structure for the management of population programmes at different executive levels.

F. PREVALENCE OF SPECIFIC METHODS

In Egypt and Jordan, where data for comparison were available, there was a tendency to change in the current use of IUDs on the account of oral pills. In Jordan, female sterilizations accounted for 20 per cent of current users in 1985, while in Egypt, the level stayed about 5 per cent.

In Iraq in 1974 and in the Syrian Arab Republic in 1978, pill users were about the level (60 per cent) in Jordan in 1972 and in Egypt in 1984.

In the Syrian Arab Republic, the fertility survey in 1987 found that even in the absence of national policy to promote family planning, contraception was fairly widely practised, as 33 per cent of ever-married women under age 50 had used contraception at some time. Also, 3 out of 10 currently married women that were capable of having more children were currently practising contraception (Syrian Arab Republic, 1982).

NOTES

[1] On 22 May 1990, Democratic Yemen and Yemen merged to form a single State. Since that date they have been represented as one Member of the United Nations with the name "Yemen". For some statistical data which predate the merger, it has been necessary to refer occasionally to the former States of Yemen and Democratic Yemen.

[2] The mufti of Al Azher was the Grand Sheikh Abedl-Majid Saleem (Fahmy, 1981, p. 30).

[3] Religious endowment.

[4] In addition, devoting more attention to the demographic concept to be included in the school curricula at all educational levels.

REFERENCES

Egypt (1962). *The National Charter, May 1962.* Cairo: Government Press.

_____ , Ministry of Health (1977). *A Proposal for a Community Based Family Planning.* Cairo.

Egypt, National Population Council (1991). *Annual Analytical Statistical Report, 1991.* Cairo.

_____ (1992). *Population Studies* (Cairo), vol. 14, No. 75 (July-September).

Egypt, Supreme Council for Population and Family Planning (1980). *National Strategy Framework for Population Program.* Cairo.

Fahmy, M. Badrawy (1981). *The Population Problems and Family Planning in Egypt.* Cairo: Al Ahram Press.

Rizk, Hanna, and others (1980). Background paper for Population Assistance Needs Assessment Mission, vol. I. Cairo.

Salas, Rafael M. (1979). *International Population Assistance; The First Decade.* New York: Pergamon Press.

Sayed, Hussein Abdel-Aziz, and others (1989). *Egypt Demographic and Health Survey, 1988.* Cairo: Egypt National Population Council; and Columbia, Maryland: Institute for Research Development/Macro Systems, Inc.

Syrian Arab Republic, Office of the Prime Minister (1982). *Syrian Fertility Survey, 1978: Principal Report,* vol. I. Damascus: Central Bureau of Statistics in collaboration with the World Fertility Survey.

United Nations (1979). *World Population Trends and Policies, 1979 Monitoring Report*, vol. II, *Population Policies*. Population Studies, No. 70. Sales No. E.78.XIII.4.

_____ United Nations (1982). *World Population Trends and Policies, 1981 Monitoring Report*, vol. II, *Population Policies*. Population Studies, No. 79/Add.1. Sales No. E.82.XIII.3.

_____ (1987). *World Population Policies*, vol. I, *Afghanistan to France*. Population Studies, No. 102. Sales No. E.87.XIII.4.

_____ (1989). *World Population Policies*, vol. II, *Gabon to Norway*. Population Studies, No. 102/Add.1. Sales No. E.89.XIII.3.

_____ (1990). *Global Population Data Base, 1989.* Population Policy Paper, No. 28. ST/ESA/SER.R/99.

United Nations Fund for Population Activities (1985). *Jordan: Report of Second Mission on Needs Assessment for Population Assistance.* Report No. 83. New York.

Zou'bi, Abdallah Abdel Aziz, Sri Poedjastoeti and Mohamed Ayad (1991). *Jordan Population and Family Health Survey, 1990: Preliminary Report.* Amman, Jordan: Ministry of Health, Department of Statistics; Columbia, Maryland: Institute for Resource Development/Macro International, Inc.

XXX. POPULATION POLICIES AND PROGRAMMES IN ASIA AND THE PACIFIC

Economic and Social Commission for Asia and the Pacific[*]

Population policies have long formed part of the national development plans of countries in Asia and the Pacific. Many countries first became aware of population problems in the 1960s and initiated official family planning programmes during that decade to try to overcome them. These programmes were significantly strengthened in the 1970s, as a result of the heightened national and international concern about the negative implications of high rates of population growth. The success of many national population policies in reducing levels of fertility became ever more apparent in the 1980s, mainly because of the efforts of their family planning programmes.

At the beginning of the 1980s, most countries of Eastern Asia had completed the transition from high to low fertility (Leete, 1992). With few exceptions, fertility has also fallen sharply in many of the countries of South-eastern Asia. In contrast, fertility in Southern Asia has remained high, except in Sri Lanka and a few of the states in India, in spite of long-standing programmes of government intervention (table 42). Similarly, in the small island countries and territories of the Pacific, only modest declines have been achieved: high fertility remains a problem (table 43). Overall, the region of the Economic and Social Commission for Asia and the Pacific (ESCAP) is falling short of the target of achieving replacement-level fertility by the year 2000, set at the Third Asia-Pacific Population Conference in Colombo in 1982, which has now been reset to be met by the year 2010, at the Fourth Asian and Pacific Population Conference held in Bali in August 1992.

In general, the pattern of mortality in the ESCAP region is closely related to the pattern of fertility (table 42). All countries have shown improvements in mortality, but very marked differentials still persist. For example, in the Eastern Asian countries, infant mortality rates are well below 30 per 1,000 live births, while most countries of Southern Asia have infant mortality rates (IMR) of more than 100. Infant mortality in the South-eastern Asian countries is closer to that of

Eastern Asia. In the majority of the Pacific States, especially in Polynesia, infant mortality has fallen to low levels. But in the larger Melanesian countries of Papua New Guinea, Solomon Islands and Vanuatu, infant mortality remains relatively high (table 43). What is clear is that despite the similarity in patterns, fertility has declined at markedly different levels of infant mortality in different countries.

Although quantitative targets for reducing population growth still retain central importance in some ESCAP countries, in others the emphasis of family planning programmes has shifted to different aspects of the relation between population and development. The focus here is on the key issues that confront national family planning programmes and the future directions of the programmes.

A. FAMILY PLANNING PROGRAMME SUCCESSES AND FAILURES

Government family planning programmes have played an extremely important role in the substantial fertility reduction that has occurred in several large Asian countries, particularly in China, Indonesia, the Republic of Korea and Thailand (Leete and Alam, 1992). Although it is plausible to argue, at least in the cases of the Republic of Korea and Thailand, that socio-economic changes played a more important part in lowering family size and that the role of the family planning programme in these two countries was secondary, it is beyond any doubt that the national programmes were the major forces behind the fertility declines in China and Indonesia.

The Chinese and Indonesian programmes shared common challenges and experience, despite their being important differences in political and cultural contexts between the two countries. The people of both these vast countries were, and continue to be, predominantly poor and rural, relying heavily upon subsistence farming. There was little motivation to adopt family plan-

---

[*]Bangkok, Thailand.

Region and country or area	Total population (thousands)	Growth rate (percentage)	Total fertility rate (per woman)	Infant mortality rate (per 1,000)	Maternal mortality (per 100,000 live births)	
					Rate	Year
Eastern Asia	1 350 517	1.3	2.3	25	55	1983
China	1 153 470	1.4	2.3	27	50	1982
Hong Kong	5 709	0.8	1.5	6	4	1987
Japan	123 537	0.4	1.8	5	16	1988
Mongolia	2 190	2.6	4.7	60	140	1989
Rep. of Korea	43 377	0.8	1.8	21	26	1987
South-eastern Asia	444 062	1.9	3.5	55	420	1983
Cambodia	8 336	2.5	4.5	116	500	1981
Indonesia	184 283	1.8	3.3	65	400	1987
Lao People's Democratic Republic	4 202	3.0	6.7	97	300	1991
Malaysia	17 891	2.4	3.7	14	26	1988
Myanmar	41 825	2.1	4.2	81	150	1982
Philippines	62 437	2.1	4.0	40	74	1989
Singapore	2 710	1.0	1.8	7	10	1988
Thailand	54 677	1.3	2.3	26	30	1986
Viet Nam	66 688	2.0	4.0	36	120	1989
Southern Asia	1 191 362	2.2	4.4	90	650	1983
Afghanistan	16 556	6.7	6.9	162	600	1981
Bangladesh	113 684	2.4	4.8	108	600	1985
Bhutan	1 539	2.3	5.9	129	773	1983
India	846 191	1.9	3.9	88	460	1984
Iran (Islamic Republic of)	58 267	2.7	6.0	40	120	1985
Nepal	19 571	2.5	5.5	99	833	1986
Pakistan	118 122	2.7	6.2	98	600-750	1985
Sri Lanka	17 217	1.3	2.6	24	80	1987

Sources: *World Population Prospects: the 1992 Revision* (United Nations publication, Sales No. E.93.XIII.7).
For regional maternal mortality, World Health Organization, *Maternal Mortality: A Global Factbook*, compiled by Carla AbouZahr and Erica Royston (Geneva, 1991), table 2.1. For maternal mortality in China, Hong Kong, Mongolia, Republic of Korea, Lao People's Democratic Republic, Malaysia, Philippines, Singapore, Thailand, Bangladesh, India, Islamic Republic of Iran and Sri Lanka, *Maternal Mortality: A Global Factbook*, civil registration data and government estimates. For maternal mortality in Japan, *Democratic Yearbook, 1989* (United Nations publication, Sales No. E/F.90.XIII.1). For maternal mortality in Cambodia, Indonesia, Myanmar, Viet Nam, Afghanistan, Bhutan, Nepal and Pakistan, *Maternal Mortality: A Global Factfook* and other unpublished sources.

ning and have small families when the programmes were initiated at the beginning of the 1970s. Unlike the situation in Thailand, there was no "latent demand" among the masses, and economic development lagged behind that of many other Asian countries. In order to help overcome these problems, the Governments of both countries provide firm central leadership in support of their family planning programmes and ensure that the programmes shall be strongly promoted and enforced at all administrative levels. Local family planning targets receive strong political and bureaucratic support, and the programmes have received support from a majority of public. The strategies adopted entail local family planning workers taking the programme messages and

providing the means of birth control directly to the rural communities. Both programmes rely upon modern methods of birth control and evolve effective distribution systems. The Chinese promote the use of intra-uterine devices (IUDs) and encourage sterilization for couples that already have one or two children. The Indonesian programme offers the pill, IUDs and injectables: each method is used by a significant proportion of married women. There is little use of sterilization because it is generally less acceptable to Muslims.

In contrast, although the populous countries of Southern Asia have a long history of promoting family planning, their programmes have so far been character-

Region and country or area	Total population (thousands)	Growth rate (per cent)	Total fertility rate (per woman)	Infant mortality rate (per 1000)
Melanesia	5 239	2.2	4.6	48
Fiji	726	1.0	3.0	23[a]
Papua New Guinea	3 875	2.3	4.9	54
Solomon Islands	320	3.3	5.4	27
Vanuatu	150	2.5	6.5a	94[a]
Micronesia	424	2.5	4.4	36
Kiribati	71	2.2	4.9a	82[a]
Marshall Islands	46	3.6	7.2a	63[a]
Micronesia (Federated States of)	103	3.5	6.5a	51[a]
Nauru	10	2.2	..a	31[a]
Palau	15	2.2	3.5a	28[a]
Polynesia	549	1.3	4.0	25
Cook Islands	17	-0.13	5.2a	28[a]
Niue	2	-4.58	4.3a	11[a]
Tonga	96	0.6	4.9a	41[a]
Tuvalu	12	2.9	2.8a	43[a]
Western Samoa	158	0.2	4.9a	33[a]

Sources: *World Population Prospects: the 1992 Revision* (United Nations publication, Sales No. E.93.XIII.7).

For total fertility rate in Vanuatu and in all individual countries in Micronesia and Polynesia; and for infant mortality in Fiji and Vanuatu and in all individual countries in Micronesia and Polynesia, M. L. Bakker, *Population of the South Pacific: An Overview of Demographic Levels, Patterns and Trends. Demographic Report No. 1, Population Studies Programme* (Suva, Population Studies Programme (Suva, Fiji, University of the South Pacific, 1990).

Updated using information from available evidence from recent censuses.

ized by very limited success. The slow secular rise in contraceptive prevalence rates cannot be entirely explained by the unfavourable socio-economic settings in which these poor and predominantly rural populations live. The weak rural health infrastructure has impaired the setting-up of adequate supply and distribution networks. More importantly, the programmes have lacked sustained committed leadership resolve at the different levels of administration. Political instability and lack of resources have been important contributory factors. These observations are further supported by the recent study undertaken by Mauldin and Ross (1991), which assessed the Asian family planning programmes based on an index of programme effort which compared the situation in 1989 with that prevailing in 1982. In constructing the index, 30 separate measures were used, grouped into four categories: policy and stage setting; service and service-related activities; record-keeping and evaluation; and availability and accessibility of contraceptive methods. They found that between 1982 and 1989, countries moved significantly towards improved programme effort scores. Effort scores improved not only in every country but also across each of the four categories. In general, programme effort scores were shown to be much higher in Asia than in Africa. Strong programme effort scores were noted in China (84 per cent), the Republic of Korea (80 per cent); Indonesia, Thailand and Sri Lanka (scores close to 80 per cent); and India, Bangladesh and Viet Nam (about 70 per cent). However, these latter three countries had comparatively weaker social settings. Weak scores were noted in Afghanistan, Myanmar and the Lao People's Democratic Republic. The authors show that overall programme effort predicts contraceptive prevalence, past reduction in fertility rates and current level of fertility. The socio-economic setting is also predictive of fertility; it and programme effort are shown to have both separate and joint effects. But it is the availability of contraceptive methods that acts as the most important predictor of contraceptive prevalence in the population.

371

Furthermore, Sathar (1992) points out that the successes among the Asian programmes are largely for those that began quietly and with little fanfare, with experimental programmes or with programmes directed to specific subgroups. In contrast, the less successful programmes too easily became standardized, inflexible and uniformly applied, often regardless of local readiness, local conditions and availability of qualified personnel. A major reason for the lack of success of family planning programmes has been inadequate accessibility of services to the majority of the rural population and, related to that factor, the lack of suitably trained personnel.

B. FAMILY PLANNING AND COMMUNITY PARTICIPATION

In most countries, family planning programmes have traditionally been implemented by approaching individual couples. This strategy has proved successful in several Eastern and South-eastern Asian countries, but it has had very limited impact in the large and predominantly rural countries of Southern Asia. A differing and potentially more beneficial approach is through the implementation of community-assisted family planning programmes. In some countries, particularly those of Southern Asia, without a societal change in attitudes towards family size, widespread acceptance of family planning is unlikely. Programmes need to take account of the sensitivities and cultural characteristics of local communities. Changes in attitudes are much more likely if programmes are accepted and promoted by local community leaders. Another factor favouring a community approach is that in some of the poorer countries, the resource requirements of family planning programmes are so great that Governments cannot meet them. It is therefore necessary to mobilize local level resources; and that objective is much more readily achieved when the local people, especially community leaders, are actively involved in the decision-making processes. Approaches that encourage community involvement, even if only to help sanction the use of birth control, lessen the burden on family planning organizations.

However, in a recent ESCAP study on community participation in China, the Philippines, the Republic of Korea and Thailand, it was found that community participation with "stand alone" family planning programmes does not always succeed (ESCAP, 1988). One factor acting against broad community participation is that family planning *per se* is only directly relevant to a small proportion of a community at any point of time. Family planning is a private matter and people may not want to act collectively. Hence it may be necessary to conceptualize family planning in a context broader than simple birth control, to highlight its relevance to communal life. Ideally, family planning services should be provided as part of an integrated package of health, education and welfare services to local communities.

C. FAMILY PLANNING AND MATERNAL AND CHILD MORTALITY

Maternal mortality constitutes a serious health problem in the least developed countries and merits more attention in family planning programmes. This is particularly so given that medical health and social services are weakest in rural areas where most people live. The widespread provision of improved family planning services can provide an effective way to minimize maternal mortality by reducing high-risk pregnancies, such as those under age 18 or over age 35, after four births and at very short birth intervals.

Child deaths are even more common than maternal deaths and are especially high during the first year of life. Many child deaths could be prevented if all women had access to family planning services and used contraception to space their births at least two years apart. One study found that infants born less than 12 months after a preceding birth are three times more likely to die before age 5 than are infants born 14-27 months after the preceding birth (Hobcraft, McDonald and Rutstein, 1983). Infants at highest risk are those born at very short birth intervals to teenage mothers. James P. Grant, Executive Director of the United Nations Children's Fund (UNICEF), has argued that a substantial proportion of the millions of infant and child deaths that occur annually could be prevented if all women had access to family planning services and used contraception to space their birth at least two years apart (Reich, 1987). Policies promoting birth-spacing, including the encouragement of breast-feeding, could have a crucial bearing on further reducing infant mortality (United Nations, 1987).

In assessing the impact of birth spacing, it has been argued that delaying the first birth and increasing the time between births can also effectively slow rates of population growth (Trussell, 1986). Furthermore, Bongaarts and Greenhalgh (1985) contend that China could abandon its one-child policy and permit two children per family if it could persuade women to postpone their first birth until they are 28 years old and to maintain an interval of four or five years between their first and second births. Unfortunately, strategies to promote better spacing of pregnancies, especially through the provision of appropriate contraceptive methods, have not been developed and implemented in as many countries would appear justified.

D. FAMILY PLANNING PROGRAMMES AND UNREACHED GROUPS

An important target for family planning programmes is to provide services for the so-called "unreached". Family planning programmes have been progressively reaching younger low-parity mothers in the process of achieving higher acceptance. However, contraceptive use is low among young married women under age 20, and only a small proportion of young couples use contraception between marriage and first pregnancy. Currently, in many of the developing countries in the ESCAP region, more than 70 per cent of women that marry at a young age have at least one child before age 20. In general, the percentage of married women under age 20 using contraception is about half as high as the percentage for all married women of reproductive age. Early pregnancy and child birth can disrupt the physiological and the intellectual development of young girls and can deprive them of education and skill development.

In some countries, premarital sexual activity is common and is increasing. Estimates of the percentage of births conceived out of wedlock are in the range of 10-15 per cent in some countries of the region (ESCAP, 1985). Throughout the world, but especially where rapid urbanization and modernization are occurring, young people are breaking away from constraints applied by their families and communities. Mass media entertainment and advertising are filled with presentations of sex as glamorous and exciting. The taboo against premarital sex is gradually weakening. Moreover, the age at first marriage has risen and continues to rise rapidly. When men and women postpone the age at which they enter marriage, they are more likely to be sexually active before marriage. One can therefore assume that rising proportions of young men and women have become sexually active. Apart from the possibilities of contracting sexually transmitted diseases, including the acquired immunodeficiency syndrome (AIDS),

the risk of an unwanted pregnancy is very high in the absence of the use of contraception.

Surveys undertaken in some developing countries outside the ESCAP region indicate that fewer than half of sexually active youths report that they have ever used contraception. Sexually active men and women cite lack of information as the main reason for not using contraception (Liskin and others, 1985). Young people find it more difficult to obtain contraceptives than older married couples. In most countries, laws restrict young people's access to family planning information and services much more than that for older men and women. Only a very few countries or areas allow all distribution of contraceptives to the unmarried or to young people. For example, in Hong Kong and Thailand, contraceptives are now available to everyone regardless of age. Given the negative consequences of early unplanned motherhood, it is important to recognize the contraceptive needs of sexually active youth. Unfortunately, most family planning programmes do not make special efforts to do so.

Another "unreached" category is sometimes referred to as the "hard core" group, or Pongeem in the Republic of Korea (Ahn and others, 1987). This category consists of couples that want no more children and yet are not currently using any contraceptive method due to lack of social support or dissatisfaction with contraceptive methods. The hard core group often includes poor, minority and disadvantaged groups. Even with a very successful family planning programme, this group is frequently not fully reached. Special efforts are required to identify and reach this group. In summarizing the socio-economic and demographic differentials relating to unmet need, Westoff and Pebley (1981) report that in many countries, particularly in Asia, working women experience a relatively high level of unmet need.

From a historical perspective, in Western countries and in Japan, male methods have played a greater role in fertility control than have female methods; yet they have been largely neglected by most official family planning programmes. Gallen, Liskin and Kak state succinctly the need to involve men in the programmes: "It takes two. For years, many family planning decision-making and practice programmes forgot that" (1986, p. J-889). Obviously, men also play a major role in family planning decision-making and practice. It is estimated that only approximately 8 per cent of the world contraceptive budget is spent on the development of male methods

(IPPF, 1988). Regardless of which partner actually uses a family planning method, the man often has a major say in decisions on child-bearing and family planning. Studies conducted in Hong Kong, Indonesia and Thailand have found that attitudes of the husbands influence the wives' decision as to whether to use family planning (Gallen, Liskin and Kak, 1986). In Indonesia, focus-group research suggests that the husband's influence on use of family planning is strong, especially in early marriage.

Apart from the obviously limited choice of male methods that are currently available, there appear to be two possible reasons that men are not being reached by family planning programmes. First, there is the stereotype that Asian men are not responsive to family planning and that they oppose it. However, the limited evidence suggests that many men do take the responsibility for family planning when they have the information and the means. Secondly, there is reluctance among many health-care professionals and family planning personnel to discuss birth control matters with men. Thus, men usually learn about contraceptives from their wives, friends or the mass media. This situation reflects the primary focus on women by health and family planning professionals. But evidence suggests that there is an interested clientele for family planning programmes that offer men easily accessible high-quality services or encourage men to support their wives' use of contraception.

E. FAMILY PLANNING AND THE QUALITY OF LIFE

In countries that have achieved their targeted fertility levels, the emphasis of population policy has now shifted away from concerns related to population growth to issues of human resource development and the quality of life. Governments are increasingly expressing their determination to improve the educational attainment and socio-economic conditions of the people, particularly the underprivileged groups, and are giving added recognition to planned parenthood as a means by which the quality of life can be improved. In particular, there is concern to improve the position of women, to safeguard and sustain the family value and culture and to alleviate extreme poverty. The exclusive emphasis on fertility reduction, which characterized the early phase of many Asian programmes, has evolved into a wider concern embracing facets of social and family life as well as with environmental issues.

For example, a feature of the current Malaysian programme is the replacement of the traditionally narrower concept of family planning by a comprehensive programme dealing with family health, especially that of children and mothers, responsible parenthood, provisions of kindergartens and nurseries to allow women to combine their dual roles of worker and mother, individual well-being and family planning. Some of the Malaysian initiatives are paralleled in the programme in Thailand, where, for example, nurseries are being encouraged in both the private and public employment sectors.

Concern with the quality of life must also take account of the interrelations between population, environment, resources and development. Traditionally, people lived in harmony with the environment. But that harmony is being disrupted in all countries by increasing population numbers and unplanned development. The undesirable consequences—seen, for example, in the spread of squatter settlements which frequently occurs with rural to urban migration—are well known to family planning workers who visiting communities where government facilities and services are absent. People living in such circumstances need clean water, environmental sanitation, parasite control, nutrition, basic health services—and, of course, family planning. There is now plenty of evidence that family planning and environmental protection, taken together, make good sense and are compatible with the current ideas about developing local self-reliance through popular participation. Family planning should increasingly be placed in the larger framework of population, environment, resources and sustainable development.

F. ROLE OF NON-GOVERNMENTAL ORGANIZATIONS

Non-governmental organizations have long played an useful role in supporting family planning and in complementing government efforts. Gaps in government services remain, especially in remote rural areas, among minority groups and in urban slums. Reaching these underserved populations can be difficult and sometimes politically or otherwise sensitive. The non-governmental organizations, with their more flexible programmes, can provide pragmatic solutions and help pioneer new approaches. They have often focused on community organizations. In addition, non-governmental organizations have also been responsive, albeit on a necessarily limited scale, to the needs of the adolescents and youth. Many of them have in the past acted as important pressure groups for Governments. They have the potential to influence Governments to recognize the problems of youth and adolescents and try to help them establish services for these groups. Similarly, some non-governmental organizations have been found more successful in providing contraceptive services to men than have been official programmes. Their experiences should be transferred to the official programmes in order to strengthen efforts to reach men on a much wider scale.

G. PACIFIC ISLANDS

Except for Papua New Guinea, the Pacific islands and their populations are very small. The island are characterized by their remoteness, their smallness, the social cohesiveness of their communities and their heavy dependence upon subsistence farming and fishing to meet basic needs. Three ethnic groups predominate. Melanesians are the largest group, covering most of the populations of Fiji, Papua New Guinea, Solomon Islands and Vanuatu. Exception for Fiji, the Melanesian countries are characterized by poorly developed physical infrastructure, low literacy and poor health. The Polynesian countries, including Cook Islands, Niue, Western Samoa and Tonga, differ from Melanesia in that they are more cohesive culturally, socially and ethnically. Literacy is high even though economic development is low, and health and other services are well established. Micronesians, the third major group, are mainly inhabitants of the former Trust Territories of the Pacific, that have adopted features of both Melanesian and Polynesian culture.

Fiji stands as an exception among the Pacific populations in having experienced considerable fertility decline, particularly among its Indian population. Much of this decline occurred during the 1970s but slowed during the 1980s. However, the annual growth rate in Fiji is still about 2 per cent. The demography of the other countries in Melanesia can be described as typical of the period of early transition. Fertility remains high, with total fertility about 6.0 (table 43). As there is little overseas migration, rates of growth are high. Polynesian countries have slightly lower fertility, but the rate still remains at almost 5.0. Although death rates are significantly lower than in Melanesia, population growth is very low, being strongly influenced by large net out-migration. In Micronesia, rates of natural increase are among the highest in the Pacific.

While the boldest population programme is in Fiji, there has been a far wider concern that population issues will need to be faced. Resistance to aggressive contraceptive distribution still persists in some Pacific countries, but Papua New Guinea has recognized that the important part health and maternal and child health (MCH) will play in tackling some of the major problems of malnutrition and high infant death rates. Several countries, including Vanuatu and the Federated States of Micronesia, have included strong references to population elements in national development plans, but population programme development and their implementation have not been vigorous.

With high demand on the limited resources of many of the Pacific countries, there is a need for even greater emphasis on integrating population policies into national development. Population programmes to be effective will require strong political commitment. For some time into the future, most of the Pacific countries will require international technical and financial assistance in developing programmes. Various activities will be needed, including revising the relevant legal provisions, developing national family planning programmes and infrastructure, improving data collection and analysis and establishing intergovernmental and agency coordinating machinery. Most important of all these strategies is the strengthening of the skills of national staff in developing and implementing population programmes. This will involve a major effort in training, critically needed to develop the potential of the human resources of the Pacific region.

H. FUTURE PROGRAMME DIRECTIONS

New family planning programmes initiatives are needed for the 1990s and beyond. Such initiatives must take into account two quite different circumstances: first, the very limited progress existing programme strategies have made in curbing high population growth rates in some countries, particularly the poor countries of Southern Asia; secondly, the need to reorient programme strategies in those countries which have succeeded in lowering their rates of population growth.

Although strategies to target individual couples will still play a vital role in family planning programmes, community-oriented approaches should also be encouraged in the poorer developing countries where continued rapid population growth exacerbates many other endemic problems. In such countries, there is a need to motivate couples to adopt family planning practice and to provide regular services of safe and acceptable contraceptive methods. Awareness creation and community campaigns could help create a better understanding of the benefits of small families and thereby increase motivation for family planning acceptance.

Breast-feeding should be vigorously promoted because it is important for infant health and contributes to child-spacing. Proper emphasis should be placed on the benefit of child-spacing, particularly among younger women. It is also necessary to ensure that contraceptive methods shall always be available and accessible. The provision of services to young people needs to be improved to minimize the incidence of illegitimate and unwanted births.

New programmes should be developed to reach young working men and women, particularly at their workplaces, and should include a variety of family planning activities, such as lectures and group meetings. Special efforts are needed to establish family planning and MCH services for vulnerable and underprivileged groups so as to improve their reproductive health. Fresh attempts should also be made to reach men by strengthening information, education and communication and by improving the male methods through more vigorous research. In each of these areas there is potential to gain from the experiences of non-governmental organizations, which should continue to persuade Governments to encourage the wider application of their innovative approaches and methods.

The priority measures must be country-specific and will depend upon the demographic and socio-economic contexts and political commitment, as well as upon the available resources. However, there are some common objectives which cut across all situations, such as the need for family planning programmes to reach the underprivileged groups, to encourage and promote birth-spacing and breast-feeding. Judging from the lessons learned so far, a key factor in determining whether future measures are likely to succeed in the least developed countries is the strength of political commitment and support for the programmes.

I. CONCLUSION

Population policies and family planning programmes in the countries of the ESCAP region have passed through three distinct phases during the past three decades. With much reduced rates of population growth in several countries, not surprisingly population policies and programmes now include a broader range of areas than mere population control. They also cover the implications of changes in the age structure, particularly the anticipated rise in the numbers and proportions of the elderly, migration and the excessive growth of large urban centres, the health and welfare of women and children; and, most recently, the interactions between population, resources, environment and sustainable development.

However, it must be reiterated that policies to reduce rates of population growth are still of prime importance in several ESCAP countries. In these countries, the priority is to lower fertility levels, and new strategies in their national family planning programmes are urgently required. In countries that have already succeeded in lowering their population growth rates, the emphasis of programmes will need to change and cover issues concerning the development and well-being of the family, women, youth and the underprivileged.

Serious efforts by national Governments as well as international organizations willl be needed to help define and deal with various population issues in the 1990s and beyond. Research on fertility, family planning and other demographic issues will remain important to help keep policy makers and planners informed about current and prospective population trends and implications for sustainable development.

REFERENCES

Ahn, Kye-Choon, and others (1987). The "unreached" in family planning: a case study of the Republic of Korea. *Asia-Pacific Population Journal* (Bangkok), vol. 2, No. 2 (June), pp. 23-44.

Bakker, M. L. (1990). *Population of the South Pacific: An Overview of Demographic Levels, Patterns and Trends*. Demographic Report No. 1, Population Studies Programme. Suva, Fiji: University of the South Pacific.

Bongaarts, John, and Susan Greenhalgh (1985). An alternative to the one-child policy in China. *Population and Development Review* (New York), vol. 11, No. 4 (December), pp. 585-617.

Gallen, Moira E., Laurie Liskin and Neeraj Kak (1986). *Men: New Focus for Family Planning Programs*. Population Reports, Series J, No. 33. Baltimore, Maryland: The Johns Hopkins University, Population Information Program.

Hobcraft, John, John W. McDonald and Shea Rotstein (1983). Child-spacing effects on infant and early child mortality. *Population Index* (Princeton), vol. 49, No. 4 (Winter), pp. 585-618.

International Planned Parenthood Federation (1988). *Medical Bulletin* (London), vol. 22, No. 4 (August), pp. 1-4.

Leete, Richard (1992). Determinants of fertility behaviour and change in Asia. In *Family Planning Programmes in Asia and the Pacific: Implications for the 1990s*. Asian Population Studies Series, No. 116. Bangkok, Thailand: Economic and Social Commission for Asia and the Pacific.

_____, and Iqbal Alam (1992). *The Revolution in Asian Fertility: Dimensions, Causes and Implications*. New York: Oxford University Press; and Oxford, United Kingdom: Clarendon Press.

Liskin, Laurie, and others (1985). *Youth in the 1980s: Social and Health Concerns*. Population Reports, Series M, No. 9. Baltimore, Maryland: The Johns Hopkins University, Population Information Program.

Mauldin, W. Parker, and John A. Ross (1992). Management lessons. In *Family Planning Programmes in Asia and the Pacific: Implications for the 1990s*. Asian Population Studies Series, No. 116. Bangkok: Economic and Social Commission for Asia and the Pacific.

Reich, Julie (1987). The international conference on better health for women and children through family planning. *International Family Planning Perspectives* (New York), vol. 13, No. 3 (September), pp. 86-89.

Sathar, Zeba A. (1992). Determinants of successful family planning/welfare programmes. In *Family Planning Programmes in Asia and the Pacific: Implications for the 1990s*. Asian Population Studies Series, No. 116. Bangkok: Economic and Social Commission for Asia and the Pacific.

Trussell, James (1986). The impact of birth spacing on fertility. *International Family Planning Perspectives* (New York), vol. 12, No. 3 (September), pp. 80-82.

United Nations (1987). *World Population Policies*, vol. I, *Afghanistan to France*. Population Studies, No. 102. Sales No. E.87.XIII.4.

_____ (1990). *Demographic Yearbook, 1980*. Sales No. E/F.90.XIII.1.

_____ (1993). *World Population Prospects: The 1992 Revision*. Sales No. E.93.XIII.7.

_____ (1985). Consideration of emerging issues and regional activities: adolescent fertility. Report submitted to the Committee on Population at its fourth session. E/ESCAP/POP.4/13.

_____, Economic and Social Commission for Asia and the Pacific (1988). *Report of the Study on theOrganizational Issues in Community Participation in National Family Planning Programmes: A Comparative Analysis of Five Countries in the ESCAP Region*. Asian Population Studies Series, No. 87. Bangkok.

Westoff, Charles F., and Anne R. Pebley (1981). Alternative measures of unmet need for family planning in developing countries. *International Family Planning Perspectives* (New York), vol. 7, No. 4 (December), pp. 126-135.

World Health Organization (1991). *Maternal Mortality: A Global Factbook*. Compiled by Carla AbouZahr abd Erica Royston. Geneva.

XXXI. FUTURE CONTRACEPTIVE REQUIREMENTS: THE POTENTIAL ROLE OF LOCAL PRODUCTION IN MEETING THE NEEDS OF DEVELOPING COUNTRIES

Program for Appropriate Technology in Health[*]

Family planning programmes in the developing countries have made a great deal of progress during the past 20 years. Looking ahead to the next decade, however, it is clear that maintaining their momentum will be difficult. On the one hand, there will be a greatly increased demand for contraceptives, due in part to the increased effectiveness of family planning education. On the other hand, the international donor community, aware of the tremendous cost of the commodities required to satisfy this expected demand, realizes its limited ability to provide what is needed. Governments of developing countries and donors need new strategies to provide efficiently for family planning programmes, and they are working to develop a specific plan for meeting future contraceptive demand. This paper discusses the recent estimates and projections of commodity requirements that have been developed as part of this plan and assess the current and potential role of local production in meeting those requirements.

A. OVERVIEW OF DONOR INVOLVEMENT IN LOCAL PRODUCTION

One strategy that has a record of achievement in several developing countries is that of developing the capability for local production of contraceptives. Manufacturing contraceptives locally would not be appropriate everywhere, and there are some countries where demand is not high enough to warrant the investment. In many developing countries, however, contraceptive production is appropriate; and the Governments of these countries are interested in exploring how, with donor assistance, they can achieve it. International donor agencies, for their part, see support of local production as a way to encourage self-sufficiency, and they are willing to play a catalytic role as well as provide direct support. Over the past two decades, both multilateral funding and bilateral funding have been used for feasibility studies, which have been catalysts for action,

as well as for implementation of local production projects. International organizations that have been involved in local production projects include the United Nations Population Fund, the United Nations Development Programme, the United Nations Industrial Development Organization, the World Health Organization and the World Bank. They have been able to cooperate on these projects with a variety of national Governments and bilateral agencies, including the international development agencies of Australia, Denmark, Canada and the United States of America. Other organizations that have been active in local production activities include the Population Council and the Program for Appropriate Technology in Health/Program for the Introduction and Adaptation of Contraceptive Technology (PATH/PIACT). A wide range of support has been given to local production, including funding for studies of supply and demand in the public sector, studies of availability of raw materials, financial feasibility studies and technical assistance for establishing full or partial production of a variety of contraceptives (see table 44).

B. CONTRACEPTIVE NEEDS AND LOCAL PRODUCTION IN 16 CORE COUNTRIES

The capacity exists for a large percentage of international contraceptive needs to be satisfied by locally produced commodities. An analysis of the populations of all developing countries shows that 16 countries represent 90 per cent of current contraceptive consumption in the developing world: Bangladesh; Brazil; Cameroon; China; Colombia; Egypt; India; Indonesia; Mexico; Pakistan; the Philippines; Republic of Korea; Thailand; Turkey; Viet Nam; and Zimbabwe. In 1990, 5 of these 16 countries had the capacity (or were nearing the capacity) to produce sufficient contraceptive commodities to meet their own requirements. These five—Brazil, China, India, Indonesia and Mexico—are among the most populous developing countries: they

---

[*] Seattle, Washington, United States of America.

TABLE 44. CONTRACEPTIVE PRODUCTION IN SELECTED COUNTRIES, BY METHOD AND DONOR INVOLVEMENT, SINCE 1970

	Contraceptive method				Donor and/or executing agency involvement	
Country	Oral contraceptives	Intra-uterine device	Condom	Injectables	UNFPA	Other[a]
Bangladesh	Multinational	—	Private (under consideration), Government (under consideration)	—	Oral contraceptives and condom feasibility	PATH/PIACT
Brazil	Multinational	Private local	Private local, multinational	Private local, multinational	—	The Population Council, USAID (preliminary condom feasibility)
Cameroon	—	—	—	—	Condom feasibility	—
China	Government	Government	Government	Government	Production: all methods	The Population Council PATH/PIACT
Colombia	Multinational	—	—	Multinational	—	—
Cuba	Government	—	—	—	Oral contraceptive production	PATH/PIACT
Democratic People's Republic of Korea . . .	—	Government (under consideration)	—	—	IUD feasibility	PATH/PIACT
Egypt	Government	Government (under consideration), private (under consideration)	—	—	IUD feasibility	The Population Council; GTZ (raw materials); USAID (Lippes Loop,[a] oral contraceptive feasibility); PATH/PIACT
India	Government multinational	Government (under development), private (under development)	Government multinational	—	IUD and condom feasibility IUD and condom production	The Population Council USAID (Lippes Loop[a] oral contraceptive feasibility); PATH/PIACT
Indonesia	Government multinational	Government	Government	Multinational	IUD feasibility IUD production	Netherlands; the Population Council; USAID (Lippes Loop[a] oral contraceptive production); PATH/PIACT

TABLE44 (*continued*)

Country	Contraceptive method				Donor and/or executing agency involvement	
	Oral contraceptives	Intra-uterine device	Condom	Injectables	UNFPA	Other[a]
Mexico	Multinational private local	Private local	Private local (manual dipping), local screening and packaging	Multinational private local	—	USAID (condom packaging)
Pakistan	Multinational	Private local	Government (under consideration)	Multinational	—	The Population Council; USAID (Lippes Loop[a] condom, injectables, oral contraceptive feasibility); PATH/PIACT
Philippines	Private local	—	—	—	—	PATH/PIACT (condom, oral contraceptive pre-feasibility)
Republic of Korea	Multinational	Private local	Multinational, local	—	—	—
Thailand	Multinational	—	Private local	Private local	—	—
Turkey	Multinational	—	Private (under consideration)	—	Condom, IUD opportunity study	UNIDO (condom feasibility)
Viet Nam	Multinational (under consideration	Government (under consideration)	Government	—	IUD and condom feasibility, condom production	FINIDA/AIDAB; PATH.PIACT
Zimbabwe	Multinational (under consideration	—	—	—	—	USAID (oral contraceptive feasibility)

NOTES: Private = private ownership. Multinational = generally either export their products to developing countries for local packaging or carry out partial or complete manufacture in developing countries; in both instances, operations are carried out by subsidiaries or in joint ventures. Government = Government-controlled. Local = owned by business people from the developing country (some minor amounts of foreign capital may be involved).

IUD = intra-uterine device; PATH = Program for Appropriate Technology in Health; PIACT = Program for the Introduction and Adaptation of Contraceptive Technology; UNFPA = United Nations Population Fund; UNIDO = United Nations Industrial Development Organization; USAID = United States Agency for International Development.

[a]Late 1960s and early 1970s.

represent 71 per cent of the total combined commodity requirements for the 16 countries mentioned above. The aggregate capacity for contraceptive production therefore seems to be nearing the point of meeting the commodity requirements of a large part of the developing world. Thus, capacity itself is not the major problem in local production. The problems, or areas where assistance is needed, are:

(a) Quality of the final product. There are problems of products not meeting standards, of outmoded contraceptive technologies, of ineffective or in some cases unsafe products and of formulas that are no longer recommended.

(b) Availability of a range of method choices to family planning programmes within each country. This step requires procurement and distribution of commodities both in countries where local production is taking place and in locations where it is not feasible.

Data have been collected on commodity requirements in 1990 and projected requirements in the year 2000 for these 16 countries for four contraceptive methods: oral contraceptives; intra-uterine devices (IUDs); injectables; and condoms. For three of the methods, estimated production capacity for 1990 and for 2000 exceeds the estimated method-specific commodity requirements for all 16 countries combined. Only the production capacity for oral contraceptives is projected to fall short of the required amounts. The figures suggest that local production is currently a viable factor in the supply of contraceptives to developing countries and that strategies to enhance local production by encouraging expanded or improved production, better quality assurance techniques and more advanced regulatory capability could help ensure contraceptive supplies in the future.

C. FEASIBILITY OF LOCAL PRODUCTION

Each country has a unique set of variables that affect the feasibility of local production, and economic and political conditions may often override all other variables for a period of time. One of the key elements that decides feasibility of local production is demand. Countries with a small total population size and/or insufficient use of a specific contraceptive method would have little long-term prospect for local production of that method because the demand would probably not amount to the minimum annual production volumes needed to cover investment and operating costs. Even for those countries, however, local production cannot be completely ruled out. The combined trends of increasing numbers in the target population, an increase in the number of potential contraceptive users, a changing contraceptive method mix and product diversification could eventually result in local manufacture of contraceptives in a country that currently appears to be an unlikely candidate. To determine feasibility of future local production, a series of studies could be done, progressing from an initial inquiry to in-depth analysis, including opportunity studies (level of interest, contraceptive need), pre-feasibility studies (technological capability and potential, local resources) and feasibility studies (identification of market, materials and financial resources, national will). Adequate planning is key to the long-term sustainability of local production.

D. KEY LESSONS LEARNED AND PLANNING OF FUTURE PROJECTS

Several factors have proved to be important considerations during the past 10 years of international donor support of local production of contraceptives. Careful, long-term planning is required in order to ensure the success of a project, including assessment of: *(a)* long-term demand for a given method; *(b)* in-country technical capability specific to the product under consideration; *(c)* financial feasibility; *(d)* degree of success of similar projects in this country; *(e)* capacity to sustain necessary inputs and to purchase and distribute the product.

All parties involved in local production need to be consulted as early as possible during the planning process. Care must be taken to build a consensus among all of those affected—government and non-governmental organization family planning providers, social marketing programmes, private and government pharmaceutical and medical device manufacturers, regulatory agencies, financial institutions and interested donor agencies.

The contraceptive method and/or product to be produced should be selected based on a thorough analysis of product safety and efficacy, production costs and user preferences. Information on safety can be obtained from clinical data from comparative trials conducted in the country and/or elsewhere. Information on acceptability and user preferences can be obtained using qualitative research methodology. Clinicians and government officials also should have an opportunity to provide input.

The issue of demand for the output of a local production facility should be resolved before further resources are invested in assessing the feasibility of local production. Prior to embarking on a production project for a particular product, an essential requirement is for the manufacturer to know that, assuming the product to be produced meets standards and specifications, a buyer is assured. Where the public sector is crucial to the success of a local production project, the manufacturer needs an expression of intent from the Ministry of Health (or other responsible government agency) to purchase the quantities required for its family planning programmes.

During the project formulation stage, appropriate sources of funds to cover operating costs should be identified. In general, from 20 to 40 per cent of operating costs must be paid with foreign currency; from 60 to 80 per cent can be paid with local currency. The availability of foreign currency is often a major constraint and can cause production to slow or halt altogether. Foreign currency will certainly be required for spare parts and accessories, and possibly for on-site vendor repair and/or maintenance services. Depending upon local resources, it may be necessary to import raw materials and/or packaging material.

A thorough review of anticipated cost may show donors and local planners that lower unit costs for labour will be offset by higher costs for utilities, raw materials and packaging materials. Therefore, the locally made product may only be marginally cheaper or even more expensive than products procured from established commodity suppliers. This higher cost should be reviewed and compared partially on the basis of the reduced foreign-exchange requirements for locally produced products.

Technical support to facilitate local production can be provided in several different stages during the manufacturing process. Support from donors could range from funding of opportunity, pre-feasibility and feasibility studies to upgrading and/or expanding existing production facilities and quality assurance institutions, to initiation of production. Establishment of a new facility would be feasible in countries where existing and projected demand are high enough; and such may be the case in Bangladesh (condoms), Egypt (IUDs and eventually condoms), Mexico (condoms), Pakistan (condoms),

Turkey (condoms and eventually IUDs), Viet Nam (IUDs) and Zimbabwe (oral contraceptives). However, most countries with sufficient demand to warrant the capital investment to establish local production already have manufacturing plants in operation.

There is scope for a wide variety of technical assistance in countries with existing production of contraceptives. For example, donor funds could be used to upgrade production by supporting technical assistance in product reformulation (such as upgrading 21- or 22-day pill package formats to 28-day package formats), technical training (such as training and audits related to good manufacturing practices for sterile medical device manufacture in countries that are current or potential manufacturers of IUDs) or purchase of imported production equipment and analytical instruments. Donor funds could also be used to expand production capacity, primarily through the purchase of imported equipment.

Quality assurance is a key area where donor support can contribute to contraceptive self-reliance in developing countries. Before developing countries can depend upon local production as a major source of commodities for their family planning programmes, they must develop the institutional capability to monitor the quality of both imported and locally produced contraceptives to ensure that these commodities shall meet internationally accepted standards. Building institutional capacity for quality assurance not only increases the certainty that locally procured contraceptives are safe and effective but also protects users from poor-quality imported products that otherwise might enter the market. Technical assistance can be provided at the level of the national Government to ensure that the infrastructure for regulatory oversight of contraceptive quality shall be sufficient. Other opportunities exist to provide technical assistance to both private and Government-owned facilities for their internal quality control programmes, for example, through audits and training for good manufacturing practices and good laboratory practices and by ensuring compliance with health, safety and environmental regulations.

REFERENCES

Bergsman, Joel, and Wayne Edisis (1988). *Debt-equity Swaps and Foreign Direct Investment in Latin America*. International Finance Corporation Discussion Paper, No. 2. Washington, D.C.: The World Bank.

Chafetz, L., and E. Parrott (1987). Assessment of the technical and economic feasibility of manufacturing oral contraceptives in Zimbabwe. Prepared for the United States Agency for International Development, Bureau of Science and Technology, Office of Population.

Free, Michael J. (1982a). Copper-T 380 Ag intrauterine device: quality control procedures. Seattle, Washington: Program for the Introduction and Adaptation of Contraceptive Technology.

_____ (1982b). Local production of contraceptives in Bangladesh: a study of options, impact, and cost. Report to the United Nations Fund for Population Activities. Seattle, Washington: Program for the Introduction and Adaptation of Contraceptive Technology.

_____ (1982c). Options of IUD production capability in developing countries. Seattle, Washington: Program for the Introduction and Adaptation of Contraceptive Technology.

_____ (1985). Options for condom production capability in developing countries. Seattle, Washington: Program for the Introduction and Adaptation of Contraceptive Technology.

_____ , R. T. Mahoney and G. W. Perkin (1984). Transfer of contraceptive production technology to developing countries. *PIACT Paper* (Seattle, Washington), No. 9 (February).

Free, Michael, and others (1984). Local production of contraceptives in developing countries. *International Family Planning Perspectives* (New York), vol. 10, No. 1 (March), pp. 2-7.

Gerofi, J. (1988). Draft report on an exploratory mission: condom manufacture in Bangladesh. Seattle, Washington: Program for the Introduction and Adaptation of Contraceptive Technology.

Gillespie D. G., and others (1988). Financing the delivery of contraceptives: the challenge of the next twenty years. Paper presented at the National Academy of Sciences Conference on the Demographic and Programmatic Consequences of Contraceptive Innovation. Unpublished.

Goldberg, Howard I., and others (1989). Knowledge about condoms and their use in less developed countries during a period of rising AIDS prevalence. *Bulletin of the World Health Organization* (Geneva), vol. 67, No. 1, pp. 85-91.

Hutchings, J., and L. Saunders (1985). Assessing the characteristics and cost-effectiveness of contraceptive methods. *PIACT Paper* (Seattle, Washington), No. 10 (August).

International Science and Technology Institute (1988). *Population Technical Assistance Project: Contraceptive Social Marketing Assessment*, vol. 1, *Worldwide Review;* vol. 2, *Six Country Reports*. Prepared for the United States Agency for International Development. Washington, D.C.

Kabalikat Ng Pamilyang Pilipino (1980). The technical and economic feasibility of manufacturing condoms in the Philippines to supply the national population program. A report to the Commission on Population. Manila.

Kleinman, Ronald L. (1988). *Directory of Hormonal Contraceptives.* London: International Planned Parenthood Federation.

Kocher, J. E., and B. C. Buckner (1989). Estimates of global resources required to meet population goals by 2010. Unpublished. Research Triangle Park, North Carolina: Research Triangle Institute.

Kuppuswamy, K. (1989). Personal communication.

Lach, J. L., P. H. Bronnenkant and L. J. Bronnenkant (1982). Contraceptive manufacturing in India. A report commissioned by the United States Agency for International Development, New Delhi.

Lee, Luke T. (1975). Laws regulating contraceptive supply, demand and procurement: country profiles, checklists and summaries. Prepared for the International Contraceptive Study Project, United Nations Fund for Population Activities.

Lewis, Maureen A., and Genevieve Kenney (1987). *The Private Sector and Family Planning in Developing Countries: Its Role, Achievements and Potential.* Washington, D.C.: The Urban Institute.

Mahoney, R. T. (1982). Production and distribution capabilities for new fertility planning technologies over the next two decades: world population and fertility planning technologies, the next 20 years. Washington, D.C.: Congress of the United States, Office of Technology Assessment.

Population Services International (1988). *Social Marketing Forum* (Washington, D.C.), No. 15 (Fall).

_____ (1989). *Social Marketing Forum* (Washington, D.C.), No. 16 (Spring).

Program for Appropriate Technology in Health (1989). Target countries for World Health Organization global programme on AIDS condom quality management in Africa: a preliminary assessment. Seattle, Washington.

Program for the Introduction and Adaptation of Contraceptive Technology (1979). Quality control procedures for contraceptive products: a manual. Seattle, Washington.

_____ (1980). Production of IUDs in Indonesia. Consulting report to the Badan Koordinasi Keluarga Berencana Nasional (BKKBN). Unpublished. Seattle, Washington.

_____ (1981). Condom production in the Socialist Republic of Vietnam. Report to the United Nations Fund for Population Activities. Seattle, Washington.

_____ (1987). Copper T 200B intrauterine device quality control procedures. Seattle, Washington.

_____ (1988). The feasibility of production of IUDs in Egypt. Seattle, Washington.

_____ (1988b). Long-life Copper-T intrauterine devices: test procedures for manufacturing quality control and independent quality audit. Seattle: Washington.

_____ (1990). Testing of condoms in the field: a handbook. Seattle, Washington.

Schwartz, J. B., and others (1989). The effect of contraceptive prices on method choice in the Philippines, Jamaica, and Thailand. In *Choosing a Contraceptive: Method Choice in Asia and the United States*, Rodolfo A. Bulatao, James A. Palmore and Sandra E. Ward, eds. Boulder, Colorado: Westview Press.

Sebastian, K., and J. Gerofi (1988). Draft prefeasibility study for condom production in Turkey. Seattle, Washington: Program for Appropriate Technology in Health.

Sherris J., and G. W. Perkin (1988). Introducing new contraceptive technologies in developing countries. Paper presented at the National Academy of Sciences Conference on the Demographic and Programmatic Consequences of Contraceptive Innovation. Unpublished.

United Nations Development Programme (1975). Final report and recommendations of international contraceptive study project. New York.

United Nations Industrial Development Organization (1978). Manual for the preparation of industrial feasibility studies. New York.

United States Agency for International Development (1986). A.I.D. policy determination implementing A.I.D. privatization objectives. Washington, D.C.

_____ (1987). Privatization: technical assessment. Prepared for the Bureau for Program and Policy Coordination, Office of Policy Development and Program Review. Washington, D.C.

_____ (1989). A.I.D. announces debt for development initiative. Washington, D.C.

_____ (1989). Communication to A.I.D. missions. Subject: new funding: private provision of social services. Washington, D.C.

_____ (1989). *Users' Guide to the Office of Population.* Washington, D.C.

_____ (1990). Overview of A.I.D. asssistance, commodities and program support. Prepared by Commodities and Program Support Division, Office of Population, Bureau for Science and Technology. Washington, D.C.

XXXII. DIFFUSION OF INNOVATIVE BEHAVIOUR, AND INFORMATION, EDUCATION AND COMMUNICATION

Scott Wittet and Elaine Murphy[*]

[*]Technology Management Department, Program for Appropriate Technology in Health, Seattle, Washington, United States of America.

A. CONTEMPORARY COMMUNICATION APPROACHES: SEEING THROUGH ANOTHER'S EYES

Information, education and communication (IEC) activities are often characterized as having three basic purposes: raising awareness; motivating for behaviour change; or teaching appropriate behaviour (such as correct condom use). All of these activities are directed to influencing the knowledge, attitudes and actions of current and potential contraceptive users. The underlying assumption of traditional communication programmes is that central planners, or family planning service providers, know what is good for their patients and that the patients share the same needs and goals as programme staff. Most clients or potential clients are assumed to be like empty pots waiting to be "filled" with useful knowledge that they will then act on it in a rational manner. When patients do not accept the information or help offer them or do not correctly adopt new behaviour, they are labelled "difficult" or "non-compliant."

Over the past decade or more, there has been a growing recognition that health and family planning programmes cannot afford to make such assumptions if they wish to succeed. There is an understanding that rather than being passive recipients of instructions, clients are active decision makers motivated by a variety of logical, emotional and physiological forces. Many of these motivations do not appear reasonable to others, especially people that are culturally or socio-economically different from the clients. Individuals judge the value of behaviour, for example, having many children or choosing to limit family size, in a broad social context which includes all types of personal considerations. Although all people face some constraints in their behaviour, most have some degree of personal power over many aspects of their lives and will act in their own interests as they see them. They will reject information or recommendations deemed irrelevant, inappropriate or not credible. Often they will even reject behaviours that they know to be in their best interests because other

forces override the desire to promote good health and long life ("I am going to stop smoking . . . one of these days"). Health programmers, service providers and communicators often find themselves at a loss when dealing with such "irrational" actions.

Successful communicators—whether politicians, advertisers or health behaviour change agents—find ways to understand people's family health needs and desires (and constraints on their ability to act), and create means to help people meet those needs. Research models, such as Dervin's "sense-making approach (Dervin, 1989 and 1992), and related qualitative and quantitative methods for gathering data useful for programme design and evaluation, focus on the interior experience of clients, not the perceptions or goals of others. These models posit that people make sense out of life as they move through different situations and face different types of questions or problems. Understanding how people make sense, and for what purposes, can help define communication programme direction. As Dervin explains, sense-making rests on a complex set of assumptions for which the bottom line is the development and implementation of a methodological perspective that tries to see and interpret people as they see and interpret themselves. Thus, assessment of needs and accountability can be based on useful foundations rather than on the myths about people arising from the bureaucratic perspectives implemented in most current research approaches. One premise of sense-making is that failures in system and programme design result from faulty research approaches which treat bureaucratic definitions of people as concrete forms. Such definitions can only succeed as frameworks if the bureaucracy has complete control over people, an untenable assumption in most cases.

One use of sense-making research techniques is to generate descriptive findings which portray the needs, assessments, thoughts, questions etc., of persons involved in a particular context. Thus, for example, a sense-making study of women's acceptance and management of contraceptives in Kenya and Zambia found that some women's sense-making is governed by fear (of neighbours knowing she is using contraceptives or of her husband refusing to support method use) and loneliness (not having anyone with whom to discuss family planning issues) (Dervin, 1992).

B. IMPORTANCE OF QUALITY OF CARE AND EFFECTIVE INTERPERSONAL COMMUNICATION IN FAMILY PLANNING PROGRAMMES

Progressive family planning programme managers have begun to broaden programme evaluation criteria beyond measures of quantities of service provided (number of clients seen or number of intra-uterine devices (IUDs) inserted) and have begun to include a focus on the quality of services. Quality is defined not only in terms of improved clinical skills but also in terms of the personal experience of the client using the system (e.g., reduced waiting times, pleasant interactions with staff and satisfaction with the services provided).

The quality of the client's "communication experience" is an important aspect of this new focus. Research findings such as those mentioned in the African example suggest that although mass media and impersonal communication channels continue to have an important role in family planning IEC, interpersonal communication and counselling play a crucial role in effectively coping with individual fears by exploring personalized coping strategies and providing a sympathetic listener and credible, interactive information sources. Some persons, especially those that exhibit more authoritarian communication styles or who resent "irrational" behaviour from clients, find the interpersonal communication focus on careful listening, compassionate understanding and creative counselling to be too "soft" for their tastes. However, experience shows that even in traditionally hierarchical family planning programmes (such as those in China and Viet Nam) new interpersonal communication styles can be successfully taught and implemented, once the benefits become evident to practitioners.

C. IMPLICATIONS FOR IEC AND TRAINING PROGRAMME AND MESSAGE DEVELOPMENT

The Program for Appropriate Technology for Health (PATH) has drawn the following conclusions from its long history of working in family planning communication.

Rather than asking how one can motivate the public to behave in ways that will help providers meet programme objectives, one should be asking how the programme and the larger social context can be changed to better relate to the needs of people, to provide them with better quality of service and to improve access to relevant information and care.

IEC and training programmes (which can be thought of as IEC for staff) should be based on findings of audience research methods keyed to the world view of the client or the trainee, in addition to the programme focus of the administration. Training and IEC media materials have as their objective cultural appropriateness, while interpersonal efforts should target individual appropriateness.

Clients will ignore information that is too difficult for them to cope with and will reject behaviour too challenging to implement. Although negative messages (fear appeals, threats and warnings) may have their place in a set of IEC messages, they should not overwhelm the audience. Positive and feasible recommendations for action should outweigh negatively toned information. A series of acquired immunodeficiency syndrome (AIDS) prevention workshops for prostitutes in Thailand included a brief section in which a "doctor" showed frightening pictures of AIDS-related diseases; in general, however, the sessions emphasized types of behaviour for avoiding infection and helped the sex workers build skills for negotiating condom use and safer sex with customers.

Individuals most often act in their own immediate interests; they rarely find appeals to national goals and objectives convincing. Demographic arguments for family planning have proved less persuasive than arguments related to an individual's day-to-day needs and experience. Research conducted in Nepal found strong support for the concept of birth-spacing to improve maternal and child health but little interest in changing behaviour on the basis of the demographically oriented "small family, happy family" approach.

Each communication medium has its advantages and disadvantages. Providing a mix of media has proved to be most effective for maximum impact. Each medium should be chosen according to the purpose of the intervention. Media choices include printed materials for literate and/or illiterate audiences, broadcast media, video, cassettes and traditional or performance media. Interpersonal communication and counselling, currently the only medium that can provide the interaction needed to answer questions as they arise, calm fears and develop creative solutions to unique problems, should be the foundation of every IEC programme. Unfortunately, building strong staff interpersonal skills is challenging, and activities to improve the quality of this medium are often overlooked or underbudgeted.

"Edutainment" (packaging educational information in entertaining formats, such as songs, dramas and films) has been popular since the days of the first storytellers. It is now being implemented for health and family planning purposes.

D. IEC AND TRAINING PROGRAMME EVALUATION

Evaluating communication programmes is extremely challenging. The "bottom line" is always to relate IEC efforts to increases in couple-years of contraceptive protection, which is difficult without establishing expensive research programmes. However, it is relatively easy to gather qualitative data documenting people's reactions to a given message or to use surveys to record changes in knowledge or reported behaviour. Furthermore, many of the interventions one might seek to measure, the effectiveness of counselling, for example, have not yet been adequately defined. What is meant by good counselling? Can counselling take place in a group setting or is that "education"? How can counselling be broken down into measurable units?

The long process of resolving some of these important evaluation issues has begun, but much additional work needs to be done. Acceptable standards for quality of interpersonal counselling and other communication interventions must be developed along with check-lists for data collection. Evaluators must be trained with a focus on reliability between evaluators. Lastly, and most importantly, ways must be found conceptually to link quality of communication and levels of contraceptive acceptance, continuation and compliance. With quantitative scores and a sufficiently large sample, one could try to ascertain which communication interventions, and interpersonal communication and counselling behaviour, are best able to bring about desired outcomes. These outcomes might then be linked to couple-years of contraceptive protection.

E. FUTURE DIRECTIONS

It is proposed that the efforts described below are worthy of continuing or future support.

Through training programmes, staff perceptions of clients as passive beneficiaries must be changed. Instead. clients should be respected as the active, empowered decision makers they are (at least in some compliance situations).

More health and family planning programmes should include objectives and evaluation criteria related to quality of care, including quality of communication, in addition to reporting service units or number of clients served.

Staff training courses in interpersonal communication and counselling are needed, along with administrative support for caring, quality-oriented IEC and service attitudes.

Sources of interpersonal health and family planning information outside the normal clinic and health fieldworker channels are being tapped in many programmes, but much more creative work needs to be done. Mothers-in-law and "aunties" have been recruited as health promoters in some programmes, but not to the extent possible. Gossip networks have proved effective in spreading "bad news" about family planning, perhaps they could also be used to spread the good word. In Nepal, adult literacy programmes provide access to villagers that attend schools or enter hospitals. Family planning programmers can make use of literacy outreach in other countries as well.

Innovative means of interacting with clients and encouraging clients to interact with one another should also be explored. In Peru, colouring books linking common domestic and societal problems (such as domestic violence, unemployment and strikes) were found to be wonderful means for getting women to talk about their life and their needs and to explore solutions to their problems. Family planning interventions naturally arose out of these discussions.

Programme staff must be trained in research techniques appropriate to their abilities and resources. Not all studies require high levels of funding, time and staff involvement. Qualitative techniques are relatively easy to implement (once staff gain experience) and can yield a wealth of data useful for programme design and IEC and training materials development.

Access to services and information must be improved at all levels. This includes everything from increasing availability of family planning counsellors in village clinics to making computers more "user friendly". Soon it will be common to work with electronic books containing libraries full of information in a lightweight package. New, intuitive software will be needed to help people navigate through the oceans of information at their fingertips.

F. CONCLUSION

Health and family planning IEC has evolved rapidly during the past few decades. Innovative ways of helping clients get information and increase control over their life are being invented almost every day. Although some family planning IEC programmes still focus on awareness-building, others have moved beyond that early stage to address more complex issues of behaviour change and provide more detailed information to a sophisticated populace. The current mandate is to build on the successes of the past and to focus on providing better services and communication in the future.

REFERENCES

Dervin, Brenda (1989). Audience as listener and learner, teacher and confidant: the sense-making approach. In *Public Communication Campaigns*, Ronald E. Rice and Charles E. Atkins, eds. 2nd ed. Newbury Park, California: Sage Publications.

_____ (1992). Personal communication.

Hirstiio-Snellman, Paula (in press). Acceptance and management of modern contraceptives by Kenyan and Zambian women. In *Methodology between the Cracks*, vol. 2, *Sense-making Issues and Exemplars*. Cresskill, New York: Hampton Press.

XXXIII. INSTITUTION-BUILDING FOR QUALITY SERVICES

The Center for Development and Population Activities*

A. RATIONALE

Quality of care is important to family planning programmes for two reasons: (*a*) it enables clients to exercise their basic right to control their reproductive life; and (*b*) it contributes to increased adoption and sustained use of contraception. Quality services enable a client to reach and implement a family planning decision that meets her or his reproductive intentions. Women are the chief beneficiaries of quality services because their low status in society is perpetuated by early pregnancies, high fertility and limited sexuality education.

Meeting the client's personal family planning needs is the major focus of a quality family planning programme. Key elements of a quality service are represented by the acronym ACCESS: accessibility/acceptability; choice; continuity of method; effective and competent providers; sensitivity to client needs and interpersonal relations; and sharing information (for specific indicators, see annex I). Each of these elements contributes to increased contraceptive use by increasing clients' options, ability to use contraception effectively and desire to return in the future. Satisfied users generally help recruit new clients.

A focus on improving the quality of family planning services to meet individual needs is consistent with meeting national objectives of fertility reduction because of their impact on continuation rates. In many countries, contraceptive prevalence rates rise to roughly 35 per cent as services become more accessible, but prevalence then levels off because new adopters merely replace those discontinuing use. To raise contraceptive prevalence to the higher levels needed for fertility reduction, improvements in quality of care are necessary in order to retain current users while reaching out to new clients.

Promoting quality services may have other benefits to family planning agencies, such as improved staff morale, reduced staff turnover, better community relations and increased programme efficiency.

Institutionalizing quality of care

Policy makers and programme managers increasingly recognize the importance of improving the quality of family planning services. Nevertheless, much work remains to be done to ensure that quality services shall become the norm throughout each service network.

B. RECOMMENDATIONS FOR GOVERNMENTS

Governments play a pivotal role in ensuring quality services, because they determine policies, enforce regulations, are major providers of health and (usually) family planning services and often regulate mass media coverage of family planning topics. Specific areas for action are described below:

(*a*) *Expansion of role of non-governmental organizations.* Non-governmental organizations can play an important role in promoting quality services by providing complementary services, testing new approaches, training staff at all levels, educating the public about child-bearing decision-making and contraceptive methods and advocating appropriate changes in regulations and protocols. Women's groups can be particularly effective in broadening service coverage and information sources;

(*b*) *Elimination of restrictive regulations.* In many countries, the range of contraceptive methods available is limited due to the drug regulatory process and overly conservative medical guidelines;

(*c*) *Loosening of media restrictions.* By permitting contraceptive advertising and discussion of specific contraceptive methods in the media, Governments can facilitate the flow of information needed for clients to make an informed choice regarding contraception;

(*d*) *Inclusion of quality as an indicator of success.* Instead of measuring success only in terms of number of new acceptors and overall contraceptive prevalence,

---

*Washington, D.C., United States of America.

decision makers should also look at continuation rates and other indicators of client satisfaction.

C. RECOMMENDATIONS FOR SERVICE PROVIDERS

Both government and private agencies that provide family planning services can do much to improve service quality. An integral part of such initiatives consists of strengthening existing institutions, not only at national and regional offices but down to the field level. Staff members at all levels must understand the principles of quality of care, must acquire the necessary technical and interpersonal skills and must be committed to changing current practices.

Some recommendations for service providers are given below.

Service delivery systems

Service providers should:

(a) Make services accessible by expanding service outlets to include health facilities, community posts, stores and other sites, even at the risk of duplication. Young adults and rural residents are especially disadvantaged in terms of access to services. More extensive outreach activities can help clients to locate services;

(b) Make services attractive to clients by ensuring that service facilities shall be well maintained and have supportive staff, convenient hours, short waiting times and affordable fees. Operations research on client satisfaction and effective counselling should be encouraged;

(c) Expand method choice by reassessing factors that lead to limited method selection, including overly conservative medical guidelines, inadequate staffing and staff training, logistics management and provider bias. The range of available methods should include temporary as well as long-acting and permanent methods, female and male methods, and medical and non-medical methods. Development of efficient commodity logistics systems is essential to ensure the continuous availability of all methods at service outlets;

(d) Increase the number of female providers because woman-to-woman counselling and services are especially popular with clients. Community-based, non-professional female health workers are highly effective in providing services to rural women. In remote areas with poor transport, community workers may be the only source of family planning information and services;

(e) Develop referral systems by creating linkages with other agencies providing specialized services, such as voluntary sterilization, natural family planning, maternity care and treatment for sexually transmitted diseases and reproductive tract infections, service providers can ensure that clients' reproductive health care needs shall be met. Staff at all levels, especially fieldworkers, must be able to provide appropriate referrals to clients.

Human resource development

With regard to human resource development service providers should:

(a) Improve staff performance by recruiting qualified staff, training and retraining staff to ensure competency in both technical skills and interpersonal communication, providing adequate supervision and rewarding high-quality work. Fieldworkers, in particular, can benefit from close supervision by experienced outreach workers, who can provide on-the-job training, while leaving paperwork to higher level supervisors. Well-trained staff are vital to the delivery of quality family planning services;

(b) Develop ongoing training programmes to train and retrain staff on quality of care, interpersonal communication (counselling techniques, listening skills, small-group discussions and presentations) community participation and informed choice. On-the-job training and technical assistance can ensure consistent implementation of quality of care principles;

(c) Sensitize managers to quality of care and gender-equity issues, so that they will become aware of the ways in which the institutional system can promote quality of care and address inequities within the institution and the larger community that limit women's opportunities. Male managers must understand that women are a valuable asset. Female fieldworkers, in particular, can make a major difference in contraceptive use rates.

Relations with clients

As concerns relations with clients, service providers should:

(*a*) Insist on client-centred services so that clients may make their reproductive choices voluntarily, without coercion or incentives that unduly influence their decisions. Clients have a right to confidential services, privacy, comfort and dignity (Huezo, 1991).

(*b*) Increase information flow to clients through improved client counselling and education, community outreach and mass media coverage. Communication activities should be expanded to raise awareness about contraceptive options, generate interest in the benefits of family planning and placate traditional sources of opposition to family planning. Provision of understandable, accurate and culturally appropriate materials can enhance the client's ability to make an informed choice regarding contraception. Sexuality education must be available to expand understanding about sexuality, personal responsibility and sexual behaviour.

(*c*) Promote continuity of use by clear instructions to users, follow-up of drop-outs and support for method-switching.

Community involvement

Promote community involvement. In areas of diverse geographical, cultural and religious populations, involving local and regional leaders and community groups ensures culturally sensitive and relevant programmes and approaches to reach target communities.

Operational systems

For their operational systems, service providers should:

(*a*) Develop indicators of quality, because programmes need to measure continuation and client satisfaction and to assess staff performance based on these findings, not just on the number of new acceptors. Management information systems should collect data on the number and percentage of continuing users as well as other indicators of quality (see annexes I-III);

(*b*) Strive for constant improvement of service quality. Such improvement is a continuous assessment process—reviewing indicators, setting up systems to fix problems and training staff and volunteers. Supervision and monitoring systems should facilitate the continuous assessment and improvement of service quality.

Providing high-quality services should not be seen as a luxury but rather as a basic component of service delivery. Once the appropriate procedures and systems are in place, service quality becomes a regular part of programme operations.

ANNEX I

The ACCESS framework

Element	Indicators
Accessibility/ acceptability	1. Service is conveniently located;
	2. Service staff are available;
	3. Facility is adequate: waiting room, examination area, clean water and sanitation facilities;
	4. Hours/days of service provision are convenient;
	5. Waiting time is acceptable;
	6. Service is affordable;
	7. Staff is acceptable in terms of sex, ethnic group and age;
	9. Frequency of outreach is adequate.
Choice	1. Number of methods approved;
	2. Number of methods available at service site;
	3. Referral for methods unavailable at service site;
	4. Percentage of sessions where provider asks about reproductive intention and preferred method;
	5. Percentage of sessions where provider offers all methods that are appropriate to reproductive intentions;
	6. Percentage of restrictions that are excessive in relation to national or local guidelines;

Element	Indicators
Choice (*continued*)	7. Percentage of clients satisfied with method received; 8. Percentage of clients receiving a method medically appropriate to reproductive intention.
Continuity of method	1. Mechanism exists and is used to contact clients past due for follow-up; 2. Percentage of users that do not return due to dissatisfaction with programme or method; 3. Percentage of sessions in which provider informs client of timing and sources for resupply/revisit; 4. Percentage of clients continuing using method or changing methods as needed.
Effective and competent providers	1. Percentage of staff meeting job descriptions and qualifications; 2. Use of written guidelines on family planning methods; 3. Percentage of new staff trained in protocols of institution; 4. Percentage of all staff undergo periodic refresher/in-service training; 5. Percentage of providers capable of explaining contraceptive benefits, correct use, mode of action, contraindications andmanagement of side-effects and complications; 6. Percentage of providers that demonstrate skill at clinical procedures (according to guidelines, including asepsis); 7. Reported complication rates for specific methods; 8. Capability for diagnosing/referring clients with sexually transmitted diseases (STDs) and reproductive tract infections.
Sensitivity to client needs and interpersonal relations	1. Percentage of sessions where provider questions client about client needspotential problems (cultural, lifestyle, personal) related to method use; 2. Percentage of clients reporting: ease/diffi-culty in answering questions; staff/providers were polite/rude; privacy was acceptable/unacceptable; they were treated with respect (culturally defined);
Sharing of information	1. Method-specific informational materials available (e.g., printed, model, sample); 2. Percentage of cases in which consent form is explained to and signed by the client, when consent is required; 3. Percentage of clients that can correctly explain how to use their chosen method, its possible side-effects, what to do if side-effects occur and when to return to provider; 4. Percentage of clients referred by existing users; 5. Information on STDs and referrals is given as necessary.

ANNEX II

Indicators for assessing quality of care: client programme

Elements	Management level	Provider level	Client level
Choice of methods	1. Wide range of methods are available including IUD, referrals for sterilization, injectables (if available within country). 2. Adequate and continuous supplies of contraceptives are available. 3. Management system projects method mix and tracks utilization of data.	1. All personnel, especially clinicians, nurses and counsellors offer choices to clients. 2. Referrals are made and follow-up provided for methods not offered. 3. Providers discuss method preferences with managers if methods are not available.	1. Clients choose method and can explain why they chose a method. 2. Clients can discuss at least one other method. 3. Clients understand medical reasons why method may not be suitable.

Elements	Management level	Provider level	Client level
Technical competence	1. Clinicians and medical staff receive technical updates once a year at a minimum. 2. Observation of clinician performance is done at least once. 3. Written guidelines for family planning practice are developed and approved. 4. Training of clinicians and approval of skills is documented. 5. A medical supervisor is designated to overview system. 6. A supervision schedule with clinical observation is followed. 7. Medical records are reviewed. 8. Job descriptions are clear.	1. Clinicians and medical staff demonstrate good knowledge of all methods, use, benefits and side-effects. 2. Clinicians and medical staff follow guidelines for family planning practice. 3. Clinicians and medical staff demonstrate good knowledge of infection control procedures. 4. Clinicians demonstrate good clinical examination skills. 5. Clinicians perform simple laboratory tests as appropriate. 6. Equipment is properly used and maintained. 7. Infections and complications are properly handled. 8. Referrals are made as appropriate. 9. Proper screening is done for clinical methods.	1. Clients experience minimal physical and emotional discomfort. 2. Clients understand about other health problems. 3. Clients can explain the benefits and risks of chosen method. 4. Clients know about common side-effects and how to manage them.
Informing and counselling clients	1. Training on counselling is built into clinician training plan. 2. Time is provided for clinician to do client counselling.	1. Clinicians and medical staff demonstrate good communication and counselling skills. 2. Clinicians and medical staff provide accurate and adequate information for client decision-making.	1. Clients understand their method and how it works. 2. Clients receive appropriate materials and instructions about side-effects and contra-indications.
Interpersonal relations	1. Selection of clinician and medical staff includes attention to interpersonal skills. 2. Supervision includes review of interpersonal skills.	1. Clinicians and medical staff develop trust and rapport with client. 2. Clinicians and medical staff listen to client and address their concerns.	1. Client feels comfortable in talking with clinician and medical staff. 2. Clients are satisfied with service. 3. Good continuation rate.
Mechanisms to encourage continuity	1. Formal follow-up plan is written and clear. 2. Referral system is developed and utilized. 3. Record-keeping system for follow-up visits is developed. 4. Supervision system is in place to track follow-up cases.	1. Clinicians follow the same clients if possible. 2. Clinician maintains good record-keeping system. 3. Manager ensures follow-up between clinic and outreach community-based distribution.	1. Client continues using method or changes as needed. 2. Client returns to clinic for follow-up care as needed.
Appropriateness and acceptability of services	1. Clinic is in accessible, convenient location. 2. Clinic is personal, private, clean and attractive. 3. Hours are convenient and varied as needed.	1. Clinician and staff have client orientation. 2. Clinician and staff are well organized and clients are not made to wait for unusually long periods.	1. Clients are satisfied with services and return as needed. 2. Clients tell others about clinic services. 3. Community makes referrals to clinic.

Elements	Management level	Provider level	Client level
Appropriateness and acceptability of services (*continued*)	4. Clinic has adequate examination and supplies, equipment, running water etc. 5. Client flow plan is organized and well supervised. 6. Outreach, community education plan is well defined. 7. Increased access to family planning services.	3. Staff work in coordination as a team. 4. Staff understand and work to achieve clinic goals.	4. Increase in users.

ANNEX III

Indicators for assessment of quality of care community-based distribution programmes

Elements	Management level	Provider level	Client level
Choice of methods	1. Methods are available and supply is continuous. 2. Record-keeping system tracks commodities distributed. 3. Supervision system tracks field-worker goals and activities.	1. Fieldworker offers choices to clients without bias. 2. Referrals are made for methods not available through community-based distribution. 3. Fieldworkers are motivated to recruit clients.	1. Clients choose method and can explain why they chose their method. 2. Clients can describe other methods
Technical competence	1. Refresher training for fieldworkers is provided at least annually. 2. Consultation by medical person to discuss cases. 3. Written guidelines are provided for screening and distribution of methods. 4. Fieldworker receives training and supervision in record-keeping and follow-up. 5. Fieldworker job descriptions are clear.	1. Fieldworkers are knowledgeable about methods, proper use and side-effects. 2. Fieldworkers follow guidelines in follow-up methods. 3. Fieldworkers complete record-keeping system. 4. Fieldworkers know how to discuss and help clients manage side-effects.	1. Clients can explain the benefits and risks of their chosen method. 2. Clients know about common side-effects and how to manage them. 3. Clients know where to go for serious complications.
Informing and counselling	1. Training on educational counselling approaches are provided at least annually. 2. Written material or pamphlets are given to fieldworkers.	1. Fieldworker is able to communicate clearly about methods and answer client questions. 2. Fieldworker uses written materials appropriately.	1. Clients feel their questions have been answered. 2. Clients receive accurate information about methods.
Interpersonal relations	1. Staff selection is based on good interpersonal skills. 2. Training includes interpersonal communications skills building. 3. Supervision is based on periodic observation of client interaction.	1. Fieldworker can build trust with clients and gain their respect. 2. Fieldworker demonstrates good listening skills and sensitivity to clients.	1. Clients feel comfortable in discussing family planning and other health issues. 2. Clients are satisfied with service.

Elements	Management level	Provider level	Client level
Mechanisms to encourage continuity	1. Referral linkages and procedures are developed. 2. Transportation plan is in place. 3. Follow-up guidelines and system is clear and in writing.	1. Fieldworker follows system for follow-up visits. 2. Fieldworker maintains accurate records.	1. Clients receive supplies as scheduled. 2. Clients have opportunity to discuss and change methods. 3. Good continuation rates.
Appropriateness and acceptability of services	1. Community leaders and health agencies support CBD programme. 2. Informal and formal IEC plan promotes programme. 3. Increased access to services.	1. Fieldworker provides services in an appropriate, private setting. 2. Fieldworker understands and works towards goals of programme. 3. Fieldworker keeps community informed and involved in programme.	1. Clients are satisfied with service. 2. Clients tell others about programme. 3. Community makes referrals to programme. 4. Increase in users.

NOTE: CBD = community-based distribution; IEC = information, education and communication.

REFERENCES

Bruce, Judith (1990). Fundamental elements of the quality of care: a simple framework. *Studies in Family Planning* (New York), vol. 21, No. 2 (March/April), pp. 61-91.

Calla, Cynthia (1991). Translating concepts of total quality management to improve quality of health care in family planning service delivery programmes in developing countries. Washington, D.C.: International Science and Technology Institute.

DiPrete, Lori (1992). User's guide: PHC management advancement programme: Module 5, Service quality assessment. Draft. Bethesda, Maryland: Aga Khan Foundation, Center for Human Services.

_____ , and others (1992). *Quality Assurance of Health Care in Developing Countries*. Bethesda, Maryland: Aga Khan Foundation, Center for Human Services.

Family Planning Service Expansion and Technical Support (1991). The quality of family planning services in field projects: a workshop report. Arlington, Virginia: John Snow, Inc.

Hardee-Cleaveland, Karen, Maureen Norton and Cynthia Calla (1992). *Quality of Care in Family Planning Service Delivery: A Survey of Cooperating Agencies of the Family Planning Services Division*. Washington, D.C.: United States Agency for International Development, Office of Population.

Huezo, Carlos (1991). *IPPF Medical and Service Delivery Guidelines*. London: International Planned Parenthood Federation.

Jain, Anrudh K., ed. (1992). *Managing Quality of Care in Population Programs*. West Hartford, Connecticut: Kumarian Press.

Karim, Raj (1992). Policies and programmes for fully involving women in the development process. E/ESCAP/POP/SFAP/5. New York: United Nations Economic and Social Council. 7 July.

Klitsch, Michael, and Julia A. Walsh (1988). Finding the keys to success: what makes family planning and primary health care programs work? *International Family Planning Perspectives* (New York), vol. 14, No. 1 (March), pp. 20-24.

Service Delivery Working Group/The Evaluation Project (1992). Service delivery working group minutes of meeting, 3-4 June 1992; Subcommittee on quality assurance service delivery working group minutes of meeting, 17 June 1992. Chapel Hill, North Carolina: University of North Carolina at Chapel, Carolina Population Center.

Simmons, Ruth, and George Simmons (1990). Implementing the quality of care: challenges for management. Paper presented at the Twelfth International Council on Management of Population Programmes International Conference, Kuala Lumpur, 12-15 November.

Wells, Elisa S. (1992). Contraceptive method mix: the importance of ensuring client choice. *Outlook* (Seattle, Washington), vol. 10, No. 1 (May).

XXXIV. ELEMENTS OF FAMILY PLANNING IN POPULATION EDUCATION PROGRAMMES

United Nations Educational, Scientific and Cultural Organization[*]

A. BACKGROUND

Population education is essentially an educational response to the social, cultural and economic aspects of demographic problems. It is directed to highlighting awareness and understanding of the demographic process and related problems by encouraging responsible behaviour while contributing to the improvement of the quality of life for both individuals and society.

Since its inception at the end of the 1960s, population education has developed rapidly. Unlike most subjects, however, it did not evolve as a standard element in the curricula of schools and colleges. It emerged as a topic to be incorporated within educational curricula, largely as a response to awareness of the rapidity of world population growth and its increasing necessity to be controlled. Efforts were made to associate closely population education with family planning programmes, which had been seen by many as the principal answer to rapid population growth. The approach was to teach schoolchildren about population issues, thereby encouraging smaller families.

Over the years, research in population science has shown the multitude of interrelated variables affecting and affected by population growth and of the rapidity of changes; and as a result demography has broadened. Long regarded as a discipline, it is becoming increasingly practised as an interdiscipline with strong interrelations with many other psychological, biological, social, economic and environmental sciences. Therefore, the population education concept has been broadened accordingly, becoming interdisciplinary as well; family planning has remained one element of an extended population education content involving teaching such subjects as social studies, geography, home economics, biology and mathematics.

Meaning of "elements of family planning"

A typical population education programme usually organizes its content around the following four major areas: (*a*) sociodemographic framework, with emphasis on sociodemography; (*b*) an environmental ecosystem framework with concern about population and environment relations; (*c*) a sexuality and personal development framework, which includes the human reproduction issue and fertility mastery; (*d*) a family welfare framework, with emphasis on family structures, family roles and women's concerns.

Family planning elements are usually part of, and are dealt with, in population education programmes within the framework of fighting against high mortality rates in favour of maternal and child health care, but more often within the sex and family education components of these programmes. Indeed, the need to give children, adolescents and adults sex and family education is not denied by anyone, even though opinions differ with regard to the content of this education and who should be the one to impart it. As concerns family planning, what is provided, however, is often only scientific knowledge on contraceptive methods and sometimes, as in certain Asian countries, for example, encouragement to use them in order to reduce family size.

In general terms, if one considers the totality of population education programmes, one finds that the sex and family education component is insufficient, both quantitatively and qualitatively. This education, which includes family planning, is still too often limited to simple information on biological aspects and rarely constitutes true education with regard to sex life encompassing all its dimensions: emotional; family; social; and reproductive.

Importance of family planning elements in population education

The importance of family planning elements in a population education programme is subject to various factors, among them: (*a*) a favourable national education policy; and (*b*) the existence of a strong official population policy.

[*]Paris, France.

Furthermore, and despite the fact that the objectives of population education are inspired by a main concern for all population programmes, that of the mastery of the population dynamics and related problems, they do vary from region to region and from country to country. Indeed, some countries seek to reduce demographic growth rate by decreasing fertility, others concentrate on improving family health and environment conditions, while still others want to control distribution of the population and urbanization growth and/or population migration. Depending upon where the emphasis is laid, provision for family planning elements is more or less important.

The content of population education also varies according to the audience, as well as the level and type of education; and according to those differences, the importance given in this content to family planning elements varies. Indeed, one cannot address this subject in the same manner to children, youth or adults, and men or women. In the same way, one cannot provide the same type of information in literacy and post-literacy classes nor for basic education, secondary or post-secondary education. Within this framework, family planning could also, when included, be limited to a presentation of the different contraceptive methods as a corollary to the study of the human reproductive process or be directed towards the changing of attitudes, thereby encouraging smaller families.

During the 1970s, the population education programmes in the Asia region[1] had no sex education; by the late 1980s, only Thailand, some of the Philippine islands and South Pacific countries had incorporated family life and sexuality into their programmes. In the Latin America region, population education began through work in sex education, although ties to formal education programmes through education ministries were loose. Nevertheless, this early orientation influenced the approach of that region to population education, so that balanced attention was given to demographic, ecological and sex education issues. In the Arab region, since rapid population growth is perceived as a problem in the more populated countries, population education programmes deal, in priority order, with population and development, environmental issues and family life education. In sub-Saharan Africa, though concern about problems of adolescent fertility was evident, there were few elements of family planning in programmes. More recently, improved pedagogical skills have permitted a sharper focus on attitudinal and behavioural change, with increasing attention to the prevention of adolescent pregnancy, rapid population growth and the acquired immunodeficiency syndrome (AIDS).

Resistance to family planning

In most countries, when national authorities turn to education to disseminate one or other family models in the name of collective interest, the general public, considering this an invasion of privacy, is somewhat reluctant. Occasional resistance, or even flat refusal, can sometimes be found among educational officials, teachers and parents themselves. It is and always will be difficult to converge between individual values and national objectives to harmonize the State's duty to dispense education to young people with the rights of parents to do it.

Several impact evaluations of population programmes conducted in various countries have demonstrated valid knowledge of family planning, exemplifying an evolution in mentalities towards this subject in target groups. Nevertheless, it appears that there is a notable gap between knowledge and contraception acceptance. In Tunisia, for example, a survey among secondary-school pupils found that 74 per cent of those questioned were in favour of controlling demographic growth and 66 per cent considered that family planning did not constitute a limitation on individual freedom. In Bangladesh, results of various tests indicated that 75 per cent of pupils were currently aware of the negative consequences of having a large family. In Nepal, 45 per cent of students in the education faculty thought that it was better to wait until age 24 or 26 before marrying and 86 per cent were in favour of family planning. However, further examination of replies to surveys indicates that such declarations of principle are not necessarily deeply enough implanted to put "theory into practice". In effect, while the idea of family planning currently seems to be accepted by more than two thirds of those surveyed, attitudes towards contraception and towards equality between men and women remain very conservative.

Providing knowledge and information and inducing a certain evolution in mentalities is not enough to produce a change of behaviour. The knowledge, attitude and practice (KAP) model, which has dominated numerous educational programmes, for example, has often proved quite inoperative because it is far too simplistic. Each person tends to adapt his behaviour to sociocultural representation. To the weight of sociocultural representation, among those factors which determine the choice of a given behaviour by an individual are to be added the expected benefits and the estimated exertion required to achieve a result.

Population education in the Pacific region

There are currently eight operational population education projects in the Pacific region. Even though population education began there in 1982, it is still struggling to establish its own identity, acceptance and place in the education programme for students and adults. One reason for this situation seems to be the lack of commitment at higher levels. As declared by one of the directors of Population Education Projects, this may be due to "the fear of people at these levels, especially if they are politicians, to advocate measures which might be designed to influence reproductive behaviour. While population education is not the same as family planning or sex education (a common misconception), it will, intended or not, provide a rationale for family planning".

It is interesting to note that several countries, Fiji, Marshall Islands and Kiribati, have included family life/sex education in their school curricula. In fact, the focus of the project in Fiji is on family life/sex education to address problems of high teenage pregnancy, sexually transmitted diseases and illegitimacy rates. In Kiribati, the churches have strongly opposed the teaching of sex education in class 9. Western Samoa has tried it in the secondary Teacher Training College. In most other countries, however, sex education in schools is still a very controversial topic, and educators are reluctant to introduce it into schools.

*Population education in francophone
sub-Saharan African countries*

If sub-Saharan African countries were at first very cautious about participating in population education programmes, during the past decade, many of them have begun to support demographic and development policies.[2]

Although these programmes are specific to each country, they do have many common characteristics, of which, *inter alia*, are the following elements which do not work in favour of family planning:

(*a*) The concern to safeguard positive cultural traditions and moral values of the society linked to family and community life is constant and generalized;

(*b*) The notion of responsible parenthood is not limited to choosing the size of the family to match available family resources and tends to be approached within a larger perspective linked to economic development prospects and improvement of the quality of family and community life. Thus, a family limited in size is not considered a panacea but more a factor favouring rehabilitation of responsible parenthood as concerns adequately supporting the family, educating the children and safeguarding family health. It also contributes to avoidance of pregnancies at too early an age and too close together.

Fertility is not a priority in population education programmes in Africa. When the topic is approached, it is usually in relation to maternal and infant mortality or the status of women. Given the value attached to children in African society, a high rate of fertility is akin to a high social status of women. Consequently, African women do not perceive their fertility—even when high—as a burden or a calamity but rather as a factor of personal and social fulfilment. Thus, the ambition of each woman is to get married and have children. For this reason, education that conveys only messages promoting a reduction in the size of the family have very little impact on the public opinion.

C. CONCLUSION

In general, it can be affirmed that the country population education programmes which have been implemented over the past 20 years have influenced the thinking, if not the action, of the target groups with respect to the global population challenge to be faced. They have induced individual concerns which did not previously exist; people are, for example, more inclined to consider that each person has a responsibility to participate in solving the problems of society, such as those deriving from high rates of population growth.

However, if it stands alone, educational action will not suffice to attain the objectives of a population family planning programme and produce behavioural change.

The most important factor in changing attitudes towards fertility, for example, is the education of girls. An important lacuna remains to be overcome in this field, nowhere more prevalent than in many of the least developed countries experiencing rapid population growth and severe poverty, where the role and status of women need serious improvement.

To be efficient, education must be supported by other measures and must be introduced into integrated development policies and "strategic planning" which touch upon the most diverse domains, which presumes the mobilization of all political, economic and social resources in a given country along with the participation of many partners in each community. However, information, education and training are starting-points for all activities in this domain.

NOTES

[1]The countries included in the regional divisions used in this chapter do not in all cases conform to those included in the geographical regions established by the Population Division of the Department for Economic and Social Information and Policy Analysis of the United Nations Secretariat.

[2]In the 1970s, UNESCO assisted only five programmes in the region. Today there are almost 40.

XXXV. INTERNATIONAL FAMILY PLANNING: CHARTING A NEW COURSE

Werner Fornos*

A. THE IMPACT OF FAMILY PLANNING

The past 20 years have seen the institutionalization of family planning. Indeed, in 30 countries where strong family planning programmes have been established and implemented, population growth has declined.

A more difficult job lies ahead. The next 20 years require that family planning become an integral part of individual aspirations for improving the quality of life. Efforts by governmental, non-governmental and multilateral service providers cannot slacken, but rather must be intensified to incorporate family planning as a means to a healthier life, improved educational and employment opportunities and family well-being.

Couples everywhere, and especially the women, must be introduced to family planning within the broader contexts of improvement of the human condition and ensurance of basic human rights. Universal availability and accessibility of family planning must become a priority for the achievement of sustainable development.

Any discussion of international family planning needs for the future and possible responses to these needs must begin with an assessment of the effectiveness of family planning programmes. An impressive and growing body of evidence shows that family planning is an important component of improving maternal and child health, protecting the environment, preserving finite resources and enhancing opportunities for women.

Although family planning efforts have not been uniformly successful, in countries where government leadership has actively and consistently supported well-managed, innovative programmes emphasizing information, education and service delivery—such as in China, Colombia, Costa Rica, Indonesia, Sri Lanka and Thailand—population growth rates have declined substantially.

A recent United Nations report (1992) observes that the availability and accessibility of family planning worldwide has resulted in a world population with 400 million fewer people than there might have been. The report further notes that 51 per cent of women of reproductive age in the developing world currently use a method of birth control. That figure is unacceptable when one considers that four fifths of all people live in developing countries—those least able to accommodate rapidly expanding human numbers. In the foreseeable future, these same countries will account for 9 of every 10 persons added to the world.

However, while contraceptive use by little more than half the women of reproductive age in the poorest countries of the world is far from satisfactory and, in fact, serves as a disturbing reminder of how much needs to be done, it is also a clear sign of the tremendous strides that have been made in family planning acceptance.

Only 21 years ago, a mere 12-14 per cent of the women of reproductive age in developing countries used a method of family planning. During their reproductive lifetime, these women averaged 6.0 children. In the developing world today, women average 3.8 births.

There is even more reason to be encouraged about the progress in family planning in the poorest countries of the world. From 20 to 25 years ago, some leaders of developing countries were opposed to family planning programmes, and others were sceptical that these programmes would have much of an impact on the population growth of their country. An underlying feeling persisted that lower fertility rates might actually deter rather than bolster development; there were suspicions that programmes designed to reduce these rates could be a devious ploy perpetrated by the industrialized countries to sap the strength and vitality of poorer countries and prevent them from achieving their development goals.

---

*President, The Population Institute, Washington, D.C., United States of America.

In this regard, the sea change in attitudes is best illustrated by the fact that despite worsening economic conditions in recent years, Governments and individuals in developing countries are paying for well over 70 per cent of their family planning costs.

Moreover, United Nations demographers have concluded that if the current trend towards wider contraceptive use continues, the result by the year 2050 will be 3 billion fewer people in the world than called for by current population projections.

B. THE COST OF STABILIZATION

Accelerated family planning programmes can reduce the current 2 per cent annual population growth of the developing world to 1 per cent by the year 2020, according to the United Nations Population Fund (UNFPA). The cost of attaining this goal would be moderate compared with the toll in human misery, morbidity and mortality combined with the costs of environmental degradation and loss of finite resources resulting from unchecked population growth.

A number of studies have shown that family planning reduces the need for future expenditures on maternal and child health care. Instituto Mexicano del Seguro Social (IMSS), the social security institute of Mexico, found that it saved 8 Mexican pesos for every peso spent on family planning in urban areas. IMSS estimated that by 1984 the family planning programme had averted expenditures in maternal and child health care equal to 8.5 per cent of its total health budget—funds that were then available for other IMSS health services.

Similarly, Tata Steel at Jamshedpur, India, has calculated that the benefits of the family planning programme it initiated for its employees in 1960 far outweigh the costs. According to company calculations, since the programme began, each Indian rupee (Rs) invested has yielded an overall savings of Rs. 2.39.

The World Bank estimates that if annual spending to provide improved family planning and maternal health services in developing countries were increased by only $1.50 per capita—from $9 to $10.50—the maternal mortality rate would drop by half within a decade and the infant mortality rate would also decline. For even one third that amount, considered to be a more realistic investment for some Governments, there would be a substantial beginning in decreasing the number of maternal deaths.

But it would be irresponsible to ignore the fact that there is a price tag on substantially reducing world fertility.

The expenditures needed to achieve the best possible scenario for stabilizing world population were considered by ministers and senior officials from 79 countries attending the International Forum on Population in the Twenty-first Century, held in Amsterdam in 1989.

Their deliberations focused on the cost of an increase in contraceptive prevalence in developing countries "so as to reach at least 56 per cent of women of reproductive age by the year 2000 in view of the considerable unmet needs in family planning, thereby expanding the currently estimated 326 million user couples to 535 million user couples". These experts concluded that accomplishing this goal would require, at a minimum, a doubling of annual international population and family planning resources from the 1987 level of $4.5 billion to $9 billion by the year 2000.

Would the results be worth an investment of this magnitude? Compared with the astronomical costs of stocking and maintaining superpower arsenals with state-of-the-art machinery for destruction during some 45 years of the cold war, $9 billion seems a rather modest outlay to avoid or alleviate the apocalyptic consequences of rapid demographic growth. There was an assumption that the large sums that had previously been poured into the arms race—so-called "peace dividends"—would easily cover the cost of substantially broadening family planning efforts worldwide. But the vagaries of the global economy have turned this hopeful prospect into a matter that requires considerable thought.

Competition for "peace dividends" is already intense. Lengthy lists of humanitarian projects, many of them highly worthwhile, are presented almost daily to Governments that had left a number of vital human needs relatively unattended for so long. From the dead, gray ashes of four and a half decades of the politics of paranoia, there is hope for the emergence of a flock of phoenixes—social, educational, environmental and health agendas designed to improve the human condition.

Few of these, however, hold the far-reaching promise of a vast expansion of family planning services. A 50 per cent decline in population growth in the developing world would, in fact, pave the way for stabilizing population at approximately 10 billion by the middle of the twenty-first century. Failure to continue the current trend towards greater access to family planning will still lead to population stabilization but only after human numbers reach 15 billion or even 20 billion, according to the United Nations medium- and high-variant projections. The difference then between what can be attained by stepping up family planning efforts, as opposed to failing to take such action, is from 5 billion to 10 billion people. Moreover, it is the difference between reducing the number of people affected by virtually any conceivable condition the "peace dividends" might be called upon to correct, or unconscionably multiplying the direct human consequences of deprivation, poverty, unemployment, hunger and environmental deterioration.

The substantial increase in family planning acceptance over the past two decades amounts to nothing less than an international revolution in family planning. In a great many instances, the acceptance of family planning may have been little more than a matter of the basic logistics of supply and demand: merely providing methods of birth control that allowed couples to have only the number of children they desired. Much of the evidence to support this supposition can be found in the results of the World Fertility Survey, which did much to dispel the old northern hemisphere myth that couples in the southern hemisphere overwhelmingly favour larger families. The preliminary findings of the World Fertility Survey indicated that 50 per cent of the women in the developing world either wanted no more children at all or at least wanted to delay their next pregnancy but did not have either the information, education or means to obtain family planning. The 1992 report on reproductive health published by the World Health Organization (WHO) maintains that approximately 300 million couples in the developing world do not want more children but still lack access to family planning.

C. CHANGING PERCEPTIONS

Over the past 25 years, much of the effort of advocates of population stabilization has been directed towards convincing national leaders and senior government officials of developing countries that the adoption and implementation of a policy to reduce population growth is instrumental to the attainment of economic progress.

Besides the wariness with which a number of leaders in the developing world viewed this kind of advice, coming, as it mostly did, from more affluent countries, there were other reasons for third world leaders to be less than receptive to family planning messages.

First, there was the question of priorities. Even when leaders trusted and accepted the suggestion that rampant population growth was seriously eroding the development progress of their country, they were confronted with the matter of balancing scarce resources with their most pressing needs. In terms of priorities, those which require long-range attention are nearly always slotted for the back-burner, no matter what form of government is making the decisions. And, in the case of leaders of the least affluent countries, the most urgent issues typically involved health, hunger and poverty, followed by employment and education. Rapid population growth, of course, has an impact on each of these concerns—either as the underlying cause or a primary factor in their exacerbation. However, few leaders could seriously contemplate prioritizing the allocation of sufficient resources for family planning clinics in a country where even the most basic services were woefully inadequate or totally lacking, and where there was pervasive hunger, disease, illiteracy and abject human deprivation. It seemed logical enough to many leaders of countries with limited resources that an impoverished mother of from 8 to 10 ill and malnourished children might well need birth control, but her immediate needs were food and medicine.

Another consideration that prompted leaders of some poor countries to back away from family planning programmes was the question of government involvement in the most private matters that couples can decide: the size and spacing of their families. There was a particular reluctance among leaders of countries where prevalent religious, cultural or traditional beliefs were, or seemed to be, opposed to birth control.

Over the years, however, the hurdles and obstacles in the path of establishing family planning programmes in developing countries have, by and large, been cast aside. A notable exception has been male resistance to birth control in many areas of the world, particularly in Islamic regions. According to a WHO analysis, surveys indicate that at least one third of men believe that family planning should be a joint decision. The remaining two thirds feel the male should make the decision. Although male contraceptive methods have been limited to the condom, vasectomy, abstinence and withdrawal, more attention is currently being directed to the male role in family planning because of: (*a*) the importance of the condom in the battle against the acquired immunodeficiency syndrome (AIDS); and (*b*) the advent of the no-scalpel vasectomy method. Still, it is universally agreed that much more research is needed in order to come up with additional effective male methods of contraception. Most other barriers in the way of establishing family planning programmes have been broken down by the willingness of private non-voluntary organizations and multilateral agencies to establish programmes in countries where Governments, for whatever reasons, refused to act or fully to implement programmes on their own behalf. In case after case, leaders of such countries came to learn that couples were interested in limiting their family size or at least spacing the births of their children. Rarely was family planning anywhere near as controversial as a leader at first believed.

The transformation in perceptions about family planning, where before there had been lingering doubt in some parts of the developing world, is all but complete. Experience, circumstances and time have established a consensus in developing countries that population must be brought into balance with resources and environment. The vast majority of poor countries with high fertility rates have adopted policies directed to reducing their population growth.

This consensus marks perhaps the first major milestone in the struggle towards population stabilization.

D. FOCUS ON NEW DIRECTIONS

The remainder of the 1990s will be crucial in deciding the number of people there will be in the world when population stabilizes. The actions taken or not taken between now and the end of the twentieth century will have far-reaching consequences. The Population Council, for example, has estimated that if all unwanted pregnancies could be avoided, the populations of developing countries could be stabilized at about 7.8 billion; if not, they will stabilize at 10 billion or higher. Even someone as optimistic as the present author could not suggest that there is any chance of preventing all unwanted pregnancies. But there is little doubt that, given the political will, the world can prevent most unwanted pregnancies.

The Honourable Lucille Mathurin Mair, Ambassador of Jamaica to the United Nations and a trustee of the Population Council, observed that the principal lessons learned in the delivery of family planning programmes to the developing world were:

1. Family planning programmes work best when they are voluntary and when they offer services of good quality, as seen from the perspective of the user;

2. Contraceptive prevalence tends to rise with the number of reversible contraceptive methods offered in the programme: people that are given wider contraceptive choices are better able to avoid having unwanted children;

3. Family planning services meet people's needs better when they are integrated with other reproductive health services, such as antenatal and post-partum care, and the prevention and cure of reproductive tract infections and sexually transmitted diseases. They are more likely to be used regularly and effectively when they meet people's needs better.

Now that virtually all Governments of the world accept family planning as a fundamental human right, the world must move into the next phase of the struggle: ensuring the accessibility of this right. In many ways, this goal may be more difficult to achieve than it was to win the support and active involvement of Governments. The difficulty derives mainly from the sheer numbers involved—hundreds of millions of women scattered throughout the world. Many of these women live in the remotest rural areas of the world; most of them are illiterate and substantial numbers of them are dominated by husbands and families vehemently opposed to family planning.

International family planning efforts must be directed towards:

(*a*) Improving communication between population assistance and family planning service providers—including multilateral organizations and governmental and non-governmental agencies—as well as coordination of their efforts, in order to both ensure that specific problems in a country are being adequately addressed and that some services are not being replicated while other needs are unaddressed;

(*b*) Establishing improved lines of communication between developing countries regarding programmes and projects, especially among countries situated in the same region and those with similar problems. Often, it has been found that projects that succeed in one country can, with relatively minor adjustments and modifications, work elsewhere;

(*c*) Reaching the women in greatest need through the most innovative, resourceful and expansive efforts of information, education and communication (IEC) and service delivery ever conceived. All previous efforts to establish social marketing and community-based distribution programmes in the farthest reaches of the poorest countries of the world pale in comparison with the efforts that will be required to fulfil the unmet need for family planning;

(*d*) Offering the widest possible range of modern contraceptives in order to give these women the opportunity to select the method most suited to their personal preference. The confidence level concerning these methods must be raised considerably, in terms of both effectiveness and safety. This goal can only be achieved by a continuation and expansion of contraceptive research to improve vastly the existing methods, with the goal of reducing failure rates and health risks to the absolute minimum;

(*e*) Developing new and improved contraceptives, with an emphasis on efficiency, safety, ease of use and cultural appropriateness, as well as developing safe, effective and easy to use male contraceptives. In the United States of America, once the leader in the development of contraceptive technology, there must be a reversal of the wholesale shift away from research and development in the field. (Only one pharmaceutical firm remains involved in the field.) The movement away from contraceptive research was precipitated by: (i) an increasingly litigious society where lawsuits are almost routinely filed to collect damages on grounds of product failure; and (ii) the fact that it can take years, even decades, before a new product gains approval of the United States Food and Drug Administration (FDA). The significance of these detriments is twofold: the United States was among the leaders in contraceptive technology and the Government is prohibited from exporting contraceptives that have not been approved by FDA. A recent report in the *Journal of the American Medical Association* recommends the following remedies: (i) alteration of the FDA approval process for

contraceptives so that approval may be given if the benefits of using the contraceptives significantly outweigh the health risk of pregnancy for an identifiable group of users; and (ii) passage of federal legislation granting manufacturers of contraceptives the use of FDA approval as a limited defense in product liability suits;

(*f*) Introducing family planning into government maternal and child health services, where they are not yet available; and where some family planning services are already provided, expanding the locations, days, hours and types of methods offered to ensure that services shall be available and convenient to all requiring them, and improving the quality of services to promote higher acceptance and continuation rates;

(*g*) Increasing the availability of family planning offered by the private sector. Avenues for private sector involvement include: family planning associations; commercial marketing of contraceptives; and the inclusion of family planning in health services offered by employers or insurance companies;

(*h*) Placing strong emphasis on IEC activities through the use of mass media, person-to-person counselling and group discussions;

(*i*) Educating women and health providers about high-risk pregnancies and how to avoid them by using family planning, as well as clear information on the use, benefits and risks of various family planning methods;

(*j*) Developing culturally sensitive family planning information, services and counselling for persons with special needs, including men, teenagers, unmarried and newly married women, and new mothers;

(*k*) Developing programmes to encourage full and prolonged breast-feeding, which significantly reduces a mother's chance of becoming pregnant and the same time is beneficial to the health of her infant;

(*l*) Providing information, education and testing on AIDS as part of family planning programmes, and promoting the use of condoms to prevent the transmission of the human immunodeficiency virus (HIV).

While the future of family planning must focus on accommodating individuals and substantially raising family planning acceptance, the concentration on IEC and delivery of services cannot neglect correlative development factors. By far the most important of these is elevation of the status of women.

In far too many countries, women seem to be regarded as little more than chattel, farm-hands and "baby factories" rather than as persons with vital contributions to make to the development process.

In her address to the United Nations Conference on Environment and Development, held at Rio de Janeiro in June 1992, Dr. Nafis Sadik, Executive Director of UNFPA, correctly noted that: "In the international community the words "family planning" have a clear and clearly understood meaning. But whether we talk of family planning or of responsible planning of family size, we have to ensure the availability of full information and services which will enable women and men to make voluntary, free and informed choices in the matter of family size."

With very little variance, studies and surveys in a number of developing countries have shown that more educated women have fewer children than less educated women and that women employed outside the home have fewer children than those who are not. The more readily that poorer countries open greater employment and education opportunities for women, the greater are the chances that these countries will reach a smaller family norm. Additional dividends will doubtless surface as educated and employed women become vital and viable participants in development.

REFERENCES

Finger, William R. (1992). Getting more men involved. *Network: Family Health International* (Durham, North Carolina), vol. 3, No. 1 (August), pp. 4-6.

Fomos, Werner (1990). *Gaining People, Losing Ground: A Blueprint for Stabilizing World Population.* Washington, D.C.: The Population Institute; and Ephrata, Georgia: Science Press.

_____ (1992). *Testimony Before Foreign Operations Subcommittee of the United States House of Representatives Committee on Appropriations.* Washington, D.C.

International Planned Parenthood Federation (1992a). The lack of contraceptive research in the USA. IPPF Open File (London) (August), p. 21.

_____ (1992b). WHO report on family planning world-wide. IPPF Open File (London) (August), p. 2.

Meadows, Donella, Dennis L. Meadows and Jorgen Randers (1992). *Beyond the Limits: Confronting Global Collapse or Envisioning a Sustainable Future.* Post Mills, Vermont: Chelsea Green Publishing Co.

Mair, Lucille Mathurin (1992). Speech at the United Nations Population Award Ceremony. New York.

The Population Institute (1992a). Four hundred million people use family planning. *Popline* (Washington, D.C.), vol. 14 (July-August), p. 2.

_____ (1992b). Many advantages of small families cited. *Popline* (Washington, D.C.), vol. 14 (March-April), p. 4.

_____ (1992c). U. S., U. K. scientists stress the importance of population factor. *Popline* (Washington, D.C.), vol. 14 (March-April), pp. 1-2.

Sadik, Nafis (1992a). Cooperation, not confrontation. *Populi* (New York), vol. 19, No. 2 (July-August), p. 14.

_____ (1992b). Statement at the United Nations Conference on Environment and Development, Rio de Janeiro, 8 June.

United Nations (1992). *Long-range World Population Projections: Two Countries of Population Growth, 1950-2150.* Sales No. E.92.XIII.3.

United Nations Population Fund (1992). The good, the bad, and the surprising. *Populi* (New York), vol. 19, No. 2 (July-August), pp. 4-5.

XXXVI. POTENTIAL CONSTRAINTS TO AND PROSPECTS OF IMPROVING QUALITY OF CARE IN FAMILY PLANNING PROGRAMMES IN DEVELOPING COUNTRIES

*Anrudh K. Jain**

Over the years, a number of concepts (for example, programme effort, availability, accessibility and density of workers) have been used to describe family planning programme features and to measure their impact upon contraceptive use and fertility (see, for example, Mauldin and Lapham, 1985; Hermalin and Entwisle, 1985). Some of these concepts and indices measure programme input at the national level and others at the subnational level, and a few review programme features from the client's perspective. They emphasize policy commitment and/or quantity and distribution of services. Most of them, however, do not observe or define the service-giving process and therefore do not overlap much with the concept of quality of care (for comparisons of these concepts, see Jain, Bruce, and Kumar, 1992).

Quality is a dimension that every programme has; yet, quality of services has not received the same degree of attention as other features of the programme, such as availability. It is defined in terms of the way individuals (or clients) are treated by the system providing the services. Bruce (1990) has evolved a working definition of quality that incorporates six elements: choice of contraceptive methods; information given to clients; technical competence; interpersonal relations; mechanisms to encourage continuity; and appropriate constellation of services (see box 2). These elements provide a framework through which the quality of a given programme can be viewed, that is, described, monitored and evaluated.

This note identifies some of the factors that may inhibit attention to improving quality of care being rendered through family planning programmes in developing countries and discusses steps that can be taken to rectify the situation.

A. POTENTIAL CONSTRAINTS

The constraints to improving quality of care in developing countries are based on the erroneous perception that the concept may not be relevant in these countries, scepticism that improving quality of care would make a difference, the erroneous perception that improving quality of care is costly and the lack of a specified process for improving quality.

Lack of relevance to developing countries

An emphasis on quality of care, which emerged recently in the United States of America, is derived both from a consumer orientation and recently from a feminist perspective. The concept of quality, therefore, may be perceived as completely foreign in countries where consumers' needs in general get low priority and where feminism has yet to take hold. However, quality is as much a Western concept as, for example, the reduction in population growth rate. Attention to rapid population growth rates in most of the developing countries did not emerge from within. Yet, an overwhelming majority of developing countries do provide services for contraceptive methods through organized family planning programmes. Very few population professionals reject the need for population stabilization or the need for the developing countries to reduce their population growth rates. Why then should the concept of quality be brushed aside as a Western concept?

In the author's view, quality of care is as relevant in developing countries as it is in developed countries. However, one way to address this issue is to evolve a definition of quality appropriate to a country or programme. This can be done by collecting information from managers, providers and clients. The author's colleagues at the Population Council have developed an instrument to collect information from programme managers about the degree of emphasis a programme should place and actually places on a particular attribute of high quality. The annexed questionnaire has been sent to managers in about 100 developing countries and their responses would help both to evolve a normative definition of quality and to encourage the managers to articulate what their programmes are actually doing.

*Senior Associate and Deputy Director, The Population Council, New York, New York, United States of America.

BOX 2. COMPONENTS OF PROGRAMME QUALITY

Choice of methods refers to both the number of contraceptive methods offered on a reliable basis and their intrinsic variability. Which methods are offered to serve significant subgroups as defined by age, gender, contraceptive intention, lactation status, health profile, and—where cost of method is a factor—income group? To what degree will these methods meet current or emerging need (for example, adolescents)? As contraceptive choice is an ongoing process requiring negotiation between partners, are there alternatives for men and women, for spacers and limiters and for clients discontented with a given choice or with a specific formulation of a method?

Information given to clients refers to the information imparted during service contact that enables clients to choose and employ contraception with satisfaction and technical competence. It includes: *(a)* information about the range of methods available, their scientifically documented contraindications, advantages and disadvantages; *(b)* screening out of unsafe choices for the specific client and provision of details on how to use the method selected, its possible impacts on sexual practice and its potential side-effects; and *(c)* an often neglected element, explicit information about what clients can expect from service providers in the future with regard to sustained advice, support, supply and referral to other methods and related services, if needed.

Technical competence involves, principally, such factors as the competence of the clinical technique of providers, the observance of protocols and meticulous asepsis required to provide clinical methods, such as intra-uterine device (IUD), implants and sterilization. This element overlaps with "information given to clients" to the extent that clinical information about methods is transmitted accurately and clients are appropriately screened for contraindications. It overlaps with "follow-up to the extent that medically indicated follow-up is conducted.

Interpersonal relations are the personal dimensions of service, principally the received effected content of exchanges between providers and clients or potential clients. How do individuals feel about the service system, particularly the technical capacity and social attitude of the personnel with whom they interact? Relations between providers and clients are strongly influenced by the programme mission and ideology, management style and resource allocation (for example, patient flow in clinical settings); the ratio of workers to clients and the supervisory structure.

Mechanisms to encourage continuity indicate programme interest in promoting—and its ability to promote—a continuity of contraceptive use, irrespective of the method used, whether well-informed users manage that continuity on their own or the programme has formal mechanisms to assure it. It can rely upon community media or upon specific follow-up mechanisms, such as forward appointments or home visits by workers.

Appropriate constellation of services refers to situating family planning services so that they are convenient and acceptable to clients, responding to their natural health concepts, and meeting pressing pre-existing health needs. There is no one appropriate constellation of services. Family planning services can be appropriately delivered through a vertical infrastructure, or in the context of maternal and child health initiatives, post-partum services, employee health programmes or other means.

Source: Judith Bruce, "Fundamental elements of the quality of care: a simple framework", *Studies in Family Planning* (New York), vol. 21, No. 2 (January-February 1990), pp. 61-91.

This approach can easily be adapted to evolve a definition of quality appropriate to a particular country or programme. A sample of providers and clients of a programme can be contacted informally through focus groups or formally through a survey to solicit their views about the importance of each of the attributes of quality and to identify other attributes not included in the questionnaire.

Scepticism that improving quality would make a difference

The provision of services and information about contraceptive methods through organized family planning programmes is based on a variety of rationales, including meeting the needs of individuals and reducing population growth rates. The relative emphasis placed on each of these and other rationales, however, varies from country to country. In countries where implementation of the family planning programme is driven mainly by a demographic rationale and among professionals primarily interested in macrolevel fertility reduction, there may be scepticism that improving quality would help them to achieve these macrolevel objectives.

One way to overcome this constraint is to re-emphasize the goal of family planning programmes in terms of helping persons achieve their reproductive intentions and, at the same time, to synthesize and review the literature on this subject. Another way is to initiate field studies to demonstrate the fertility impact of improving quality of care. The international literature on this subject has been reviewed elsewhere (Bruce, 1990; Jain, 1989). Similar reviews need to be commissioned and undertaken at the country level. The international literature, though limited, strongly suggests that improvements in quality of care will lead to an increase in contraceptive use and a decrease in fertility. Four propositions, formulated on the basis of this review, can be taken as the basis for improving quality of care as well as for developing hypotheses to be tested by country-specific field studies. These propositions are listed below (Jain, 1992):

(a) Providing a choice of methods will increase effectiveness of family planning programmes, raise contraceptive prevalence and reduce fertility;

(b) Taking individuals' needs and preferences into account while prescribing a contraceptive method can increase its continuity of use;

(c) Recruiting a small number of acceptors each year and taking good care of them is a better strategy than trying to recruit a large number of acceptors whose needs cannot be met by the programme; and

(d) Following the individual/woman/couple rather than any particular method will increase the impact of family planning programmes.

Improvement in quality of care is erroneously perceived to be costly

It is true that improvements in certain elements of quality will add to the cost of delivering services. For example, adding a method to the programme will most likely increase the overall budget of the family planning programme. However, the marginal cost of improving quality in most cases is likely to be much lower than the original investment. Moreover, improvements in certain elements of quality will not add to the cost of delivering services. Treating clients in a humane fashion, for example, is unlikely to cost more than treating them simply as mere numbers.

It is wrong to focus on the absolute cost of improving quality of care. Instead, one should consider the cost effectiveness of these improvements. If, for example, addition of a method also increases the contraceptive prevalence rate and helps more persons achieve their reproductive goals, then the benefits may outweigh the increase in cost. It is an empirical question and must be tested empirically.

The underutilization of service delivery points (SDPs), found in many developing countries, is costly. For example, a situation analysis study conducted in Kenya showed that 52 per cent of SDPs visited did not have any new client on the day the team visited (Miller and others, 1991). Another study in Nigeria showed that 75 per cent of the clients were accounted for by only 19 per cent of SDPs; and 6 per cent of SDPs had no client during the entire year (Nigeria, 1992). Such statistics are not limited to countries in sub-Saharan Africa. SDP underutilization may in part reflect the lack of demand for contraceptive methods in the particular area served. However, the contribution of poor quality of services—for example, unavailability of contraceptive methods—to the underutilization of SDPs cannot be ruled out.

It is costly to expand the number of SDPs that are not used. Improving quality of services offered by SDPs currently underutilized may be more cost-effective than expanding the number of SDPs that might be underutilized. Whether improving quality of services is more cost-effective than expanding the number of SDPs that provide poor quality of services is again an empirical question that must be tested empirically.

Lack of specified process for improving quality of care

The process of improving quality of care is unlikely or desirable to be uniform. It would depend upon a particular setting. An attempt to identify various steps that can be considered by programme managers and population professionals has been made elsewhere (Bruce and Jain, 1991; Jain, 1992). The process of improving quality of care can begin by addressing any one or all of the following interrelated issues:

(a) Explicit specification of standards or norms of quality that the family planning programme should meet;

(b) Assessment of the capacity of the programme to offer services of the intended quality;

(c) Assessment of the extent to which the programme in fact offers services of the intended quality; and

(d) Assessment of the extent to which the individual clients are receiving services of the intended quality.

One of the best ways to improve quality, learn from the experience and document the cost effectiveness of the improvements is to initiate field studies in a country. Such studies will help document the quality of care being received by persons, to identify gaps between the quality of care intended by the programme and received by the clients and identify the reasons for the gaps. Various designs can be followed in such studies. A typical approach would include field studies in limited geographical areas and would consist of the following steps:

(a) A diagnostic study of service delivery points in the selected geographical area(s) to describe quality of services being offered and to identify elements that need to be improved (for guidelines of a diagnostic study, see Fisher and others, 1992);

(b) A baseline survey of clients to describe the quality of services being received and desired by them and to establish the level of contraceptive use in the selected geographical area(s);

(c) Design of an intervention based on the diagnostic and baseline studies to improve quality of care;

(d) Implementation of this intervention and monitoring of its cost;

(e) Follow-up of SDPs to document changes in quality of care; and

(f) Follow-up survey of clients to document changes in contraceptive use dynamics.

The basic design can be adapted in various ways to suit the features of a particular setting and interest. First, a survey of providers and clients can be added as a part of the diagnostic study to evolve a definition of quality appropriate to the setting. Secondly, the intervention can be thought of in terms of, for example, expanding choice of contraceptive methods, in which case methods not available in the geographical area can be added simultaneously or sequentially. Thirdly, the quality of services can be improved only at underutilized SDPs. Fourthly, a sample of clients included in the baseline survey also could be included in the follow-up survey in order to understand the process of change and to assess the extent to which the intervention has helped persons to achieve their reproductive goals. Fifthly, a control area will be required if the interest is in assessing the relative cost effectiveness of the intervention for improving quality of care.

B. PROSPECTS OF IMPROVING QUALITY

The prospect of improving quality of care in a country or programme will depend upon the degree of commitment among the top management and population professionals to improve the quality of care provided through the programme. An emerging emphasis on macrolevel global issues, such as the environment, is likely to strengthen the demographic rationale of family planning programmes. It may weaken the commitment to improving quality of care unless managers are convinced that such improvements will help them to achieve these macrolevel demographic goals. In the absence of a strong commitment, there must at least be some curiosity among the managers and providers to determine the extent to which improvements in quality of care will help them achieve the macrolevel objectives of the programme. In the absence of any commitment and any curiosity, the prospect of improving quality of care in a country or programme will depend upon the degree of emphasis placed by donors and international agencies and upon the emergence of a consumer-oriented movement which will educate clients to demand and expect services of high quality.

ANNEX

QUALITY OF CARE: DEFINITION OF ASSESSMENT

Anrudh Jain, Barbara Mensch and Judith Bruce

Family planning programme managers in most countries do intend to provide services of adequate quality. It is understood that political realities and resource constraints must be considered while implementing their desire to provide services of high quality and to plan improvements in a logical sequence. The definition of high quality may itself vary from setting to setting. The authors would like your assistance in identifying important attributes of high-quality pro-grammes that are relevant in most developing countries.

To achieve this objective, a set of attributes has been identified that may be used to define a programme of high quality. Two questions are asked for each attribute. The first question refers to the emphasis or importance a programme should place, and the second question refers to the emphasis your programme actually places on a particular attribute. Please feel free to circle 0 if a particular attribute is not relevant in your setting or if your programme places no emphasis on it. Please circle 3 if a particular attribute is most important or if your programme places most emphasis on it. Please feel free to add any other attributes(s) that you think are most im-portant for a high-quality family planning programme.

A. How much emphasis should family planning programmes place on the attributes included in the enclosed table.

0.	No emphasis	2.	Moderate emphasis
1.	Minor emphasis	3.	Considerable emphasis

B. How much emphasis does your programme actually place on the attributes included in the enclosed table.

0.	No emphasis	2.	Moderate emphasis
1.	Minor emphasis	3.	Considerable emphasis

Attributes of family planning programmes of high quality	Ideal emphasis	Actual emphasis
1. (a) Providing an appropriate choice of methods to a significant proportion of clients;	0 1 2 3	0 1 2 3
(b) Not promoting any particular method;	0 1 2 3	0 1 2 3
(c) Not restricting any particular method.	0 1 2 3	0 1 2 3
2. Ensuring that providers are technically competent in:		
(a) Screening clients for contraindications;	0 1 2 3	0 1 2 3
(b) Supplying "clinical" methods;	0 1 2 3	0 1 2 3
(c) Applying effective aseptic techniques.	0 1 2 3	0 1 2 3
3. Ensuring that clients shall receive information about:		
(a) Method options appropriate to client needs;	0 1 2 3	0 1 2 3
(b) Contraindications of method selected;	0 1 2 3	0 1 2 3
(c) Common side-effects of method selected;	0 1 2 3	0 1 2 3
(d) Follow-up requirements of method selected;	0 1 2 3	0 1 2 3
(e) Duration of effective use of method selected;	0 1 2 3	0 1 2 3
(f) Possibility of switching the method if it turns out to be unsuitable;	0 1 2 3	0 1 2 3
(g) Possibility of switching the source of supply.	0 1 2 3	0 1 2 3
4. Ensuring that providers shall assist client's choice process by soliciting information from clients about client's:		
(a) Background (age, number of children);	0 1 2 3	0 1 2 3
(b) Reproductive goals (timing of next desired child);	0 1 2 3	0 1 2 3

(continued)

Attributes of family planning programmes of high quality	Ideal emphasis	Actual emphasis
(c) Attitudes and preferences for contraceptive methods	0 1 2 3	0 1 2 3
(d) Prior experience with contraceptive methods.	0 1 2 3	0 1 2 3
5. Ensuring that clients shall make a specific appointment for a follow-up visit or a specific plan for resupply with providers	0 1 2 3	0 1 2 3
6. Ensuring that clients shall receive visual and physical privacy for:		
(a) Information sharing and personal interviews;	0 1 2 3	0 1 2 3
(b) Physical examination/method provision.	0 1 2 3	0 1 2 3
7. Ensuring that providers shall treat clients with dignity and respect	0 1 2 3	0 1 2 3
8. Other (please specify)_____	0 1 2 3	0 1 2 3

REFERENCE

Bruce, Judith (1990). Fundamental elements of the quality of care: a simple framework. *Studies in Family Planning* (New York), vol. 21, No. 2 (March/April), pp. 61-91.

_____, and Anrudh Jain (1991). Improving the quality of care through operations research. In *Operations Research: Helping Family Planning Programs Work Better*, Myrna Seidman and Marjorie C. Horn, eds. New York: Wiley-Liss.

Fisher, Andrew A., and others (1992). *Guidelines and Instruments for a Family Planning Situation Analysis Study*. New York: The Population Council.

Hermalin, Albert I., and Barbara Entwisle (1985). Future directions in the analysis of contraceptive availability. *International Population Conference, Florence, 1985*, vol. 3. Liège, Belgium: International Union for the Scientific Study of Population.

Jain, Anrudh K. (1989). Fertility reduction and the quality of family planning services. *Studies in Family Planning* (New York), vol. 20, No. 1 (January-February), pp. 1-16.

_____ (1992). *Managing Quality of Care in Population Programs*. West Hartford, Connecticut: Kumarian Press.

_____, Judith Bruce and Sushil Kumar (1992). Quality of services, program efforts and fertility reduction. In *Family Planning Programs and Fertility*, James Phillips and John Ross, eds. Oxford, United Kingdom: Clarendon Press.

Mauldin, W. Parker, and Robert J. Lapham (1985). Measuring family planning program effort in developing countries, 1972 and 1982. In *The Effects of Family Planning Programs on Fertility in the Developing World*, Nancy Birdsall, ed. World Bank Staff Working Paper, No. 677. Population and Development Series. Washington, D.C.: The World Bank.

Miller, Robert A., and others (1991). The situation analysis study of the family planning program in Kenya. *Studies in Family Planning* (New York), vol. 22, No. 3 (May/June), pp. 131-143.

Nigeria (1992). *Nigeria: The Family Planning Situation Analysis Study*. Issued by Federal Ministry of Health, Primary Health Care Unit; Obafemi Awolowo University, Family Health Services Project, Operations Research Unit and Network; and the Population Council, Africa OR/TA Project.

XXXVII. EXTENDING FAMILY PLANNING SERVICES TO UNREACHED POPULATION GROUPS

United States Agency for International Development[*]

During the past 25 years, the developing world has experienced unprecedented changes in the availability and use of modern contraception. In 1965, fewer than 10 per cent of couples in the developing countries were using any form of contraception; by 1983, the figure had risen to about 45 per cent (United Nations, 1989). Today, the contraceptive prevalence rate for developing countries may be as high as 50 per cent.

However, this overall trend masks significant differentials in contraceptive use that persist between and within countries. In Eastern Asia and Latin America, for example, effective national family planning programmes have been in place for more than two decades in most countries, and contraceptive use in many of these countries (e.g., Republic of Korea, Singapore, Thailand, Brazil and Colombia) exceeds 65 per cent of married couples. In many African countries, on the other hand, national programmes have been under way for only a decade or less, and both the availability and the demand for contraception are much lower. The contraceptive prevalence rate in these countries commonly is fewer than 10 per cent of married couples.

In most developing countries, important intra-country socio-economic and demographic differentials in contraceptive use also persist. Contraceptive availability and use may be very high among some subgroups of the population, while other subgroups are much less likely to use contraception, often because quality family planning services are not fully available. Three underserved subgroups deserve special attention by policy makers and programme administrators during the next decade: rural and peri-urban populations; males; and adolescents.

The scope of the problem and possible solutions related to contraception and unwanted fertility among adolescents are well summarized in other papers prepared for this Expert Group Meeting (see Mohamud,

1992; and WHO, 1992). The present authors heartily endorse the various recommendations for policy action given in these excellent papers, particularly the call for improved family life education and family planning services. For the remainder of this paper, however, attention is focused on the need for better programme outreach to rural and peri-urban populations and males.

A. RURAL AND PERI-URBAN POPULATION GROUPS

Approximately 2.6 billion people live in rural areas in developing countries, and many millions more live in marginal peri-urban areas. Despite the enormous diversity that exists among these populations throughout the world, they share one common attribute: they endure significantly disadvantaged conditions compared with those in modern urban areas. There is limited access to basic infrastructure, health and social services, and education and employment opportunities for these populations.

Access to modern family planning services is also more limited in rural areas, even though in many countries demand for contraception in rural areas is not very different than that in urban areas. The result is that in some regions, particularly Latin America and Northern Africa, the unmet need for contraception in rural populations is considerably higher than in urban areas—where services are more widely available (Westoff and Ochoa, 1991). In Peru and Bolivia, for example, 18 and 30 per cent, respectively, of married women in urban areas have an unmet need for contraception; but for married women in rural areas, the figure for both countries is over 40 per cent.

The programmatic challenges of providing quality family planning services in rural and peri-urban areas are daunting. Existing health facilities in these areas are frequently poorly staffed, poorly equipped and under-

---

[*]Office of Population, Washington, D.C., United States of America.

utilized. Client counselling and follow-up are generally weak. Sociocultural and linguistic barriers present an additional challenge in many areas. Nevertheless, innovative family planning service delivery programmes, including the use of community-based distribution (CBD) and mobile teams, have been utilized effectively in some countries to improve outreach to underserved populations in rural areas. Where quality services have been made available, they have been widely utilized. What, then, are the most important priorities for reaching rural and peri-urban populations more effectively?

Strategic planning to expand service delivery

Sound strategic planning must be the foundation of any agenda for action. Constraints to service delivery and programmatic responses must be identified. Analysis of recent survey data, situation analysis, operations research, market research and focus group studies are all valuable tools in formulating a service delivery strategy for underserved rural and peri-urban populations.

Effective coordination of public and private sectors

Greater public and private sector collaboration is an excellent way to improve service delivery in rural areas. In many countries, strong non-governmental organizations can assist in training staff of public sector health posts in rural areas. The commercial sector can also do more to provide contraceptives at affordable prices. The collaboration of social marketing and CBD efforts has been effective in increasing the availability of contraceptives in rural areas.

Measures to ensure high-quality services

Several aspects of quality of service delivery to rural and peri-urban populations are likely to need improvement. One aspect is expanding the range of contraceptive methods available. Currently, pills and condoms are the most widely available methods in most rural areas. Introduction of injectables into outreach programmes would expand contraceptive choice and increase client satisfaction. In addition, referral systems for long-acting or permanent methods need to be strengthened for the benefit of women that have already reached their desired family size.

Another key component of quality of care is better trained and supervised staff that are responsive to client concerns. Rural service providers must be technically competent and provide accurate information and good counselling to clients.

Expanded promotional activities

Much more work needs to be done in family planning information, education and communication (IEC) programmes for rural and indigenous populations, tailoring messages to their distinct needs and cultural traditions. Vehicles that have been effective recently include: promotional ads on local radio; service promotion on market day; mobile caravans; audio cassettes on long omnibus routes.

Attention to programme sustainability

In extending services to underserved rural and peri-urban populations, cost/benefit concerns must be kept in mind. The relative cost and impact of reaching the most remote rural areas must be weighed against expanding services in more densely populated rural areas. Expansion of outreach must be accompanied by efforts to improve efficiency. In addition, the potential for partial cost recovery must be examined.

B. Males

Despite evidence that men play a pivotal role in reproductive decision-making in many developing countries, few family planning programmes throughout the world focus adequate attention on reaching men with family planning information or services. There are many reasons that this approach may be regarded as short-sighted.

First, in many developing countries (particularly in more traditional societies), women's attitudes and behaviour with regard to fertility and family planning are strongly influenced by the husband. Often, there is very little husband-wife communication or joint decision-making on such matters, but where there is disagreement on these issues, cultural norms dictate that a wife is expected to conform to the views of her husband (Ezeh, 1992)

Data from the Demographic and Health Survey (DHS) of Mali in 1987, illustrate the problem: fewer than 20 per cent of the men surveyed approved of family planning, compared with 70 per cent among their spouses. Two thirds of couples reported that they had never discussed family planning together, which may account for the fact that nearly 60 per cent of wives thought that their husbands approved of family planning—more than twice the actual level (Traoré Konaté and Stanton, 1989). If these findings are at all typical, they may offer a partial explanation of why 15-35 per cent of married women in developing countries report a desire to space or limit child-bearing and yet are not using any form of contraception.

A second reason that men deserve more attention in family planning programmes is that they are an untapped reservoir of potential clients. Currently, four family planning methods are available to men (in addition to total abstinence): vasectomy; condoms; withdrawal; and periodic abstinence. Among these methods, condoms are the most widely used method, but many men use condoms mainly as a prophylaxis against the human immunodeficiency virus (HIV) or sexually transmitted diseases. Only 4 per cent of men in developing countries use condoms as a family planning device (FHI, 1992). Withdrawal and periodic abstinence are traditional methods that are not widely practised in most countries, and these methods are also characterized by high failure rates. Female sterilization is the most commonly used family planning method in the developing world. By comparison, use of vasectomy—a procedure that is safer and just as effective—is rare in developing countries: only in India and China is vasectomy used by more than 5 per cent of married men (FHI, 1992). However, several small-scale vasectomy promotion programmes (for example, in Brazil and Colombia) have demonstrated that prevalence of vasectomy use can increase rapidly if high-quality services are offered. The acceptability of vasectomy may be increased as a result of the new no-scalpel" vasectomy procedure, which is quicker than traditional vasectomy, with fewer complications (Family Health International, 1992)

Male involvement in family planning will happen only if there is a concerted effort by family planning programmes to target men. Three immediate priorities are: (a) to develop IEC materials that promote smaller family size desires and support for family planning among men; (b) to promote open husband-wife communication on family planning; and (c) actively to promote male methods of family planning. Vasectomy information and services, in particular, should be promoted vigorously and made widely available. Family planning clinics should also encourage couples to obtain counselling on contraceptive methods together whenever possible, so that husbands and wives will be fully informed about contraceptive options.

Programme managers seeking guidance on how to reach males more effectively may find the husband component of DHS, now available for a number of countries, to be a useful resource (Lacey, 1992). These surveys can help identify gaps in male knowledge and use of family planning, determine whether they approve of family planning or of the methods their wives are using, establish objectives for male-oriented IEC and service delivery efforts, develop different strategies to reach different segments of the male population, and monitor and evaluate male-oriented efforts.

A long-term goal is the empowerment of women to enable them to exercise greater control over all aspects of their lives, including their own fertility. In many countries, this will require efforts to reach males and females of all ages to change gradually deeply rooted social norms and to elevate the role of women in family decision-making.

REFERENCES

Ezeh, Alex Chika (1992). Family planning in Ghana: why bother about men? Paper presented at the 1991-92 OPTIONS II Fellows Programme, April 1992.

Family Health International (1992). Men and family planning. *Network* (Durham, North Carolina), vol 13, No. 1 (August).

Lacey, Linda (1992). Use of DHS to design family planning programs oriented towards men. Draft. Chapel Hill, North Carolina: University of North Carolina, Carolina Population Center.

Mohamud, Asha A. (1992). Adolescent fertility and adolescent reproductive health. Chapter IX om the present volume.

Traoré, Baba, Mamadou Konaté and Cynthia Stenton (1989). *Enquête démographique et de santé au Mali, 1987*. Bamako, Institut du Sahel, Centre d'études et de recherches sur la population pour le développement; and Columbia, Maryland: Institute for Resource Development/Macro Systems, Inc.

United Nations (1989). *Levels and Trends of Contraceptive Use as Assessed in 1988*. Population Studies, No. 110. Sales No. E.89.XIII.4.

Westoff, Charles F., and Luis H. Ochoa (1991). *Unmet Need and the Demand for Family Planning*. Demographic and Health Surveys Comparative Studies, No. 5. Columbia, Maryland: Institute for Resource Development/Macro International, Inc.

World Health Organization (1992). Problems and prospects of integrating family planning with maternal and child health with special emphasis on adolescents. Chapter XLII in the present volume.

XXXVIII. COMMUNITY-BASED DISTRIBUTION AND CONTRACEPTIVE SOCIAL MARKETING

United States Agency for International Development*

Both community-based distribution (CBD) of contraceptives and contraceptive social marketing (CSM) grew out of the need to provide family planning services to populations whose access to traditional clinic services was limited.

In CBD, a number of approaches are used, but a key element involves identifying, recruiting and training members of the community to become family planning workers. Distribution typically takes one of two approaches: household distribution in which workers systematically canvass neighbourhoods; or, in the later stages of programme development, community depots, which require the user to take the initiative to go to the depot (a CBD worker's home or a small shop) to obtain supplies, usually pills, condoms or spermicides.

In contrast, CSM programmes use commercial marketing, advertising and distribution techniques to increase awareness and use of contraceptive products among low- and middle-income groups. Each CSM programme is designed within the country environment to achieve a level of sustainability through the establishment of cost-recovery schemes and sound business plans. CSM programmes have recently expanded to include long-term contraceptive methods, such as the intra-uterine device (IUD), injectables and Norplant implants.

Although this discussion note gives separate attention to each of these major approaches to delivering family planning, it also shows that the two approaches can and do overlap with each other in a number of instances. The observations and examples presented here draw on the experience of projects and programmes in developing countries funded by the United States Agency for International Development (USAID).

A. COMMUNITY-BASED DISTRIBUTION

CBD programmes have varied greatly both in their design and in their effectiveness, depending upon the country and the situation. Some of the dimensions along which CBD models differ include the following: workers may be volunteers or paid staff; training ranges from minimal to extensive; and some CBD workers provide only family planning while others may include primary health care services. For a programme manager contemplating the use of CBDs, the organizational options and choices are many; and often it is not clear which model, if any, might work best. In Kenya, some type of CBD approach is used by 23 different organizations to deliver services. A particular CBD model may work successfully in one area but not in another. Considerable resources have been wasted because programme managers introduced a CBD approach without first fully considering (and field-testing) the various options. No single model is necessarily the best one. Thus, whenever CBD is to be introduced, the specific model being implemented should be field-tested.

Although there is a continuing need to test CBD approaches in specific settings, it is no longer necessary to demonstrate the feasibility of using non-medical, community workers to distribute contraceptives. The experience of family planning programmes with CBD has been well summarized elsewhere and is not repeated here. (Bertrand, 1991; Gallen and Rinehart, 1986; and Lewis and Keyonzo, 1990). Also, this paper does not address implementation issues, such as approaches to training, supervision strategies, target-setting and so on, as they can often be handled more appropriately in specific country settings. Instead, this note focuses on selected issues related to the future development of CBD and points to the need for CBD approaches to adapt to changing circumstances.

Government policies

Although Governments increasingly accept the general idea of community-based distribution of contraceptives, policy barriers often remain which affect the implementation of CBD. Areas of potential conflict may relate to regulations concerning medical examinations or

*Office of Population, with the assistance of the United States Agency for International Development Cooperating Agencies, Washington, D.C.

laboratory tests, restrictions on the categories of personnel permitted to dispense certain contraceptives and classification of some contraceptives as restricted and requiring a prescription.

Governmental policies or practices with regard to collaboration between public sector and non-governmental organization projects also affect improvements in CBD programmes. Greater cooperation between government and non-governmental organizations potentially strengthens the contribution of each to CBD activities. One approach is for CBD agents from non-governmental organization programmes to act as extension agents of government programmes, while those programmes in turn provide backup and referral services for long-term and permanent family planning methods. Such a strategy might entail supervision of CBD agents, provision of commodities and access to client lists by government health workers.

Response of CBD programmes to maturation of family planning programmes

Experience in Asia and Latin America suggests that CBD programmes may have a limited life-span. At first, CBD workers provide education, referral and limited commodities to clients in their homes or through depots, and potential family planning users seek their assistance. As clients become more experienced with family planning and are more committed to controlling their fertility, they may begin to seek other sources of contraceptives. Some clients may desire more effective methods that are not available from CBD programmes. Community-based family planning programmes may bias the method mix away from more effective clinical methods.

As prevalence increases, and as Norplant, injectables, IUDs and sterilization are added to the method mix, the role and functions of CBD workers are also likely to change. Thus, attention might shift from resupply to recruiting clients for other long-acting methods. This would imply a greater focus by CBD workers on education and referral, as well as a need for closer links with clinics and hospitals.

With the maturation of the family planning programme, some clients may prefer the privacy and convenience of the commercial sector—formal or informal—for resupply. In fact, as CBD programmes develop, it may be appropriate for them to move to more cost-effective models, including greater emphasis on depots for contraceptive supply and modified social marketing strategies. Questions that arise in this context concern: how this type of transition can be encouraged and implemented; and how the issue of fee-for-services for workers can be handled in a setting where health services have traditionally been provided without charge. These questions also relate to a key concern of family planning programmes in general and CBD approaches in particular—sustainability.

Sustainability

The sustainability of CBD programmes is a central topic for any discussion of the long-term usefulness of the approach. This topic encompasses a host of other issues, including the merits of paid versus volunteer workers, the introduction of user fees or other income-generating strategies and the extent of community participation.

The payment of workers is one of the thorniest issues in developing and implementing a CBD programme. The use of paid workers is often avoided because of the high recurrent costs. On the other hand, volunteer workers are often difficult to supervise, turnover tends to be high and volunteers may be unresponsive to performance targets. Thus, it is useful to consider the role that incentives to CBD workers can play in influencing the success of the CBD project. Are such incentives cost-effective? Can CBD projects be sustained if workers receive incentives or other payments? What is the impact on the project if worker incentives, once provided, are later discontinued?

An illustration of the difficulties of using volunteer workers with no incentives is the experience of CBD programmes using traditional health practitioners (THPs), including traditional birth attendants as distributors. In all parts of the world, THPs (herbalists, birth attendants, rural traditional doctors) of one type or another exist. For years, family planning programmes have assumed that these groups represented a vast, relatively inexpensive source of rural personnel for delivering services. Countless training programmes have been conducted and numerous projects using THPs have been funded and implemented. Nevertheless, the impact of THPs on service delivery is probably marginal and very likely not cost-effective. Since these projects typically rely upon volunteers, any initial success may quickly decline into ineffectiveness over the long run because of the absence of incentives, as well as the lack of supervision and supplies. This approach has been popular within CBD programmes but perhaps it needs to be re-examined.

One approach to the problem of worker incentives has been the introduction of user fees or other payment schemes, such as modified contraceptive social marketing. Such payments can provide some income to the CBD workers and, at the same time, help make programmes more sustainable. User fees or payments raise further questions, however. If CBD workers receive a percentage of the sales of certain contraceptives, will they actively refer clients for other methods? How viable is this approach in countries where Governments are committed to free provision of health care? Will clients be able to pay for methods obtained through CBD workers? For example, since CBD workers may visit households only periodically, perhaps every three months, clients would need to purchase a three-month supply each time. Even though there may be a willingness to pay, clients may not be able to accumulate that much cash.

Quality of care

There is much variation between as well as within countries in the ability and willingness of clients to pay for services. In some countries, the shift to a cash economy may give clients the resources to purchase medical services, including family planning. The ability to pay for services may confer social prestige, and clients may perceive such services to be of higher quality than CBD because of their higher cost. The concept of quality of care is most often applied in medical or highly developed clinic settings. Nevertheless, service quality improvement should be of concern in CBD programmes as well, with particular attention given to training of CBD agents in a wide range of family planning methods and counselling techniques, and to ensuring linkages with clinical services to offer the broadest possible method mix. A major challenge is to develop training curricula, supervision protocols and other elements of CBD programmes in such a way as to ensure adequate quality of care.

Integrated service delivery

Often, CBD programmes include other primary health care services. The challenge in integrating service delivery is to ensure sufficient attention to family plan-ning. Recently, the role of CBD programmes in responding to the acquired immunodeficiency syndrome (AIDS) and other sexually transmitted diseases (STDs) has become a major concern. What is the appropriate role of CBD programmes in AIDS/STD education and treatment? How can programmes better address what should be natural overlaps between family planning and AIDS/STD prevention efforts? As with many other questions concerning the application of CBD, operations research can help to field test new approaches.

Gender considerations

CBD programmes have shown that a woman-to-woman approach has been the most effective for reaching women about family planning services. Given the extensive participation of women in these programmes as community-based family planning providers, it is of some interest to consider the impact of this experience on their lives. At the same time, it may be that men are the most effective outreach workers for communicating with other men, and thus more attention might be given to the use of male workers in CBD programmes. It is likely that gender issues will receive increasing attention in CBD programmes, along with focused training to heighten gender awareness among programme designers and managers as well as fieldworkers.

B. CONTRACEPTIVE SOCIAL MARKETING

Private sector participation

CSM projects have undergone significant changes since the inception of the first large-scale efforts in 1969. CSM programmes today are an effective vehicle to help users make the transition from public sector to private sector resources, thereby freeing public resources for populations with special needs (Lande and Geller, 1991). Recent studies in a number of countries where CSM projects have been in place for four or more years show that the costs per couple-year of protection decline significantly as projects mature (Stover and Wagman, 1992).

The role of the private sector in CSM has dramatically increased over the past 10 years and is an important element in allowing CSM projects to achieve self-sufficiency. The establishment of partnerships within existing private sector infrastructures lessens the burden

416

of public sector investment and improves the sustainability of projects. In recent CSM projects, private sector investment contributes to covering substantial costs for advertising, promotion, management, commodities, distribution and training. For example, for the first time in any CSM project in Turkey, a commercial distributor independently purchased and imported condoms for promotion in the project, constituting a commodity savings of over $200,000 in the first year. In Papua New Guinea, an oral contraceptive manufacturer in the private sector recently donated products for the initiation of the project. The manufacturer is currently collaborating with the distributor on efforts to expand the commercial market.

Due to the increasing level of private sector participation in CSM, it is estimated that 13 CSM projects (among those funded by USAID through the social marketing project of The Futures Group) will have fully self-sufficient products by the end of 1993. Since 1984, four projects have attained completely self-sufficient products: Mexico (Protector condom); Eastern Caribbean (Panther condom); Dominican Republic (Microgynon oral contraceptive); and Indonesia (Dualima Red condom).

CSM programmes are successful in reaching new contraceptive users in lower income groups. USAID data show that "C" and "D" class users constitute approximately 60-98 per cent of all CSM programmes. In addition, information taken from user profile studies indicate that 32-47 per cent of CSM product users are new acceptors of contraceptive methods.

Alternative distribution networks

CSM programmes often seek alternative distribution systems in order to maximize the availability of products in those areas where traditional systems are unavailable or are less effective in reaching the target market. Several innovative distribution networks are being used, and preliminary studies indicate that this strategy has increased total CSM sales.

In Indonesia and Peru, CBD networks have proved successful in reaching the target markets. Alternative networks are used to distribute CSM products in Ghana, where market women distribute to urban and rural communities. In Malawi, a private sector beer distributor was recruited in 1992 to provide distribution of CSM condoms to bars, hotels, rest-houses and other alternative distribution centres. In the Dominican Republic, Rwanda and Uganda, individual promoters are hired to reach other outlets to further the acceptance and sales of CSM products.

Regional branding

In an effort to optimize the cost efficiency of CSM projects, a regional Pan-African communications strategy for the CSM condom was launched in 1991. Advertising pre-test research showed that consumers of countries across regions were able to positively identify with a single advertising behavioural message. With minor adjustments to accommodate to language and cultural characteristics, the campaign theme and product packaging were identical in each country, thus reducing development and production costs. The Pan-African campaign has tested successfully in nine countries in the region—Benin, Ghana, Lesotho, Malawi, Swaziland, Togo, Uganda and Zimbabwe.

With the proven success of the Pan-African condom campaign, the regional branding and communications strategy concept was tested in Asia and Latin America. In Papua New Guinea, the campaign was used to launch condom sales in September 1991. A regionally oriented campaign was also recently tested successfully in Mexico.

Contraceptive social marketing and AIDS prevention

In recent months, projects funded by USAID have been communicating the message of "protection" for use in family planning as well as in prevention of AIDS. The campaign does not specifically mention either family planning or AIDS but leaves the interpretation of protection to the audience.

The campaign projects a positive message overall and a positive image of the condom in particular. According to the data provided, the campaign continues to be successful for audiences seeking family planning and those seeking AIDS prevention. This strategy of using one campaign to address separate issues is extremely cost-effective. To reduce costs even further, these projects provide an important and sustainable avenue for integrating AIDS awareness and prevention activities in areas where CSM projects already exist.

C. RECOMMENDATIONS

Recommendations concerning community-based distribution

With regard to community-based distribution, it is recommended that:

(*a*) CBD should be considered a primary means of expanding access to family planning in both rural and marginal urban areas;

(*b*) Policy makers should seek to remove barriers to utilization of CBD workers, such as requiring unnecessary medical tests and examinations before permitting supply by CBD workers or limiting CBD workers to distributing condoms or spermicides;

(*c*) Non-governmental organizations should be widely utilized to extend the reach of government programmes, especially for referral services;

(*d*) CBD programmes should seek to expand the capacity of CBD workers to provide education and referral for long-acting and permanent contraceptive methods;

(*e*) Gender analysis should be included in programme design and the role of women as decision makers and managers should be expanded; women should be better represented at all levels of family planning programme design and management;

(*f*) AIDS and STD counselling and education should be included in CBD programmes, where appropriate.

Recommendations concerning contraceptive social marketing

The following recommendations are based on lessons that have been learned in recent years from various contraceptive social marketing programmes:

(*a*) CSM projects must be designed with realistic cost expectations. Cost recovery, even at the lowest level, must be integral to the system design;

(*b*) CSM projects should be designed to maximize the use of existing private sector infrastructures, prod-

ucts, expertise and resources. Private sector participation in training, detailing, advertising and promotion increases efficiency and lowers cost;

(*c*) In low prevalence areas, mass media messages must be supported by already existing networks, such as outreach workers, community-based distribution networks, theatre groups, and other unconventional media;

(*d*) CSM systems and techniques should be used to increase the contraceptive utilization levels of service delivery outlets as well as the cost effectiveness of cost recovery strategies;

(*e*) Regional campaigns for CSM projects are effective in promoting a single theme that reaches audiences of different countries within a particular region. The strategy substantially reduces development and production costs for CSM projects;

(*f*) CSM projects can be an invaluable and cost-effective tool in jointly communicating family planning and AIDS prevention messages. CSM projects have effectively integrated AIDS awareness and prevention activities in areas where condom social marketing activities are already in place. These existing projects should be used to maximize efficiency and avoid duplicating programme activities.

REFERENCES

Bertrand, J. (1991). Recent lessons from operations research on service delivery mechanisms. In *Operations Research: Helping Family Planning Programs Work Better*, Myrna Seidman and Marjorie C. Horn, eds. New York: Wiley-Liss.

Gallen, Moira, and Ward Reinhart (1986). *Operations Research: Lessons for Policy and Programs*. Population Reports, Series J, No. 31. Baltimore, Maryland: The Johns Hopkins University, Population Information Program.

Lande, Robert E., and Judith S. Geller (1991). *Paying for Family Planning*. Population Reports, Series J, No. 39. Baltimore, Maryland: The Johns Hopkins University, Population Information Program.

Lewis, G., and N. Keyonzo (1990). Community based distribution of family planning services: the international experiences with selected issues. Paper presented at the National Workshop on Guidelines for CBD Programs in Kenya. Unpublished. Nairobi, Kenya: The Population Council.

Stover, John, and Anne Wagman (1992). *The Costs of Contraceptive Social Marketing Programs Implemented through the SOMARC Project*. Special Study, No. 1. Washington, D. C.: The Futures Group.

XXXIX. SUSTAINABLE COMMUNITY-BASED FAMILY PLANNING PROGRAMMES

Japanese Organization for International Cooperation in Family Planning[*]

A. HUMANISTIC FAMILY PLANNING

The Japanese Organization for International Cooperation in Family Planning (JOICFP) has been promoting humanistic family planning since its establishment. By humanistic family planning is meant the following concept:

The family planning concept can be promoted only after humans awaken to rationalism and realize that they must take necessary actions to protect their lives and bring health and happiness to their families. Family planning programmes should begin with respect for humankind, and their ultimate aim should be to bring happiness to individuals.

B. WHY JOICFP PROMOTES HUMANISTIC FAMILY PLANNING

Family planning is fundamentally a very private matter. People will resent or disregard family planning if it is forced on them in a top-down manner for the purpose of curbing population growth. Hence, family planning can only be promoted if the community people themselves are motivated. In Japan, this lesson was learned during the post-war period when the country experienced rapid population increase. JOICFP was established in Japan in 1968 as a non-governmental organization to promote international cooperation in family planning and has been implementing pilot projects with one question in mind: how family planning activities can be implemented with the full and active support and participation of the people at the grass-roots.

C. THE JAPANESE EXPERIENCE WITH FAMILY PLANNING

The Japanese Government began promoting family planning in 1952. In 1954, the Japan Family Planning Association (JFPA) was established as a non-govern-

mental organization to carry out a massive family planning campaign in close cooperation with the Government. Under this arrangement, JFPA conducted information, education and communication (IEC), community-based distribution (CBD) and training activities and gained much experience. The lessons learned are described below.

First, family planning programmes must be based on a principle that is both acceptable and understood by the people. Family planning should be promoted as a means by which each and every citizen's family can attain health and happiness. If the programme confronts people with the population problem, the people will not only find the concept difficult to understand but the programme will sometimes provoke resentment.

Secondly, family planning workers must be trusted and well recognized by people in the community and be persons with whom they can openly discuss their concerns. Family planning is a very private matter because it concerns sex, and it is important that the workers are trusted.

One of the main reasons that Japan could spread the family planning message across the country in such a short time was that members of the established network of midwives and public health nurses were trained as family planning workers so that they could provide this service within their package of health services. These people were already veterans of baby delivery, maternal and child health (MCH) and parasite and infectious disease control and they had long-standing relationships with community people. Therefore, they could easily teach family planning concepts.

Thirdly, to involve the community, it is necessary to appeal to people's natural desire to avoid illness and to live happy and healthy lives with their families. To ensure that a family planning programme becomes deeply rooted in the community and therefore becomes long-lasting, it is essential that it be combined with an

---

*Tokyo, Japan.

activity that enlightens the people. The people must realize that the activities exist for their health and happiness, and must be mobilized into action.

Next, to foster the community spirit and gain support to expand family planning activities, active participation of groups of people is the most effective. In Japan, community-based activities were conducted in many localities throughout the country. Subunits of 30-50 households grouped together and voluntarily began to conduct MCH, preventive health, environmental hygiene and self-reliance activities, such as income generation. Most of these activities were conducted by women (housewives), who played a very active role in improving the life in the village and community development.

Lastly, family planning projects should not be conducted in a disjointed fashion by the Government and non-governmental organizations. They should be conducted under the tripartite cooperation of government (central and local), private organizations and expert groups (academics). For that, it is necessary to set up a system in which each group has a fully recognized role and each can have a maximum say in its area of expertise, and one in which the groups can cooperate and give feedback to one another.

D. JOICFP INTEGRATED FAMILY PLANNING PROJECTS: EXPERIENCES IN AFRICA, ASIA AND LATIN AMERICA

JOICFP first began implementing the Integrated Family Planning, Parasite Control and Nutrition Project based on the concept of humanistic family planning in Nantow Province in Taiwan Province of China, in 1974. Since then, the JOICFP project has been implemented in 24 countries in Africa, Asia, Latin America and the South Pacific. When one compares the people's attitudes and behaviour towards family planning and measures the acceptance rates in project and non-project areas, one finds that the project has definitely had a significant impact. As with any project, there have been some failures, but they were due to management problems and not because the concept is unworkable.

E. WHAT JOICFP LEARNED FROM THE INTEGRATED PROJECT

Trust must exist between family planning workers and the people in the community before there can be success.

Grass-roots communities are very realistic. They only actively participate in something that clearly demonstrates/guarantees benefits for their lives and health. Once they decide voluntarily to join in the activities, the collective energy of the people can be utilized to promote the activities. For example, once people accept the programme, they will develop new ideas themselves and new ways of financing the activities will be sought and pursued. A very effective approach is required to capture the attention of illiterate people deprived of health care in developing countries. From the JOICFP experience, parasite control activities, in particular ascariasis (roundworm infection) control, have an enormous effect on the people. Such activities have an immediate impact on health to instantly capture the attention of the people and heighten their concern about health matters.

Family planning promotion is more effective when it is presented as an integral part of MCH and other public health centre activities.

Establishment of local steering committees has proved effective in promoting the Integrated Project. This committee must include members that can take a leadership role. For instance, in Ghana, each project area has a local steering committee, and its members (usually ranging from 9 to 18) include schoolteachers, pastors, representatives of mothers' clubs, farmers, "market mammies" (women market vendors), cooperative representatives etc.

Women play a major role in family planning promotion. Once motivated and given the opportunity, women will be an energetic force in the society and can exert influence on men and encourage their participation.

Technical cooperation between developing countries has worked well for the Integrated Project because the countries that share experiences have a common ground.

All international cooperation projects must stress self-reliance to ensure continuity. From the very beginning of activities, people should be asked to pay for services, even token amounts.

The tripartite cooperation of Government, non-governmental organizations and experts is a key to success.

The unique role of non-governmental organizations must be recognized by the Government. The partnership of these bodies should not be sought solely for the purpose of cost-sharing. They must be able to fully serve their advocacy and pioneering role in the society. Non-governmental organizations can also reach special groups of people, such as minorities, indigenous people and slum-dwellers, who would otherwise be missed by the government system. In many cases, family planning promotion works better if non-governmental organizations are at the front line of programme promotion.

XL. FAMILY PLANNING FOR THE UNDERSERVED: AN IPPF PERSPECTIVE

*International Planned Parenthood Federation**

Family planning for the underserved: this is a large subject, one of the biggest in the world, in fact. When it comes to family planning, more people are underserved than are properly served. In 60 per cent of developing countries, half the people do not have easy access to contraceptive services. In Latin America, three out of four women that are not planning their family would like to do so. In Africa, in particular, there is a real unmet need for family planning, especially in the cities: there are illegal abortions and the mortality and infertility associated with them, adolescent pregnancies; abandoned children and even infanticides.

The largest single group of underserved people worldwide is undoubtedly the adolescent population aged 15-19 years. Not all are sexually active, of course, but in all regions, large and increasing numbers are and high rates of adolescent pregnancy are found in both developed and developing countries. One reason that the contraceptive needs of adolescents are ignored is that single women are excluded from unmet needs surveys, so they do not appear in statistics. What is worse, in most developing countries, family planning clinics only cater to married women—and most teenagers are unmarried.

The family planning movement has often been criticized for wanting to address the problems arising from adolescent sexuality and even accused of encouraging precocious sexual behaviour. But no serious research of which the author is aware has suggested that providing education for young people about their sexuality has had the effect of making them more sexually active. On the contrary, if they are not given correct information and advice, the chances are that they will pick up erroneous information about their bodies and fertility. Their sexuality exists anyway, regardless of whether they receive correct information about it; and if they are sexually active, it is most important that they should understand the facts of conception and contraception.

Adolescent sexuality and adolescent pregnancy are not restricted to the third world. In the United States of America alone, there are currently 17 million young people in age group 15-19, and over 600,000 unintended pregnancies (over half of which end in abortion) occur in that age group every year. In Eastern Europe and the former Union of Soviet Socialist Republics, there are nearly 30 million adolescents, most of whom are unlikely to have access to contraceptive services (United Nations, 1989a; Jones and others, 1986).

In much of the developing world, there is an even greater need. in Asia and the Middle East,[1] there are some 300 million teenagers; and in some countries, adolescent pregnancy and premature child-bearing is a major problem. Adolescent pregnancy rates are generally even higher among the 100 million aged 15-19 years in Latin America and sub-Saharan Africa, most of whom have no access to family planning because few clinics serve unmarried women. Abortion, though illegal in most of these countries, is used with often tragic results: in 1988, a study in Nigeria found that abortion complications accounted for 72 per cent of all deaths to young women under age 19 (United Nations, 1989b).

The needs of young people can be met through sensitive and non-directive programmes. Through a project called Youth for Youth: Promotion of Adolescent Reproductive Health, already under way in Colombia, Egypt, Jamaica, Senegal, Sierra Leone and Sri Lanka, the International Planned Parenthood Federation (IPPF), with the support of the United Nations Population Fund (UNFPA), is trying to involve young people in meeting the needs of their peers.

An example of a successful programme of this kind is Gente Joven (young people), run by the Mexican Family Planning Association, Mexfam, which is intended to provide sexuality education to young people, delay parenthood until age 20 and target in-school, working and street youth. In 1989, 400,000 births, one fifth of the national total, were to mothers under age 20; the average age at first intercourse is 16. In 1988, Mexfam closed all its adolescent centres and went out to look for

---

*Fred Sai, London, United Kingdom of Great Britain and Northern Ireland.

teenagers on the streets: they set about training selected young people as distributors of information and contraceptives to their peers in the community. They are now working in 52 urban areas throughout Mexico and have recently extended services to the most marginalized youth, including street gang members (Valdés-Smith, 1992).

In other countries of Latin America, family planning associations run telephone hotlines (in Brazil and Guatemala) to provide information and referrals, which are especially effective in reaching out to young men. Others have special hours for adolescents in an existing family planning clinic or have special teenage clinics, sometimes combined with recreation or other health services; while still others have organized teenage theatre groups or helped young people make films or videos to express their views of sexuality issues.

There are fewer programmes of this type in Africa, although the need there is great. An example is the Youth Counselling Project run by the Ethiopian Family Planning Association with the Ethiopia Youth Association at Addis Ababa, where teenage pregnancy and illegal abortion are increasing rapidly. Here the aim is to reach in-school and out-of-school youth and college students, as well as young couples and young people working in factories and workshops. This programme uses reading material, film shows and drama to attract young people: a play about the consequences of unwanted pregnancies produced by young volunteers was seen by 30,000 adolescents, mainly secondary-school students. In this as in similar programmes, the approach, personality and communication skills of the project staff and the creation of a friendly atmosphere are important factors in getting the message across to the young people.

There are many groups that are underserved because they have no easy access to existing clinics or distribution systems. For some years the Thai Family Planning Associaton has been trying to provide family planning services to the hill tribe people, who number some 500,000 in the northern region bordering on China and Myanmar (formerly Burma). Family size is large and infant mortality is high. With the support of village elders, the Association has recruited and trained local health workers from the hill tribe communities in basic health care and family planning, so that they can provide general first aid, basic drugs, immunization and condoms to people in their area.

Another example from within the IPPF family is the programme set up by the Viet Nam Family Planning Association to improve family planning services to the families of 36,000 miners in northern Viet Nam. One aim of the project is to reduce the almost total reliance of these families upon the intra-uterine device (IUD), which has been virtually the only method available. The Association has trained 12 mobile teams and had given family planning training to the 70 midwives working at the mine health stations, focusing on the importance of interpersonal communication and counselling in gaining the confidence of potential clients.

Community-based distribution of contraceptives is used in many countries to reach people that cannot or will not use a clinic-based service. The Moroccan Family Planning Association has set up a network of community agents, who may be Red Crescent nurses or housewives in apartment blocks or even shanty towns, who keep stocks of pills and condoms to sell cheaply to their clients or neighbours. Respected women in remote rural communities are also appointed. Some training and instruction on referral of problem clients is given, and the agents are visited at least every three months for replenishment.

Often, as in Honduras, illiteracy rates are much higher in rural areas and contraceptive use is that much lower. The Honduras Family Planning Association has made considerable progress in rural areas by training "promoters", who make house-to-house visits and set up village distribution posts, supported by promotional campaigns on local radio and loudspeaker vans.

Most family planning programmes target women, no doubt because they are most directly concerned by decisions on child-bearing, are most closely involved in family health issues and, frankly, are easier to reach. But successful family planning does depend upon positive male attitudes, and many family planning associations are making special efforts to reach men, especially since the human immunodeficiency virus (HIV) epidemic has created a new and powerful argument for the use of the condom. In the author's country, Ghana, the family planning association has for some years run successful "Daddies Clubs" to help increase men's share in parental responsibility and child-bearing decisions; and it has trained plantation managers to support family planning initiatives among their workers. The Kenyan Family Planning Association has improved its outreach to men through training male community-based distribution agents.

Lastly, among the underserved one must, as a conscientious provider, include those that are reached by existing services but are dissatisfied with them. Recent Demographic and Health Surveys in 12 countries discovered that over half the women they studied had discontinued the contraceptive method they were using because of failure or dissatisfaction: 58 per cent discontinued the pill; 57 per cent discontinued IUD; 63 per cent, injectables; and 47 per cent, the condom. If these discontinuation rates are applied to the 200 million current users of contraception in developing countries, it seems likely that over hal, about 111 million, will end up unsuccessful or dissatisfied (IPPF, 1992).

What many of these women need is certainly a higher quality of family planning care. They need appropriate counselling about methods and their possible side-effects, they need reassurance, they need quick but pleasant service with streamlined procedures, or they may just need kind and sympathetic treatment.

In some areas of the developing world, and in the former Soviet Union, doctors are available, but because of insufficient training, they lack the knowledge and involvement to make them good family planning providers. In some areas again, continuity of contraceptive supplies is a problem.

To help family planning associations and other service providers to a better focused "user perspective",

IPPF and its International Medical Advisory Panel have been developing medical and service delivery guidelines. The basic principles and objectives for quality of care are presented in the form of 10 rights of the client: information; access; choice; safety; privacy; confidentiality; dignity; comfort; continuity; and opinion. These clients' rights must remain as a benchmark for all family planning services.

NOTE

[1] The countries included in the regional divisions used in this chapter do not in all cases conform to those included in the geographical regions established by the Population Division of the Department for Economic and Social Information and Policy Analysis of the United Nations Secretariat.

REFERENCES

International Planned Parenthood Federation (1992). *IPPF Annual Report, 1991-92.* London.

Jones, Elise F., and others (1986). *Teenage Pregnancy in Industrialized Countries.* New Haven, Connecticut: Yale University Press.

Valdés-Smith, Cecilia (1992). Breaking barriers with youth. *Planned Parenthood Challenges* (London), No. 1 (October), pp. 22-23.

United Nations (1989a). *Adolescent Reproductive Behaviour,* vol. I, *Evidence from Developed Countries.* Population Studies, No. 109. Sales No. E.88.XIII.8.

_____ (1989b). *Adolescent Reproductive Behaviour,* vol. II, *Evidence from Developed Countries.* Population Studies, No. 109/Add.1. Sales No. E.89.XIII.10.

XLI. MEDICAL QUALITY ASSURANCE THROUGH DEVELOPMENT OF LOCAL SYSTEMS

Association for Voluntary Surgical Contraception[*]

The Association for Voluntary Surgical Contraception (AVSC) has recently adopted a strategic plan to the year 2000 to guide it in helping to meet the demand for permanent and long-term contraception—voluntary sterilization (male and female), intra-uterine devices, implants and injectables—that is projected for the rest of this decade (Mauldin and Ross, 1992).[1]

The first thing that this new plan does is to expand the AVSC mission to include, along with the voluntary sterilization services with which AVSC has traditionally worked, IUDs, implants and injectables. Including these long-term methods in its mission will allow AVSC to ensure that clients shall have a broad array of methods to choose from and enables clinics to offer more methods to more people at a low marginal cost in equipment, training, space and staff. This plan also allows AVSC to apply the skills and experience it has gained in infection control, training and provision of equipment to these other important methods.

The plan builds on the three principles that have characterized AVSC work through the years: (a) the right of men and women to have access to permanent and long-term contraception services that are (b) safe and effective; and (c) through free and informed choice.

Operating within these principles, AVSC will centre its work on services; training, information and education, and research will all be based in services and carried out in support of services. AVSC work will be based in the field, with the principal authority and responsibility resting with its field staff. Lastly, AVSC programmes must be based on what the countries themselves want and must be rooted in local systems and be responsive to local circumstances.

A. DEVELOPMENT OF A NEW APPROACH TO MEDICAL QUALITY ASSURANCE

AVSC is developing an approach to medical quality assurance that grows out of these principles and its service-centred, field-based and country-driven approach. It is part of a systematic approach to provision of quality services that is being developed in Kenya. It is based on COPE, a technique that family planning clinics use to assess their services and to make them client-oriented and provider efficient (hence COPE). COPE consists of instruments that clinics use themselves to analyse client flow, to check for problems in service provision and to set up a follow-up plan of action for solving identified problems (Dwyer and others, 1991). COPE has been successfully used in nine countries and in over 30 family planning service sites since 1990.

The key to the success of COPE is that it turns over the tasks of assessment of a service and of solving problems to the services themselves. AVSC is now working on the application of the COPE approach to broader aspects of quality in family planning services, including medical quality.

The projected numbers of sterilizations, IUDs, implants and injectables mentioned in note 1 are staggering and suggest the magnitude of the task of medical quality assurance: innumerable clinics will be providing these services. Even if it were appropriate for a foreign organization like AVSC to attempt to ensure medical quality in the services it supports or assists, it would be physically impossible to undertake the task of doing this at the level of services that is currently projected. And yet it must somehow be done. Respect and concern for the well-being of the clients of these services demand it and the continued acceptability of family planning services depends upon it. How can technical assistance organizations like AVSC help ensure that these services shall be delivered in a way that does not expose clients to risk of death or injury?

A first step is the development of medical standards. With the use of internationally recognized guidelines (such as those of the World Health Organization) and others (like those of AVSC), local medical leaders work to develop guidelines appropriate to the circum-

---

*New York, New York, United States of America.

stances of the country involved. Nigeria, for example, has been divided into four zones for the purpose of medical quality assurance. Medical leaders, based in medical schools, have been identified and are jointly developing service standards and are taking the lead in medical monitoring and quality assurance. These persons are leading academic physicians who are also involved in training the service providers they work with in quality assurance.

With this approach, quality assurance and monitoring become and are more likely to be perceived as a supportive effort rather than as a policing effort merely to be tolerated. This approach provides the opportunity for follow-up and for the development and fostering of a mentoring relation with the service providers that is crucial for sustaining quality services. The approach demands more time and travel on the part of scarce medically trained persons than the usual system of elaborate reporting and check-lists, but is, in the judgement of AVSC, more likely to achieve the end goal, which is to ensure that clients of these services shall not be exposed to undue risk from infection (especially important in view of the growing and invisible threat of human immunodeficiency virus (HIV) and hepatitis B infection) and that techniques shall be appropriate. It is ideally linked to training (the first step in medical quality assurance) because the trainer is likely to have the trust of his or her trainees and is likely to have the most influence.

AVSC is just beginning to apply the training-connected, service-based and locally managed approach to medical quality assurance, and it is too early to be able to report on results. It is clear that the application of these principles will vary from country to country, according to such circumstances as the approach to training, the style of service delivery (whether by government or non-governmental organization, or a mix),

the existing approach to quality assurance etc. Even so, it is believed that given the task to be accomplished and the importance of assuring that services offered are safe and effective, these principles need to be applied.

As the connection to training mentioned above suggests, the quality of services is best assured through a systems approach rather than through individual, vertical interventions. AVSC is now working to develop a broader application of the COPE approach to take in such areas as infection control, staff training and IUD asepsis, involving all staff in prenatal clinics, maternity wards, obstetrics-gynaecology clinics and outlying maternity centres to information about all family planning methods and to include the entire perinatal period and post-partum contraception in their family planning focus. This systems approach will be undertaken by staff of the service, after orientation and training, and with the provision of the necessary materials. The assessment and the follow-up will depend upon them.

NOTE

[1]Mauldin and Ross (1992) project that service providers will have to perform 150 million sterilizations, insert 310 million IUDs, implant 31 million sets of Norplant and give 663 million injections between 1990 and 2000.

REFERENCES

Dwyer, Joseph, and others (1991). COPE: a self-assessment technique for improving family planning services. AVSC Working Paper, No. 1. New York: Association for Voluntary Surgical Contraception.

Mauldin, W. Parker, and John A. Ross (1992). Contraceptive use and commodity costs in developing countries, 1990-2000. *International Family Planning Perspectives* (New York), vol. 18, No. 1 (March), pp. 4-9.

XLII. PROBLEMS AND PROSPECTS OF INTEGRATING FAMILY PLANNING WITH MATERNAL AND CHILD HEALTH, WITH SPECIAL EMPHASIS ON ADOLESCENTS

*World Health Organization**

A. SITUATION ANALYSIS

The problem

The prevention of pregnancy in adolescence is an issue of great importance for both health and population reasons. It has been given increasing priority by both government and non-governmental agencies in recent years (WHO, 1989a and 1989c). The heightened biomedical risks of maternal and child morbidity and mortality, especially in early adolescence, are accompanied by stunted social, educational and economic development, particularly of the young mother (WHO, 1991). The child may suffer from having a parent or parents who are just emerging from childhood themselves. An early beginning of child-bearing also increases the likelihood that a woman will have a larger number of children, exacerbating population growth, and possibly having them too close together as well. Currently, more than 50 per cent of the world's people are under age 25 and 80 per cent of the 1.5 billion young people (between ages 10 and 24) live in developing countries (United Nations, 1991). Increased telecommunications across cultural boundaries, travel, tourism, migration, urbanization (United Nations, 1989b) and a general decline in social control are contributing to an increase in and an earlier beginning of unprotected sexual relations before marriage, with adverse consequences in the young (Friedman, 1989b; United Nations, 1989a). The World Health Organization (WHO), the United Nations Children's Fund (UNICEF) and the United Nations Population Fund (UNFPA) have policy commitments to prevent too early pregnancy; and this stand has been endorsed at major conferences on population and family planning, women's health and status, safe motherhood and the health of young people. Although progress has been made in both policy and action, far more is needed for impact. One major area of importance is service provision, in its broadest sense, which is rarely adapted to meet adolescent needs nor integrated across key areas, including maternal and child health (MCH), family

planning services and services to prevent sexually transmitted diseases (STDs), including human immunodeficiency virus (HIV) infection leading to the acquired immunodeficiency syndrome (AIDS).

Family planning, or more precisely, the prevention of too early, unwanted and unplanned pregnancy in adolescence is somewhat different in nature for the married and unmarried adolescent. The young married adolescent will most commonly be found in highly traditional, rural societies, where an arranged marriage by agreement of two families is the norm and where the first child will be excepted soon after cohabitation begins. For contraception to be used requires changing the attitudes of the elders in the family, the community and the husband (as well as the young woman). Although she may be relatively safe from hazardous induced abortion, STD and HIV leading to AIDS, she remains at great risk for pregnancy and childbirth. Antenatal care may not be adequate to meet her needs, and she and her child will be at great risk of illness, injury and death, particularly in early adolescence.

The young unmarried adolescent girl (and boy) will face different obstacles to effective contraception, dependent upon the society in which they live, but the following obstacles are common. Little or nothing will be taught about sexuality or sexual behaviour, nor will sound and specific information be given about what methods of contraception exist, how to obtain and use them, what their degree of effectiveness is or possible side-effects. Where there is education on family life, for example, in the school system, it is more likely to deal with biological issues of reproduction and moral rules governing sexual behaviour before marriage.

The unmarried adolescent is likely to anticipate correctly a negative attitude on the part of family planning service providers if he or she shows interest in contraception, thereby indicating the possibility of current or future sexual relations. The adolescent will

---

*Division of Family Health, Geneva, Switzerland.

have less information about where to find services and how to use them, will be constrained from asking about them and is likely to have less money to expend on services of contraceptives than the adult. There will also be uncertainty about the legal status of seeking help with contraception, or abortion, the degree of confidentiality that will obtain and the extent to which parents or others will have to consent to their use of services. The net effect of these factors is that they will have less access to existing contraceptive services, to antenatal care and to abortion even in circumstances where it can be legally obtained. Those that do use services are likely to come later than adults, increasing their health risks.

Early sexual encounters by unmarried adolescents are less likely to be planned. In most developing countries, a contraceptive method is not likely to be used at first in sexual relations. Nor will either partner take conscious action to prevent STD or HIV infection, leading to AIDS, through the use of a condom or safe sex practices. This sexual activity is likely to be kept secret from a girl's family. If she suspects a pregnancy, she is more likely to turn to her boyfriend or to a close girlfriend for advice, rather than to either the family or health services. In many circumstances, she may well try to induce an abortion herself or go to a non-medical practitioner, clandestinely, often with tragic consequences.

Although the male adolescent is not vulnerable to pregnancy, he is equally and often more exposed to STD than the girl, especially in societies where it is common for initial experiences to be with sex workers. Even if the adolescent male is interested in using contraceptive methods to prevent pregnancy, he is unlikely to make use of family planning services catering predominantly for married women. Research also suggests that he may attribute more knowledge about contraception to the adolescent female than she actually has, and there is likely to be very little communication between them on that subject or STD prevention, even if it is on their minds.

Although because of the AIDS pandemic, there is much more public communication about the use of the condom in many societies, that information is often not specific enough to tell the young adolescent how to use a condom nor to overcome embarrassment about asking for one or purchasing one at pharmacy. If he does use it, he is likely to purchase it from a vending machine (without instruction) or to obtain it from a friend.

Obstacles to overcome

Broadly speaking, there are four major obstacles to overcome in order to facilitate better pregnancy and STD prevention in adolescence.

(a) A lack of knowledge about maturation, sexual behaviour, pregnancy, contraception, STD and AIDS among young people, accompanied by a lack of information about sources of help, how to use them and their rights to them;

(b) A lack of services adapted to meet adolescent needs which are accessible, effective and integrated in approach to maximize their timely utilization;

(c) A lack of training among health providers in MCH and family planning services, particularly in subjects of adolescent sexuality and maturation, and interpersonal communication and counselling skills for working with the young;

(d) A lack of policies and legislation that affect adolescent health care in such a way as to facilitate the provision and accessibility of services for young people.

B. Action needed

Education and information

The lack of knowledge and information from which young people suffer needs to be addressed from multiple sources, including schools, youth organizations, women's organizations and religious institutions, as well as the family. This can be done in partnership with health and family planning establishments which have expertise on specific subjects. The mass media are another major channel of knowledge and information which can be both unidirectional, as in the case of brief cogent information presented to a mass audience, and participatory, as in question-and-answer columns in magazines and newspapers, and on radio and television programmes. A third important means of imparting information and knowledge is through telephone "hot-lines", which are feasible in towns with public telephone kiosks and which provide both an anonymous and confidential service as well as a personalized communication system, although it is important that such services be appropriately supervised.

Training and sensitization

For such education to be provided, however, it must be relevant to the young people participating in it and appropriate within the cultural context. For this purpose, training in communication skills of those who teach is essential. Such interaction, which permits young people to put forward their questions and ideas, is essential for the integration of information into young people's attitudes and behaviour and also assures the relevance and culture specificity of information. It is also important that an understanding of adolescent sexuality and development be part of training so that those who impart knowledge will be able to encourage and answer questions without undue embarrassment and on the basis of sound information. Such training can be part of the professional preparation, for example, of nurses, doctors, midwives, pharmacists, teachers and others that are likely to interact with the young, as well a part of continual in-service training in such professions, at least for a portion of those willing and able to work with young people.

Service provision

The provision of information and education by trained people must be backed up by service provision to those adolescents who need help. Services can take a variety of forms, including guidance and counselling; but ultimately, for the sexually active young person, there must be help with contraceptive provision, antenatal care when needed and help with unwanted pregnancy within the context of the culture. Counselling needs to be a part of all such services, particularly counselling provided through effective listening skills. WHO has developed a module for such training (Friedman and Hedlund, 1991). For such services to have an impact, they must, first of all, be accessible to young people. They must be legally mandated or at least not run strongly counter to laws which make them inaccessible to young (or unmarried) people. To be accessible they must meet certain characteristics for adolescents: they must be, and be seen to be, confidential so that young people will not be deterred from going to them for help. They must be run at hours when young people can conveniently get to them, have a low cost to the young client and provide the maximum degree of privacy so that a young person may approach them without excessive fear of exposure. They must be advertised in such a manner that information about them reaches young people. Their procedures of admitting a young person for help must be simple and clear, and to the extent possible quick, because adolescents may be anxious and grow increasingly uncomfortable when they are not certain how they will be received.

The reproductive health problems of young people—too early or unwanted pregnancy and childbirth, induced abortion in hazardous circumstances, STDs and now HIV infection leading to AIDS—have as a root cause unprotected sexual behaviour. For multiple reasons, it is difficult for adolescents to use any such services. The more compartmentalized such services are, the less likely it is that they will use them and use them in a timely fashion. There is a growing consensus on the need for a holistic approach for services to be effective (WHO, 1989c). A young woman who comes for contraceptive help is just as likely to need protection from STD as from pregnancy as, say, a young man who goes for treatment for STD is in need of contraception to protect his sexual partner(s) from pregnancy. STD is particularly insidious both because it is often asymptomatic in the young woman and because it is likely to heighten the risks of AIDS (as well as being a major cause of infertility).

The adolescent girl who comes for contraceptive help may, in fact, already be pregnant (or suffering from STD). She may need antenatal care rather than contraception help at this juncture, though she will need help in protecting herself in the future. The knowledge of a pregnancy may lead her to seek an abortion and she will need counselling. If the atmosphere of the service inspires her confidence she is more likely to be candid about her intentions and benefit from all the help available.

It is greatly to the advantage of an adolescent to have integrated services which optimize the likelihood of getting help both for care and for future problem prevention. Helping the young person deal with the factors that push them, perhaps prematurely, into sexual activity needs to be permitted to be addressed at any clinic providing contraceptive or antenatal care, as well as treatment and control of STD. And those services which make it feasible, within the cultural context, for both sexes to be served will have a considerable advantage in helping the young.

There are a number of different models for health services for young people, including those which: (a) provide special services for adolescents within a service for adults, by, for example, setting aside special hours, or especially trained staff to deal with young people; (b) have a separate service for young people alone (a costlier approach and not always practical); and (c) provide a health service for young people in the context of a youth or community service.

Any model that fits the community resources can work, if the criteria for accessibility, confidentiality and appropriate trained staff are met. From what has been learned in the field, it is also clear that the more young people themselves are involved in the planning, implementation and evaluation of services, the more likely they are to be acceptable and effective.

Policy and legislation

In order for education, information, training and service provision to take place, it is essential that there be public support both at the policy-making level and within local communities. It is important that advocacy takes place, but to be effective in any given culture it is essential that sound information be provided about the health needs of young people, existing problems and how they are being met in that society. The views of key people needs to be elicited, particularly with respect to how they would like to resolve problems and meet the new needs which are being generated by changes in behaviour and social mores, so that they become partners for change consistent with their cultural values.

Legislation that affects the health and behaviour of young people in this sphere is often inconsistent, not known or misunderstood and unequally applied (Paxman and Zuckerman, 1987). Legislation that affects, for example, the age of consent for sexual relations, in regard to sexual abuse, for marriage, for contraceptive provision, for pregnancy termination, for reporting of STDs, for tracing of partners, for parental or partner consent for the use of family planning or maternity services etc. may be inconsistent and markedly different for males and females. Most of all, there will be often confusion about what the law is and how it is applied among the professional health community as well as among adolescents. An understanding of what the law is and how it is being applied would be helpful in determining whether there is a need for change in legislation.

Research and evaluation

Although much of what is needed for action is known, there remains a considerable need for research, particu-

larly at the country level, on a number of issues. These issues include:

(a) Epidemiological research which describes the reproductive health and STD problems among young people in a given society and provides a baseline for measuring trends and potential evaluation of impact;

(b) Behavioural research which shows the patterns of adolescent sexual and reproductive health behaviour and the use of existing services by young people and also provides a baseline for measuring future trends for the potential measurement of the impact of action. WHO has developed a special method for such research (Friedman, 1989a).

(c) Operational research which contributes to the understanding of how services are currently functioning, including the involvement of young people themselves in the planning, implementation and evaluation of services, in the broadest sense;

(d) Policy/legislation research which describes the current status and how implementation of law and policy takes place;

(e) Biomedical research to continue to find contraceptive methods that better meet the needs of young people, including efficiency, effectiveness, ease of use, lack of side-effects and long-term negative consequences, low cost, low embarrassment level and effectiveness for both STD and pregnancy prevention.

C. CONCLUSION

The overall approach to the promotion of adolescent reproductive health requires an interactive approach in which each sector of the community provides what it can do best. All societies want the best for their children, and it is on that basis that appropriate behaviour and health can best be promoted. There is common ground that can be elicited through a consensual rather than a confrontational approach, which draws upon the best in people for a common cause. The need for promoting and protecting the health of young people has never been greater both for their own good and for that of their societies. A concerted effort and cooperation is needed, not only of agencies and organizations but of the public at large.

REFERENCES

Friedman, H. L. (1989a). Address to the Society for Adolescent Medicine on behalf of WHO: 1989 Recipient of the Hilary Millar Award for Innovative Approaches to Adolescent Health Care, San Francisco, March. Geneva: World Health Organization.

_____ (1989b). The health of adolescents: beliefs and behaviour. *Social Science and Medicine* (Tarrytown, New York), vol. 29, No. 3, pp. 309-315.

_____, and D. E. Hedlund (1991). Counselling skills training for adolescent health: a WHO approach to a global need. *International Journal for the Advancement of Counselling* (Dordrecht, Netherlands), vol. 14, pp. 59-69.

Paxman, John M., and Zuckerman, Ruth Jane (1987). *Laws and Policies Affecting Adolescent Health*. Geneva: World Health Organization.

United Nations (1989a). *Adolescent Reproductive Behaviour*, vol. II, *Evidence from Developing Countries*. Population Studies, No. 109/Add.1. Sales No. E.89.XIII.10.

_____ (1989b). *Prospects of World Urbanization, 1988*. Population Studies, No. 112. Sales No. E.89.XIII.8.

_____ (1991). *World Population Prospects, 1990*. Population Studies, No. 120. Sales No. E.91.XIII.4.

World Health Organization (1989a). The health of youth. Background document of the 1989 technical discussions. Geneva.

_____ (1989b). *The Health of Youth*. Final report of the 1989 technical discussions. Geneva.

_____ (1989c). *The Reproductive Health of Adolescents: A Strategy for Action*. Joint WHO/UNFPA/UNICEF statement. Geneva.

_____ (1993). Resolutions 38.22 and 42.41. In *Handbook of Decisions and Resolutions of the World Health Assembly and Executive Board*, vol. III, *1985-1990*. Geneva.

_____ (1991). *Maternal Mortality: A Global Factbook*. Compiled by Carla AbouZahr and Erica Royston. Geneva.

_____ (1992). *A Study of the Sexual Experience of Young People in Eleven African Countries: The Narrative Research Method*. WHO/ADH.92.5. Geneva.

XLIII. FAMILY WELL-BEING: AN INTERNATIONAL YEAR OF THE FAMILY PERSPECTIVE

*United Nations Office at Vienna**

The family has been recognized as the basic unit of society. In all parts of the world, families continue to be the social institution entrusted with the responsibility for population renewal and the rearing of children. As it is within families that reproduction, in general, takes place, they are a central object of focus in addressing population issues and population policies that have a direct impact on families.

The close interrelatedness of the substantive concerns and the complementarity of the International Conference on Population and Development and the International Year of the Family, 1994, are obvious. It is imperative that various family aspects of population issues are addressed in the preparation, observance and follow-up of the International Year of the Family. It is also essential that the Population Conference and its expert deliberations take account of the International Year of the Family, particularly in terms of reinforcing an integrated family perspective to population issues.

The purpose of this discussion note is: (*a*) to present the basic substantive orientation of the International Year of the Family; (*b*) to provide an analysis, from that perspective, of the impact of changes in family size and forms on family well-being and the effects of decline in fertility and mortality rates on family support systems, as well as to identify their policy and programme implications; and (*c*) to suggest some recommendations with regard the family and population policies.

A. THE INTERNATIONAL YEAR OF THE FAMILY

The United Nations General Assembly, in its resolution 44/82 of 8 December 1989, proclaimed 1994 as the International Year of the Family, with the theme of "Family: resources and responsibilities in a changing world". The proclamation resulted from an ever-increasing global concern over the precarious situation of families and the future of that basic unit of society.

A major objective of the International Year is to create among policy makers and the public a greater appreciation of the family as the fundamental unit of society, leading in turn to increased governmental and voluntary action on its behalf. The Year should encourage a better understanding of family functions and problems; promote knowledge of the economic, social and demographic processes affecting families and their members; and focus attention on the rights and responsibilities of all family members. With its primary focus on action at the local and national levels, to be supported by the United Nations and its system of organizations, the Year should strengthen national capabilities to formulate, implement and monitor policies on behalf of families; enhance the effectiveness of local, regional and national efforts to respond to problems affecting, and affected by, the situation of families; and improve collaboration among national and international non-governmental organizations in support of multi-sectoral activities relating to families. The strengthening of the family as a primary social group should take place in the context of full enjoyment of each individual's basic human rights. Hence the motto for the Year: "Building the smallest democracy at the heart of society".

An important contribution of the International Year should be fostering the development of a family impact consideration in all development activities. A first goal must therefore be to encourage organizations and agencies, governmental or non-governmental, national or international, to recognize that their decisions and actions usually have an impact on families, for example, on how families will be formed, whether they will survive, and how well they function as nurturers and providers. A second goal might then be to improve the formulation and implementation of family-sensitive policies and to devise appropriate means to deal with a broad and varied range of specific problems related to families. The Year also offers an opportunity to reinforce an integrated strategy in social policy and develop-

*Secretariat for the International Year of the Family, Social Development Division, Centre for Social Development and Humanitarian Affairs, Vienna, Austria.

ment, as the subject of families offers a comprehensive and, at the same time, synthesizing approach.

The International Year of the Family programme identifies three specific issues as starting-points for the identification of local and national priorities:

(a) Strengthening the family's ability to meet its own needs. The family should be aided and encouraged to fulfil its important functions for the benefit of all society;

(b) Clarifying and understanding the balance between how the family can satisfy its needs and what it can expect through public provision of services. When making decisions about providing or cutting back services, consideration should be given to how these decisions will affect families, directly or indirectly;

(c) Recognizing the effect of societal ills on family relationships and acknowledging that government policy intervention may be needed to counter negative behaviour or exploitation in the family. Because of the intimate nature of family relationships, negative behaviour or exploitation is only too often tolerated within families. In line with the concepts of equality between women and men and the rights of all individual family members, it is imperative to promote the development and strengthening of perceptions and perspectives regarding intra-familial relationships that are consistent with basic human rights and fundamental freedoms, as well as internationally accepted social policy standards and principles.

The programme of the Year recognizes that familial well-being may depend in large measure upon the ability of families to make informed and sensitive choices concerning fertility. Such choices are important in diminishing maternal and infant morbidity and mortality. Full, informed and joint participation in family planning decisions by both spouses is recognized to be essential for a responsible choice and a wider sharing of familial roles and responsibilities. Increased efforts are required to ensure adequate family life education concerning reproduction, sexuality, birth-spacing, the impact of the acquired immunodeficiency syndrome (AIDS), parenting skills and responsibilities, as well as access in rural and urban areas of family planning and fertility services. Family life education is required also to promote a deeper understanding of responsibilities in a familial and interpersonal context, as well as the promotion of family

values. Increased attention is called for to promote the role of families in meeting the health requirements of all their members, in primary health care and in maternal and child health.

B. FAMILY PLANNING AND FAMILY WELL-BEING

The International Year of the Family takes a broad view of family well-being, which includes the physical, emotional, economic, social and psychological elements necessary to strengthen and support the family's ability to perform its functions. What differentiates families from other social institutions are the emotional, social and legal relationships between spouses, parents and children, siblings and relatives. The main functions of families can be best described according to the relationships that exist between various family members. Thus, the primary functions of all families are: establishing emotional, social and economic bonds between the spouses; regulating procreation and sexual relations between the spouses; giving name and status, especially to children; providing basic care for children, as well as elderly and disabled members; socializing and educating children; protecting family members; providing emotional care and recreation of family members; and exchanging goods and services (United Nations Office at Vienna, 1992a).

Family well-being is seen as the foundation of the well-being of society. It is the family that provides the primary social, physical, emotional, psychological and economic training for its members and serves as a social safety net for them during times of crisis. Social and economic policies must be directed to strengthening the family in carrying out its functions, especially during times of rapid change or crisis. Although all societies have norms, traditions, laws, policies, benefits, services and programmes that affect family functions, careful planning to support and strengthen the functions of families is scare. As a result, many families have had to create their own support systems, often adapting to the lack of external support by having a large family.

Family size

There is a direct correlation between the size of the family and the well-being of its members. As family size decreases, the well-being of its members increases and the family is better able to perform its functions. It has been clearly shown that when families are supported externally, they have fewer children and provide better care for them. This improved family well-being contributes to an improvement in overall social well-being and leads to reduced need for government spending on rehabilitating family members that did not receive proper care from their family.

Although the reduction in family size has had an overall positive effect on well-being, there have been some important negative consequences associated with smaller family size. For example, the reduction of family size has reduced the number of people in the family who can provide care or emotional support. The influence of older siblings was often an important component in the socialization of younger children in larger families.

Smaller families have also enabled more women to participate in the labour market and spend more years there, enabling them to meet economic needs. However, despite working full time, most working women still are required to fulfil the nurturing role inside the family. Unless there is greater sharing of family responsibilities between the spouses, the emotional and nurturing functions of the family are dispersed to people or institutions outside the family, affecting family well-being.

Migration of people in search of work often physically separates families from their extended family support system, which traditionally shared the care for children, elderly and disabled. In single-parent families the situation is even worse, because they are almost always headed by women that have to work and support themselves and their children, and often have very few resources available to them. In families where these mothers cannot find work or cannot earn enough to pay for the basic needs of their children, these children may be physically abandoned.

Family equilibrium is best ensured when all family members share in the care and emotional support functions by helping with meal preparation, household chores and listening to each other's problems. It is important that men take equal responsibility for these functions in order to reduce the pressure in the family for working mothers. In single-parent families, there is a danger that the parent may be overburdened or that the children may be forced to assume adult responsibilities.

Changes in family form

As the size of the family has been reduced, there have been increased opportunities for increased material and economic well-being. Reduction in the size of the family often brings with it rapid changes in the form of the family. These structural changes are often accompanied by emotional, psychological and social stresses which may counterbalance the material and economic gains.

The extended family has been replaced by the nuclear family in more industrialized and urbanized societies and the nuclear family itself is changing substantially (United Nations, 1989). Divorce, desertion, migration, unwed mothers and death of a spouse due to war have created many single-parent families, mostly headed by women and existing at or below poverty level. Kinship families, usually consisting of more than three generations, have also declined due of migration.

One of the recent changes in family form has been the rise of reorganized families. Reorganized families occur when couples remarry or decide to cohabit. Another form of family appearing more frequently in developed countries is cohabitation between young people that decide to live together without getting legally married. More and more couples are also choosing to marry or cohabitat and remain childless.

Effects of declining fertility and mortality on families

The positive effects of fertility decline on family support systems can be offset by the added burdens of the care of aged parents that live longer, when not adequately supported. With the breakdown of extended, kinship and tribal family systems, the responsibility for elderly care falls to the children and their families. Even though many developing countries have successfully reduced their birth and death rates, they have not provided enough external support for families that have to care for elderly or disabled parents. There is a need for public support mechanisms to help families cope with the rapid social, economic, political and technological changes which are occurring in many countries.

In addition, there is another structural problem to overcome. Welfare and human services are usually provided in two ways: functional programmes; and categorical programmes. Functional programmes are problem-oriented and individually focused, and may focus on the problems of women, men or children, but not usually on families. Categorical programmes often target the needs of certain categories of the population, such as the disabled, the elderly or the economically disadvantaged. Again, their problems are not usually viewed from a family perspective, except for families that are chronically disadvantaged. Public policy, laws, benefits, programmes and services must be refocused on the needs of all families and must develop ways to strengthen families so that they can perform their functions more effectively.

Family planning programmes must also be broadly based so they can support and strengthen families and avail of the resources they offer. They should have a broad perspective and relate to other programmes. Individual problems should be examined in the context of the family as a social unit and not just as problems of individuals that happen to be family members. For example, the educational and emotional support functions of families in the prevention of teenage pregnancy and AIDS are of vital importance.

Family well-being: a prevention model

A major problem with public welfare and support programmes for families is that they are usually too little too late. State welfare services usually seek to remediate problems when families have already broken down. Very little attention is given to designing preventive programmes that could strengthen the family's capabilities to handle predictable crises. Attention should be directed to developing cost-effective preventive approaches to family support.

Prevention programmes and services are cost-effective and less intrusive on family autonomy. Such services as parent education, nutritional education, health support, prenatal and perinatal care, family planning, medical care, marriage counselling or family therapy; school courses in communication and human relationships, conflict management, sexuality, home economics and child development; and government policies that support and strengthen families are all crucial components in a prevention-oriented model of service delivery. As part of a prevention-oriented model of service delivery, greater attention must be given to creating and strengthening indigenous support networks.

It is necessary to bring needed services and programmes to the people rather than expect the people to obtain them from centralized offices. Neighbourhood schools, clinics, religious and community centres could be utilized as family resource centres to provide easily accessible local support for families. These centres could develop programmes and services in family planning, family life education, prenatal and perinatal care, nutrition, family recreation and so forth with the help of professionals as well as trained volunteers.

The most important area of primary prevention is prenatal and perinatal care programmes and services. Early intervention is the best way to prevent health, developmental and learning problems. By providing free or low-cost services to prospective parents (both men and women), children can be given the nutritional support and medical care they need from the very beginning of life in order to grow and develop in normal healthy ways. Perinatal services are also important.

Equal education rights for the girl child and women need to be emphasized, as there is a direct correlation between the education of mothers and the health of the family, the family size, the spacing of children and the economic well-being of the family. Mothers also often need education and supportive services to help them properly bond with their children and to know how to support a gradual and healthy psychological separation of the infant. If this vital individuation process is not properly supported, the child will be unable to function effectively as an autonomous adult (Weinhold and Weinhold, 1992). It is far more effective to teach parents or prospective parents how to bond effectively with their children and inform them about the dangers of prolonged separation than to try to repair damage years later.

Policy and programme implications

Throughout the world, families are undergoing drastic changes. Although these changes differ in each region, there are some commonalities: smaller families; an increase in divorces; the longevity of family members; and the transformation of relationships due to changes in values as well as in industrial and post-industrial economics. Also, changes in the roles of men and women and in the forms of families are taking place everywhere in the world.

It is important to take into account policy and programme implications for creating more effective support for all families. It is obvious that the reasons for "family problems" do not lie solely in families. Neither are the solutions to these problems solely in their hands. Families "at risk" should not be viewed as "risky families," but instead "families in risky situations". This point highlights the need to develop effective legislation, family policies, services and benefits targeted to strengthen the basic family functions. The following areas need to be addressed in developing effective preventive legislation, family policies, services and benefits for families (United Nations Office, at Vienna, 1992b).

Social security programmes and policies

A significant decline in fertility takes place only when families perceive that their security can be assured by other means than by maintaining large families. The provision of social security systems, to the extent feasible, is one of the most effective way to ensure a rapid yet orderly demographic transition.

Social assistance programmes and policies

Notwithstanding the limits imposed by their financial implications in developing countries, for those people not eligible for assistance under a contributory programme, non-contributory social assistance can be crucial to break the self-perpetuating cycle of poverty. Because of the vital role that women play in maintaining the internal family support system, they should be the recipients of any direct social assistance payments. Assistance should not, however, entrust them with the sole responsibility of performing the function. These payments can be tied to participation in prenatal and perinatal programmes or other preventive programmes.

Local accessibility of services

Every effort must be made to bring the necessary programmes and services closer to the families that need them. This means the creation of a decentralized service delivery programme for families, utilizing neighbourhood facilities.

Development of indigenous support networks

In any given neighbourhood or community indigenous helpers are already performing valuable family support services. They are usually well known by the family members and are often sought out for advice or assistance. Governmental social welfare programmes usually do not make use of these people in the design of social safety nets for families. These agencies must begin to identify, train and coordinate the efforts of these people to create indigenous support networks for families. Families usually already know and trust these people, making it easier for them to intervene or provide services to families than the welfare department professionals. Moreover, where resources lack for social security or social assistance programmes, indigenous support networks represent a valuable alternative.

General objectives of preventive family policies

In the development of sound preventive family policies, policy makers may make use of the following guidelines:

(a) Identify and monitor all existing indigenous support systems of social welfare and social security, including an evaluation of the effectiveness of these support systems;

(b) Promote and develop all possible means of articulation between public social services (central and local) and all indigenous support systems. The informal and non-traditional relationships that make these indigenous support networks effective must be honoured and respected. Any temptation to reduce their diversity or formalize their roles should be resisted;

(c) Provide direct support in areas where the indigenous system is unable to do so. Support should strengthen the self-help capability of families rather than make them dependent upon the support. It also should have preventive potential and be given to the family member who can most directly provide help or care for those family members needing it. It is preferable to giving direct support to a dysfunctional family member whenever possible;

(d) Constant monitoring of social conditions is required in order to identify potential and actual processes that may increase the level of family or individual dysfunction or put added stress on the family or indigenous support systems. Analysing potential family problems related to AIDS is an example of this type of monitoring;

(e) Constant reviewing of family policies is required to identify gaps, overlap and changes needed because of changing social conditions, demographic transitions, economic fluctuations etc. Family policy must be able to change and adapt to rapidly changing conditions that adversely affect families;

(f) Public welfare agencies must develop and utilize flexible and innovative methods when working with indigenous support systems. The traditional methods of articulation which are usually top-down, may not work well in dealing with indigenous support systems. Professionals must be able to create peer relationships with indigenous helpers;

(g) Create a database of relevant demographic and research information to help guide family policy decisions. Without accurate information that permits a trend analysis, it is difficult to do any effective long-range policy planning. Much of the information needed for this database may have been gathered for other purposes and will have to be reinterpreted in relation to family issues and problems. It must also be continually updated as new information and research findings become available.

C. THE FAMILY AND POPULATION POLICIES: SUGGESTIONS FOR RECOMMENDATIONS

To a large extent, the perception, attitudes, aspirations and decisions of individuals with regard to fertility and migration, as well as nutrition, sanitation and labour, that are relevant to morbidity and mortality, are developed in the context of the family and broader kinship-based micro-support systems. They are affected by the pattern of rights, expectations and responsibilities of individuals as members of these systems. It is the aggregate of demographically relevant decision-making and behaviour in the context of family membership that makes up the demographic condition of a society. The concern of population policies is to bring this demographic condition into harmony with broad societal conditions and goals. In turn, changes in fertility, mortality and migration influence the size and structure of populations from which family support systems can be drawn. Moreover, demographic conditions may affect, directly or indirectly, the capability of Governments to provide support for families and may influence the economic condition of families. Therefore, careful consideration must be given to the need to achieve close coordination between population and family policies and harmonization of their goals and measures.

From a social policy and development perspective on the family, and in the context of the International Year of the Family, attention may be given to the following suggestions in formulating recommendations for consideration of the International Conference on Population and Development in 1994:

(a) Recognizing the fundamental role of the family in procreation and socialization as well as in providing economic, social and emotional support essential to the well-being of the individual members, in particular, children, elderly and the disabled, a "family impact" consideration should be promoted in the formulation and implementation of population and demographic policies and programmes;

(b) It is essential to undertake reviews of national family laws and to initiate family legislation projects in order to ensure family-oriented policies and programmes. In these efforts, laws and legislation influencing family formulation and fertility should receive special attention;

(c) Families offer valuable resources in achieving population policy objectives. Policies and programmes should therefore seek to support the functions of the family with regard to procreation, socialization and caregiving. In the observance of and follow-up to the International Year of the Family, special attention should be given to promoting family life education, responsible parenthood and, in particular, responsible fatherhood and equal rights and responsibilities of both spouses with regard to family planning, as well as increased access to education and health for both sexes;

(d) Families can positively influence adolescent reproductive behaviour. Families should be encouraged and supported in educating adolescents on reproductive behaviour and on the risks associated with unprotected sexual activities, particularly the increased exposure to sexually transmitted diseases and the human immunodeficiency virus (HIV) and AIDS.

REFERENCES

United Nations (1989). *Report on the World Social Situation*. Sales No. E.89.IV.1.

United Nations Office at Vienna (1992a). *Families: Forms and Functions*. Centre for Social Development and Humanitarian Affairs, International Year of the Family Secretariat. Occasional Paper Series, No. 2.

_____ (1992b). Relationships between demographic and social processes and social policy interventions at different stages of the demographic transition. Background paper for the Seminar on the Social Consequences of Population Growth and Changing Social Conditions with Particular Emphasis on the Family, Vienna, 21-25 September 1992. Centre for Social Development and Humanitarian Affairs, Developmental Social Welfare Unit.

Weinhold, Janae B., and Barry K. Weinhold (1992). *Counter-dependency: The Flight From Intimacy*. Colorado Springs, Colorado: CICRCL Press.

XLIV. ECONOMICS OF FAMILY PLANNING

*Barbara Janowitz**

As the demand for contraceptive protection continues to grow throughout the developing world, donor resources for family planning have stagnated. Although forecasts of the cost of family planning services vary, all projections show substantially higher costs in the year 2000. Where will the resources for family planning programmes come from? If larger contributions from donors or local governments are unlikely to materialize, the other alternatives are to institute or increase client fees for family planning and/or other services or to reduce the costs of service provision.

Many countries and programmes are faced with the phasing out of population assistance. Such countries must put major emphasis on activities that encourage efficiency and sustainability. Other countries and programmes need to begin planning for eventual reductions in donor funding.

In order to assess the potential for cost savings through increases in efficiency and cost recovery, family planning programmes should be encouraged to:

(*a*) Compare cost/output ratios of various services in order to provide the information needed to improve programme efficiency and to establish pricing policies;

(*b*) Explore options for reducing dependence upon donors to the greatest extent possible, given the constraints faced;

(*c*) Evaluate new methods and delivery systems in terms of their impact on incremental costs and contraceptive use;

(*d*) Weigh the health benefits and economic costs of medical requirements which may be unnecessary and may actually reduce quality of services.

These four recommendations translate directly into corresponding sets of research questions:

(*a*) What are the costs of method-specific contraceptive services and how do costs vary with how methods are delivered (clinic, community-based distribution (CBD) or social marketing)? What are the implications for overall programme costs when different combinations of methods and delivery systems are selected? How is the cost of a family planning service distributed among programmes, clients and donors?

(*b*) What options do family planning programmes have to raise revenues? What impact do price increases have on the demand for family planning services and on total revenues? What is the potential for "instalment financing" of long-acting and permanent methods? What is the potential for cross-subsidization of family planning services?

(*c*) What does it cost to provide new methods (or methods new to countries) or new ways of delivering methods? What is the impact on contraceptive use?

(*d*) How do medical barriers affect costs to programmes and to users? If barriers are removed, what are the resource savings and health consequences?

The following sections develop each of these four areas in greater detail.

A. COSTS OF METHODS AND DELIVERY SYSTEMS

With information on costs, programmes can quantify resource needs, determine if they should emphasize different methods or ways of providing them and establish cost recovery targets.

Costing methodology should be based on the fundamental economic concept of opportunity costs. This concept requires cost analyses to focus on full programme costs, not just those costs which are currently paid by the programme. One important rationale for this approach is that programmes may eventually have to pay

*Director, Economics Unit, Family Health International, Research Triangle Park, North Carolina, United States of America.

all their costs; thus, they need information on what the total cost burden would be.

Studies of the costs of family planning have been completed in the Dominican Republic, Ecuador and Morocco. Studies are currently underway in Bangladesh and Honduras. The Dominican Republic project produced estimates of the full costs of methods provided through clinics, CBD and a social marketing programme. The findings indicate that Norplant had the highest cost per couple-years of protection (CYP), as well as the largest proportion of its costs covered by donors.

If comparisons of method and delivery specific costs are to be made, programmes need to use comparable methodologies. With support from the United Nations Population Fund (UNFPA), Family Health International is preparing a manual for family planning programmes to use in calculating their costs.

B. COST RECOVERY

The potential of a family planning programme to cover a significant share of its costs depends upon several factors, including the demand for services, the socio-economic status of clients and the existence of competing service providers. Basically, programmes can try to earn or increase revenues in two ways: *(a)* charge fees for family planning services; or *(b)* cross-subsidize family planning services through sales of other goods and services.

Fees for family planning services

The precise impact of an increase in clinic fees is difficult to predict. Demand for services probably would decline at first, but could rebound after clients became accustomed to the higher fees. Clinic revenues could increase or decrease, depending upon the magnitude of the price increase and the decline in demand. The most important issue for many pro-grammes is the impact of fees on the poorest clients; will the new fees impose a barrier for those women who may be most in need of contraceptive protection?

The impact of price increases may be limited by setting prices according to income level, but such a scheme may be difficult to implement. Another option is to charge higher prices for scheduled appointments than for unscheduled visits or for evening rather than for daytime clients. Such ideas can capitalize on different abilities to pay but may not work unless clients perceive that they are getting higher quality services for the higher fees.

It is easier to collect revenues for "pay as you go methods", such as oral contraceptives and condoms than for long-acting and permanent methods. But in the light of the United Nations Agency for International Development interest in encouraging a shift to long-acting and permanent methods, what are the possibilities for "instalment" or other financing arrangements to spread the payments for these methods over longer time periods?

Cross-subsidization

The potential for cross-subsidization of family planning services depends upon several factors: *(a)* what health services the clinic provides and at what cost; *(b)* at what other places those services are sold; *(c)* the volume of sales; *(d)* the differential in quality of services at various sites; *(e)* the potential of sales of such services to raise revenue; and *(g)* whether resources will be needed to increase quality to attract new customers and, if so, at what cost.

C. COSTS AND IMPACT OF INTRODUCING NEW METHODS OR DELIVERY SYSTEMS

Programmes should evaluate whether it makes economic sense to introduce a new method or a new delivery system, given the context in which the programme operates. If the addition increases contraceptive use and lowers costs, the decision is easy. However, the programme must often weigh offsetting effects, such as a negative impact on costs and a positive impact on contraceptive use.

Research has been carried out to compare the cost of Norplant with that of other methods providing similar protection. This research also focused on the potential of Norplant to raise contraceptive use. Findings suggest that in countries with high levels of contraceptive prevalence, Norplant introduction results in higher programme costs. Most acceptors are previous users of other methods.

The impact of introducing a new distribution system, namely, social marketing, has been examined in Honduras. Results showed that the introduction of social marketing did not raise contraceptive use nor did it decrease costs. However, costs could have been reduced if the family planning programme had decreased resources invested in competing programmes at the same time that sales of the social marketing programme were expanding.

D. MEDICAL SERVICES: COSTS AND QUALITY OF SERVICES

Some clinic practices that medical personnel regard as ensuring high quality may actually discourage contraceptive acceptance or continued use, reduce service quality and raise programme costs. For example, laboratory tests for acceptors of hormonal methods or a clinic visit requirement for an acceptor in a CBD programme may have little or no impact on health of women, and yet such practices may lead to crowded facilities and disgruntled clients who must wait long hours.

Cost savings could potentially be realized if unnecessary medical services were removed. However, programmes may be reluctant to eliminate these practices if they think that such services ensure high-quality care and low medical risk to contraceptive users.

In many countries, for example, the vast majority of clients at clinics are making revisits; most of these are routinely scheduled visits. If the number of revisits could be reduced, women would benefit by saving time and money travelling to the clinic and time waiting at the clinic for services. Clinics would benefit by having more time to serve women with medical needs.

Programmatic research is being carried out by Family Health International and the Population Council in Ecuador and Mexico examine the costs and benefits of reducing the number of revisits for acceptors of an intra-uterine device.

XLV. BARRIERS TO CONTRACEPTIVE DEVELOPMENT

*J. Joseph Speidel**

Universal access to family planning is crucial with the current high rates of unintended pregnancy, unsafe abortion, poor maternal health, sexually transmitted diseases (STDs) and unprecedented growth in human numbers. Although the first priority must be to expand access to existing contraceptive methods and improve the quality of family planning services, there is also an urgent need to develop new and better contraceptives.

There is no "perfect" contraceptive method. There are trade-offs among currently available birth control methods in terms of efficacy in preventing pregnancy, health risks and benefits, and convenience. But the more contraceptive options there are to choose from, the better the fit between contraceptive user and method, based on individual priorities and concerns. A growing body of evidence suggests that each new contraceptive method attracts some persons that did not previously use a method and contributes to increased overall levels of family planning use.

The process of developing a new contraceptive is complicated, time-consuming and expensive, and it requires a supportive societal environment. Unfortunately, the current climate for contraceptive development in the United States of America is unfavourable, if not hostile. Contributing to this situation are inadequate levels of public funding for contraceptive research, combined with a lack of financial incentives for the private sector; the controversy among the American public surrounding abortion and, more generally, issues of sexuality; notions of acceptable risk and safety assurance for contraceptives which influence the stringent regulatory procedures of the United States Food and Drug Administration (FDA); and the risk of product liability litigation. To improve the climate for contraceptive development, these economic, cultural, political and legal barriers must be addressed.

A. NEED FOR NEW CONTRACEPTIVES

Current levels of access to family planning methods and services worldwide are grossly inadequate. An estimated 3 million infants and children worldwide die each year because they were born too soon, too late or spaced too closely together in their mother's reproductive life. Women themselves die from the complications of pregnancy and childbirth at the rate of one every minute —500,000 deaths each year. Approximately 125,000 women die annually attempting to terminate unwanted pregnancies with unsafe abortions, and another 500,000 men and women die each year from STDs. The number of women and children physically impaired by unsafe and unplanned pregnancies greatly exceeds the number that die. The social, economic and emotional costs of unintended pregnancies are also great.

New and improved methods of contraception are clearly needed. Many individuals and couples perceive current birth control methods to have too many side-effects, to be too difficult or inconvenient to use, to be too costly or to require too much involvement by medical professionals. This perception leads, in turn, to non-use and ineffective use of contraceptives and high rates of discontinuation. Many existing methods, even when used correctly, have high failure rates. And even for those methods with low annual failure rates, the cumulative risk of an unintended pregnancy over the course of a woman's reproductive life is high.

In the United States alone, about half of the 6 million pregnancies that occur each year are unintended and 1.6 million end in abortion. American teenagers have the highest rate of adolescent pregnancy in the industrialized world. If current trends continue, two thirds of women in the United States will have an unintended pregnancy and 45 per cent will have an abortion during their lifetime.

A number of factors have combined to slow the development and availability of new birth control methods in the United States. Moreover, fewer contraceptive methods are available in the United States than in most other developed countries, or even compared with some developing countries.

*President, Population Action International (former Population Crisis Committee), Washington, D.C., United States of America.

Several methods marketed elsewhere are not yet available in the United States. FDA has not yet approved the antiprogestin abortion pill RU486, hormonal compounds used for post-coital contraception or the injectable drug Depo-Provera for contraceptive use in the United States. Several new formulations of combined oral contraceptives using new progestins are still awaiting approval by FDA, although they have been widely available in Europe since the early 1980s. The contraceptive implant Norplant was approved in many other countries prior to approval in in the United States in 1990, even though the method was originally developed by an institution in the United States, the Population Council. Only two intra-uterine devices (IUDs) are currently on the United States market, and several IUDs popular in other countries remain unavailable to American women.

B. POLITICAL BARRIERS

One important reason that the development of new methods of fertility control is lagging in the United States is that research on new contraceptives and especially abortifacients has become highly politicized. Impediments to contraceptive development in this country include not only practical obstacles, such as the lack of funding and difficult regulatory procedures, but major moral and political controversies.

First, the level of acceptable risk and assurance of safety required of contraceptives tends to differ greatly from that required of most other drugs or medical devices. Secondly, contraceptive development is enmeshed in issues of human sexuality, an arena, especially in the United States, where there are vast differences in values.

Preventive versus curative medicine

The average person accepts a certain level of risk when using a drug or device or surgical procedure to cure a disease. But methods of fertility control are used by "healthy" people to prevent a condition, and society tends to tolerate very little risk in medical technologies used for prevention. This perception is particularly true for prevention of pregnancy since it is not considered a disease, although at times it is a potentially life-threatening event for women.

In the United States, preventive medicine seeks the impossible: perfect safety. The mother whose baby has fever convulsions after a vaccination for whooping cough may not be comforted to know that thousands of babies receiving the same immunization have no side-effects and that the vaccine prevents thousands of serious illnesses and deaths—even perhaps in her own infant. Her concern is that the doctor who gave the vaccine, the drug company that manufactured it and the local authorities that required the vaccination all had a role in making her baby sick.

Reflecting these social attitudes towards preventive medicine, FDA has often placed more stringent requirements on testing of contraceptives, compared with other drugs. Although these requirements have been recently eased, FDA has long justified its standards on the grounds that contraceptives are used for long periods of time by healthy men and women. There is very little political risk to FDA in keeping a contraceptive off the market for extensive testing, whereas there is substantial political risk in allowing a drug or device into the marketplace which might possibly cause some difficulties.

At times FDA has been subjected to, and has responded to, strong political pressures on the drug approval process. Pressure from the United States Congress, from the anti-abortion lobby and feminist health and consumer groups undoubtedly had a role in the very cautious historical stance of FDA on the injectable contraceptive, Depo-Provera. On two separate occasions, FDA expert advisory committees recommended its approval for use by certain limited patient populations in the United States. However, responding to political pressures and its own sense of caution, on both occasions the FDA refused to approve Depo-Provera for contraceptive purposes.

When the Upjohn Company requested a public hearing on Depo-Provera, the FDA convened an expert panel. Testimony at the hearing indicated that although serious side-effects appeared in early tests in beagle dogs and rhesus monkeys given very high doses of Depo-Provera, no important health risks for humans had been detected over 15 years of large-scale use in other countries. However, the panel concluded that the data were not adequate to prove safety. If this safety standard were applied to all drugs, 20 years of studies would be needed in each case to prove there were no previously unrecognized, long-term side-effects. This is a standard that is not applied to other drugs and one that has not been applied to Depo-Provera in the roughly 90 countries where it is used.

The Upjohn Company has now resubmitted an application for Depo-Provera approval to FDA. Approval appears likely on the basis of new data from long-term human studies establishing the lack of an overall increased risk of cancer of the breast and endometrium. The prior controversy over cancer has also diminished, since FDA has determined that beagle and monkey tests are not relevant to humans and no longer requires them.

Contraceptives: controversial medicine

The second major political burden that afflicts birth control is its relation to human sexuality. Contraception and especially abortion raise a broad spectrum of issues relating to human values and morality. Decisions concerning the use and development of new methods go beyond a simple medical decision or an informed choice on the part of the consumer. Societal beliefs influence family planning acceptance, sometimes in a negative manner.

Here in the United States and elsewhere, religious conservatives discourage easy access to contraceptives, especially on the part of young people, claiming this encourages promiscuity. Catholic leaders, although not most Catholics, oppose development of and access to methods that are not based on periodic sexual abstinence. Increasingly, the anti-abortion movement has overtly stated its opposition to contraception. Anti-abortion activists oppose methods that might even remotely be related to abortion, with scientifically unsubstantiated claims that birth control pills, IUDs, injectables and most recently, Norplant, routinely work as abortifacients.

Developments relating to the French abortion pill, RU486, illustrate how the climate surrounding the development of birth control technology in the United States has become fraught with controversy. Anti-abortion leaders have threatened to boycott any company that attempts to market RU486 in the United States. Currently, there is an FDA-imposed ban on the importation of RU486 into the United States for personal use, a restriction that is widely considered to be the outcome of political pressure from abortion opponents, rather than a reflection of genuine medical or scientific concerns. The import ban has had a chilling effect on RU486 research, because some scientists believe the ban applies to importing the drug for research purposes.

As a result of the political climate in the United States, Roussel Uclaf, the French company which manufactures the drug, remains reluctant to file an application to market the drug in this country or even to make it available to American scientists for research on abortion. The company has, however, agreed to provide RU486 for research purposes other than abortion. Thus, although FDA has granted permission for testing RU486, there have been only a few small clinical trials on RU486 use for abortion in the United States.

It is clear that the best way to reduce the incidence of abortion is to develop improved contraceptive techniques which are easier to provide and more acceptable to potential users. But policy makers must recognize that more research on abortion technology, safety and epidemiology is also needed.

C. THE KEY PLAYERS

Contraceptive research and development are carried out by three major types of organizations: government agencies that support and conduct research; universities and non-governmental and international organizations that conduct research; and private industry, consisting of both large and small pharmaceutical companies.

The history of successful contraceptive development suggests that for maximum progress, vigorous support is needed from a variety of sources—Governments, foundations, international donor agencies, private organizations and large multinational pharmaceutical firms. Both the public and the research community in the United States have often underestimated the time and cost of contraceptive development. Development of a new method of birth control appears to take from 5 to 15 years and to cost between $20 million and $70 million. If the costs of pursuing unproductive research leads are also included, each new method costs from $200 million to $250 million to develop.

United States leadership on contraceptive research and development has declined dramatically, in large part due to the withdrawal of large pharmaceutical companies from such research. According to Stanford University professor Carl Djerassi, in 1970 there were 13 major drug companies worldwide, including 9 in the United States, carrying out broad programmes of research and development on contraception. By 1987, this number had fallen to four—with only one company in the United States.

As the pharmaceutical industry has gradually withdrawn from contraceptive development efforts, government agencies supporting this research, such as the National Institutes of Health (NIH) and the United States Agency for International Development (USAID), similar governmental bodies overseas and private foundations have become a relatively more important source of support for these efforts.

Total United States government support for contraceptive research is currently about $165 million. The bulk of these funds—about $135 million—goes to the basic research in reproductive physiology necessary to provide leads for new contraceptive development. Government funding for basic research is particularly important because private industry is unlikely to invest in research that is not closely linked to development of a potential, profitable product. In addition, USAID and NIH provide approximately $30 million per annum for more applied contraceptive development research, including clinical trials. Smaller amounts of funds are available from private foundations, which have the considerable advantage of not being as subject to political considerations.

Currently, AID and NIH are barred, either by executive policy or by law, from supporting research on fertility regulation methods that relate to or cause abortion. Obviously, the political goals of a minority of Americans are being served by this government ban on a very important means of fertility control. With some 1.6 million abortions in the United States each year, abortion is one of the most commonly performed medical procedures. It is unconscionable that safer and more effective abortifacients, as a matter of policy, should not be a subject of medical research sponsored by the United States government sponsors of contraceptive research.

During the 1980s, the influence of anti-abortion activists on both the legislative and executive branches led not only to restrictive research policies but also to stagnating levels of financial support for contraceptive research. The political will to represent the interests of the less vocal majority is clearly lacking. Bright, young scientists are turning their attention to other more generously funded fields of research.

University programmes and non-governmental and international organizations

Contraceptive research and development is carried out in a number of universities (such as the programme at the Eastern Virgina Medical School supported by USAID) and small research institutes throughout the world, and by a few major international organizations, such as the World Health Organization (WHO), the Population Council and Family Health International. These organizations are also affected by the political pressures experienced by United States Government sponsors of contraceptive research.

Based on its anti-abortion stance, the Government of the United States has chosen not to support the WHO programme for research on human reproduction, because the programme supports work on anti-progestins, such as RU486 and other methods that act after fertilization.

AID provides a substantial level of support to the Population Council for contraceptive development, but none of these funds can be used to develop abortion-related methods. The Population Council, however, continues to support a limited programme of abortion research with private funds.

At the Population Council, a shortage of funds has made it impossible to adequately staff some aspects of contraceptive development. In particular, the small staff involved in monitoring clinical studies and preparing submissions to FDA to satisfy the requirements of its regulatory review and approval process contrasts with the much larger teams assigned to such activities by private industry. As a result, there have been long delays in the completion of studies and the submission of Council requests for United States approval of new methods of birth control. It took the Population Council 20 years to develop Norplant, and the Council submission for FDA approval was delayed by a lack of staff and funds. Lack of funds has also stalled the Council's application for FDA approval of the new levonorgestrel IUD.

Other than the Population Council, most of the university-based and other small private research organizations lack the expertise, critical mass and funding needed to carry out all the necessary steps to bring a new contraceptive from the laboratory to clinical trials and ultimately to the market-place. The millions of dollars needed to create a contraceptive research programme which pursues leads in many areas and handles all phases of the contraceptive development process are simply not available. Even the Population Council, which has the most sophisticated contraceptive research effort in the world outside of private industry, must rely upon private companies to manufacture and distribute new birth control technologies.

A crucial bottleneck in the overall contraceptive development process is the "hand-off" from universities and private research organizations to private industry. A number of factors inhibit the adoption of promising leads by pharmaceutical companies. For example, most university and private research groups receive government support and are bound by rigid and bureaucratic regulations limiting confidentiality and patent and licensing rights. These regulations often have the effect of making promising research leads unattractive to private industry for commercial development.

The pharmaceutical industry

The re-engagement of the private pharmaceutical industry is essential to the revitalization of contraceptive research and development in the United States. Historically, an estimated 92 per cent of all new drugs developed in the United States have been developed by private industry, compared with only 8 per cent for drugs developed through publicly supported research. There is no substitute for the magnitude of funds and scientific expertise the private, for-profit sector can potentially apply in this area.

The picture in private industry is complex. At least five major factors influence decisions with respect to contraceptive development by pharmaceutical firms.

Are the research leads promising?

The relatively small investment in both private and public sector reproductive research means that there are a limited number of promising scientific leads to pursue, compared with other medical fields. For example, not enough is known about male reproductive physiology to permit selection of good leads for applied research which could lead to a practical contraceptive for men. However, more leads can and should be pursued than are now being investigated. Recent dramatic increases in knowledge about immune processes could potentially be exploited to develop safe and effective contraceptive vaccines. However, the financial and scientific resources required to explore these leads thoroughly and quickly are inadequate.

Will the method be profitable?

Estimates of profitability must consider market size and potential income, compared with the cost of manufacturing and distribution and other financial risks. In addition, the profit potential must be evaluated in comparison to the other drugs a company might develop. Increasingly, pharmaceutical firms focus research and development efforts on drugs with sales potential of over $50 million per annum, such as a new antibiotic or a new drug to treat heart disease. Contraceptive sales are often half of that level.

Some methods of fertility control may be so inexpensive to make and market or used so infrequently—for example, once a year—that they would generate little profit. There would be little incentive for a pharmaceutical firm to develop the "perfect contraceptive" that could be used one time, would provide protection from pregnancy for many years, would be easily reversible and cost very little.

The risk of product liability litigation

Profits may be compromised by the risk of lawsuits; and for contraceptive manufacturers, this risk is substantial. Product liability lawsuits against the Ortho and G. D. Searle pharmaceutical companies led them to stop selling their widely used IUDs in the United States, although the companies won most of the lawsuits. On balance, it was the cost of litigation, rather than problems with product safety, that prompted these decisions. Because United States sales of IUDs totalled only about $12 million annually, there was relatively little profit that could be used to defray the cost of the lawsuits. As a result, American women were, for a period of about two years, denied access to safe and highly effective IUDs.

The threat of liability litigation also endangers the development of new spermicides, which could potentially prevent STDs, including the acquired immunodeficiency syndrome (AIDS), as well as pregnancy.

One reason the birth control pill remains available is its large volume of sales and profits—profits which can support liability awards and a legal defense. In addition, the very complete disclosure on pill labelling has made it difficult to sue successfully when side-effects or health problems occur.

The $750 million of annual sales in the United States help keep the pill on the market and spin off substantial profits that could be reinvested in new contraceptive development. These profits also encourage the pharmaceutical industry to stay in the birth control business. But as a result of concerns about potential litigation, the American consumer pays between $10 and $20 per cycle of oral contraceptives, when the actual manufacturing cost is less than a dollar. Oral contraceptives bought in bulk by USAID for use in the United States foreign aid programme cost between 17 and 27 cents per cycle.

Pharmaceutical firms now typically find liability insurance severely limited or unobtainable. At one time, the NIH Centre for Population Research had four contraceptive products stalled in research laboratories because the liability insurance needed to begin human testing was unobtainable from private sources, and the Government was unwilling to assume the financial responsibility for product liability. At least one firm has resorted to the purchase of a captive insurance agency to ensure continuing access to product liability insurance; other firms have been forced to self-insure.

Drug company executives have witnessed a $5 million jury award to a spermicide user based on scientifically unsupported claims that it caused a birth defect. They have witnessed the bankruptcy of the A. H. Robbins company, based on the avalanche of lawsuits over the Dalkon Shield. And although most companies would market a more thoroughly tested and better designed product than the Dalkon Shield, they know that if a contraceptive caused some totally unexpected side-effect—for example, if the method caused cancer after a decade of use—it might cost them their company. Fear of lawsuits is another (although probably less important) reason RU486 is likely to become available in other countries long before it reaches the United States.

Whether the level of controversy will be tolerable

Contraceptive development and marketing has been dogged with controversy. The 1970 Nelson hearings in Congress, which pilloried the birth control pill, so discouraged at least one company that it dropped major research on new contraceptives.

Politicians and drug company executives have been caught between liberal and conservative critics. Critics from the consumer movement, especially feminist health groups, became alarmed when it was discovered that such contraceptives as the pill and IUDs occasionally had serious and sometimes even life-threatening side-effects. They became suspicious that physicians and the pharmaceutical industry were knowingly promoting unsafe contraceptive methods and justifiably pointed out the lack of adequate consumer information to allow truly informed consent regarding their use.

In the past, many consumer advocates failed to acknowledge the trade-off between risks and benefits intrinsic in every contraceptive drug or device, and too often they were not fully knowledgeable about the science involved. More recently, their increased knowledge of the safety and side-effects of various birth control methods has contributed to a more sophisticated approach to safety issues. Although consumer activists still oppose many contraceptive methods, they generally support the need for expanded contraceptive research to develop a broader array of improved methods.

Anti-abortion ideologues, on the other hand, represent a very serious source of opposition to contraceptive development. The tactics used by anti-abortion groups include legislative initiatives, boycotts, and picketing and threats against drug company executives. Some have even threatened to bomb factories that manufacture IUDs, as they have bombed family planning clinics. Pharmaceutical firms, especially those with multiple product lines which could potentially be subject to anti-abortion boycotts, continue to be reluctant to undertake research on new methods of birth control—especially methods relating to abortion technology. Opposition from anti-abortion groups undoubtedly played a role in the Upjohn Company decision to scale back prostaglandin research and marketing, and in their eventual retreat from contraceptive development efforts, even though there is no evidence that boycotts actually affected company profitability.

The drug regulatory climate

As already noted, FDA, to some extent, reflects the laudable but probably unrealistic American penchant for perfection when it comes to preventive medicine. Too often, the quest for what is perfect has become the enemy of what is good.

Over the past few years, FDA has made laudable progress in streamlining testing requirements and the approval process for contraceptive methods. They have

446

discontinued or shortened the use of some of the inappropriate animal models which unfairly tainted the reputation of Depo-Provera. But experts note that although many improvements have occurred in the approval process for contraceptive drugs, the regulatory process for contraceptive devices is still excessively cumbersome.

Even so, in a regulatory climate that at least previously demanded proof of safety beyond that required for other drugs, and beyond that required in other countries and by such authorities as WHO, drug companies have been reluctant to commit resources to contraceptive development. And because FDA is perceived in many countries to be one of the most rigorous drug regulatory agencies in the world, its decisions may cause regulatory bodies in other countries to be unnecessarily conservative.

D. A PRESCRIPTION FOR PROGRESS IN CONTRACEPTIVE DEVELOPMENT

It is clear that improving the climate for contraceptive development in the United States requires vigorous action on several fronts. Very substantial increases in both private and public financial support are essential, but changes in the legal system, in current institutional arrangements for contraceptive development and in the drug regulatory process are also important.

Increased investment in contraceptive development

Information about the current level of worldwide investment in research on reproduction is incomplete, but the total is probably somewhat over $300 million per annum. However, it is likely that only about half of this amount is devoted to applied research to develop new contraceptives. Experts estimate that expanded basic research and applied research to explore promising, existing scientific leads warrant expenditures of $500 million per annum. Over the past decade, however, the funding trend in constant dollars has been downward.

Current United States government outlays for applied contraceptive research are almost trivial, at about $30 million annually, channelled mainly through USAID and NIH. More money for these existing government programmes should be a high priority. NIH should get a total of $100 million more, equally divided between basic research and applied research on contraceptive

development. USAID should get $50 million more for applied research on new and improved contraceptives. This level of funding would make it possible for research on new methods, such as vaginal rings and microsphere injectable contraceptives, to be revitalized.

New institutional arrangements

An additional $100 million in public funds is needed annually for a coordinated programme of applied research to explore the many promising contraceptive leads that already exist but lack follow-up, to accelerate necessary testing and to expedite regulatory review of such products. To accomplish this objective, it may be necessary to revamp existing organizations or create new organizations, which could carry out all of the steps of contraceptive development. Such an arrangement would facilitate the currently difficult process of handing off promising developments in university laboratories to the toxicology and clinical testing stages of drug development.

Such an institutional arrangement would also facilitate development of such methods as a once-a-month pill or a once-a-year injectable that drug firms may never find profitable. Such methods are unlikely to be developed without greater public-private collaboration. Moreover, increased public funding for research by private organizations is necessary to maintain a "pipeline" of promising leads for private industry, as well as to facilitate the hand-off from the non-profit research institutions to private industry.

Improved patent and product liability laws

More attractive conditions are needed to encourage the recommitment of the pharmaceutical industry, with its multimillion dollar annual research budgets, to the field of contraceptive research and development. To strengthen financial incentives for contraceptive development, a 1984 Congressional Act extended patent protection for up to five years in recognition of lengthy drug-testing requirements. Patent protection on new drugs should be extended further if necessary to allow companies adequate time to recoup the costs of testing and regulatory review prior to market introduction, as well as to earn a reasonable margin of profit.

New liability laws need to be formulated that provide adequate recompense to injured parties but impose greater predictability and rationality on what is currently

447

a "lottery" in which a few injured parties receive huge awards and others nothing. There is need to evolve a system that recognizes and expedites valid claims, but also recognizes that not all risks can reasonably be identified during testing and that individual decisions, even made after full and informed consent, may still entail a degree of risk.

One possible scheme put forward by the National Research Council and the Institute of Medicine suggests that full compliance with FDA regulations should be considered an adequate defence against charges of negligence or design flaws. This defence could not be used if critical information was unavailable to FDA, withheld or presented fraudulently. The same study called for new ways to compensate those injured by a contraceptive drug or device, perhaps through a system of arbitration and a fund for compensation.

A streamlined regulatory process

Some recent changes are favourable. FDA has modified its stringent animal toxicology tests and made them more sensible. Still, drug regulatory procedures need to be reviewed for possible further simplification. The FDA review of new drug applications for contraceptives still requires voluminous data which often take years to assemble, and the review process at FDA typically takes one to two years. The approval process for contraceptive devices in particular needs to be reconsidered.

In recent years, FDA has placed appropriately increased emphasis on the post-marketing surveillance needed to provide early and accurate information about the safety and side-effects of contraceptives under actual use conditions. But experts believe current United States drug regulatory procedures still overemphasize pre-marketing testing compared with post-marketing monitoring.

Although FDA has taken a number of important steps towards smoothing the contraceptive approval process, it needs to do a better job of communicating these changes to private industry. For years, the FDA double standard for approval of contraceptives compared with other drugs discouraged drug companies from investing in research on fertility regulation. For the companies to shift research directions and reassign staff to contraceptive development will be an expensive and long-term process, which FDA needs to encourage through positive signals. Like other parts of the federal Government, FDA needs to become pro-active on behalf of a broader array of safe and effective reproductive choices for Americans.

Twenty-five years of experience with family planning has taught us that couples are more willing and able to practise family planning when they have a wide range of contraceptive choices. The time has come to initiate a major, coordinated and accelerated effort to develop new and better choices.

XLVI. MARKET-BASED SERVICES: STRATEGIC ROLE IN FAMILY PLANNING SERVICE EXPANSION

Janet M. Smith[*] and Vijay Rao[**]

The challenge posed by rapidly escalating demand for family planning services will require that every resource available be mobilized in response. Dramatic growth in need can best be served by an effective division of labour involving both private and public sectors. Both sectors have distinct, complementary roles to play. The commercial sector has its niche and can do what it does best—serve consumers that can afford to pay by providing responsive services that are priced accessibly and competitively.

The commercial sector is already a major resource and has great untapped potential. Millions of couples in the developing world turn to these sources. Millions more would use the private commercial sector if changes in market conditions and government policies could be effected.

Policy or operational constraints may be limiting the role of the private sector. Demand may be constrained by income, which deters consumers that want to use private services. Secondly, government provision of free or subsidized services may curb consumer demand for private services; without perceived demand, providers will not offer services. Thus, public services may be crowding out private provision. On the supply side, legal and regulatory barriers, such as high tariffs, stringent licensing procedures and restrictions on entry of providers into the market, constitute significant disincentives.

Government has the responsibility to lay the foundation for the total service delivery system in which the private sector is an essential ingredient. Government can be an active partner to the private sector and assure the flow of quality services through licensing and regulation, provision of population-based information to the private sector, dissemination of information to consumers and strategic planning. Government also has the fundamental responsibility for allocating resources to the needs of users who cannot afford to pay for family planning services in the private market. Strategic planning for the service system should examine whether direct service provision is needed or whether the Government could serve as financier in procuring private sector services.

With leadership and practical help, donors can support Governments in the effort to forge successful partnerships with the private sector. Policy analysis and consensus-building are essential to Governments building effective new relations with the commercial sector. Policy analysis can focus on targeting of subsidies, demand and supply analysis and examination of existing regulatory and legal framework.

The private sector has enormous potential to help meet escalating demand for family planning services. In a future where every resource must be mobilized for service expansion, the Government may find the private sector a willing and able contributor.

A. DEFINITION OF THE PRIVATE COMMERCIAL SECTOR

The private commercial sector may be defined as consisting of individuals and organizations that produce, distribute, finance or deliver family planning services and products for profit, and whose very existence and growth are determined by market forces. The sector may be segmented into four different categories:

(a) *Individual and group practices.* This group includes physicians, midwives and traditional birth attendants, and health service institutions, such as clinics, dispensaries and hospitals;

---

[*]United States Agency for International Development, Options for Population Policy Project, Washington, D.C., United States of America.

[**]The Futures Group, Washington, D.C., United States of America.

(*b*) Manufacturers and distributors. They produce, package or distribute contraceptives and other health-care products;

(*c*) *Retail outlets*. This category includes pharmacies that sell contraceptive products and often also offer information on their use; and

(*d*) *Health financing institutions*. This group includes insurance companies and health maintenance organizations that offer indemnity coverage and prepaid health plans.

B. CURRENT IMPORTANCE OF THE PRIVATE COMMERCIAL SECTOR IN FAMILY PLANNING SERVICES DELIVERY

The private commercial sector provides family planning services to millions of couples worldwide. A study of 13 Demographic and Health Surveys (DHS) countries in the late 1980s found that 31 per cent of all users turned to this sector for their family planning needs. For some countries, the proportion was over 50 per cent (Cross and others, 1991). Again, it is apparent that significant numbers of users rely upon the commercial sector, although there is wide divergence between countries. In Bolivia, Brazil and Egypt, from 60 to 70 per cent of users are served by the private commercial sector; the proportions for other countries are smaller.

There is considerable variation in use of the private commercial sector, according to urban or rural residence and level of education. Although the rural population does rely upon private commercial providers, on balance, urban residents are more likely to rely upon the commercial sector. This situation is to be expected for two reasons: rural incomes tend to be lower, on average, than those in urban and peri-urban areas; and, with some exceptions, the degree of penetration of commercial sector providers into the rural areas may be less (e.g., Indonesia). For most countries, private sector utilization also rises with level of education, indicating additional potential for commercial providers as the numbers of the educated increase (Cross and others, 1991).

The private commercial sector is especially active in the provision of non-clinical methods, as shown in tables 45 and 46. In most countries, users of non-

clinical methods (such as oral pills, barrier methods and condoms) depend upon commercial providers to a greater extent than those using clinical methods. This situation partially reflects the policy environment in most developing countries where the commercial sector faces a number of legal and regulatory barriers to its entry into provision of clinical methods.

The importance of the private commercial sector in family planning service delivery varies considerably by country and region. It plays a relatively small role in sub-Saharan Africa and Asia and a much larger role in Latin America. There is general agreement, however, on the potential for increased provision of commercial services. Considering a target market of all couples that need family planning services, can afford to pay for them and have access to reliable trained sources, it is estimated that the 15 million couples currently buying contraceptives from pharmacies or other retail outlets would increase to 87 million if changes in market conditions and government policies could be effected (Lande and Geller, 1991).

C. THE STRATEGIC ROLE OF THE PRIVATE COMMERCIAL SECTOR

This section highlights the assets and the issues involved in making the private commercial sector a partner in family planning service delivery. It is important to note that the private commercial sector is not a panacea to the problems associated with expanding services. However, it has some vital strengths to assist Governments in the formidable task of satisfying all unmet need.

Assets

The private commercial sector has a number of assets that make it ideally suited to be involved in service delivery. First, it is responsive to existing effective demand, that is, demand from consumers that are ready, willing and able to pay for services. Since the primary goal of the sector is to make a profit from the sale of its services, the private commercial sector is quick to respond to these consumers. This speed of response is accentuated by the lack of bureaucratic rules and procedures. Private providers are also willing to tailor services to meet consumer preferences so that they get what they want.

TABLE 45. DISTRIBUTION OF SOURCES OF CLINICAL CONTRACEPTIVES, CURRENTLY MARRIED
WOMEN AGED 15-49, SELECTED COUNTRIES

| Country | Contraceptive source | | | |
	Private	Non-governmental organization	Public	Other
Africa				
Botswana	9.9	0.0	89.7	0.3
Burundi	2.5	0.0	92.6	5.0
Egypt	52.0	1.2	45.2	1.7
Ghana	4.4	13.3	51.9	2.2
Kenya	7.2	15.0	74.3	1.4
Liberia	7.6	29.1	61.0	2.3
Mali	0.0	15.6	54.5	30.0
Morocco	25.2	1.8	72.8	0.2
Nigeria (Ondo State)	8.7	0.0	91.3	0.0
Senegal	28.0	0.0	64.0	8.0
Togo	2.9	17.1	80.0	0.0
Tunisia	7.5	0.0	92.0	0.1
Uganda	6.9	14.0	79.5	0.0
Zimbabwe	19.3	4.5	70.5	5.6
Asia				
Indonesia	9.2	0.0	89.7	1.1
Sri Lanka	3.1	0.0	96.7	0.0
Thailand	7.0	0.1	92.9	0.0
Latin America and the Caribbean				
Brazil	42.9	1.0	54.1	2.0
Bolivia	57.5	0.9	40.9	0.7
Colombia	12.6	62.1	25.0	0.2
Dominican Republic	52.3	0.2	46.7	0.4
Ecuador	31.7	13.2	51.9	3.2
El Salvador	3.0	10.8	85.1	1.1
Guatemala	21.4	40.4	36.5	1.7
Mexico	20.0	0.0	78.2	1.8
Peru	30.8	2.1	58.9	7.7
Trinidad and Tobago	16.7	23.9	58.2	1.2

Source: Demographic and Health Surveys.

451

TABLE 46. DISTRIBUTION OF SOURCES OF NON-CLINICAL CONTRACEPTIVES, CURRENTLY
MARRIED WOMEN AGED 15-49, SELECTED COUNTRIES

Country	Contraceptive source			
	Private	NGO	Public	Other
Africa				
Botswana	7.1	0.0	92.3	0.0
Burundi	2.1	0.0	83.9	14.0
Egypt	89.8	0.2	7.7	2.1
Ghana	33.6	23.0	22.1	21.2
Kenya	5.4	17.3	70.3	1.4
Liberia	21.2	52.7	26.1	0.0
Mali	1.9	5.7	81.1	11.3
Morocco	19.2	1.0	74.7	4.8
Nigeria (Ondo State)	27.1	0.0	71.8	1.2
Senegal	59.6	0.0	36.2	4.3
Togo	46.3	7.3	26.8	7.3
Uganda	12.2	43.1	39.5	5.1
Tunisia	58.0	0.0	39.5	2.3
Zimbabwe	2.7	1.7	90.4	5.1
Asia				
Indonesia	14.2	0.0	75.1	10.7
Sri Lanka	24.2	0.3	69.5	5.3
Thailand	21.6	1.4	75.5	1.2
Latin America and the Caribbean				
Brazil	93.1	1.0	4.4	1.5
Bolivia	77.2	1.3	15.7	5.8
Colombia	71.9	4.6	19.3	3.3
Dominican Republic	29.5	2.6	55.2	11.7
Ecuador	37.1	14.3	34.9	13.7
El Salvador	38.3	16.0	36.2	4.3
Guatemala	39.9	35.4	20.2	4.5
Mexico	65.9	0.0	32.4	1.7
Peru	38.2	3.3	47.4	8.5
Trinidad and Tobago	57.8	11.0	30.1	0.4

Source: Demographic and Health Surveys.

452

Secondly, the perception of quality among its consumers also constitutes a significant asset to the private sector. Since private providers charge for their services, they are often seen as providing a higher quality of care than public providers. Considerable evidence supports the view that many consumers associate price with quality. For instance, in both India and Jamaica, public sector services are widely perceived to be of inferior quality, whereas private services are highly valued and respected. This suggests that the private sector has an important role to play in service delivery.

A third asset of market-based services has to do with the greater efficiency with which it supplies its services. Given the profit motive underlying private sector services, the incentives to keep costs under control are high. It is this bottom line orientation and the ever present risk of failure that drives these providers to cut costs. Lewis and Kenney (1988) cite evidence from the United States of America and elsewhere that public health care is consistently more expensive to deliver than private services.

Fourthly, since private sector services are financially self-sufficient, they are also likely to be more sustainable. Once in the market with a product that consumers want and that is profitable to provide, services are likely to be continuously available. This is important *vis-à-vis* the escalating demand for services because it means that Governments can count on their private sector partners. This characteristic also may protect family planning programmes from shifts in donor policy. For example, in Haiti, despite a change in donor policy towards assistance to the Government, a commercially sold oral pill originally launched as a donor-supported social marketing activity has stayed in the market and even increased its share.

Private sector services typically should not require ongoing subsidy. In the case of insufficient effective demand (too few consumers able to pay the going rate), subsidies may be needed to allow price reductions. Some social marketing programmes are designed that way, where donated products are used to build the market, demand and a capital base. Morocco is a case in point, although long-term planning is now addressing whether, when and how to phase out these donated commodities and shift to self-sufficient programmes.

Fifthly, the private commercial sector can help Governments to better target services to the poor and needy by attracting those that can afford to pay for private family planning services, thus ensuring that public subsidies shall flow to persons that truly need them.

Lastly, private services and private purchases add financial and human resources to the total pool available for family planning. This helps countries bring larger resources to bear to meet family planning goals.

Key issues in commercial sector family planning

The private sector has a distinct role to play in the provision of family planning services and is an essential ingredient in building a strong, broad-based system. But there are several issues in commercial sector family planning that help define its niche in the development of service delivery systems.

The fact that the market responds only to consumers willing to pay for its services is the first consideration to be kept in mind by Governments when engaged in strategic planning. Governments will have to allocate resources for those segments of the market that cannot pay for private sector services. Planners must then address whether Governments should finance these services through private providers or provide them directly.

Secondly, the commercial sector follows market incentives which may not always be in the public interest. Therefore, the commercial sector needs to be properly regulated to assure quality and availability. Governments can monitor and carry out inspections of these providers to ensure this. Since lack of information on the part of users is often conducive to private providers acting against the public interest, it is incumbent on Governments to remedy the situation. In the Dominican Republic, the price of the social marketing of oral pills was advertised so that consumers would know what to pay through the legitimate distribution system and not be faced with exorbitant prices for informal sector supply.

Thirdly, the commercial sector may be limited in method availability, particularly for longer term methods. For example, traditional practitioners would never be tasked with delivery of advanced clinical methods. However, the assumption that the private sector cannot offer certain services should be carefully examined. As described below, the Republic of Korea and Taiwan Province of China found that private sector physicians could play a major role in performing sterilizations and intra-uterine device (IUD) insertions.

D. CONSTRAINTS

On its face, it would appear that as urbanization, education and income rise over time, reliance upon the private commercial sector for family planning services would show a steady increase. However, DHS trend data for 13 countries indicate otherwise. In as many as seven countries, use of the private commercial sector has actually declined. For the remainder, growth has been negligible. Since contraceptive supplies to the private sector in many of these countries were heavily subsidized, one would expect to see some evidence of growth. The explanation for this anomalous situation lies in both demand and supply factors.

Demand constraints

One of the single most important factors responsible for poor growth of the private commercial sector is the "crowding out" of their services by the public sector (Lewis and Kenney, 1988; Cross and others, 1991). This term refers to a situation in which publicly provided services are heavily subsidized and untargeted, so that their benefits flow indiscriminately to both upper and lower income groups. As a result, private commercial providers, that are ready to cater for the section of the market that is willing to pay for their services, are priced out of the market.

In Brazil, a government initiative dramatically expanded family planning services in Piaui State. Yet, an assessment of the initial impact of the programme showed no change in pill use, although female sterilizations did increase. Many women that had been purchasing contraceptives from pharmacies switched to the free supplies offered in health facilities. The proportion of pill users obtaining their supplies from a pharmacy dropped from 56 to 34 per cent between 1979 and 1984, while the proportion relying upon health facilities increased from 20 to 49 per cent (Arruda, Thome and Morris, 1983). Thus, much of the money invested in the state programme had the effect of undermining the existing commercial market for contraceptives while failing to expand the base of family planning users.

Declining economic conditions have also forced users to move away from the private commercial sector (Cross and others, 1991). This has been true in Peru and could also happen in sub-Saharan Africa, where the past decade has seen setbacks to economic growth in many countries. It may be necessary to turn to reductions in prices for services. For example, manufacturers have reduced the price of oral pills in several countries to expand market share. It may also be necessary to address the lack of third-party payment mechanisms, such as health insurance, which could relieve the burden for many consumers (Griffin, 1989). Large-scale employers are often unaware of the potential savings from providing family planning services to their employees and their families. Communicating the costs and benefits of such interventions can encourage employers to turn to commercial providers to supply these services.

The final aspect of the demand side of the equation is the fact that commercial providers must perceive that demand exists before they will be prepared to invest in training, equipment, supplies etc. to deliver services. Anecdotal evidence suggests that the private sector in India may not offer oral contraceptives because providers do not perceive a demand for private sector provision. Without information on the consumer market, private providers are often unaware of the concept and magnitude of unmet need other than on a case-by-case basis.

Supply constraints

There are also supply-side constraints that hamper the development of the private sector. First, many countries may have de facto restrictions on growth of the sector. By virtue of better training, equipment and supplies, the public sector may possess a comparative advantage in the delivery of long-term methods, such as IUDs and sterilizations, forcing the commercial sector to concentrate on temporary methods. Moreover, as users change their method mix in favour of longer term methods, further declines in the commercial sector may occur.

This need not always be the case. In Taiwan Province of China, the government reimburses private providers for voluntary sterilizations and IUDs provided to low-income couples. As a result, approximately 80 per cent of all sterilizations financed by the government are carried out by private providers. Essentially, the government contracts with commercial providers to offer these services to the majority of users. In the Republic of Korea, the public sector network operates with similar contractual arrangements (Lewis and Kenney, 1988).

Legal and regulatory barriers to the growth of the private commercial sector constitute a major impediment. Tariff and non-tariff barriers (such as local content laws), complicated licensing procedures, value-added taxes, denial of access to commodities and restrictions on entry of providers into the market all constitute significant disincentives. Mexico reduced import duties on condoms from 45 to 10 per cent between 1988 and 1991, which contributed to a 25 per cent increase in condom sales (Lande and Geller, 1991). Egypt currently allows only obstetrician-gynaecologists to provide injectable contraceptives. As the programme evolves, it may wish to consider extending that method to general physicians, if the right mix of licensing, training and counselling materials could be made available to providers.

Lastly, private commercial providers may require some assistance from government in the form of loans and start-up funding, as well as training skills. In Mexico and the Dominican Republic, there are programmes to help doctors just beginning to set up clinics in underserved areas and provide family planning and child health services (Lande and Geller, 1991). In the Philippines, the Integrated Maternal Child Care and Social Development Institute carried out in-service training for pharmacists and private midwives.

Pre-service training can also equip providers with the skills to offer family planning services. For example, in the United Republic of Tanzania the medical school attached to the University of Dar es Salaam recently expanded its family planning curriculum to include comprehensive training with courses on community health and paediatrics so that graduates entering private practice will be better able to provide these services. Indonesia plans to increase the number of trained midwives from 8,000 to 34,000 over the next five years, and each will be permitted to operate private practices while they work for the Government.

E. THE ROLE OF GOVERNMENT

Policy support to facilitate private sector service expansion

The private sector can serve those that can afford to pay if a supportive policy climate exists. There are a number of ways in which government can facilitate private sector participation through policy support. As described above, it can remove constraints that are impeding the development of private services. A major constraint is crowding out—where the availability of Government-subsidized services to consumers that can afford to pay deters them from using the private market. This is an irony of many successful public sector family planning programmes (e.g., Jamaica), that a situation of unequal competition may develop as direct service delivery in public programmes grows. Private providers have little incentive to enter the market under these conditions.

Other supportive functions for government include: provision of information about population; strategic planning; information dissemination; and licensing and regulation. These are social goods where the benefits accrue at the social level, not to individual users or to private providers *per se*. Thus, government is required to step in to perform these functions. But once performed, the private sector as a partner will benefit from their accomplishment.

Population-based information

Population-based information on health and family planning may take the form of DHS. Private providers of various types may be unaware of the magnitude of unmet need and the preference and ability of groups of users to pay for private services. Data collection efforts of this type are frequently used to support new initiatives with the private sector. In Bolivia, for example, additional questions were added to DHS specifically to provide data for design of social marketing initiatives. Periodic data about personal consumption can also be used for these purposes.

Strategic planning

Governments can and must undertake strategic planning to assure that the needs of everyone are met, that appropriate resources are being allocated and that subsidies are properly targeted. Note that population-based information (and other consumer information, if possible) is essential for strategic planning, as the examples given below reflect. In the course of strategic planning, Governments may also examine their own role and whether they are crowding out private services; the private sector may then benefit from reduced competition from subsidized services.

Indonesia is facing this type of challenge now: with a contraceptive prevalence rate of 49 per cent, the oral pill is the most frequently used method, with one fourth of users relying upon it. According to the Indonesia DHS in 1991, the public sector distributes 90 per cent of pills, despite the fact that the pill is a very good method to supply through commercial channels. The large public sector role has important recurrent cost implications in view of the expense of resupply of the pill (Smith, 1992).

Egypt is facing a somewhat different challenge in strategic planning. The programme has a moderately high prevalence (47 per cent contraceptive prevalence) and significant private sector participation. According to the Egypt DHS in 1991, approximately 70 per cent of services were provided in the private sector. Private sector involvement is a result of an incentive system where all methods are paid for in the public sector at a token price, and the private sector has access to subsidized contraceptives. But the donor that has previously supplied the contraceptives is phasing out this function. The issue for strategic planning is to try to preserve the favourable participation of the private sector. It will be important (again using population-based information) to study consumers and try to determine where they will seek services under different pricing scenarios.

Dissemination of information

The Government can also help to disseminate information to generate demand for private sector services. If consumers are not sufficiently informed (and this can be determined using population-based data like DHS), Governments have many ways to get the word out—mass media advertising, community information networks and counselling in public-health programmes. Again, population-based information can be used to identify target groups for various information activities. The Government can adjust policy restrictions on types of material which may be included in advertising in order to better inform the population of where information and services may be obtained. Social marketing programmes typically seek approval to do this; for example, programmes in the Dominican Republic, Egypt and Indonesia have helped to position service providers as sources of information.

Government also has the responsibility to assure that the private sector is providing safe services. One mechanism for assuring this is through licensing and regulation of private providers. Certain groups of users could be reached by certain types of practitioners that have not previously participated. In expanding services to those providers, licensing and regulation provisions that prohibited their involvement may be rewritten to require them to have certain types of training, registration etc. to assure that they can properly support the delivery of safe family planning services.

Assistance to the private sector

Just as licensing and regulation provisions might be changed to increase the number and variety of private sector providers, assistance from the Government might be necessary to launch them.

Private providers may need access to training sessions, information materials for use in service delivery and access to affordable methods to include in their services. Part of the recent success story in Egypt has been that these types of input have been available through the Regional Coordination and Training Programme with the Egyptian Young Doctors' Association.

Assistance should be designed with regard to the market basis of the services to be delivered. These services will ultimately be profitable to the provider. Therefore, to the greatest extent possible, the practitioner should pay for what is received. Affordable contraceptives can be made available through social marketing programmes, as in the Dominican Republic, Haiti and Indonesia, instead of being provided at no cost. The Government's necessary function, therefore, is to make the input available, not necessarily to subsidize it.

Selected types of assistance should be available to all providers. It will not help to provide input items to a select group of providers, who can provide them on a monopoly basis. Competition keeps prices low, makes providers focus on service quality and expands availability.

Resource allocation and the government role as financier

Not only does the Government need to facilitate private sector services to consumers in the market, it must also be concerned about the needs of users that cannot be served in the market. The Government's role is to ensure that these groups shall be targeted and have access to subsidized public services. There are many ways for the Government to do this.

The challenge is for Governments to target subsidies to their market segment. In many countries, public sector programmes are swamped by the current needs of the general public. As programmes expand, new users will also typically be those unable to pay for services. Where there is no effective division of labour with the private sector, Governments will have difficulty meeting the needs of its target population. They may need to move political systems (and certainly manage user expectations) to steer the private sector target market to it and to reserve public sector resources for those that need them. Jamaica is struggling with just these issues. In that high-prevalence country (54 per cent), 60 per cent of services are public sector; and most private sector service takes the form of sales of donated oral pills and condoms (again, donor resources are public sector resources). The economy of Jamaica is collapsing, and the Government can no longer afford to be the provider of first resort.

Many Governments interpret their charge to serve the poor as requiring direct service provision, but this is not necessarily so. Analysis of population data can shed light on whether direct service provision is needed or whether other mechanisms, such as contracting for service and vouchering, can be used to procure private sector services.

There is a growing body of knowledge about government contracting and reimbursing for family planning services. Even advanced clinical methods may be so financed, though conventional wisdom holds that public sector programmes have a comparative advantage to provide these services in their existing networks of hospitals. Securing these services from the private sector, however, takes advantage of the ability of the private sector to gain efficiency through specialization.

Government or other financing entities that procure services from the private sector can stimulate a powerful supply response from the market. In response to reimbursement mechanisms, private sector providers will begin to offer these services, not just to users entitled to them under the rules but more generally to others desiring these services. This is one of the important consequences of the presence of insurance schemes and financing/reimbursement mechanisms in the market. Anecdotal evidence from the Philippines suggests that if the employment insurance system (Medicare) begins to reimburse for family planning services on an out-patient basis, then private providers will respond by offering these services to the employed population and to other consumers.

This expansion of supply is meaningful because the private sector can offer a range of prices for services according to the consumer's ability to pay. Griffin (1989) cites the example of rural areas in the Philippines, where surveyed physicians mentioned that they could not price services without knowing the income group of the consumer. Thus, the new supply could be expected to respond to needs of a large range of income groups preferring private sector services.

The financing and licensing/regulatory functions of government are powerful mechanisms for ensuring that quality services shall actually be delivered. Governments have both a carrot and a stick: if quality standards are not maintained, the provider can be shut down or prohibited from taking part in reimbursement programmes. In contrast, public sector services have only command and control mechanisms to assure quality.

F. CONCLUSION AND RECOMMENDATIONS

The private sector has enormous potential to help meet the escalating demand for family planning services. Government can take advantage of this potential if it establishes a supportive policy environment with the private commercial sector as a full partner.

Governments should adopt an appropriate division of labour between the public and private sectors, where the latter group meets the needs of those that can afford to pay for family planning services and the former targets its subsidies to those that cannot.

Donors should provide technical assistance to Governments of developing countries seeking to develop the role of the private commercial sector.

REFERENCES

Arruda, José Maria, A. M. Thome and Leo Morris (1983). *Pesquisa sobre Saude Materno-Infantil e Planejamento Familiar, Piaui - 1982*. Rio de Janeiro: Sociedade Civil de Bem-Estar Familiar no Brazil.

Cross, Harry E., and others (1991). Contraceptive source and the for-profit private sector in third world family planning. Paper presented at the Annual Meeting of the Population Association of America, Washington, D.C., 21-23 March.

Griffin, Charles C. (1989). *Strengthening Health Services in Developing Countries Through the Private Sector*. IFC Discussion Paper, No. 4. Washington, D.C.: The World Bank.

Lande, Robert E., and Judith S. Geller (1991). *Paying for Family Planning*. Population Reports, Series J, No. 39. Baltimore, Maryland: The Johns Hopkins University, Population Information Program.

Lewis, Maureen A., and Genevieve Kenney (1988). *The Private Sector and Family Planning in Developing Countries: Its Role, Achievements, and Potential*. Washington, D.C.: The Urban Institute.

Smith, Janet M. (1992). *Trends in Contraceptive Sales and Social Marketing in Indonesia*. Washington, D.C.: The Futures Group.

كيفية الحصول على منشورات الأمم المتحدة

يمكن الحصول على منشورات الأمم المتحدة من المكتبات ودور التوزيع في جميع أنحاء العالم . استعلم عنها من المكتبة
التي تتعامل معها أو اكتب إلى : الأمم المتحدة ، قسم البيع في نيويورك أو في جنيف .

如何购取联合国出版物

联合国出版物在全世界各地的书店和经售处均有发售。请向书店询问或写信到纽约或日内瓦的
联合国销售组。

HOW TO OBTAIN UNITED NATIONS PUBLICATIONS

United Nations publications may be obtained from bookstores and distributors throughout the
world. Consult your bookstore or write to: United Nations, Sales Section, New York or Geneva.

COMMENT SE PROCURER LES PUBLICATIONS DES NATIONS UNIES

Les publications des Nations Unies sont en vente dans les librairies et les agences dépositaires
du monde entier. Informez-vous auprès de votre libraire ou adressez-vous à : Nations Unies,
Section des ventes, New York ou Genève.

КАК ПОЛУЧИТЬ ИЗДАНИЯ ОРГАНИЗАЦИИ ОБЪЕДИНЕННЫХ НАЦИЙ

Издания Организации Объединенных Наций можно купить в книжных магазинах
и агентствах во всех районах мира. Наводите справки об изданиях в вашем книжном
магазине или пишите по адресу: Организация Объединенных Наций, Секция по
продаже изданий, Нью-Йорк или Женева.

COMO CONSEGUIR PUBLICACIONES DE LAS NACIONES UNIDAS

Las publicaciones de las Naciones Unidas están en venta en librerías y casas distribuidoras en
todas partes del mundo. Consulte a su librero o diríjase a: Naciones Unidas, Sección de Ventas,
Nueva York o Ginebra.

Litho in United Nations, New York
18107—August 1996—5,270
ISBN 92-1-151308-1

United Nations publication
Sales No. E.96.XIII.12
ST/ESA/SER.R/131